n below.

Oral and Maxillofacial Surgery

VOLUME

4

Temporomandibular Disorders

Oral and Maxillofacial Surgery

VOLUME

4

Temporomandibular Disorders

Edited by
Raymond J. Fonseca, D.M.D.

Dean
University of Pennsylvania
School of Dental Medicine
Philadelphia, Pennsylvania

Volume Editors

Robert A. Bays, D.D.S.

Peter D. Quinn, D.M.D., M.D.

Illustrated by William M. Winn, Medical Illustrator

Saunders
An Imprint of Elsevier Science

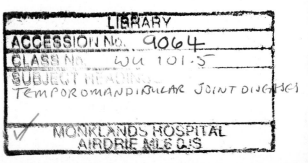

SAUNDERS
An Imprint of Elsevier Science
The Curtis Center
Independence Square West
Philadelphia, PA 19106

Library of Congress Cataloging-in-Publication Data

Oral and maxillofacial surgery/editor, Raymond J. Fonseca.—1st ed.

p.   cm.

Contents: v. 1. Anesthesia/dentoalveolar surgery/office management/volume
editors, David E. Frost, Elliot V. Hersh, Lawrence M. Levin   v. 2. Orthognathic
surgery/volume editors, Norman J. Betts, Timothy A. Turvey   v. 3. Trauma/
volume editors, Robert D. Marciani, Barry H. Hendler   v. 4. Temporomandibular
disorders/volume editors, Robert A. Bays, Peter D. Quinn   v. 5. Surgical
pathology/volume editors, Thomas P. Williams, Jeffery C. B. Stewart   v. 6. Cleft,
craniofacial, cosmetic surgery/volume editors, Raymond J. Fonseca, Stephen B.
Baker, Larry M. Wolford   v. 7. Reconstructive and implant surgery/volume
editors, Michael P. Powers, H. Dexter Barber.

ISBN 0–7216–9631–7

1. Mouth—Surgery.   2. Maxilla—Surgery.   3. Face—Surgery.
 I. Fonseca, Raymond J.
 [DNLM: 1. Surgery, Oral.   2. Face—surgery.   3. Facial Bones—surgery.
 4. Maxilla—surgery.   WU 600 0633 2000]

RK529.0662 2000   617.5′2059—dc21

DNLM/DLC   99-11886

Editor: Judith Fletcher
Developmental Editor: Arlene Chappelle
Production Manager: Natalie Ware
Supervisory Copy Editor: Carol DiBerardino
Illustration Coordinator: Peg Shaw
Designer: Ellen Zanolle

ISBN Volume 1 0–7216–9632–5
Volume 2 0–7216–9633–3
Volume 3 0–7216–9634–1
Volume 4 0–7216–9635–X
Volume 5 0–7216–9636–8
Volume 6 0–7216–9637–6
Volume 7 0–7216–9638–4
(set) 0–7216–9631–7

ORAL AND MAXILLOFACIAL SURGERY

Permissions may be sought directly from Elsevier's Health Sciences Rights Department in Philadelphia, USA: phone: (+1)215-238-7869, fax: (+1)215-238-2239, email: healthpermissions@elsevier.com. You may also complete your request on-line via the Elsevier Science homepage (http://www.elsevier.com), by selecting 'Customer Support' and then 'Obtaining Permissions'.

Printed in the United States of America.

Last digit is the print number: 9   8   7   6   5   4   3   2

To Marilyn, you make it all possible!!!

RAYMOND J. FONSECA

To Beth, who fills up my senses like a night in a forest.

ROBERT A. BAYS

Volume Editors

Robert A. Bays, D.D.S.

Professor and Chief
Division of Oral and Maxillofacial Surgery
Emory University School of Medicine
Chief of Oral and Maxillofacial Surgery and Dentistry
Emory University Hospital
Chief of Oral and Maxillofacial Surgery and Dentistry
Crawford Long Hospital
Chief of Oral and Maxillofacial Surgery and Dentistry
Henrietta Egleston Hospital (Children's)
Chief of Oral and Maxillofacial Surgery and Dentistry
Grady Memorial Hospital
Consultant
Veterans Administration Medical Center
Atlanta, Georgia

Peter D. Quinn, D.M.D., M.D.

Chairman
Department of Oral and Maxillofacial Surgery
University of Pennsylvania School of Dental Medicine
Chairman
Department of Oral and Maxillofacial Surgery
Hospital of the University of Pennsylvania
Philadelphia, Pennsylvania

Contributors

A. Omar Abubaker, D.M.D., Ph.D.

Associate Professor, Department of Oral
and Maxillofacial Surgery, Virginia
Commonwealth University Medical College
of Virginia School of Dentistry; Department
of Surgery, Medical College of Virginia
Hospitals, Richmond, Virginia
*Diagnosis and Management of Dentoalveolar
Injuries*

Leonard F. Allen, D.M.D., M.D.

Clinical Instructor, Department of Surgery,
West Virginia University; Private Practice,
Charleston, West Virginia
Treatment of the Complex Facial Trauma Patient

Brian Alpert, D.D.S.

Professor of Oral and Maxillofacial Surgery
and Chair, Department of Surgical and
Hospital Dentistry, University of Louisville
School of Dentistry; Chief, Oral and
Maxillofacial Surgery and Dentistry,
University of Louisville Hospital, Louisville,
Kentucky
Reconstruction of Developmental Deformities

Douglas R. Anderson, D.D.S., M.S., J.D.

Adjunct Clinical Professor, Ohio State
University, Columbus, Ohio
*Accreditation of the Oral and Maxillofacial Surgery
Office*

Quentin N. Anderson, M.D.

Associate Professor of Radiology, University
of Minnesota; Chief of Radiology, Hennepin
County Medical Center, Minneapolis,
Minnesota
*Temporomandibular Joint Imaging: Treatment
Planning*

G. William Arnett, D.D.S., F.A.C.D.

Assistant Professor of Oral and Maxillofacial
Surgery, Loma Linda University, Loma
Linda, California; Orthognathic Surgery
Clinical Instructor, UCLA School of
Dentistry, Department of OMS, Los Angeles,
California; Orthognathic Surgery Clinical
Instructor, University of California at Los
Angeles, Valley Medical Center, Fresno,
California; Clinical Assistant Professor,
Department of Orthodontics, USC School of
Dentistry, Department of Orthodontics, Los
Angeles, California; Courtesy Staff, St.
Francis Medical Center, Santa Barbara,
California Courtesy Staff St. Francis Medical
Center, Santa Barbara, CA
*Morphologic Changes of the Temporomandibular
Joint Associated with Orthognathic Surgery*

Leon A. Assael, D.M.D.

Dean and Professor, College of Dentistry,
University of Kentucky, Professor of Oral and
Maxillofacial Surgery, Department of Oral
Health Science, College of Dentistry and
Professor, Department of Surgery, College of
Medicine, University of Kentucky, Lexington,
Kentucky
*Unusual Maxillofacial Soft Tissue Malignancies:
Sarcomas, Mucosal Melanoma, and Lymphoma*

L'Tanya J. Bailey, D.D.S., M.S.

Associate Professor, Department of
Orthodontics, University of North Carolina
at Chapel Hill School of Dentistry, Chapel
Hill, North Carolina
Patient Selection for Orthognathic Surgery

H. Dexter Barber, D.D.S.

Clinical Associate Professor, Department of

Oral and Maxillofacial Surgery, University of
Medicine and Dentistry of New Jersey,
Newark, New Jersey; Private Practice Oral
and Maxillofacial Surgery, Philadelphia,
Pennsylvania

*Coordination in the Comprehensive Diagnosis and
Treatment of the Implant Patient: The Relationship
between the Implant Surgeon and the Restorative
Doctor; Preprosthetic Surgery: An Overview and Soft
Tissue Procedures; Principles for the Surgical
Placement of Endosseous Implants; Surgical Implant
Failures*

Manraj Bath, D.D.S.

Former Chief Resident, Department of Oral
and Maxillofacial Surgery, Case Western
Reserve University, Cleveland, Ohio;
Associate in Private Practice, Jewish Hospital
Outpatient Care Center, Louisville, Kentucky
Basic Exodontia

Robert A. Bays, D.D.S.

Professor and Chief, Division of Oral and
Maxillofacial Surgery, Emory University,
School of Medicine; Chief of Oral and
Maxillofacial Surgery and Dentistry, Emory
University Hospital; Chief of Oral and
Maxillofacial Surgery and Dentistry,
Crawford Long Hospital; Chief of Oral and
Maxillofacial Surgery and Dentistry,
Henrietta Egleston Hospital (Children's);
Chief of Oral and Maxillofacial Surgery and
Dentistry, Grady Memorial Hospital;
Consultant, Veterans Administration Medical
Center, Atlanta, Georgia
Surgery for Internal Derangement

Barry W. Beck, D.D.S., M.D.

Former Chief Resident, Department of Oral
and Maxillofacial Surgery, Case Western
Reserve University School of Dentistry,
Cleveland, Ohio; Private Practice, Nashville,
Tennessee
Soft Tissue Considerations

Robert Beideman, D.M.D.

Director of Radiology, University of
Pennsylvania School of Dental Medicine,
Philadelphia, Pennsylvania
*Imaging for Maxillofacial Reconstruction and
Implantology*

William H. Bell, D.D.S.

Oral and Maxillofacial Surgery, Plano, Texas
*Model Surgery; Intraoral Distraction Osteogenesis;
Rehabilitation after Orthognathic Surgery*

M. Elizabeth Bennett, Ph.D.

Adjunct Assistant Professor, University of
North Carolina School of Dentistry, Chapel
Hill, North Carolina
Psychological Ramifications of Orthognathic Surgery

James E. Bertz, A.B., M.S., D.D.S., M.D., F.A.C.S.

Lecturer, Visiting Professor, UCLA School of
Dentistry, Los Angeles, California; Visiting
Professor, Northwestern University, Chicago,
Illinois; Lecturer, Visiting Professor, LSU,
School of Dentistry Medical Center, New
Orleans, Louisiana; Attending Staff,
Scottsdale Healthcare, Scottsdale, Arizona
Nasal Injuries

Norman J. Betts, D.D.S., M.S.

Associate Professor and Chairman,
Department of Oral and Maxillofacial
Surgery, University of Medicine and
Dentistry of New Jersey–New Jersey Dental
School; Chief of Service, Department of
Dental Medicine, University Hospital,
University of Medicine and Dentistry of New
Jersey, Newark, New Jersey
*Surgically Assisted Maxillary Expansion; Soft
Tissue Changes Associated with Orthognathic
Surgery; Preprosthetic Surgery: An Overview and
Soft Tissue Procedures*

Mark L. Billy, D.D.S.

Chairman, Department of Dentistry and Oral
and Maxillofacial Surgery, Forum Health,
Youngstown, Ohio
Avulsive Hard Tissue Facial Injuries

John Birbe, M.D., D.D.S.

Staff Surgeon, Institut Universitari Dexeus,
Barcelona, Spain
Zygomatic Complex Fractures

John R. Blakemore, D.D.S.

Assistant Clinical Professor, Case Western
Reserve University Dental School, Cleveland;
Chief, Oral and Maxillofacial Surgery, St.
John Westshore Hospital, Westlake, Ohio
Subperiosteal Implants

George H. Blakey, D.D.S.

Clinical Assistant Professor, Department of
Oral and Maxillofacial Surgery, University of
North Carolina at Chapel Hill, North
Carolina
*Surgical Uprighting and Repositioning; Model
Surgery*

William S. Blood, D.D.S., M.D.

Assistant Clinical Professor, Oral and Maxillofacial Surgery, Case Western Reserve University School of Dentistry, Cleveland, Ohio

Subperiosteal Implants

Hans Bosker, D.D.S., Ph.D.

Chief, Department of Oral and Maxillofacial Surgery, Martini Hospital, Groningen, The Netherlands; Visiting Professor, Department of Oral and Maxillofacial Surgery, Case Western Reserve University School of Dentistry; University Hospitals of Cleveland, Cleveland, Ohio

The Transmandibular Implant Reconstruction System

Scott B. Boyd, D.D.S., Ph.D.

Professor and Chairman, Department of Oral and Maxillofacial Surgery, Vanderbilt University, Nashville, Tennessee

Rehabilitation after Orthognathic Surgery

Jon P. Bradrick, D.D.S.

Associate Professor of Surgery, University of Texas—Houston Dental Branch; Director, Division of Oral and Maxillofacial Surgery, Hermann Hospital, Houston, Texas

Avulsive Hard Tissue Facial Injuries

Pablo Bringas

Senior Research Technician and Laboratory Manager, Center for Craniofacial Molecular Biology, University of Southern California, Los Angeles, California

Embryogenesis and the Classification of Craniofacial Dysmorphogenesis

James R. Bruno, D.M.D., M.D.

Chief Resident, Hospital of the University of Pennsylvania, University of Pennsylvania, Philadelphia, Pennsylvania

Preoperative Evaluation

Michael J. Buckley, D.M.D., M.S.

Associate Professor and Director of Research, Department of Oral and Maxillofacial Surgery, University of Pittsburgh; Director, Department of Dental Medicine, University of Pittsburgh Medical Center, Pittsburgh, Pennsylvania

Total Mandibular Subapical Osteotomy

Robert L. Campbell, D.D.S.

Professor, Oral and Maxillofacial Surgery, Professor of Anesthesiology, Medical College of Virginia, Virginia Commonwealth University, Richmond, Virginia

Ambulatory Anesthesia for Orthognathic Surgery

Lionel M. Candelaria, D.D.S.

Diplomate of the American Board of Oral and Maxillofacial Surgery; Private practice, Oral Maxillofacial Surgery Associates, Albuquerque, New Mexico

Head and Neck Infections

Stephen B. Cantrell, D.D.S., M.D.

Director, University Craniofacial Center of New Jersey; Asssistant Professor, Oral and Maxillofacial Surgery; Clinical Assistant Professor, Plastic and Reconstructive Surgery, University of Medicine and Dentistry of New Jersey, Newark, New Jersey

Orbital Pathology and Secondary Reconstruction; Micrognathia and Mandibular Hypoplasia

Jeffrey O. Capes, D.M.D., M.D.

Private Practice, Oral and Maxillofacial Surgery, St. Simon's Island, Georgia; Former Chief Resident, Oral and Maxillofacial Surgery, University Hospitals, Cleveland, Ohio

Complications of Dentoalveolar Surgery

Robert P. Carmichael, DMD, MScD, MRCDC

Coordinator of Prosthodontic Services, The Hospital for Sick Children, The Bloorview MacMillan Centre; Assistant Professor, Faculty of Dentistry, The University of Toronto, Toronto, Ontario, Canada

Orbital Hypertelorism

Jeffrey B. Carter, M.D., D.M.D.

Clinical Assistant Professor of Oral and Maxillofacial Surgery, Vanderbilt University; President, Oral Surgical Institute, Medical Director, Oral Facial Surgery Center, Oral Surgical Institute, Oral Facial Surgery Center, Nashville, Tennessee

Surgical Implant Failures

Cameron M. L. Clokie, D.D.S., Ph.D., F.R.C.D.C.

Associate Professor and Chairman, Division of Oral and Maxillofacial Surgery, Faculty of Dentistry, University of Toronto; Head, Division of Oral and Maxillofacial Surgery, Toronto General Hospital, University Health Network, Toronto, Ontario, Canada

Orbital Hypertelorism

Bernard J. Costello, D.M.D., M.D.

Chief Resident, University of Pennsylvania Medical Center, Department of Oral and Maxillofacial Surgery, Philadelphia, Pennsylvania
Complicated Exodontia; Lasers in Oral and Maxillofacial Surgery; Preprosthetic Surgery: An Overview and Soft Tissue Procedures

David A. Cottrell, D.M.D.

Associate Professor, Director, Oral and Maxillofacial Surgery Residency Program; Director of Resident Research, Boston University School of Dental Medicine, Department of Oral and Maxillofacial Surgery, Boston, Massachusetts
Reactive Proliferations

L. Angelo Cuzalina, D.D.S., M.D.

Resident, Department of Oral and Maxillofacial Surgery, University of Alabama School of Dentistry, Birmingham, Alabama
Rhytidectomy (Face-lift)

Paul A. Danielson, D.M.D.

Assistant Clinical Professor, University of Vermont College of Medicine; Chief, Section of Dentistry and Oral and Maxillofacial Surgery, Fletcher Allen Health Care, Burlington, Vermont
Soft Tissue Cysts and Benign Neoplasms

William L. Davenport, D.D.S.

Chief, Department of Oral and Maxillofacial Surgery, Wilford Hall Medical Center, San Antonio, Texas
Monitoring for Oral and Maxillofacial Surgery

Kenneth H. Dawson, B.D.S., M.D.Sc., F.R.A.C.D.S.(O.M.S.)

Assistant Professor and Director of Resident Training, The University of Washington; Attending Oral and Maxillofacial Surgeon, Harborview Medical Center, Seattle, and Seattle Children's Hospital and Regional Medical Center, Seattle, Washington; Major, Royal Australian Army Dental Corps, Melbourne, Australia
Maxillofacial Injuries in Children

Alan E. Deegan, D.D.S., M.S.D.

Chairman, Risk Management Committee, AAOMS National Insurance Company, Rosemont, IL
Risk Management in Oral and Maxillofacial Surgery

Jeffrey B. Dembo, D.D.S., M.S.

Professor, Division of Oral and Maxillofacial Surgery, University of Kentucky College of Dentistry, Lexington, Kentucky
Complications in Anesthesia

Eric J. Dierks, M.D., D.M.D.

Clinical Professor and Vice Chairman, Department of Oral and Maxillofacial Surgery, Oregon Health Sciences University; Staff Head and Neck Surgeon, Legacy Emanuel Hospital, Portland, Oregon
Skin Lesions of the Maxillofacial Region

Thomas B. Dodson, D.M.D., M.P.H.

Associate Professor, Department of Oral and Maxillofacial Surgery, Harvard School of Dental Medicine; Visiting Surgeon, Director of Resident Training, Massachusetts General Hospital, Boston, Massachusetts
Epidemiology of Temporomandibular Disorders; Autogenous Temporomandibular Joint Replacement

William C. Donlon, D.M.D., M.A.

Assistant Professor, Department of Maxillo-Facial Surgery, University of Florida, Health Sciences Center/Jacksonville; Attending Surgeon, Department of Maxillo-Facial Surgery and Otolaryngology, Shands/Jacksonville Medical Center, Jacksonville, Florida
Credentialing and Privileging for Oral and Maxillofacial Surgeons

Samuel F. Dworkin, D.D.S., Ph.D.

Professor, Departments of Oral Medicine, and Psychiatry and Behavioral Sciences, University of Washington; Attending Clinical Psychologist, University of Washington Medical Center, Seattle, Washington
Biobehavioral Assessment and Treatment of Temporomandibular Disorders

Mark A. Egbert, D.D.S.

Associate Professor, Department of Oral and Maxillofacial Surgery, University of Washington; Chief, Oral and Maxillofacial Surgery, Harborview Hospital and Medical Center, Seattle, Washington
Maxillofacial Injuries in Children

Edward Ellis III, D.D.S., M.S.

Professor of Oral and Maxillofacial Surgery, University of Texas Southwestern Medical Center Oral and Maxillofacial Surgery Chief of Oral and Maxillofacial Surgery, Parkland Memorial Hospital, Dallas, Texas
Functional Outcomes Following Orthognathic Surgery

Robert W. Emery

Diplomate, American Board of Oral and Maxillofacial Surgery, Senior Attending Surgeon, Washington Hospital Center, Washington Institute for Mouth, Face and Jaw Surgery, Washington, D.C.
Aesthetic Cutaneous Laser Surgery and Chemical Peels

Kim L. Erickson, D.D.S.

Attending Surgeon, Center for Craniofacial Disorders, Spectrum Health East Hospital; Attending Surgeon, Spectrum Downtown Hospital, Grand Rapids, Michigan
Model Surgery

T. William Evans, D.D.S., M.D., M.Sc., F.A.C.S.

Adjunct Associate Professor, The Ohio State University, Columbus, Ohio; Adjunct Assistant Professor, The University of Michigan, Ann Arbor, Michigan
Endoscopic Facial Aesthetic Surgery

Claire Ferrari, D.D.S., M.S.

Teaching Fellow, University of California, San Francisco, School of Dentistry, San Francisco, California
Embryogenesis and Comprehensive Management of the Cleft Patient

R. Theodore Fields, D.D.S.

Resident, Baylor College of Dentistry–Texas A&M, University System, Dallas, Texas
Diagnosis and Treatment Planning for Orthognathic Surgery

Michael W. Finkelstein, D.D.S., M.S.

Professor, College of Dentistry, University of Iowa, Iowa City, Iowa
Sarcomas of Bone in the Maxillofacial Region

Raymond J. Fonseca, D.M.D.

Dean, University of Pennsylvania School of Dental Medicine, Philadelphia, Pennsylvania
Complicated Exodontia; Revascularization and Healing of Orthognathic Surgical Procedures; Soft Tissue Changes Associated with Orthognathic Surgery; Orthognathic Surgery in the Cleft Patient; Fibro-osseous Diseases and Benign Tumors of Bone; Reconstruction of the Edentulous Maxilla

Joseph W. Foote, D.M.D., M.D.

Assistant Professor, University of Pennsylvania School of Dental Medicine; Attending, Presbyterian Medical Center, University of Pennsylvania Medical Center, and Veterans Administration, Philadelphia, Pennsylvania
Preoperative Evaluation

Robert M. Fox, D.D.S.*

Private Practice, Florida
Distraction Osteogenesis: A Unique Treatment for Congenital Micrognathias

Troy A. Frazee, D.D.S., M.D.

Assistant Clinical Professor, Department of Oral and Maxillofacial Surgery, Case Western Reserve University School of Dentistry; Attending Surgeon, University Hospitals/Mt. Sinai Medical Center, Cleveland, Ohio
Rehabilitation of the Edentulous Mandible: Prosthetic and Surgical Concerns

James Fricton, D.D.S., M.S.

Professor, University of Minnesota School of Dentistry, Minneapolis, Minnesota
Clinical Evaluation for Temporomandibular Disorders and Orofacial Pain

James A. Giglio, D.D.S., M.Ed.

Professor, Oral and Maxillofacial Surgery, Virginia Commonwealth University Medical College of Virginia School of Dentistry; Institution Hospital, Medical College of Virginia Hospitals, Richmond, Virginia
Diagnosis and Management of Dentoalveolar Injuries

Lionel Gold, D.D.S.

Associate Professor, Jefferson Medical College; Senior Attending Oral and Maxillofacial Surgeon and Past Chairman, Department of Oral and Maxillofacial Surgery, Thomas Jefferson University Hospital, Philadelphia, Pennsylvania
Odontogenic Tumors: Surgical Pathology and Management

---

*Deceased.

Jerold S. Goldberg, D.D.S.

Dean, School of Dentistry, Professor, Department of Oral and Maxillofacial Surgery, Case Western Reserve University; Staff, University Hopsitals of Cleveland, Cleveland Veterans Administration Medical Center, Cleveland, Ohio
Implant-Retained Facial Prostheses

Douglas H. Goldsmith, D.D.S.

Assistant Clinial Professor, Oral and Maxillofacial Surgery Section, Albert Einstein College of Medicine; Attending Oral and Maxillofacial Surgeon, Montefiore Hospital and Medical Center, Bronx, New York; Chairman, Department of Oral and Maxillofacial Surgery, White Plains Hospital Center, White Plains, New York; Private Practice, Scarsdale, New York
Model Surgery

Arthur A. Gonty, D.D.S.

Associate Professor, Division of Oral and Maxillofacial Surgery, University of Kentucky College of Dentistry, Lexington, Kentucky
Management of Frontal Sinus Fractures and Associated Injuries

Marianela Gonzalez, D.D.S., M.D.

Senior Resident, Department of Oral and Maxillofacial Surgery and Pharmacology, Baylor College of Dentistry, Texas A&M University System Health Science Center, Dallas, Texas
Intraoral Distraction Osteogenesis

Lawrence Gottesman, D.D.S.

Former Director of Neuropathic Pain, Advanced Orofacial/TMD Program, Department of Oral Medicine and Pathology, Division of Basic Sciences, New York University College of Dentistry, New York, New York
Morphologic Changes of the Temporomandibular Joint Associated with Orthognathic Surgery

James D. Grady, D.M.D., M.S.

Medical Staff, East Alabama Medical Center, Opelika, Alabama
Oral and Maxillofacial Surgery: Practice and Personnel Development

John M. Gregg, D.D.S., M.S., Ph.D.

Virginia–Maryland College of Veterinary Medicine, Virginia Tech University; Chairman, Department of Surgery, and Chairman, Institutional Review Board, Columbia Montgomery Regional Hospital, Blacksburg, Virginia; Chairman, Committee Research and Technology Assessment A.A.O.M.S.
Chronic Head and Neck Pain

César A. Guerrero, D.D.S.

Director, Santa Rosa Oral and Maxillofacial Surgery Center; Consulting Professor, Department of Orthodontics, Central University of Venezuela, Caracas, Venezuela.
Intraoral Distraction Osteogenesis

Steven A. Guttenberg, D.D.S.

Chairman, OMS Training and Education Committee, Temple University School of Dentistry, Philadelphia, Pennsylvania; Diplomate, American Board of Oral and Maxillofacial Surgery; Fellow, American Academy of Cosmetic Surgery; Senior Attending Surgeon, Washington Hospital Center; Clinical Institute for Mouth, Face, and Jaw Surgery, Washington, D.C.
Aesthetic Cutaneous Laser Surgery and Chemical Peels

Daniel A. Haas, D.D.S., Ph.D.

Associate Professor and Head of Anesthesia, Faculty of Dentistry, Department Associate Professor of Pharmacology Faculty of Medicine, University of Toronto; Active Staff, Department of Dentistry, Sunnybrook Health Science Center, Toronto, Ontario, Canada
Parenteral Sedation

H. David Hall, D.M.D., M.D.

Emeritus Professor, Department of Oral and Maxillofacial Surgery, Vanderbilt University School of Medicine, Nashville, Tennessee
Vertical Ramus Osteotomy and the Inverted-L Osteotomy

Richard H. Haug, D.D.S.

Associate Professor, Case Western Reserve University, School of Medicine; Director, Division of Oral and Maxillofacial Surgery, Director of Postgraduate Training in Oral and Maxillofacial Surgery, MetroHealth Medical Center, Cleveland, Ohio
Avulsive Hard Tissue Facial Injuries

James R. Hayward, D.D.S., M.S.

Emeritus Professor and Chairman,
Department of Oral and Maxillofacial
Surgery, University of Michigan; Chairman
Emeritus, Section of Oral and Maxillofacial
Surgery, University of Michigan Hospital,
Ann Arbor, Michigan
Introduction: Historical Perspectives

John W. Hellstein, D.D.S., M.S.

Professor of Oral and Maxillofacial
Pathology, Naval Postgraduate Dental School;
Staff, National Naval Dental Center; National
Naval Medical Center, Bethesda, Maryland;
Walter Reed Army Medical Center,
Washington, DC
*Odontogenic Cysts of the Jaws and Other Selected
Cysts*

Barry H. Hendler, D.D.S., M.D.

Associate Professor, Department of Oral and
Maxillofacial Surgery, University of
Pennsylvania School of Medicine; Director,
Continuing Postgraduate Medical Education,
and Coordinator of Laser and Cosmetic
Surgery, Department of Oral and
Maxillofacial Surgery, University of
Pennsylvania Medical Center, Philadelphia,
Pennsylvania
*Basic Principles of Treatment: Hard and Soft
Tissue; Soft Tissue Injuries; Hair Restoration
Surgery: Transplantation and Micrografting; Facial
Suction Lipectomy*

Theodore B. Hennig, D.D.S., M.S.

Private Practice; Director, Saginaw Valley
Cleft Palate Clinic, Saginaw, Michigan
*Velopharyngeal Dysfunction; Reconstruction of the
Edentulous Maxilla*

Lawrence T. Herman, D.M.D.

Assistant Clinical Professor, Boston University
School of Dental Medicine; Assistant Clinical
Professor, Tufts University School of Dental
Medicine, Boston, Massachusetts; Chief,
Division of Dental Medicine, Caritas
Norwood Hospital, Norwood, Massachusetts
Reactive Proliferations

Elliot V. Hersh, D.M.D., Ph.D.

Associate Professor, Departments of Oral and
Maxillofacial Surgery and Pharmacology;
Director, Division of Pharmacology and
Clinical Therapeutics, University of
Pennsylvania School of Dental Medicine,
Philadelphia, Pennsylvania
Local Anesthetics

Jon D. Holmes, D.M.D., M.D.

Assistant Clinical Professor, Department of
Oral and Maxillofacial Surgery, Oregon
Health Sciences University; Dennis A. and
Roberta R. Youde Fellow in Head and Neck
Surgery, Legacy Emanuel Hospital, Portland,
Oregon
*Maxillofacial Surgery for Treatment of Obstructive
Sleep Apnea*

Anders B. Holmlund, D.D.S., Ph.D.

Professor and Consultant, Department of
Oral and Maxillofacial Surgery, Karolinska
Institute; Consultant, Department of Oral
and Maxillofacial Surgery, Huddinje
University Hospital, Stockholm, Sweden
Arthroscopy

John-Wallace Hudson, D.D.S.

Professor and Program Director, Department
of Oral and Maxillofacial Surgery, University
of Tennessee Medical Center, Knoxville,
Tennessee
Osteomyelitis and Osteoradionecrosis

James R. Hupp, D.M.D., M.D., J.D.

Professor and Chair, Oral-Maxillofacial
Surgery, University of Maryland; Chair,
Department of Dental and Maxillofacial
Surgery, University Hospital, Baltimore,
Maryland
*Embezzlement: Its Detection, Management, and
Prevention; Preoperative, Intraoperative, and
Postoperative Care*

Douglass L. Jackson, D.M.D., M.S., Ph.D.

Assistant Professor, University of Washington,
School of Dentistry, Seattle, Washington
Management of Acute Postoperative Pain

Francis R. Johns, D.M.D., M.D.

Fellow, Department of Plastic and
Reconstructive Surgery, University of
Virginia, Charlottesville, Virginia
Orbital Trauma

James V. Johnson, D.D.S., M.S.

Clinical Professor, UTHSC–Houston; Chief of
Services Oral and Maxillofacial Surgery, Ben
Taub General Hospital, Houston, Texas
Management of Midface Injuries

Jerry L. Jones, D.D.S., M.D.

Clinical Assistant Professor, Department of Surgery, Division of Otolaryngology/Plastic Surgery, University of New Mexico School of Medicine, Albuquerque, New Mexico
Head and Neck Infections

Richard D. Jordan, D.D.S., M.S.

Clinical Associate Professor, Northwestern University, Chicago, Illinois; Former Chair, Prosthodontics, and Associate Professor, University of North Carolina School of Dentistry, Chapel Hill, North Carolina; Private Practice, Asheville, North Carolina
Rehabilitation of the Edentulous Mandible: Prosthetic and Surgical Concerns

Leonard B. Kaban, D.M.D., M.D.

Walter C. Guralnick Professor of Oral and Maxillofacial Surgery, Harvard School of Dental Medicine; Chief, Department of Oral and Maxillofacial Surgery, Massachusetts General Hospital, Boston, Massachusetts
Autogenous Temporomandibular Joint Replacement

Gerald Kearns, M.B., B.Dent.Sc., F.F.D., F.D.S., F.R.C.S.(Ed.)

Consultant Oral and Maxillofacial Surgeon, Department of Oral and Maxillofacial Surgery, Limerick Regional Hospital, Limerick, Ireland
Pediatric Dentoalveolar Surgery

E. E. Keller, D.D.S., M.S.D.

Professor, Oral and Maxillofacial Surgery, Mayo Medical School–Mayo Medical Center; Consultant, Oral and Maxillofacial Surgery, Mayo Medical Center, Rochester, Minnesota
Maxillary Quadrangular LeFort I and Quadrangular LeFort II Osteotomy

Kevin G. Kempers, D.D.S., M.D.

Former Chief Resident, University of Pennsylvania, Department of Oral and Maxillofacial Surgery, Philadelphia, Pennsylvania; Private Practice, Boise, Idaho
Basic Principles of Treatment: Hard and Soft Tissue; Soft Tissue Injuries; Surgical Management of Langerhans' Cell Histiocytosis

Barry D. Kendell, D.M.D., M.S.

Clinical Associate Professor, Department of Oral and Maxillofacial Surgery, University of North Carolina at Chapel Hill, Chapel Hill; Attending Physician, Durham Regional Hospital, Durham, North Carolina
Computers—Practice Management Systems in the Oral and Maxillofacial Surgery Office

Brent D. Kennedy, D.D.S., M.D.

Associate Clinical Professor, Louisiana State University, New Orleans, Louisiana; Associate Clinical Professor, University of Texas Southwestern Medical Center at Dallas Medical School, Dallas, Texas; Director, Institute of Facial and Cosmetic Surgery, Murray, Utah
Cosmetic Rhinoplasty

Greg F. Kewitt, D.M.D., M.D.

Chief Resident, Department of Oral and Maxillofacial Surgery, University of Texas Health and Science Center–San Antonio, San Antonio, Texas
Bilateral Sagittal Split Osteotomy Advancement and Setback

Ashoo Khanuja, D.D.S., M.D.

Chief Resident, Department of Oral and Maxillofacial Surgery, University Hospitals of Cleveland, Cleveland, Ohio
Surgical Management of Impacted Teeth

Syngcuk Kim, D.D.S., M.Phil., Ph.D.

Louis I. Grossman Professor and Chairman, Department of Endodontics, University of Pennsylvania School of Dental Medicine, Philadelphia, Pennsylvania
Principles of Endodontic Microsurgery

Jeffrey C. Knorr, D.D.S., M.B.A.

Attending Staff, Detroit–Macomb/St. John's Hospital, Oral Surgery Residency Training Program, Detroit, Michigan
Computers—Practice Management Systems in the Oral and Maxillofacial Surgery Office

D. A. Koppel, M.B., B.A.S., F.D.S.R.C.S., F.R.C.S.

Honarary Clinical Lecturer, University of Glasgow; Consultant Surgeon, Canniesburn Hospital/Institute of Neurological Sciences, Glasgow, Scotland
High-Level Midface Osteotomy Surgery

Steven L. Kraus, P.T., O.C.S., M.T.C.

Clinic Director with Physiotherapy Associates; Clinical Assistant Professor, Department of Rehabilitation Medicine, Emory University School of Medicine, Atlanta, Georgia
Physical Therapy Management of Temporomandibular Disorders

George M. Kushner, D.M.D., M.D.

Associate Professor of Oral-Maxillofacial Surgery; Director, Residency Program in Oral and Maxillofacial Surgery, University of Louisville School of Dentistry, Louisville, Kentucky

Reconstruction of Developmental Deformities

Peter E. Larsen, D.D.S.

Associate Professor and Chairman, Department of Oral and Maxillofacial Surgery, Ohio State University College of Dentistry, Columbus, Ohio

Diagnosis and Management of Vascular Malformations

Stacey J. Law, D.D.S., M.S.

Voluntary Clinical Faculty, Division of Plastic and Reconstructive Surgery, UCSF-Stanford Health Care, Stanford University Medical Center, Stanford; Staff Orthodontist, Craniofacial Anomalies Center, Lucile Salter Packard Children's Hospital at Stanford, Palo Alto, California

Use of Orthopedic Appliances in Growth Modification

Lawrence M. Levin, D.M.D., M.D.

Assistant Professor, Department of Oral and Maxillofacial Surgery, University of Pennsylvania School of Dental Medicine; Chief, Division of Oral and Maxillofacial Surgery, University of Pennsylvania Medical Center, Philadelphia, Pennsylvania

Lasers in Oral and Maxillofacial Surgery; Surgical Management of Langerhans' Cell Histiocytosis

Daniel Lew, D.D.S.

Professor and Chairman, Department of Oral and Maxillofacial Surgery, University of Iowa College of Dentistry; Head, Department of Hospital Dentistry, University of Iowa Hospitals and Clinics, Iowa City, Iowa

Zygomatic Complex Fractures

Jeffrey S. Lewis, M.D., D.M.D.

Assistant Clinical Professor, University of Rochester School of Medicine and Dentistry, Department of Oral and Maxillofacial Surgery, Rochester; Director, Cleft Palate and Facial Deformities Team and Clinic, Cayuga Medical Center of Ithaca, Ithaca, New York

Cosmetic Surgery of the Forehead and Brow

Stuart E. Lieblich, D.M.D.

Associate Clinical Professor, University of Connecticut, School of Dental Medicine, Department of Oral and Maxillofacial Surgery, Farmington, Connecticut; Director, Ambulatory Anesthesia (Dentistry), Hartford Hospital, Hartford, Connecticut; Private Practice, Oral and Maxillofacial Surgery Avon, Connecticut

General Anesthesia for the Office Patient

Gilbert E. Lilly, D.D.S.

Professor and Head, Department of Oral Pathology, Radiology, and Medicine, College of Dentistry The University of Iowa; Oral Pathologist, Department of Hospital Dentistry, University of Iowa Hospitals and Clinics; Consultant, Veterans Affairs Medical Center, Iowa City, Iowa

Pathology of the Oral and Maxillofacial Region: Diagnostic and Surgical Considerations; Head and Neck: Medical Oncology

Scott G. Lilly

Associate in Medicine, Duke Medical Center, Durham, North Carolina

Head and Neck: Medical Oncology

Russell M. Linman, D.D.S., M.D.

Staff Oral and Maxillofacial Surgeon, USAF Hospital, Lakenheath AFB, England

Monitoring for Oral and Maxillofacial Surgery

John P. Lupori, D.D.S., M.D.

Alpine Oral and Maxillofacial Surgery, Steamboat Springs, Colorado

Bilateral Sagittal Split Osteotomy: Advancement and Setback

Gregory J. Lutcavage, D.D.S.

Attending Oral and Maxillofacial Surgeon, Department of Surgery, Wayne Memorial Hospital, Goldsboro, North Carolina

Sarcomas of Bone in the Maxillofacial Region

Mitchell Machtay, M.D.

Assistant Professor, University of Pennsylvania School of Medicine, Philadelphia, Pennsylvania

Radiation Therapy for Head and Neck Cancer

Robert B. MacIntosh, D.D.S.

Section Chief, Oral and Maxillofacial Surgery, Department of Dentistry and Oral and Maxillofacial Surgery, Sinai-Grace Hospital–Detroit Medical Center, Detroit, Michigan
Oral Malignant Disease: Management and Investigational Directions

A. K. Bobby Mallik, D.M.D.

Post Doctoral Fellow in Oral and Maxillofacial Surgery, University of Pennsylvania, School of Dental Medicine, Philadelphia, Pennsylvania
Complicated Exodontia

Allen Maniker, M.D.

Assistant Professor, Division of Neurosurgery, New Jersey Medical School, University of Medicine and Dentistry of New Jersey, Newark, New Jersey
Orbital Pathology and Secondary Reconstruction

Robert D. Marciani, D.M.D.

Professor, Division of Oral and Maxillofacial Surgery, University of Kentucky College of Dentistry; Chief, Division of Oral and Maxillofacial Surgery, University of Kentucky Medical Center; Staff, Department of Oral and Maxillofacial Surgery, Veterans Affairs Medical Center, Lexington, Kentucky
Diagnosis and Perioperative Management of Head and Neck Injuries; Mandibular Fractures; Maxillofacial Injuries in the Elderly

Richard M. Martin, D.D.S.

Private Practice, Oral Surgical Institute, Oral Facial Surgery Center, Nashville, Tennessee
Surgical Implant Failures

Joseph McManners, F.D.S.R.C.S., F.R.C.S.

Honorary Senior Lecturer, Oral and Maxillofacial Surgery; Consultant Oral and Maxillofacial Surgeon, Falkirk and District Royal Infirmary, Glasgow, Scotland
Mandibular Body Osteotomy

Karen McAndrew, D.M.D., M.S.

Assistant Professor, Department of General Practice, Virginia Commonwealth University; Private Practice, Richmond, Virginia
Single-Tooth Replacement in Oral Implantology

Leddy S. Meza, D.D.S.

Senior Resident, Department of Oral Surgery, Central University of Venezuela, Caracas, Venezuela
Intraoral Distraction Osteogenesis

Christopher C. Medley, D.D.S., M.D.

Staff Oral and Maxillofacial Surgeon, Ramstein Air Base/Landstuhl Regional Medical Center, Germany
Monitoring for Oral and Maxillofacial Surgery

S. B. Milam, D.D.S., Ph.D.

Professor and Acting Chairman, Department of Oral and Maxillofacial Surgery, University of Texas Health Science Center, San Antonio, Texas
Pathophysiology of Articular Disk Displacements of the Temporomandibular Joint; Morphologic Changes of the Temporomandibular Joint Associated with Orthognathic Surgery

Michael Miloro, D.M.D., M.D.

Associate Professor and Residency Program Director, Department of Oral and Maxillofacial Surgery, University of Maryland, Baltimore, Maryland
Combined Maxillary and Mandibular Surgery

Ronald Mizrahi, D.D.S.

Director, Orthodontics, New York Eye and Ear Infirmary; Private Practice, New York, New York,
Distraction Osteogenesis: A Unique Treatment for Congenital Micrognathias

Norman D. Mohl, D.D.S., M.A., Ph.D.

Distinguished Service Professor and Chairman, Department of Oral Diagnostic Sciences, School of Dental Medicine, University of Buffalo, Buffalo, New York
Clinical Evaluation for Temporomandibular Disorders and Orofacial Pain

Paul A. Moore, D.M.D., Ph.D., M.P.H., F.A.D.S.A., F.A.C.D.

Professor, Pharmacology, School of Dental Medicine, University of Pittsburgh, Fellow, American Dental Society of Anesthesiology, Fellow, American College of Dentistry, Adjunct Professor, Pharmacology School of Pharmacy, University of Pittsburgh, Pittsburgh, Pennsylvania
Management of Acute Postoperative Pain; Pharmacosedation for Pediatric Patients

K. F. Moos, M.B.B.S., B.D.S., F.R.C.S.(Ed.), F.D.S.R.C.S.(Eng. Ed.), F.D.S., R.C.P.S.(Glasg.)

Honorary Professor, Faculty of Medicine, University of Glasgow Dental Hospital and School–Glasgow; Consultant Oral and Maxillofacial Surgeon, Plastic and Maxillofacial Unit, Canniesburn Hospital, Glasgow, Scotland
High-Level Midface Osteotomy Surgery

Mark E. Moss, D.D.S., Ph.D.

Assistant Professor, Department of Community Preventive Medicine and Eastman Department of Dentistry, University of Rochester–Eastman Dental Center, Rochester, New York
The Role of Occlusion in Temporomandibular Disorders; Orthognathic Surgery and Temporomandibular Joint Ramifications

Arthur P. Mourino, D.D.S., M.S.D.

Associate Professor and Director, Advanced Education in Pediatric Dentistry, Virginia Commonwealth University, Richmond, Virginia
Diagnosis and Management of Dentoalveolar Injuries

Muralidhar Mupparapu, M.D.S., D.M.D.

Assistant Professor of Radiology, University of Pennsylvania School of Dental Medicine, Philadelphia, Pennsylvania
Imaging for Maxillofacial Reconstruction and Implantology

Robert W. T. Myall, B.D.S., M.D., F.R.C.D.(C)., F.D.S.R.C.S.

Professor of Oral and Maxillofacial Surgery, Adjunct Professor of Biological Structure, University of Washington; Chief, Division of Pediatric Oral and Maxillofacial Surgery, Children's Hospital and Regional Medical Centre, Seattle, Washington
Maxillofacial Injuries in Children

Masaki Nagata, D.D.S., Ph.D.

Assistant Professor, Second Department of Oral and Maxillofacial Surgery, Niigata University, Niigata, Japan
Embryogenesis and the Classification of Craniofacial Dysmorphogenesis

Talib A. Najjar, D.M.D., M.D.S., Ph.D.

Professor Oral and Maxillofacial Surgery, Clinical Professor, Pathology and Laboratory Medicine, New Jersey Dental School, New Jersey Medical School, University of Medicine and Dentistry of New Jersey; Attending, Oral and Maxillofacial Surgery, University Hospital, University of Medicine and Dentistry of New Jersey, Newark, New Jersey
Physiopathology of Osseointegration

Greg Ness, D.D.S.

Associate Professor of Clinical, Oral and Maxillofacial Surgery, College of Dentistry, Ohio State University, Columbus, Ohio
Maxillary Sinus Grafts and Implants

Joseph Niamtu III, D.D.S.

Private Group Practice, Richmond, Virginia
Marketing the Oral and Maxillofacial Surgery Practice

Glen Nuckolls,

Senior Staff Fellow, Craniofacial Development Section, National Institute of Arthritis and Musculoskeletal and Skin Diseases, National Institutes of Health, Bethesda, Maryland
Embryogenesis and the Classification of Craniofacial Dysmorphogenesis

Mark W. Ochs, D.M.D., M.D.

Associate Professor, Vice Chairman, and Director of Residency Education, University of Pittsburgh Pittsburgh, Pennsylvania
Orbital Trauma

Richard Ohrbach, D.D.S., M.S., Ph.D.

Assistant Professor, Department of Oral Diagnostic Sciences, School of Dental Medicine; Director, TMD and Orofacial Pain Clinic; Director, Advanced Education Program in TMD and Orofacial Pain, State University of New York–Buffalo, Buffalo, New York
Biobehavioral Assessment and Treatment of Temporomandibular Disorders

Robert A. Ord, D.D.S., M.D., F.R.C.S., F.A.C.S., M.S.

Professor, Department of Oral and Maxillofacial Surgery, Baltimore College of Dental Surgery, University of Maryland;

Professor, Oncology Program, Greenbaum Cancer Center, University of Maryland Medical School; Attending Surgeon, Division of Surgical Oncology, Franklin Square Hospital; Attending Surgeon and Chief of Head and Neck Surgery, Department of Otolaryngology, Maryland General Hospital, Baltimore, Maryland
Salivary Gland Disease

Todd G. Owsley, D.D.S., M.D.

Private Practice, Carolina Surgical Arts, Greensboro, North Carolina
Otoplastic Surgery for the Protruding Ear

Willie J. Parks, Jr., D.D.S., M.D.

Associate, Olympic Plaza Oral and Maxillofacial Surgery Associates; East Texas Medical Center Hospital and Trinity Mother Frances Hospital, Tyler, Texas
Temporomandibular Joint Region Injuries

James C. Perhavec, D.D.S.

Clinical Professor, Case Western Reserve University, Cleveland, Ohio
Basic Exodontia

Richard H. Perry, C.P.A.

Perry amd Varsalona CPAs LLC, Knoxville, Tennessee; Private Practice, Knoxville, Tennessee
Office Management

Ceib Phillips, M.P.H., Ph.D.

Research Professor, Department of Orthodontics, University of North Carolina, Chapel Hill, North Carolina
Psychological Ramifications of Orthognathic Surgery

Keith M. Phillips

Assistant Professor, Director, Graduate Prosthodontics, University of Washington, Seattle Washington
Posterior Implant Restorations for the Partially Edentulous Patient

M. Anthony Pogrel, M.B., Ch.B., B.D.S., F.D.S., R.C.S., F.R.C.S., F.A.C.S.

Professor and Chair, Department of Oral and Maxillofacial Surgery, University of California, San Francisco, San Francisco, California
Tooth Reimplantation and Transplantation

Stanley L. Pollock, B.S., D.M.D., M.S., Ph.D., J.D.

President and CEO. Professional Practice Planners, Inc., McKeesport, Pennsylvania
From Starting to Ending: A Guide to Professional and Personal Achievement

Alan M. Polson, D.D.S., M.S.

Professor of Periodontics and D. Walter Cohen Chair; Associate Dean for Graduate Education; Director of Periodontal Clinical Research Center, Department of Dental Medicine, University of Pennsylvania, Philadelphia, Pennsylvania
Peridontal Considerations for Oral Surgery Procedures Involving the Dentogingival Junction

Michael P. Powers, D.D.S., M.S.

Associate Professor and Chair, Department of Oral and Maxillofacial Surgery, Case Western Reserve University; Head, Division of Oral and Maxillofacial Surgery and Hospital Dentistry, University Hospitals of Cleveland, Cleveland, Ohio
Complicated Exodontia; Surgical Management of Impacted Teeth; Complications of Dentoalveolar Surgery; The Transmandibular Implant Reconstruction System; Soft Tissue Considerations; Reconstruction of the Maxillofacial Cancer Patient

David S. Precious

Professor and Chair, Department of Oral and Maxillofacial Sciences, Dalhousie University; Head, Department of Oral and Maxillofacial Surgery, Queen Elizabeth II Health Sciences Centre, Halifax, Nova Scotia, Canada
Cleft Lip and Palate

William R. Proffit, Ph.D., D.D.S.

Kenan Professor and Chairman, Department of Orthodontics, University of North Carolina at Chapel Hill, Chapel Hill, North Carolina
Patient Selection for Orthognathic Surgery

Marsha A. Pyle, D.D.S., M.Ed.

Assistant Professor, Department of Oral Diagnosis and Radiology, Case Western Reserve University School of Dentistry, Cleveland, Ohio
Rehabilitation of the Edentulous Mandible: Prosthetic and Surgical Concerns

Faisal A. Quereshy, D.D.S., M.D.

Assistant Professor, Department of Oral and Maxillofacial Surgery, Case Western Reserve University School of Dentistry; Assistant Professor, Department of Surgery, Case Western Reserve University School of Medicine; Attending Staff, Division of Oral and Maxillofacial Surgery, University Hospitals of Cleveland, Cleveland, Ohio
Reconstruction of the Maxillofacial Cancer Patient

Peter D. Quinn, D.M.D., M.D.

Chairman, Department of Oral and Maxillofacial Surgery, University of Pennsylvania School of Dental Medicine; Chairman, Department of Oral and Maxillofacial Surgery, Hospital of the University of Pennsylvania, Philadelphia, Pennsylvania
Alloplastic Reconstruction of the Temporomandibular Joint

Joe Rebellato, D.D.S.

Assistant Professor, Orthodontics, Mayo Medical School; Senior Associate Consultant, Orthodontics, Mayo Medical Center, Rochester, Minnesota
Maxillary Quadrangular LeFort I and Quadrangular LeFort II Osteotomy

Eric H. Reed, M.D., D.D.S.

Private Practice of Maxillofacial and Cosmetic Surgery, Daytona Beach, Florida
Facial Suction Lipectomy

David J. Reisberg, D.D.S.

Associate Professor, Department of Surgery, University of Illinois at Chicago College of Medicine; Medical Director, The Craniofacial Center, University of Illinois Medical Center, Chicago, Illinois
Implant-Retained Facial Prostheses

Sivakami Rethnam, B.D.S., Endo Certificate

Ph.D. Candidate, Institute of Physiology, University of Bergen, Bergen, Norway
Principles of Endodontic Microsurgery

David I. Rosenthal, M.D.

Assistant Professor, University of Pennsylvania School of Medicine; Director, Head and Neck Radiation Oncology, University of Pennsylvania Medical Center, Philadelphia, Pennsylvania
Radiation Therapy for Head and Neck Cancer

Dale M. Roberts, D.M.D., M.D., F.A.C.S.

Assistant Clinical Professor, Division of Plastic and Reconstructive Surgery, Department of Surgery, University of Louisville School of Medicine; Director Craniomaxillofacial and Cleft Palate Team, Commission for Children with Special Healthcare Needs, Louisville, Kentucky
Hemifacial Microsomia

Steven M. Roser, D.M.D., M.D.

Georg Guttman Professor of Craniofacial Surgery, Director, Oral and Maxillofacial Surgery, Columbia University School of Dental and Oral Surgery; Attending and Director, Dental Service, New York Presbyterian Hospital, Columbia-Presbyterian, New York, New York
Preoperative, Intraoperative, and Postoperative Care

Mark T. Roszkowski, D.D.S., Ph.D.

Department of Oral and Maxillofacial Surgery, University of Texas Health Sciences Center at San Antonio, San Antonio, Texas
Management of Acute Postoperative Pain

Ronald H. Roth, D.D.S., M.S.

(Adjunct) Clinical Professor of Orthodontics, University of the Pacific, San Francisco, California; (Adjunct) Clinical Professor of Orthodontics, University of Detroit/Mercy, Detroit, Michigan; Surgical Staff, Mills/Peninsula Hospital, Roth/Williams Center, Burlingame, California
Orthognathics and the Temporomandibular Joint

Ramon L. Ruiz, D.M.D., M.D.

Clinical Instructor, Department of Oral and Maxillofacial Surgery, University of North Carolina School of Dentistry; Attending, Division of Oral and Maxillofacial Surgery, University of North Carolina Hospitals, Chapel Hill, North Carolina; Fellow in Pediatric Craniofacial Surgery, Posnick Center for Facial Plastic Surgery, Chevy Chase, Maryland, and Georgetown University Medical Center, Washington, DC
Model Surgery; Craniosynostosis and Craniofacial Dysostosis

Doran Ryan, D.D.S., M.S.

Associate Professor of Surgery/Oral and Maxillofacial Surgery, Medical College of Wisconsin; Adjunct Professor, Department of Oral and Maxillofacial Surgery, Marquette

University, Milwaukee, Wisconsin; President, American Society of Temporomandibular Surgeons
Management of Failed Alloplastic Implants: Immunologic Considerations

Manaf Saker, D.M.D.

Private Practice in Oral and Maxillofacial Surgery, South Orange, New Jersey; Beth Israel Medical Center, Newark, New Jersey
Revascularization and Healing of Orthognathic Surgical Procedures

Noah A. Sandler, D.M.D., M.D.

Assistant Professor, Department of Oral and Maxillofacial Surgery, University of Minnesota–Minneapolis; Attending, Fairview University Medical Center and Hennepin County Medical Center, Minneapolis, Minnesota
Total Mandibular Subapical Osteotomy

George K. B. Sàndor, M.D., D.D.S., F.R.C.D.C., F.R.C.S.C., F.A.C.S.

Director, Graduate Residency Training Programme in Oral and Maxillofacial Surgery, Associate Professor, Faculty of Dentistry, University of Toronto; Coordinator, Oral and Maxillofacial Surgical Services, The Hospital for Sick Children and The Bloorview Macmillan Centre; Staff Plastic Surgeon, Etobicore General Hospital and Humber River Regional Hospital, Toronto, Ontario, Canada
Orbital Hypertelorism

Joseph J. Sansevere, D.M.D.

Clinical Assistant Professor, Department of Oral and Maxillofacial Surgery, University of Medicine and Dentistry of New Jersey–New Jersey Dental School, Newark, New Jersey; Private Practice, Flemington, New Jersey
Soft Tissue Changes Associated with Orthognathic Surgery

David M. Sarver, D.M.D., M.S.

Adjunct Professor, Department of Orthodontics, University of North Carolina, Chapel Hill, North Carolina
The Application of Video Imaging Technology to Orthognathic Surgery

Debra Schardt-Sacco, D.M.D., M.D.

Clinical Assistant Professor, University of North Carolina at Chapel Hill, Chapel Hill, North Carolina
LeFort I Osteotomy; Rigid Internal Fixation in Orthognathic Surgery

Robert J. Seckinger, D.M.D., M.D.S.

Clinical Associate Professor, University of Pennsylvania School of Dental Medicine, Philadelphia, Pennsylvania
Coordination in the Comprehensive Diagnosis and Treatment of the Implant Patient: The Relationship between the Implant Surgeon and the Restorative Doctor; Single-Tooth Replacement in Oral Implantology

Ichiro Semba, D.D.S., Ph.D.

Associate Professor, Department of Oral Pathology, Kagoshima University Dental School, Kagoshima, Japan
Embryogenesis and the Classification of Craniofacial Dysmorphogenesis

Shiva Shanker, B.D.S., D.D.S., M.D.S., M.S.

Assistant Professor, Orthodontics Department, The Ohio State University, College of Dentistry, Section of Orthodontics, Columbus, Ohio
Orthodontic Preparation for Orthognathic Surgery

Mohamed Sharawy, B.D.S., Ph.D.

Professor and Director, Department of Oral Biology and Anatomy, and Professor of Oral and Maxillofacial Surgery, School of Dentistry; Professor of Anatomy, School of Medicine, Medical College of Georgia, Augusta, Georgia
Developmental and Clinical Anatomy and Physiology of the Temporomandibular Joint

Lillian Shum, Ph.D.

Senior Staff Fellow, Craniofacial Development Section, National Institute of Arthritis and Musculoskeletal and Skin Diseases, National Institutes of Health, Bethesda, Maryland
Embryogenesis and the Classification of Craniofacial Dysmorphogenesis

Rebeka G. Silva, D.M.D.

Assistant Clinical Professor, Department of Oral and Maxillofacial Surgery, University of California–San Francisco; Chief, Dental Service, Veterans Administration Medical Center, San Francisco, California
Tooth Reimplantation and Transplantation

Steven J. Silverman, D.M.D., M.D.

Private Practice, Oral and Maxillofacial Surgery, Morristown, New Jersey
Preoperative Evaluation; Hair Restoration Surgery: Transplantation and Micrografting

Keith Silverstein, D.M.D., M.D.

Clinical Assistant Professor of Oral and
Maxillofacial Surgery, University of
Pennsylvania School of Dental Medicine,
Philadelphia, Pennsylvania
Arthritis of the Temporomandibular Joint

Kirt Simmons, D.D.S., Ph.D.

Adjunct Assistant Professor, Department of
Surgery, University of Askansas for Medical
Sciences; Director, Craniofacial Orthodontics,
Arkansas Children's Hospital, Little Rock,
Arkansas
Orthognathic Surgery Before Completion of Growth

Harold Slavkin, D.D.S.

Chief, Craniofacial Development Section,
National Institute of Arthritis and
Musculoskeletal and Skin Diseases, National
Institutes of Health, Bethesda, Maryland
*Embryogenesis and the Classification of Craniofacial
Dysmorphogenesis*

Brian R. Smith, D.D.S., M.S.

Associate Clinical Professor, Louisiana State
University Medical Center, Shreveport,
Louisiana
Treatment of the Complex Facial Trauma Patient

R. Gregory Smith, M.D., D.D.S.

Clinical Assistant Professor, Maxillofacial
Surgery, University of Florida, Gainesville,
Florida; Clinical Assistant Professor of
Department of Oral and Maxillofacial
Surgery, Case Western Reserve University,
Cleveland, Ohio; Private Practice, Ponte
Vedra Beach, Florida
Facial Suction Lipectomy

Thomas Sollecito, D.M.D.

Assistant Professor, Oral Medicine, Director,
Oral Medicine Residency, University of
Pennsylvania School of Dental Medicine;
University of Pennsylvania Health System,
Philadelphia, Pennsylvania
*Role of Splint Therapy in Treatment of
Temporomandibular Disorders*

Anthony M. Spina, D.D.S., M.D.

Assistant Professor, Division of Oral and
Maxillofacial Surgery, University of Kentucky,
Lexington, Kentucky
Mandibular Fractures

David C. Stanton, D.M.D., M.D.

Assistant Professor and Residency Program
Director, Oral and Maxillofacial Surgery,
University of Pennsylvania School of Dental
Medicine, Philadelphia, Pennsylvania
*Tumors of the Temporomandibular Joint; Alloplastic
Augmentation of the Maxillofacial Region*

Jeffrey W. Stearns, D.M.D.

Resident in Oral and Maxillofacial Surgery,
University of Pennsylvania Medical Center,
Children's Hospital of Philadelphia,
Presbyterian Medical Center, Philadelphia,
Pennsylvania
*Revascularization and Healing of Orthognathic
Surgical Procedures*

Scott I. Stein, D.D.S., Certificate in Orthodontics

Clinical Instructor Department of Dentistry,
Program of Orthodontics, University of
Rochester–Eastman Dental Center, Rochester,
New York
*The Role of Occlusion in Temporomandibular
Disorders*

Jeffery C. B. Stewart, D.D.S., M.S.

Associate Professor, Department of
Pathology, School of Dentistry, Oregon
Health Sciences University, Portland, Oregon
*Tumors of the Temporomandibular Joint; Fibro-
osseous Diseases and Benign Tumors of Bone;
Surgical Management of Langerhans' Cell
Histiocytosis*

Christian S. Stohler, D.D.S., Dr.Med.Dent.

William R. Mann Professor and Chair,
Department of Biologic and Materials
Sciences, University of Michigan School of
Dentistry, Ann Arbor, Michigan
Mastication Myalgias

Suzanne U. Stucki-McCormick, M.S., D.D.S.

Assistant Professor, New York Medical
College; Assistant Clinical Professor, New
York University, Mt. Sinai Medical Center;
Private Practice, New York, New York
*Distraction Osteogenesis: A Unique Treatment for
Congenital Micrognathias*

Deborah Studen-Pavlovich, D.M.D.

Director, Predoctoral Pediatric Dentistry, Associate Professor, Department of Pediatric Dentistry, University of Pittsburgh, School of Dental Medicine, Pittsburgh, Pennsylvania
Pharmacosedation for Pediatric Patients

Steven M. Sullivan, D.D.S.

Professor and Chairman, Department of Oral and Maxillofacial Surgery, University of Oklahoma; Chief, Section of Oral and Maxillofacial Surgery, University of Oklahoma College of Medicine, Oklahoma City, Oklahoma
General Procedures

Eric D. Swanson, D.M.D., M.D.

Assistant Professor, Department of Oral and Maxillofacial Surgery, Columbia University School of Dental and Oral Surgery; Attending, Division of Oral and Maxillofacial Surgery, New York Presbyterian Hospital, Columbia-Presbyterian, New York, New York
Preoperative, Intraoperative, and Postoperative Care

Ichiro Takahashi, D.D.S., Ph.D.

Research Associate, Department of Orthodontics, School of Dentistry, Sendai, Japan
Embryogenesis and the Classification of Craniofacial Dysmorphogenesis

Katsu Takahashi, D.D.S., Ph.D.

Research Associate, Department of Oral and Maxillofacial Surgery, Kyoto University School of Medicine, Kyoto, Japan
Embryogenesis and the Classification of Craniofacial Dysmorphogenesis

Ross H. Tallents, D.D.S., B.S. Pharm.D.D.S.

Professor, Department of Dentistry, Programs of Orthodontics, Temporomandibular Disorders, and Prosthodontics, University of Rochester–Eastman Dental Center, Rochester, New York
The Role of Occlusion in Temporomandibular Disorders

Dong-Ping Tan, Ph.D.

Visiting Associate, Craniofacial Development Section, National Institute of Arthritis and Musculoskeletal and Skin Diseases, National Institutes of Health, Bethesda, Maryland
Embryogenesis and the Classification of Craniofacial Dysmorphogenesis

Osamu Tanaka, D.D.S., Ph.D.

Lecturer, Department of Morphology, Human Structure and Function, School of Medicine, Tokai University, Kanagawa, Japan
Embryogenesis and the Classification of Craniofacial Dysmorphogenesis

Clark O. Taylor, M.D., D.D.S.

Assistant Professor of Surgery, Loma Linda University, Loma Linda, California; Assistant Professor of Surgery, University of Nebraska, Department of Maxillofacial Surgery; Director, Institute of Facial Surgery, Omaha, Nebraska
Cosmetic Surgery of the Forehead and Brow

Tinerfe J. Tejera, D.M.D., M.D.

Fellow in Facial Plastics and Reconstructive Surgery, Carolina Surgical Arts, Greensboro, North Carolina
Surgical Uprighting and Repositioning; Otoplastic Surgery for the Protruding Ear

Gaylord S. Throckmorton, Ph.D.

Professor of Cell Biology, University of Texas Southwestern Medical Center at Dallas, Dallas, Texas
Functional Outcomes Following Orthognathic Surgery

Paul Tompach, D.D.S., Ph.D.

Oral Surgeon, Oakdale Medical Center, Robbingdale, Minnesota
Autogenous Temporomandibular Joint Replacement

Sharon Turner, D.D.S., J.D.

Professor and Dean of Dentistry, Oregon Health Sciences University, Oregon Health Sciences University, Portland, Oregon
Insurance and Third-Party Payers

Timothy A. Turvey, D.D.S.

Professor and Chairman, Department of Oral and Maxillofacial Surgery, University of North Carolina at Chapel Hill, Chapel Hill, North Carolina
Patient Selection for Orthognathic Surgery; LeFort I Osteotomy; Orthognathic Surgery Before Completion of Growth; Orthognatic Surgery in the Cleft Patient; Craniosynostosis and Craniofacial Dysostosis

L. George Upton, D.D.S., M.S.

Professor, Department of Oral and Maxillofacial Surgery/Hospital Dentistry, University of Michigan School of Dentistry; Associate Professor, University of Michigan School Medical School; Attending Staff, University of Michigan Hospitals, Ann Arbor, Michigan

Velopharyngeal Dysfunction

Andreas H. Valentin, D.D.S., Ph.D., M.S.C.

Visiting Professor, Nippon Dental University, Tokyo, Japan

Single Tooth Replacement in Oral Implantology

Joseph E. Van Sickels, D.D.S.

Professor, Department of Oral and Maxillofacial Surgery, University of Texas Health and Science Center–San Antonio; Senior Surgeon, Texas University Hospital/ St. Luke's Baptist Hospital, San Antonio, Texas

Bilateral Sagittal Split Osteotomy: Advancement and Setback; Temporomandibular Joint Region Injuries

Robert L. Vanarsdall, Jr., D.D.S.

Professor and Chairman, Department of Orthodontics, University of Pennsylvania School of Dental Medicine; Clinical Professor, Medical College of Pennsylvania; Staff, Childrens' Hospital of Philadelphia, Philadelphia, Pennsylvania

Ectopically Positioned and Unerupted Teeth

Karin Vargervik, D.D.S.

Professor, Department of Growth and Development, University of California–San Francisco, School of Dentistry, San Francisco, California

Congenital and Developmental Temporomandibular Disorders; Embryogenesis and Comprehensive Management of the Cleft Patient

Katherine W. L. Vig, B.D.S., M.D., D.Orth., F.D.S.

Professor and Chairman, Department of Orthodontics, Ohio State University College of Dentistry; Chief of Orthodontic Services, Childrens' Hospital, Columbus, Ohio

Orthodontic Preparation for Orthognathic Surgery

Peter D. Waite, M.P.H., D.D.S., M.D.

Professor and Chairman, Department of Oral and Maxillofacial Surgery, University of Alabama, Birmingham, Alabama; President, American Academy of Cosmetic Surgery, Chicago, Illinois

Maxillofacial Surgery for Treatment of Obstructive Sleep Apnea; Rhytidectomy (Face-lift)

David L. Wells II, D.M.D., M.D.

Resident, Oral and Maxillofacial Surgery, Case Western Reserve University, University Hospitals of Cleveland, Cleveland, Ohio

Complications of Dentoalveolar Surgery

John R. Werther, D.M.D., M.D., F.A.C.S.

Assistant Professor, Department of Oral and Maxillofacial Surgery, Vanderbilt University School of Medicine; Assistant Chief, Oral and Maxillofacial Surgery, Nashville Virginia Medical Center, Nashville, Tennessee

Vertical Ramus Osteotomy and the Inverted-L Osteotomy; Special Soft Tissue Injuries; Aesthetic Blepharoplasty

Raymond P. White, Jr., D.D.S., Ph.D.

Professor, Department of Oral and Maxillofacial Surgery, University of North Carolina–Chapel Hill, Chapel Hill, North Carolina

Patient Selection for Orthognathic Surgery

Randall Wilk, D.D.S., Ph.D., M.D.

Assistant Professor, Department of Oral and Maxillofacial Surgery, New Jersey Dental School, Newark, New Jersey

Anterior and Posterior Maxillary Segmental Osteotomies; Skin Lesions of the Maxillofacial Region

Thomas P. Williams, D.D.S.

Adjunct Professor of Oral Pathology and Oral Diagnosis, University of Iowa, Iowa City; West Third Oral and Maxillofacial Surgery Associates, Dubuque, Iowa

Pathology of the Oral and Maxillofacial Region: Diagnostic and Surgical Considerations; Odontogenic Cysts of the Jaws and Other Selected Cysts

Travis A. Witherington, D.D.S.

Private Practice, Oak Ridge, Tennessee

Sit-Down Oral and Maxillofacial Surgery; Office Management

Larry M. Wolford, D.D.S.

Clinical Professor, Department of Oral and
Maxillofacial Surgery, Baylor College of
Dentistry–Texas A&M University System;
Private Practice, Baylor University Medical
Center, Dallas, Texas
*Diagnosis and Treatment Planning for
Orthognathic Surgery*

Mark E. K. Wong, D.D.S.

Associate Professor, Residency Program
Director, University of Texas Health Sciences
Center–Houston, Houston, Texas
Management of Midface Injuries

Scott Woodbury, D.M.D., M.D.

Private Practice, Saginaw, Michigan
*Velopharyngeal Dysfunction; Reconstruction of the
Edentulous Maxilla; Principles for the Surgical
Placement of Endosseous Implants*

C. MacDonald Worley, Jr., D.M.D., M.D.

Active Staff, Department of Surgery, Wellstar
Kennestone Hospital, Marietta, Georgia
*Morphologic Changes of the Temporomandibular
Joint Associated with Orthognathic Surgery*

John F. Zak, M.D., D.M.D.

Assistant Clinical Professor, Department of
Oral and Maxillofacial Surgery, Case Western
Reserve University, Cleveland, Ohio; Private
Practice, Western Reserve Center for
Orofacial and Cosmetic Surgery, Lakewood,
Ohio
Implant-Retained Facial Prostheses

Deborah Zeitler, D.D.S., M.S.

Professor of Oral and Maxillofacial Surgery,
University of Iowa; University of Iowa
Hospitals and Clinics, Iowa City, Iowa
Alveolar Cleft Grafts

Vincent B. Ziccardi, D.D.S., M.D.

Assistant Professor, Department of Oral and
Maxillofacial Surgery, and Residency
Program Director, University of Medicine
and Dentistry of New Jersey Dental School,
Newark, New Jersey
*Surgically Assisted Maxillary Expansion; Anterior
and Posterior Maxillary Segmental Osteotomies*

Barry E. Zweig, D.D.S.

Professor of Oral and Maxillofacial Surgery,
University of Medicine and Dentistry of New
Jersey–New Jersey Dental School, Newark,
New Jersey
Anterior Mandibular Subapical Osteotomy

Foreword

Gardner's story of Alexander the Great's visit with Diogenes is appropriate to the monumental work done by the editor of this seven-volume text. When Alexander asked Diogenes whether he could do anything for the famed teacher, Diogenes replied, "Only stand out of my light." Perhaps some day we shall know how to heighten industry and creativity to the level that culminated in production of these volumes. Until then, one of the best things we can do for highly creative men and women who are able to develop such a majestic tome as this is to stand out of their light.*

After review of the expansive scope and masterful job done by the editor and his volume editors and chapter contributors, one would be hesitant to find fault with this exceptional coverage of the extent of oral and maxillofacial surgery. It would take a brash soul to cast a shadow over this work.

There are excellent single title textbooks on each of the major subjects, and many of the sub-subjects written about in this seven-volume compilation. But as the editor points out, there has not been such a comprehensive text of oral and maxillofacial surgery previously published in which all titles and interests of a vocation are included under one cover. In the finest spirit of innovation and entrepreneurship at writing, if being "Fustest with the Mostest"† is the strategy to provide convenience and reliability at one source for all matters related to oral and maxillofacial surgery, these books succeed beyond expectation.

There is such a gathering of national and international and recognized and emerging authorities who have contributed as authors that there will be a universal attraction to these books. When one reads the noble words of Fonseca, Frost, Gregg, Dembo, Deegan, Hupp, Donlon, Betts, Turvey, White, Wolford, Vig, Bell, Roser, Campbell, Moos, Van Sickels, Hall, Buckley, Guerrero, McCormick, Ellis, Throckmorton, Waite, Boyd, Marciani, Lew, Ochs, Wong, Gonty, Bertz, Hendler, Werther, Haug, Smith, Myall, Milam, Fricton, Anderson, Roth, Arnett, Holmlund, Bays, Kaban, Quinn, Ryan, Dworkin, Williams, Lilly, Danielson, MacIntosh, Wilk, Dierks, Assael, Ord, Gold, Hudson, Vargervik, Precious, Takahashi, Slavkin, Kennedy, Taylor, Evans, Guttenberg, Barber, Najjar, Alpert, Powers, and others, which are complemented by those of a coming age of equally able professionals, there is no wonder why this work stands out and will endure because of the fine blending of talent. The books have the appeal of a new and satisfying symphony. One is reminded of the story of the maestro who repeatedly nodded his head listening to and enjoying a new symphony. Asked why he did this, he responded, "It is a beautiful symphony, I was merely bowing my head when I heard something from the great masters." And so it will be with this reputable achievement. We will enjoy the total work and nod in satisfaction when reading familiar and established words.

Every imposing publication within a discipline in which writing by several authors

---

*Gardner, J. W. Self Renewal. Harper & Row, Publishers, Inc. N.Y. 1963, 1964.

†Drucker, P. F. Innovation and Entrepreneurship. Harper & Row, Publishers, Inc. N.Y. 1985.

is to be done requires commitment to common goals and shared values of the initiative. Without such a commitment, the writers can wander and produce only a collection of papers. The editor has done a marvelous job in thinking through what he envisioned this extraordinary textbook was to become, and he has convinced his volume editors and contributors of the merit of participating in the production of a highly exciting and distinctive text. This close collaboration has resulted in a distinguished work that speaks for itself, and the textbook is destined to become a prime resource for students, residents, teachers, and practitioners of oral and maxillofacial surgery.

ROBERT V. WALKER, DDS, FFDRCS(I), FDSRCS(E)
Professor Emeritus and Past Chairman
University of Texas Southwestern Medical Center
Dallas, Texas

Preface

We feel privileged to have the opportunity to present *Oral and Maxillofacial Surgery,* a seven-volume text. Approximately 5 years ago, the seed of a thought was planted. It was our goal to create a multiauthored, comprehensive text of oral and maxillofacial surgery. Through the tireless efforts of our volume editors and chapter contributors, our goal has been realized. Our seed took root, and a seven-branched tree bears the fruits of our labor. We are especially proud of the growth of our specialty over the past 30 years. Thoma's fifth-edition *Oral Surgery* text was a two-volume, 58-chapter, two-author, and 1264-page representation of contemporary oral surgery at that time. Our text is a seven-volume, 151-chapter, 16-volume-editor, 282-author, and over 3500-page testament to the vibrant, exciting, and comprehensive scope of our specialty.

Volume 1 is entitled "Anesthesia/Dentoalveolar Surgery/Office Management." We placed this volume first because we believe that the subject matter covered in these chapters constitutes the foundation of the practice of oral and maxillofacial surgery. David E. Frost, Elliot V. Hersh, and Lawrence M. Levin are the volume editors and elicted contributions from authorities on these subjects.

Volume 2 is co-edited by Norman J. Betts and Timothy A. Turvey and is an excellent compilation of the body of knowledge on Orthognathic Surgery. The emphasis in this and other volumes is on surgical considerations; more detailed nonsurgical topics can be found in other subject-related texts.

Robert D. Marciani and Barry H. Hendler are responsible for organizing Volume 3, "Trauma." They have collaborated with experts in the field of facial trauma to produce a concise, surgically oriented volume.

Volume 4, entitled "Temporomandibular Disorders," is co-edited by Robert A. Bays and Peter D. Quinn. Chapters on principles of therapy, diagnosis, and surgical and non-surgical treatment are presented by experts in the field.

Volume 5 is co-edited by Thomas P. Williams and Jeffery C. B. Stewart and is on the subject of Surgical Pathology. They have brought together pathologists and surgeons to discuss comprehensively the basic principles, histopathology, and surgical management of oral and head and neck pathologies.

I had the privilege of co-editing Volume 6 with Stephen B. Baker and Larry M. Wolford. In this volume we cover three areas: Cleft, Craniofacial, and Cosmetic Surgery. We were fortunate to have contributions from an international group of experts.

Last, Volume 7 is entitled "Reconstructive and Implant Surgery" and is co-edited by Michael P. Powers and H. Dexter Barber. The principles of preprosthetic surgery, soft and osseous tissue surgical management, and implantology are discussed in detail.

Our goal was to present the specialty of Oral and Maxillofacial Surgery in its fullest scope by assembling as comprehensive a text as possible. This is our first attempt, and we hope that this text serves your needs and that in our future attempts we will present an even broader scope of our discipline!

Acknowledgments

Oral and Maxillofacial Surgery represents 5 years of 16 volume editors pestering contributors to turn in their chapters on time. Seriously, we owe a great debt to our numerous expert contributors for their comprehensive authoritative treatises in their respective areas. This book defines the scope of oral and maxillofacial surgery and could not have become a reality without the cooperative efforts of experts within and outside of our specialty.

We would also like to thank the many residents, some of whom are contributors to this text. They have provided us with friendship, dedication, intellectual stimulation, and humility, without which this book would not have been written.

Last, I would like to thank Natalie Giuliano and Bobby Mallik for their help, encouragement, and friendship.

Contents

VOLUME 2

Orthognathic Surgery

Volume Editors: Norman J. Betts • Timothy A. Turvey

VOLUME 3

Trauma

Volume Editors: Robert D. Marciani • Barry H. Hendler

VOLUME **4**

Temporomandibular Disorders

Volume Editors: Robert A. Bays • Peter D. Quinn

VOLUME 5

Surgical Pathology

Volume Editors: Thomas P. Williams • Jeffery C. B. Stewart

VOLUME **6**

Cleft/Craniofacial/Cosmetic Surgery

Volume Editors: Raymond J. Fonseca • Stephen B. Baker • Larry M. Wolford

VOLUME 7

Reconstructive and Implant Surgery

Volume Editors: Michael P. Powers • H. Dexter Barber

Principles of Temporomandibular Joint Management

CHAPTER

Developmental and Clinical Anatomy and Physiology of the Temporomandibular Joint

Mohamed Sharawy

Oral and maxillofacial surgeons must understand the functional anatomy of the temporomandibular joint (TMJ) before they can effectively diagnose and treat diseases of the TMJ. Unfortunately, two-dimensional line drawings of the human TMJ have created many misunderstandings about its anatomy. In this chapter, the anatomy of the TMJ is presented at the gross, cellular, subcellular, and molecular levels. Some of the information is based on more than 10 years of research at the author's laboratory, with the help of many faculty members, graduate students, dental students, and postdoctoral fellows.

Developmental Anatomy

The TMJ begins to develop by the 10th week of gestation from two separate blastemas (mesenchymal condensation)[1]—one for the temporal bone component, and one for the condyle. Superior to the condylar blastema, a band of mesenchymal cells develops that will eventually differentiate into the disk. The temporal and condylar mesenchymal cells will differentiate into osteoblasts, which lay down membrane bone. Soft x-ray analysis of human fetal TMJ from 12 to 32 weeks of gestation revealed high degrees of calcification of the condylar head in comparison to the temporal bone.[2] In the center

of the condyle, cartilage develops. This will become the secondary cartilage that remains in the condyle up to 27 years of age. The secondary cartilage contributes to subchondral bone formation by an endochondral mechanism, and it may contribute to the enlargement of the condyle in adulthood as part of the adaptive changes in response to overloading.[3] The developing disk is highly cellular and vascular. It continues anteriorly with the developing lateral pterygoid muscle[4] and posteriorly by a ligament with the superior end of the Meckel's cartilage, which will develop into the malleus of the middle ear.[5] Recently, it was shown that the superior fibers of the ligament insert on the anterior process of the malleus, while the inferior fibers encircle the anterior malleolar ligament, the remnant of Meckel's cartilage, and the chorda tympani and insert on the tympanic wall of the temporal bone.[6] This attachment develops into the discomalleolar ligament, which in postnatal life inserts most of its fibers into the lips of the squamotympanic fissure and apparently loses its attachment to the malleus (Fig. 1–1). In the adult TMJ, the ligament is made primarily of collagen, with elastic fibers only in its proximal two thirds (see Fig. 1–1). In contrast to the postnatal modification of the discomalleolar ligament, the anterior attachment to the superior head of the lateral pterygoid continues to exist after birth. We and others[7] have found that the

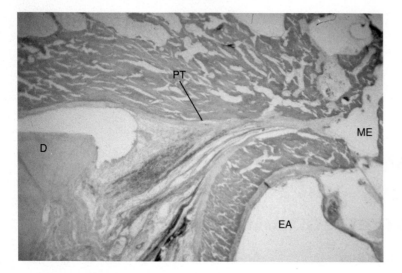

FIGURE 1–1. Most medial parasagittal section of the human temporomandibular joint at the site of the petrotympanic fissure (PT), showing the disk (D), the discomalleolar ligament stained for elastin, a portion of the malleus in the middle ear (ME), and the external auditory canal (EA). Note the absence of elastic fibers in the most distal part of the ligament and the absence of a connection between the ligament and the malleus.

developing anterior and posterior attachments of the human fetal disk are rich in elastic fibers, contradicting the idea that disk elastic develops as a result of masticatory function. The developing TMJ shows all the components of the mature joint by the 14th week of gestation. It is interesting to note that the division of the disk into anterior band, intermediate zone, and posterior band exists in the fetus, which indicates that its morphogenesis is genetically determined.[7] The fetal disk was also found to contain nerve fibers and blood vessels at its peripheries.[8] The blood vessels and nerves disappear from the disk proper but remain at the disk attachment after birth.[9] The sphenomandibular ligament, which connects the spine of the sphenoid to the lingula of the mandible in the adult, is a derivative of the sheath of Meckel's cartilage.[6]

Classification

The TMJs are bilateral, diarthrodial, ginglymoid, synovial, and freely movable. The term *diarthrodial* is used because the joint has two articulating bone components—the mandibular condyle inferiorly, and the articular eminence and glenoid fossa of the temporal bone superiorly. The term *ginglymoid* is used because the joint has a hingelike movement component. The joint is lined by synovial membrane, and it is freely movable.

Clinical Anatomy and Physiology of Temporomandibular Joint Components

The components of the TMJ are presented in the following sequence: capsule, extracapsular ligaments, articular eminence, glenoid fossa, condyle, disk, disk ligaments, and synovial membrane.

CAPSULE

The joint capsule is a fibroelastic, highly vascular, and highly innervated dense connective tissue. The lateral aspect of the capsule attaches to the zygomatic tubercle, the lateral rim of the glenoid fossa, and the postglenoid tubercle. The lateral capsule continues medially until the midsagittal plane and then become less distinct anteriorly at the site where the superior and inferior heads of the lateral pterygoids support the anterior bilaminar zone (Figs. 1–2 and 1–3). Medially, the capsule attaches to the medial rim of the glenoid fossa. The spine of the sphenoid, the sphenomandibular ligament, and the middle meningeal artery passing through the foramen spinosum are all closely related to the medial capsule. The surgeon has to be aware of these relationships and should avoid interfering with the medial capsule. Posteriorly, the capsule attaches to the petrotympanic fissure and fuses with the superior stratum of the posterior bilaminar zone.[10] Between the posterior capsule and the postglenoid tubercle, a

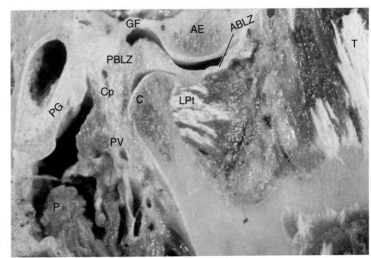

FIGURE 1–2. Midsagittal section of a human cadaveric head. The labeled structures can be identified in Figure 1–3.

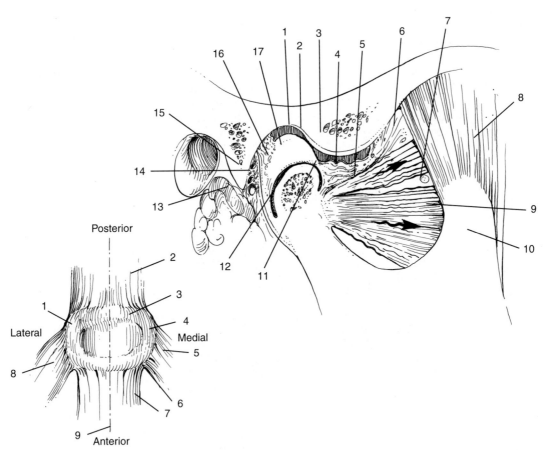

FIGURE 1–3. Midsagittal view drawn from the anatomic dissection shown in Figure 1–2. 1, Glenoid fossa. 2, Fibrous covering (NV, NI, F). 3, Articular eminence. 4, Anterior band. 5, Superior head, lateral pterygoid muscle. 6, Anterior bilaminar zone (V, I, E). 7, Long buccal nerve. 8, Temporalis muscle. 9, Inferior head, lateral pterygoid muscle. 10, Coronoid process. 11, Intermediate zone (NV, NI, F). 12, Fibrous covering of condyle (NV, NI, F). 13, Parotid gland. 14, Vascular body. 15, Postglenoid tubercle. 16, Posterior bilaminar zone (V, I, E). *Inset,* Top view of disk and attached ligaments: 1, Lateral rim. 2, Posterior bilaminar zone (V, I, E). 3, Posterior rim. 4, Medial rim. 5, Medial collateral ligament (V, I, E). 6, Anterior rim. 7, Anterior bilaminar zone (V, I, E). 8, Lateral collateral ligament (V, I, E). 9, Sagittal plane of cut shown in Figures 1–3 to 1–5. E, elastic; F, fibrous; I, innervated; NI, noninnervated; NV, nonvascular; V, vascular.

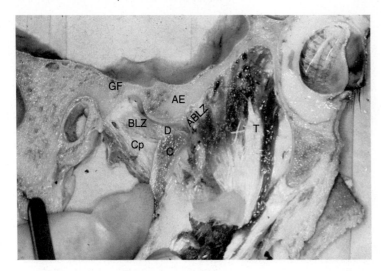

FIGURE 1–4. Midsagittal section of a human cadaver head with the mouth wide open. See Figure 1–5 for identification of temporomandibular joint structures. Note the translation of the disk in a horizontal position under the transverse ridge of the articular eminence, the marked stretch of the capsule and posterior bilaminar zone, and the downward stretch of the anterior bilaminar zone. Compare with the magnetic resonance images in Figure 1–7.

highly vascular tissue called the vascular body is found[10] (Figs. 1–2 to 1–6). Extension of a lateral capsular incision into this area without precautions will cause severe bleeding. These retrodiscal tissues are drawn into the joint by the anteriorly moving disk during jaw opening, as seen by arthroscopy. In addition to the blood vessels, parotid tissue is usually found between the posterior capsule and the postglenoid tubercle (see Figs. 1–2 to 1–6). The parotid gland extends from this location medially until it reaches the lateral wall of the pharynx. Enlargement of the parotid therefore could impinge on the posterior capsule of the TMJ and cause pain during closure of the mouth or during chewing movements. The lateral capsule is thought to be thickened to form a definite ligament known as the temporomandibular ligament. However, some recent cadaveric studies have questioned the presence of this ligament.

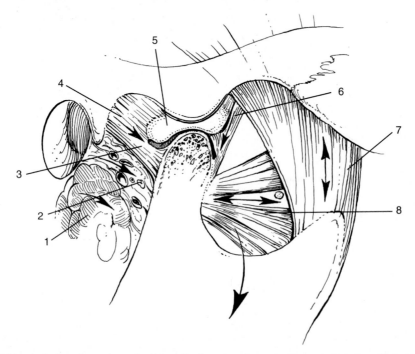

FIGURE 1–5. Midsagittal view drawn from the anatomic dissection shown in Figure 1–4. 1, Parotid. 2, Vascular body. 3, Posterior capsule. 4, Posterior bilaminar zone. 5, Disk, under the transverse ridge of the articular eminence. 6, Anterior bilaminar zone in the stretched position. 7, Temporalis. 8, Inferior head of the lateral pterygoid.

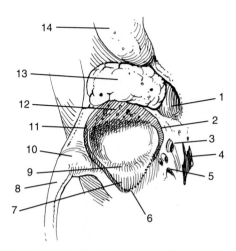

FIGURE 1–6. Inferior view of the temporal bony component of the temporomandibular joint. 1, Carotid canal. 2, Medial capsule. 3, Foramen spinosum. 4, Foramen lacerum. 5, Foramen ovale. 6, Anterior capsule. 7, Ascending slope of eminence. 8, Zygomatic arch. 9, Descending slope of eminence. 10, Zygomatic tubercle. 11, Lateral capsule. 12, Posterior capsule. 13, Parotid gland. 14, Mastoid bone.

During surgical exposure of the lateral capsule through a preauricular incision, one should protect the temporal branch of the facial nerve by having the dissection plane under the superficial layer of the deep temporalis fascia until reaching the root of the zygomatic arch and then keeping tissue reflection close to the periosteum and descending inferiorly to expose the entire lateral capsule. The capsule attaches inferiorly to the periosteum of the neck of the condyle. Lateral retraction of the capsule should allow access to the upper joint space. Incising and reflecting the capsule usually lead to the cutting of nerve fibers, which may result in a period of postoperative analgesia and relief from pain.

EXTRACAPSULAR LIGAMENTS

The main extracapsular ligaments that provide stability to the joint are the lateral temporomandibular and the sphenomandibular ligaments. The sphenomandibular ligament originates from the anterior process of the malleus, the lips of the petrotympanic fissure, and the spine of sphenoid above and inserts into the lingula of the mandibular foramen below. At its upper end, the ligament is crossed by the chorda tympani nerve. The ligament represents one of the embryonic remnants of Meckel's cartilage.

Recently, Loughner and colleagues[11] found, after gross anatomic dissection of 14 heads, that the sphenomandibular ligament has no connection to the medial capsule of the TMJ and therefore has no significance to the biomechanics of the joint. Two other ligaments are associated with the TMJ but are considered accessory to the stability of the joint—the stylomandibular ligament and the pterygomandibular raphe. The stylomandibular ligament attaches to the styloid process above and the angle and posterior border of the mandibular ramus below. The pterygomandibular raphe, when present, attaches to the pterygoid hamulus above and to the posterior end of the mylohyoid ridge of the mandible below.

ARTICULAR EMINENCE

The articular eminence consists of a descending slope, a transverse ridge that is a medial extension of the zygomatic tubercle, and an ascending slope (see Figs. 1–2 to 1–6). The superior stratum of the anterior bilaminar zone inserts on the ascending slope of the eminence and therefore limits the anterior superior recess of the joint cavity. The eminence is covered by dense, compact, fibrous tissue that consists primarily of collagen with a few fine elastic fibers. The fibrous covering is thickest at the descending slope of the eminence. Underlying the fibrous tissue covering is chondroid bone and then compact bone. Unlike the glenoid fossa, the articular eminence is subjected to loading during function.

GLENOID FOSSA

The glenoid, or mandibular, fossa is limited posteriorly by the petrotympanic fissure, which provides attachment to the posterior capsule and limits the boundary of the posterior superior recess of the joint cavity (see Figs. 1–2 to 1–6). The fossa has lateral and medial rims (see Fig. 1–6). The medial rim is just lateral to the spine of the sphenoid and the foramen spinosum with its middle meningeal artery. The lateral rim continues anteriorly into the zygomatic tubercle, which can be felt under the skin, and posteriorly into the postglenoid tubercle (see Fig. 1–6). The chorda tympani nerve appears at the medial end of the petrotympanic fissure close to the spine of sphenoid. The roof of the fossa is thin and separates the brain from the joint cavity (see Fig. 1–2); therefore, during surgical manipulation at the fossa, care should be taken to avoid perforation of the roof of fossa. The fossa is covered by a thin fibrous layer, suggesting that the area is not normally loaded.

CONDYLE

The condyle is broad mediolaterally and narrow anteroposteriorly (see Figs. 1–2 to 1–5). It has a lateral tubercle that can be felt under the skin, a joint capsule, and a medial tubercle. The tubercles provide attachments to the lateral and medial collateral ligaments. The condylar axis runs between the tubercles in a posteromedial direction and meets the axis from the opposite side at an angle that varies from zero to obtuse. The articular surface of the condyle is covered by a thick layer of fibroelastic tissue containing fibroblasts and a variable number of chondrocytes. The condylar covering is sometimes classified as fibrocartilage, and its components vary with age and with the region of the condyle—anterior, middle, or posterior. At a young age, the deepest layer of the fibrocartilage is rich in small undifferentiated cells; this is called the reserve cell layer.[3] Many of the cells in this layer become labeled with tritiated thymidine and are proliferating cell nuclear antigen (PCNA)–positive, indicative of their high proliferative activity. A recent experiment we did on the rabbit condyle using PCNA immunocytochemistry showed PCNA-positive cells at all layers of the condyle, such as in the chondrocytic layer and the hypertrophied chondrocytic layer, indicating each zone's ability to renew its own cells.[12] However, these results do not mean that the undifferentiated reserve cell layer is incapable of contributing to the chondrocytic cell layer. Between the reserve cell layer and the subchondral bone in the young condyle, a hyaline cartilage exists. It consists of several layers of chondrocytes, followed by several rows of upper hypertrophied chondrocytes, followed by a hypertrophied degenerating chondrocytic layer. The last shows a large number of apoptotic cells (unpublished observation). It appears that in the presence of cartilage, the condyle is able to adapt to excess loading by becoming hyperplastic.[3] In the aging condyle, only remnants of the cartilage remain, and it becomes calcified. At this stage, trauma from overloading may lead to degenerative joint disease.

DISK

The gross morphology, histology, immunocytochemistry, and ultrastructure of the disk are considered here. The term *disk* is preferred over *meniscus* because the latter refers to a semilunar structure that may have a central perforation. Because TMJ disk perforation is considered a pathologic condition, the term *meniscus* should not be used to describe the TMJ disk. The disk fills in the space between the condyle and the temporal bone. In the centric relation position of the mandible, the central portion of the disk is in contact superiorly with the descending slope of the articular eminence and inferiorly with the convex articular surface of the condyle (Fig. 1–7). Therefore, the disk is biconcave in shape, with anterior and posterior rims and medial and lateral rims (see Fig. 1–3 inset). In midsagittal cut, the disk consists of an anterior band, intermediate zone, and posterior band (see Figs. 1–3 to 1–5). It is described as avascular noninnervated fibrocartilage. In hematoxylin-eosin–stained sections, the disk consists primarily of collagen that runs in many directions, particularly in the thick rim parts. The majority of the cells are fibroblasts, with some chondrocytes that stain heavily with basic dyes. Resorcin-fuchsin stain, which is selective for elastin, demonstrates the presence of thin elastic fibers that run parallel with collagen bundles. Immunohistochemical techniques using polyclonal antibodies directed against type I collagen, a marker of fibroblasts, or type II collagen, a marker of chondrocytes, have revealed the predominance of type I collagen and the presence of type II collagen in the TMJ disk of many animal species.[13, 14] In addition, lectins (Fig. 1–8) (which bind to the sugar components of proteoglycans) and monoclonal antibodies directed against specific proteoglycans revealed the presence of these macromolecules as part of the extracellular matrix of the disk.[15–18] Specifically, keratan

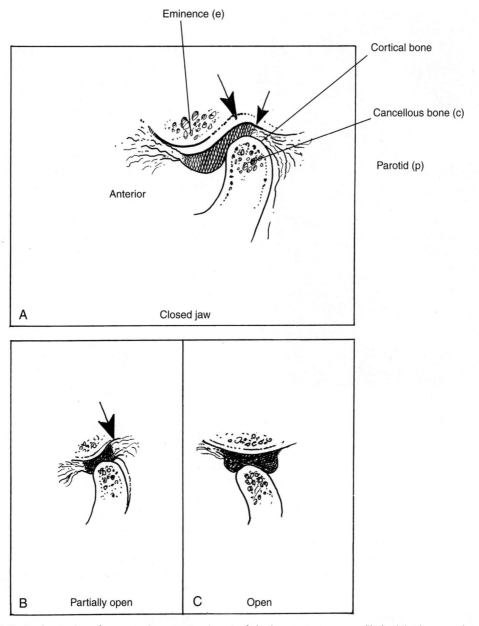

FIGURE 1–7. Overlay tracing of a magnetic resonance image of the human temporomandibular joint in a centric relation position *(A)*, partially open position *(B)*, and open position *(C)*. Note at the disk covers the condyle during all condylar movements.

sulfate (KS), chondroitin 4-sulfate (C4S), chondroitin 6-sulfate (C6S), hyaluronic acid (HA), and link protein (LP) are essential components of condylar cartilage and disk fibrocartilage.[16] These glycosaminoglycans (GAGs) are distributed mainly in the load-bearing areas. The negative charges on the GAGs attract water and allow the disk or condylar cartilage to absorb the stresses applied to it by deforming and leaking water. After relief from the compressive force, the water content is restored and the loaded tissue returns back to its original shape.[19] In an experimental model of anterior disk displacement, we demonstrated a marked loss of GAGs in condylar cartilage and the disk and the concomitant development of osteoarthritis similar to other synovial joint osteoarthritis.[16] The chondrocyte plasma membrane contains receptors for HA called CD_{44} and receptors for GAGs known as beta glycans. These receptors anchor HA or

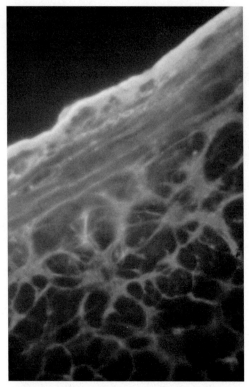

FIGURE 1–8. Frozen section of a rabbit temporomandibular joint disk showing strong binding of fluorescin-conjugated maclura pomifera agglutinin (MPA) (galactose-binding lectin) to proteoglycans in the disk matrix.

the ultrastructural characteristics of fibroblasts; a smaller number of cells appeared as chondrocytes, with their typical territorial matrices (Figs. 1–10 and 1–11). At the electron-microscopic level, the extracellular matrix consists primarily of collagens that run parallel to each other at the intermediate thin zone and in all directions at the anterior and posterior thick zones (see Figs. 1–10 and 1–11). In loaded areas, the diameter of the collagen fibrils varies, a characteristic shared by tissues that are subjected to heavy loading.[17] From the cellular, subcellular, and molecular organization of the TMJ disk, one can clearly see the disk's adaptation to its function as a shock absorber. At the end of this chapter, experimental evidence is presented to support the view that the disk is the protector of the bony components of the joint.

DISK LIGAMENTS

The disk ligaments consist of the anterior and posterior bilaminar zones or ligaments, the lateral and medial collateral ligaments, and the discomalleolar ligament. All these ligaments are vascular, innervated, and fibroelastic in nature. The anterior ligament has a superior stratum that inserts on the ascending slope of the articular eminence and an inferior stratum that inserts inferiorly at the anterior aspect of the condyle (see Figs. 1–2 and 1–3). The ligament is normally relaxed and folded on itself while the dentulous mandible is in a centric rela-

GAGs to the chondrocyte membrane and therefore contribute to the integrity of the extracellular matrix under loading. At the ultrastructural level, we were able to localize these macromolecules using a colloidal gold labeling technique (Fig. 1–9). The majority of the cells found in the disk showed

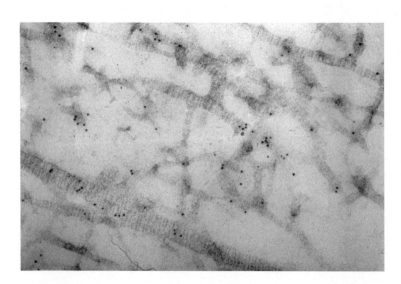

FIGURE 1–9. Electron micrograph of a portion of temporomandibular joint disk incubated with chondroitin 4-sulfate antibody conjugated to colloidal gold particles. Note the presence of chondroitin sulfate in the extracellular matrix in close relationship to collagen.

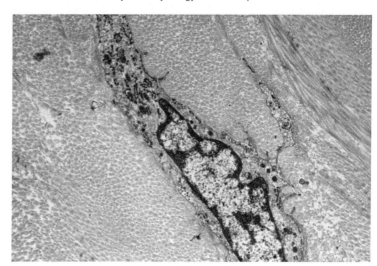

FIGURE 1–10. Electron micrograph of a rhesus monkey temporomandibular joint disk showing collagen running in different directions and a fibroblast. The fibroblast is the most common disk cell.

tion position. The ligament stretches downward as the condyle rotates during mouth opening. This can be seen in cadaveric simulation of mouth opening (see Fig. 1–4) and with magnetic resonance imaging (MRI) (see Fig. 1–7). The anterior ligament is supported by the superior and inferior heads of the lateral pterygoid muscles (see Figs. 1–2 and 1–3). The posterior ligament or bilaminar zone consists of a highly elastic superior stratum that inserts on the lips of the petrotympanic fissure and an inferior stratum that also contains elastic fibers that inserts on the posterior aspect of the condyle below. The superior stratum of the posterior bilaminar zone limits the boundary of the posterior superior recess, and the superior stratum of the anterior ligament limits the boundary of the anterior superior recess.

The anterior inferior recess is limited by the inferior stratum of the anterior bilaminar zone, and the posterior inferior recess is limited by the inferior stratum of the posterior bilaminar zone (see Figs. 1–2 and 1–3). The posterior bilaminar zone stretches considerably during jaw opening to allow the disk to continue to cover the condyle at all ranges of motion. The elastic fibers in the posterior ligament are organized at a right angle to those of the posterior capsule, suggestive of its role in allowing the anteroposterior stretch of the ligament. The cells of the disk and the ligaments secrete protease inhibitors that protect the elastin from the action of free elastase. The latter is known to be released during trauma. In our laboratory, we injected pure porcine elastase into rabbit bilaminar zones, which resulted in a

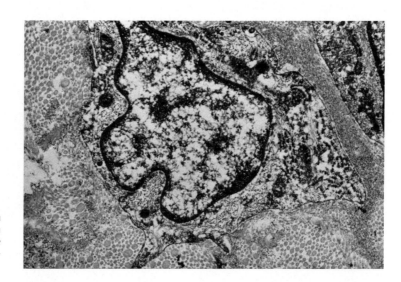

FIGURE 1–11. Chondrocytes with a typical territorial matrix are seen in the disk. Note the variation in the cross-sectional diameters of collagen, characteristic of loaded tissues.

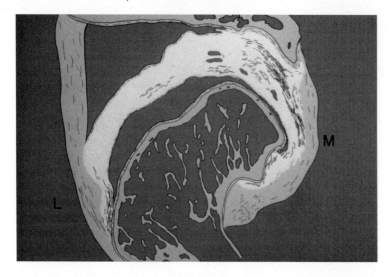

FIGURE 1–12. Camera lucida tracing of a coronal section of human temporomandibular joint stained with resorcin-fuchsin for localization of elastic fibers. The dark lines indicate the presence of elastic fibers in both the medial and the lateral condylodiskal collateral ligaments.

marked loss of elastin.[18] MRI of the injected joints revealed moderate but consistent anterior disk displacement in comparison to control sham injected joints (unpublished observation). These results point to the important role of the elasticity of the posterior ligament in maintaining the position of the disk relative to the condyle. The bilaminar zones contain only type I collagen and GAGs, similar to other fibrous connective tissue.[20] It has been reported that the posterior bilaminar zone in joints with anterior disk displacement without reduction undergo fibrotic changes and become a disklike structure referred to as a pseudodisk.[21] In an experimental model of the disease, we reported on the appearance of type II collagen and sulfated proteoglycans characteristic of fibrocartilage and disk tissue in the rabbit bilaminar zone, therefore confirming the process of pseudodisk formation under overloading.[16, 20] It was observed that the bilaminar zone blood vessels became obliterated. Whether the nerves also degenerate needs to be investigated. It is a common clinical observation that some patients who suffer from anterior disk displacement without reduction experience a decrease in their pain. It also appears that the pseudodisk may slow the development of degenerative joint disease. In some cases, the bilaminar zone responds to trauma with a perforation rather than with pseudodisk formation. Disk perforation is commonly associated with degenerative joint disease.

The medial and lateral condylodiscal or collateral ligaments are collagenous and firmly attach the disk to the lateral and

medial poles of the condyle, respectively. In our laboratory, cadaveric study of resorcin-fuchsin–stained sections revealed numerous elastic fibers that insert at right angles to the surfaces of the condyle (Figs. 1–12 and 1–13). At the electron-microscopic level, mature elastic fibers with amorphous elastin

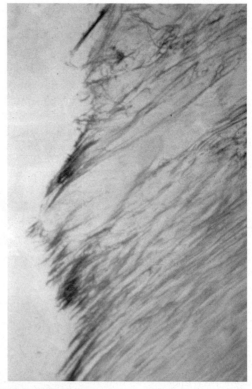

FIGURE 1–13. Human temporomandibular joint medial ligament stained with resorcin-fuchsin for localization of elastic fibers. Note the abundance of elastic fibers, their parallel orientation, and their insertion into the unstained condyle.

and microfibrillar components were consistently present. These results suggest that the elastic collateral ligaments could allow the mediolateral shift of the disk relative to the condyle during lateral chewing movements. It has been suggested, but without experimental evidence, that traumatic injury to the lateral collateral ligament could lead to subluxation and medial displacement of the disk proper. Both of the collateral ligaments are vascular and highly innervated. As discussed later, the medial collateral ligament receives fibers from the inferior head of the lateral pterygoid muscle. Although it is tempting to speculate, based on this observation, that spasm of the muscle could lead to medial disk displacement, there is no experimental evidence to support this idea.

The most medial portion of the disk is connected posteriorly to a ligament referred to as the discomalleolar or Pinto's ligament. Pinto in 1962 presented histologic evidence for the presence of a fibrous link between the disk and the anterior process of the malleus of the middle ear.[22] Because such a relationship exists in the fetus, it was accepted as an anatomic fact until further studies confirmed the presence of the ligament but disputed its consistent connection to the malleus. Loughner and colleagues in 1989 found in gross anatomic dissection of 14 cadaver heads that only one specimen showed anatomic continuity of the ligament through the petrotympanic fissure to the malleus of the middle ear.[23] We studied several histologic sections of eight TMJs from four cadavers and failed to demonstrate a connection to the malleus. Also, elastic fibers were found only in the proximal (toward the joint cavity) two thirds of the ligament. Collagen bundles were inserted on the lips of the fissures all the way to the middle ear cavity (see Fig. 1–1). The question that remains to be answered is whether these few cases in which an anatomic connection with the malleus can be demonstrated represent an anomaly that may have clinical significance to the known otic complaints of some patients with TMJ disorders.

SYNOVIAL MEMBRANE

The inside of the TMJ capsule and the nonarticulating surfaces of disk ligaments are lined with synovial membrane. Synovial villous projections can be seen grossly as hyperemic tissue in the anterior, posterior, medial, and lateral recesses of the joint cavities (Fig. 1–14). Histologically, the synovial membrane consists of intimal and subintimal layers. The intima is one to four layers deep. Two types of cells that are not connected to each other are usually differentiated by their RNA content. One cell type appears as a fibroblast under the light microscope and possesses all the ultrastructural features of a fibroblast, such as abundant rough endoplasmic reticulum and a nucleus with euchromatin and prominent nucleoli. These cells are thought to secrete subintimal collagen and proteoglycans and the glycoproteins of the synovial fluid. These cells are referred to as type B, or S cells. The second type of cell is macrophage-like and contains a large number of lyso-

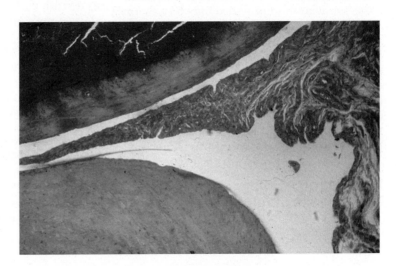

FIGURE 1–14. Human temporomandibular joint showing a well-developed synovial villus in one of the joint recesses, with surface intimal cells and vascular subintimal connective tissue.

somes, free ribosomes, and a well-developed Golgi complex. These cells are active in phagocytosis and are referred to as type A, or M cells.[24] Chronic hemarthrosis or injection of blood into rabbit synovial joint was found to activate the synovial type A cells to phagocytose the red blood cells, many of which were found intracellularly.[25] Both types of synovial cells are capable of secreting proteases such as collagenase and elastase into the synovial fluid, the purpose of which is to prevent fibrous adhesions between the joint surfaces. There is no true basal lamina that separates the intima from the subintimal connective tissue. The latter is vascular and consists of either areolar loose connective tissue containing collagen and elastin fibers (fibroareolar) or dense fibrous tissue (fibrous). Free nerve endings have been demonstrated in human subsynovium. Substance P–like immunoreactive nerve fibers were also described in the subsynovium of monkeys.[26]

In rheumatoid arthritis, synovial hyperplasia may contribute to the severity of pain, and surgical synovectomy usually leads to relief from pain. It has been estimated that the volume of synovial fluid in the superior joint compartment is 1.2 mL, whereas the inferior compartment contains 0.9 mL.[27] The fluid exists under negative intraarticular pressure.[28] The surface tension of the synovial fluid allows the spread of the fluid over the articular surfaces as a capillary film that permits the lubrication of the joint during condylar movements. The synovial fluid contains a glycoprotein known as lubricin, which serves to lubricate and minimize friction between articular surfaces of synovial joints.[29] An increase in intraarticular synovial fluid pressure may be a factor in the pathogenesis of osteoarthritis and may cause pain. Westessen and Brooks, using MRI, found synovial effusion in many patients with internal derangement. They correlated the severity of pain with the degree of synovial effusion.[30] More studies of synovial fluid, cytokines, proteoglycan content, and physical properties of healthy and pathologic human joints need to be done.

Innervation of the Temporomandibular Joint

The TMJ receives innervation primarily from the auriculotemporal nerve branch of the mandibular nerve (V3 of the trigeminal nerve), with contribution from other branches from V3, such as the masseteric and deep temporal nerves.[31] The joint capsule, the disk ligaments (anterior, posterior, medial, and lateral), and the synovium are innervated, whereas the disk proper and the fibrous coverings of the articulating surfaces and condylar cartilages are noninnervated.[32] In addition to the nerve fibers, the TMJ capsule contains three types of mechanoreceptors: Ruffini receptors, Golgi tendon organs, and pacinian corpuscles.[32] In addition, free nerve endings—referred to as nociceptors—were localized in the TMJ. Studies using retrograde axonal tracing reported that the origin of the peripheral nerves is in the superior cervical and stellate sympathetic ganglia, trigeminal ganglia, and second to fifth dorsal root ganglia. These fibers synapse centrally with second-order neurons in the subnucleus caudalis of the trigeminal nerve.[33, 34] Several studies described the presence of substance P–immunoreactive nerve fibers in the TMJ capsule and disk attachments. Other neuropeptides such as calcitonin gene-related peptides (CGRPs), neuropeptide Y (NPY), and vasoactive intestinal polypeptide (VIP) have been demonstrated in the TMJ tissues. These peptides are thought to be neurotransmitters for a pain-mediated pathway.[35–37] A recent study in the rat demonstrated the presence of the peptidergic nerves in the disk attachment at birth and their increase by functional stimuli such as sucking and mastication to the adult innervation. It is interesting to note that the nerves developed before the appearance of synovial cells, which suggests that the nerves may affect the differentiation of the synovial cells.[9] The use of nerve-specific antibodies such as neurofilaments and myelin basic proteins confirmed the absence of nerves in the disk proper, the condylar cartilage, and the fibrous coverings of the articulating surfaces and confirmed the presence of nerves in the disk attachments and the capsule.[38, 39] A change in the normal distribution of nerves can occur under certain pathologic conditions. Several studies have demonstrated the presence of higher concentrations of neurofilaments and neuropeptides in the synovium, periosteum, joint capsule, and synovial fluid of patients with rheumatoid arthritis and osteoarthritis.[40–43]

In an animal model for anterior disk displacement, fibrous adhesions and osteoarthritic cartilage were found to be innervated,[39] which may indicate a possible mechanism of nociception in diseased joints. It may also offer an explanation for patients' pain relief after joint lavage, which may disrupt adhesions and release the nerves from sites of intraarticular pressure.

Muscles Closely Related to the Temporomandibular Joint

The lateral pterygoid, temporalis, and masseter muscles are considered here. The lateral pterygoid muscle consists of two heads, upper and lower. The lower head originates from the outer surface of the lateral pterygoid plate, the pyramidal process of the palatine bone, and the adjacent portion of the maxillary tuberosity. The superior head arises from the upper third of the lateral pterygoid plate, from the infratemporal surface of the greater wing of the sphenoid lateral to the foramen ovale. The fibers from the two heads get closer and almost unite before their insertion sites. The medial half of the condylar fovea receives most of the fibers of both heads of the lateral pterygoid. The upper head inserts some of its fibers (~15%) into the medial portion of the anterior band of the disk. In sagittal sections that cut through the medial pole of the condyle, fibers that can be traced to the inferior head are clearly seen inserting into the fibrous covering of the pole (Fig. 1–15). Sagittal sections through the medial collateral ligament and the medial surface of the disk showed lateral pterygoid muscle fibers that belong to the inferior head continuing into these tissues (Fig. 1–16). This was confirmed in coronal sections (Fig. 1–17), as well as histologically (Fig. 1–18). These results point out the possibility that spasm of the inferior head of the lateral pterygoid could lead to medial disk displacement. Also, such an anatomic relationship may be important during normal medial rotation of the condyle-disk complex during chewing.

Electromyographic (EMG) studies presented evidence to support the idea that the upper head is active during closing movements while the inferior head is active during protraction, opening, and eccentric lateral movements.[44–46] Because of the presence of medial pterygoid muscle fibers lateral to the origin of the lateral pterygoid, clinical palpation of the lateral pterygoid muscle intraorally is questionable, and blind placement of electrodes into the two heads of the muscle in humans is difficult. Therefore, the results of these EMG studies need to be confirmed by placement of electrodes when the joint is open. Fibers from the posterior one third of the temporalis muscle and fibers of the deep masseter muscle were described to be attached to the anterolateral one third of the disk.[47, 48] However, the function of these muscle attachments is still unknown.

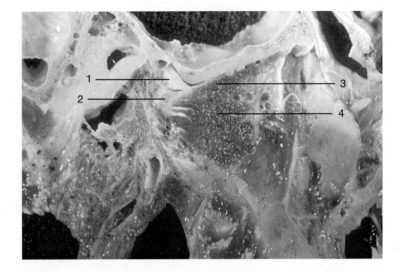

FIGURE 1–15. Sagittal section of a human temporomandibular joint at the medial pole of the condyle. Note the attachment of the superior and inferior heads to the disk and medial pole of the condyle. 1, Disk. 2, Medial pole of condyle. 3, Superior head of lateral pterygoid. 4, Inferior head of lateral pterygoid.

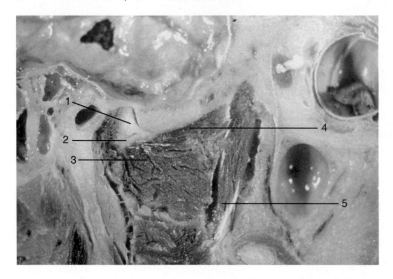

FIGURE 1–16. Sagittal section of a human temporomandibular joint at the disk and medial collateral ligament. Note the attachment of the inferior head of the lateral pterygoid to the medial collateral ligament. 1, Disk. 2, Medial collateral ligament. 3, Inferior head of lateral pterygoid. 4, Superior head of lateral pterygoid. 5, Temporalis.

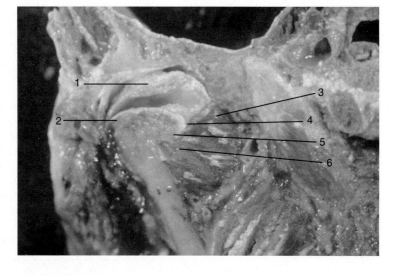

FIGURE 1–17. Coronal section of a human temporomandibular joint showing the attachment of the superior and inferior heads of lateral pterygoids to the medial pole, medial collateral ligament, and disk. 1, Disk. 2, Lateral pole of condyle. 3, Superior head of lateral pterygoid. 4, Medial collateral ligament. 5, Medial pole of condyle. 6, Inferior head of lateral pterygoid.

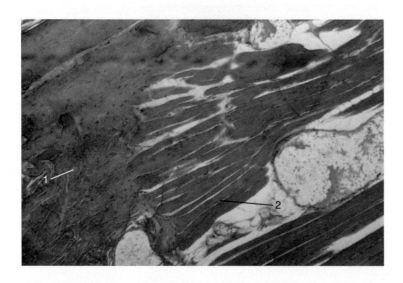

FIGURE 1–18. Histologic section of a human temporomandibular joint disk showing the insertion of lateral pterygoid muscle fibers into disk tissues. 1, Disk. 2, Muscle fibers from inferior head of lateral pterygoid.

Functions of the Temporomandibular Joint Disk

Unlike in other synovial joints, the TMJ condyle and temporal bone do not fit together in the absence of the disk. The disk fills the wedgelike gaps created by the rounded bony edges of the joint and thus stabilizes the joint during rotation and translation. The inferior concavity of the disk fits precisely onto the convexity of the condyle, while its upper concavity fits the convexity of the articular eminence in centric occlusion. Normally, there is no space between the disk and the articular surfaces, except for the anterior superior and anterior inferior recesses and the posterior superior and posterior inferior recesses. There are also medial upper and lower recesses and lateral upper and lower recesses. The recesses are filled with synovial fluid and allow the rotation of the condyle into the anterior recess during jaw movement, which squeezes the fluid back into the posterior recess and spreads a film of the lubricating synovial fluid on the articulating surfaces of the joint. A similar fluid dynamic occurs during lateral chewing movements. The maximal joint contact provided by the disk reduces the contact stress on the load-bearing surfaces of the joint. Experimental disk removal or experimental creation of disk perforation in nonhuman primates resulted in the development of histopathologic changes consistent with the osteoarthritic changes we commonly see in patients with disk perforation or with anterior disk displacement without reduction.[49, 50] Recently a rabbit model for anterior disk displacement without reduction (ADD) was developed. Two weeks following ADD, degenerative joint disease occurred, with histopathologic and immunocytochemical changes similar to those seen in osteoarthritis of other synovial joints. A marked decline in proteoglycans (essential for the shock-absorber function of the disk) and link proteins (essential for the integrity of the aggrecan molecules) was reported.[14, 51–55] It appears, at least in experimental animals such as monkeys and rabbits, that the degenerative changes can be reversed if the TMJ disk is repaired.[56] These experimental results all point to the importance of the disk as a shock absorber that protects the articulating surfaces against overloading. Unfortunately, one cannot correlate the degenerative changes following disk perforation or disk displacement with nociception in experimental animals.

In addition to the shock-absorber function, the disk reduces the space between the articular surfaces so that a capillary film of synovial fluid spreads to cover the surfaces and maintain lubrication. Also, because of the attachment of the disk to the retrodiscal tissue, the disk translation pulls the vascular tissues forward and opens the vascular elements to increase the blood flow during jaw opening.

Summary

The TMJ has a lot in common with other synovial joints, but it also has its own unique features. These unique features include (1) the articulating surfaces are covered not by hyaline cartilage but by fibroelastic tissue; (2) the condylar cartilage is considered a growth center that insignificantly contributes to the overall growth of the mandible but is important for condylar response to trauma, and it disappears by about age 25; (3) the TMJ functions bilaterally and can be influenced by dental occlusion; and (4) the TMJ has an intact disk that is movable during all joint movements and functions as a shock absorber.

REFERENCES

1. Perry HT, Xu Y, Forbes DP: The embryology of the temporomandibular joint. J Craniomandibular Pract 1985;3:126.
2. Sato I, Ishikawa H, Shimada K, et al: Morphology and analysis of the development of the human temporomandibular joint and masticatory muscle. Acta Anat 1994;149:55.
3. Carlsson GE, Oberg T: Remodelling of the temporomandibular joints. Oral Sci Rev 1974;6:53.
4. Ogutcen-Toller M, Juniper RP: The development of the human lateral pterygoid muscle and the temporomandibular joint and related structures: A three-dimensional approach. Early Hum Dev 1994;39:57.
5. Vazquez R, Velasco M, Collado J: Relationships between the temporomandibular joint and the middle ear in human fetuses. J Dent Res 1993;72:62.
6. Ogutcen-Toller M: The morphogenesis of the human discomalleolar and sphenomandibular ligaments. J Craniomaxillofac Surg 1995;23:42.
7. Valenza V, Farina E, Carini F: The prenatal morphology of the articular disk of the human tempo-

romandibular joint. Ital J Anat Embryol 1993;98:221.

8. Ramieri G, Bonardi G, Morani V, et al: Development of nerve fibres in the temporomandibular joint of the human fetus. Anat Embryol 1996;194:57.

9. Shimizu S, Kido MA, Kiyoshima T, Tanaka T: Postnatal development of protein gene product 9.5– and calcitonin gene-related peptide-like immunoreactive nerve fibers in the rat temporomandibular joint. Anat Rec 1996;245:568.

10. Rees LA: The structure and function of the mandibular joint. Br Dent J 1954;96:125.

11. Loughner BA, Gremillion HA, Mahan PE, Watson RE: The medial capsule of the human temporomandibular joint. J Oral Maxillofac Surg 1997;55:363.

12. Choi WS: Alterations in articular cartilage of the rabbit mandibular condyle following surgical induction of anterior disc displacement: Light and electron microscopic immunocytochemistry using colloid gold conjugates. Ph.D. thesis, May 1996.

13. Milam SB, Klebe RJ, Triplett RG, Herbert D: Characterization of the extracellular matrix of the primate temporomandibular joint. J Oral Maxillofac Surg 1992;49:381.

14. Ali AM, Sharawy M: An immunohistochemical study of the effects of surgical induction of anterior disk displacement of the rabbit craniomandibular joint on type I and II collagens. Arch Oral Biol 1995;40:473.

15. Sharawy MM, Linatoc AJ, O'Dell NL, et al: Morphological study of lectin binding in the rabbit temporomandibular joint disc. Histochem J 1991;23:132.

16. Ali AM, Sharawy M: Histochemical and immunohistochemical studies of the effects of experimental anterior disc displacement on sulfated glycosaminoglycans, hyaluronic acid, and link protein of the rabbit craniomandibular joint. J Oral Maxillofac Surg 1996;54:992.

17. Ghadially FN: Articular cartilage. In Ghadially FN (ed): Fine Structure of Synovial Joints. London, Butterworths, 1983, pp 42–79.

18. Sharawy M, O'Dell NL, Pennington CB, et al: Effects of elastase on the rabbit craniomandibular articular disk. J Dent Res 1992;71(suppl):237.

19. Mankin HJ, Mow VC, Buckwalter JA, et al: Form and function of articular cartilage. In Simon SR (ed): Orthopaedic Basic Science. Chicago, IL, American Academy of Orthopaedic Surgeons, 1994, pp 1–44.

20. Ali AM, Sharawy M: An immunohistochemical study of the effects of surgical induction of anterior disc displacement in the rabbit craniomandibular joint on type I and type II collagens. Arch Oral Biol 1995;40:473.

21. Blaustein DI, Scapino RP: Remodelling of the temporomandibular joint disc and posterior attachment in disc displacement specimens in relation to glycosaminoglycan content. Plast Reconstr Surg 1986;78:756.

22. Pinto OF: A new structure related to the temporomandibular joint and middle ear. J Prosthet Dent 1962;12:95.

23. Loughner BA, Larkin LH, Mahan PE: Discomalleolar and anterior malleolar ligaments: Possible causes of middle ear damage during temporomandibular joint surgery. Oral Surg Oral Med Oral Pathol 1989;68:14.

24. Dijkgraaf LC, Lambert GM, Bont DE, et al: Structure of the normal synovial membrane of the temporomandibular joint: A review of the literature. J Oral Maxillofac Surg 1996;54:332.

25. Ghadially FN: Chronic haemarthrosis (haemophilic arthropathy and experimentally produced chronic haemarthrosis). In Ghadially FN (ed): Fine Structure of Synovial Joints. London, Butterworths, 1983, pp 164–179.

26. Johansson AS, Isacsson G, Isberg A, Granholm AC: Distribution of substance P–like immunoreactive nerve fibers in temporomandibular joint soft tissues of monkey. Scand J Dent Res 1986;94:225.

27. Toller PA: The synovial apparatus and TMJ function. Br Dent J 1961;111:355.

28. Roth TE, Goldberg JS, Behrents RG: Synovial fluid pressure determination in the temporomandibular joint. Oral Surg 1984;57:583.

29. Hatton MN, Swann DA: Studies on bovine temporomandibular joint synovial fluid. J Prosthet Dent 1986;56:635.

30. Westesson PL, Brooks S: Temporomandibular joint: Relationship between MR evidence of effusion and the presence of pain and disk displacement. Am J Radiol 1992;159:559.

31. Thilander B: Innervation of the temporomandibular joint disc in man. Acta Odontol Scand 1964;22:151.

32. Wink CS, Onge MS, Zimmy ML: Neural elements in the human temporomandibular articular disc. J Oral Maxillofac Surg 1992;50:334.

33. Widenfalk B, Wiberg M: Origin of sympathetic and sensory innervation of the temporomandibular joint: A retrograde axonal tracing study in the rat. Neurosci Lett 1990;109:30.

34. Broton JG, Hu JW, Sessle BJ: Effects of temporomandibular stimulation on nociceptive and nonnociceptive neurons of the cat's trigeminal subnucleus caudalis (medullary dorsal horn). J Neurobiol 1988;59:575.

35. Ichikawa H, Wakisaka S, Matsuo S, Akai M: Peptidergic innervation of the temporomandibular disk in the rat. Experientia 1989;45:303.

36. Hanesch U, Heppelmann B, Schmidt RF: Substance P and calcitonin gene-related peptide immunoreactivity in primary afferent neurons of the cat knee joint. Neuroscience 1991;45:185.

37. Kido MA, Kiyoshima T, Kondo T, et al: Distribution of substance P and calcitonin gene-related peptide–like immunoreactive nerve fibers in the rat temporomandibular joint. J Dent Res 1993;72:592.

38. Favia G, Maiorano E: Presence of neuroreceptors in normal and diseased temporo-mandibular joints. Boll Soc Ital Biol Sper 1995;71:205.

39. Ali AM, Sharawy M: Changes in the innervation of rabbit craniomandibular joint tissues associated with experimental induction of anterior disk displacement: Histochemical and immunohistochemical studies. J Craniomandibular Pract 1995;13:50.

40. Konttinen YT, Gronblad M, Hukkanen M, et al: Pain fibers in osteoarthritis: A review. Semin Arthritis Rheum 1989;18(supp l2):35.

41. Mapp P, Kidd B, Perry P, et al: Neuroanatomical features of the synovial membrane. Br J Rheumatol 1988;27:92.

42. Buma P, Verschuren C, Versleyen D, et al: Calcitonin gene-related peptide, substance P and GAP-43/B-50 immunoreactivity in the normal and arthritic knee joint of the mouse. Histochemistry 1992;98:327.

43. Appelgren A, Appelgreen B, Eriksson S, et al: Neuropeptides in temporomandibular joints with rheu-

matoid arthritis: A clinical study. Scand J Dent Res 1991;99:519.

44. Williamson EH, Steinke RM, Morse PK, Swift TR: Centric relation: A comparison of muscle-determined position and operator guidance. Am J Orthod 1980;77:133.

45. Mahan PE, Wilkinson TM, Gibbs CH, et al: Superior and inferior bellies of the lateral pterygoid EMG activity at basic jaw positions. J Prosthet Dent 1983;50:710.

46. Gibbs CH, Mahan PE, Wilkinson TM, Mauderli A: EMG activity of the superior belly of the lateral pterygoid muscle in relation to other jaw muscles. J Prosthet Dent 1984;51:691.

47. Meyers LJ: Newly described muscle attachments to the anterior band of the articular disk of the temporomandibular joint. J Am Dent Assoc 1988;117:434.

48. Velasco JRM, Vaszuez JFR, Collado JJ: The relationships between temporomandibular joint disc and related masticatory muscles in humans. J Oral Maxillofac Surg 1993;51:390.

49. Helmy E, Bays R, Sharawy M: Osteoarthrosis of temporomandibular joint following experimental disc perforation in *Macaca fascicularis*. J Oral Maxillofac Surg 1988;46:979.

50. Helmy E, Bays RA, Sharawy M: Histopathological study of human TMJ perforated discs with emphasis on synovial membrane response. J Oral Maxillofac Surg 1989;47:1048.

51. Ali M, Sharawy M: Histopathological changes in rabbit craniomandibular joint associated with experimentally induced anterior disk displacement. J Oral Pathol Med 1994;23:364.

52. Ali AM, Sharawy M: Enlargement of the rabbit mandibular condyle following experimental induction of anterior disc displacement: A histomorphometric study. J Oral Maxillofac Surg 1995;53:544.

53. Ali AM, Sharawy M: Alteration in fibronectin of the rabbit craniomandibular joint tissues following surgical induction on anterior disk displacement: Immunohistochemical study. Acta Anat 1995; 152:49.

54. Ali AM, Sharawy M: Immunohistochemical study of the effects of surgical induction of anterior disk displacement on collagens type III, VI and IX of the rabbit craniomandibular joint tissues. J Oral Pathol Med 1996;25:78.

55. Ali AM, Sharawy M: Histochemical and immunohistochemical studies of the effects of experimental anterior disk displacement on sulfated glycosaminoglycans, hyaluronic acid and link protein of the rabbit craniomandibular joint. J Oral Maxillofac Surg 1996;54:992.

56. Sharawy MM, Helmy ES, Bays RA, Larke VB: Repair of TMJ disk perforation using synovial membrane flap in *Macaca fascicularis* monkeys: Light and electron microscopy studies. J Oral Maxillofac Surg 1994;52:259.

2

Congenital and Developmental Temporomandibular Disorders

Karin Vargervik

In infants and children, the condition of the temporomandibular joint (TMJ) is important to many essential functions, such as respiration, feeding, speech, eustachian tube function, and hearing, and for growth of the lower part of the face. Of all the characteristics associated with temporomandibular disorders, severe restriction of jaw movement has the most detrimental effects on both function and growth. In nongrowing individuals, sequelae of congenital conditions may remain but are usually without pain symptoms. In adults, temporomandibular disorders are more often associated with disk problems and degenerative processes. In this chapter the focus is on congenital disorders and those developmental disorders associated with idiopathic condylar overgrowth in adolescents and young adults.

Growth Deficiency Disorders

ETIOLOGIC FACTORS

The mandible, the TMJ, and the outer and middle ear structures are derived from the first and second branchial arches. Disruption of cell migration and/or proliferation, such as could result from a vascular insult, has been implicated as an etiologic factor in hemifacial microsomia, which is the most frequently occurring congenital anomaly affecting these structures. The

malformations seen in the mandibulofacial dysostosis syndrome are thought to be due to disturbance of migration or differentiation of neural crest cells.[1] This autosomal dominant disorder has recently been shown to be caused by mutations in gene TCOFI on chromosome 8.[2] Animal models mimicking clinical findings in humans have been developed by various experimental methods.[3–5]

DIAGNOSIS AND GENETIC COUNSELING

Establishing an accurate diagnosis is essential for predicting growth and development, for determining appropriate treatment, and for providing genetic counseling. Diagnostic tools include amniocentesis for chromosome and gene testing, ultrasound imaging to detect structural aberrations, and careful analysis of all clinical findings. A medical geneticist and genetic counselor with special training and experience in craniofacial anomalies are essential members of the craniofacial team.

SPECIFIC CONGENITAL ANOMALIES

Hemifacial Microsomia

Hemifacial microsomia (HFM) is primarily a unilateral congenital birth defect with involvement of several skeletal, neuromuscular, and other soft tissue components of the first and second branchial arches. HFM covers a wide spectrum of craniofacial anomalies and may also include ocular, renal, spinal, and cardiac involvement. Dysmorphologists and others have created a variety of terms to describe the broad spectrum of phenotypes, but HFM remains the most widely used name. Other terms include oculoauriculovertebral (OAV) spectrum, craniofacial microsomia, otomandibular dysostosis, and lateral facial dysplasia.[6–8] OAV dysplasia may be considered a separate category of HFM, also referred to as Goldenhar's syndrome. The additional characteristics of this type are epibulbar dermoids and cervical spine abnormalities. There is also a higher incidence of oronasal clefting in OAV dysplasia, and most likely there are specific etiologic factors causing this constellation of birth defects. HFM is the second most common congenital craniofacial anomaly after cleft lip and palate. The most frequently quoted incidence estimate is 1 in 5600 live births.[7, 9] There seems to be agreement that there is a male predominance of 3:2 and a right-side predominance of 3:2 as well.[10] For an extensive overview of the heterogeneous phenotypes in this spectrum, the reader is referred to Cohen and colleagues[6] and to Peterson-Falzone.[8] In the mildest form of HFM, the only clinical manifestation may be ear tags with or without malformed ears. The most severe cases may present with malformed ear; temporal bone involvement, including missing glenoid fossa; and malformed or absent joint structures and mandibular ramus, including both coronoid and condylar processes.

Classification by Phenotype

Tenconi and Hall distinguished among the classic type, microphthalmic type, bilateral asymmetric type, complex with limb deformity type, frontonasal type, Goldenhar type, and the recently added "infant of diabetic mother type."[11–14] (Fig. 2–1). Of the 67 individuals included in the Tenconi-Hall study, 14.9% had cardiac malformations, 5.9% had renal system malformations, 17.6% had microcephaly, and developmental delay was found in 13.3%. Cervical spine abnormalities were not assessed in their study, but our finding and those of others

indicate that close to 50% have some type of cervical spine abnormality.[15–18]

The OMENS classification attempts to include all the most prominent features of HFM: orbit (O), mandible (M), ear (E), facial nerve (N), and skeleton (S). Each entity is graded from 1 to 3 according to severity. Others have suggested additions, such as the presence of noncraniofacial involvement, that could be annotated by an asterisk (OMENS*).[19–21]

The SAT classification system addresses only three main features: skeleton (S), auricle (A), and soft tissue (T).[22] In this system there are five levels of skeletal deformity (S1 through S5), four levels of auricular deformity (A0 through A3), and three levels of soft tissue deformity (T1 through T3). For example, an individual with minimal deformity might be classified as S1A0T1, whereas an individual with severe deformity would be S5A3T3. It does not appear that this classification system has clear advantages over the OMENS system and falls short of including all the essential elements involved.[21]

Classification by Mandibular Involvement

In this chapter, the emphasis is on mandibular and temporomandibular bone and joint malformations and malfunctions. The classification system we use is an amalgamation of the classifications devised by several other authors.[23–26] It describes middle and lower face involvement and is based on discrete findings of the presence or absence of critical elements of the mandible and TMJ. It consists of types I, IIA, IIB, and III.

In type I, all parts of the affected side of the mandible and the attached muscles are present but are hypoplastic to varying degrees. The glenoid fossa is usually missing, and translational joint movement is minimal (Fig. 2–2). Rotational movement of the condyle is usually not impaired, resulting in hinge movement on the affected side. During jaw opening, the mandible shifts to the affected side, as translational movement occurs on the contralateral side only. Quite frequently, the contralateral condyle moves excessively during maximal jaw opening.

Type IIA is characterized by a cone-shaped, anteriorly and medially displaced

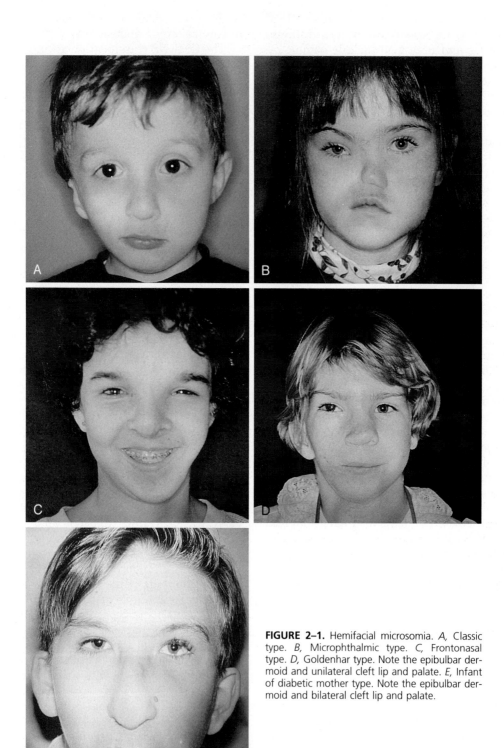

FIGURE 2–1. Hemifacial microsomia. *A,* Classic type. *B,* Microphthalmic type. *C,* Frontonasal type. *D,* Goldenhar type. Note the epibulbar dermoid and unilateral cleft lip and palate. *E,* Infant of diabetic mother type. Note the epibulbar dermoid and bilateral cleft lip and palate.

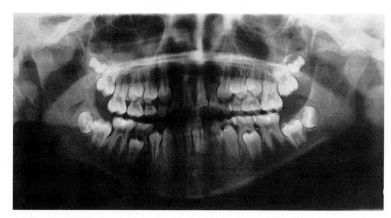

FIGURE 2–2. Hemifacial microsomia mandibular type I, at the severe end of the spectrum.

condyle; a missing glenoid fossa; and the presence of all masticatory muscles with variable degrees of hypoplasia. The jaws and face are usually very asymmetric (Fig. 2–3). In type IIB, the condyle is missing, along with the lateral pterygoid muscle. The coronoid process is usually small, and the temporal muscle hypoplastic. Jaw and facial asymmetry is usually quite marked (Fig. 2–4).

Type III represents congenital absence of the entire ramus of the mandible and most of the masticatory muscles. The mandible can be guided freely into various positions, as the movements of the affected side are not limited by either joint structures or muscles and ligaments (Fig. 2–5). All joint structures are missing, and frequently the temporal region is flat or even concave, resulting in a poor platform for the ear, which usually requires reconstruction.

Normal Mandibular Growth

In the embryo, mandibular bone formation starts in association with Meckel's car-tilage (Fig. 2–6) and around the developing tooth buds. The osseous areas expand, coalesce, and become the body of the mandible. The neuromuscular and vascular networks are well established before bone formation starts and are presumably prerequisites for osteogenesis. During these early stages of development, the mandibular structures are carried forward by the growing Meckel's cartilage. The various muscle masses become attached to or included into the developing bone, probably by the same mechanisms by which muscle reattachment occurs.[27] The posterior muscles extending into the temporal region provide the environment for development of the ramus with the condylar and coronoid processes. The condylar process and the developing TMJ structures, in association with the lateral pterygoid muscle, presumably take over the propulsive action, which up to that point had been provided by Meckel's cartilage. This new propulsive mechanism continues postnatally throughout the growth period and presumably functions by sensorimotor feedback, primarily from the

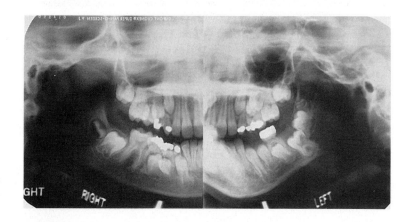

FIGURE 2–3. Hemifacial microsomia mandibular type IIA. Note the cone-shaped, anteriorly positioned left condylar process.

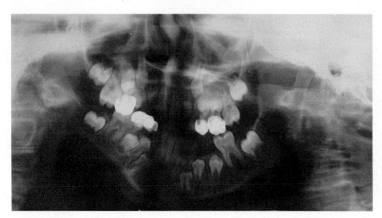

FIGURE 2–4. Hemifacial microsomia mandibular type IIB.

joint structures.[28] It appears that the periodic proliferation of condylar cartilage toward the glenoid fossa elicits activity in the lateral pterygoid muscle, which advances the condyle, thereby maintaining the optimal joint space. The various areas of the mandible remodel as the jaw is brought forward relative to its muscles and other structures. Bone apposition, which replaces cartilage in the interface between condylar cartilage and bone, appears to occur only when the cartilage is proliferating.[29] The condylar cartilage is therefore a controlling factor during growth.

Growth in HFM

In patients with HFM, the very structures that are essential to mandibular

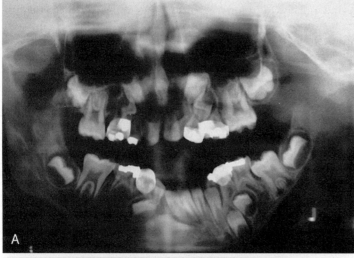

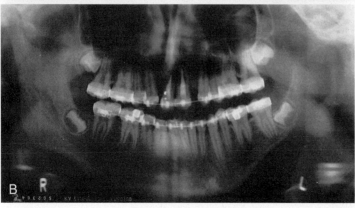

FIGURE 2–5. *A,* Hemifacial microsomia mandibular type III, with both coronoid and condylar processes missing. *B,* Eight years later, the bone has extended distally to encompass the developing third molar.

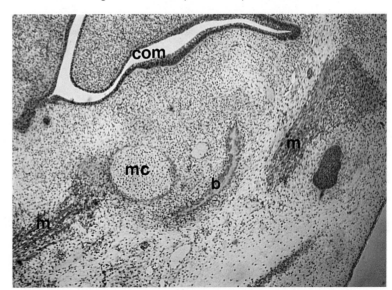

FIGURE 2–6. Coronal section through an embryo showing the mandibular bone developing lateral to Meckel's cartilage with adjacent muscle development. com, commissure of mouth; m, muscle; mc, Meckel's cartilage; b, bone.

growth are affected; impairment of mandibular growth is therefore always present, varying in degree according to the primary tissue deficiencies. Characteristically, in most individuals with HFM, the affected side of the mandible and the associated muscles grow less than the contralateral side. However, it is interesting to note that even in type III, where the entire ramus is missing, the length of the mandibular body increases as bone forms around each successively developing tooth bud (see Fig. 2–5B). This side of the mandible is gradually brought forward a small amount, presumably by the presence and function of the tongue and tissues in the floor of the mouth. Because the main propulsive factors in advancing the mandible (i.e., the condylar cartilage and lateral pterygoid muscle) are rudimentary or missing, it is understandable that jaw and facial asymmetry may increase rather than improve with growth.

Overall Management

The overall team management for a child with HFM involves attention to respiration, hearing, speech and language development, and psychosocial issues and management of associated problems such as cervical spine fusions, scoliosis, and epibulbar dermoids. Every child with HFM should have a renal sonogram, cardiac evaluation, spinal radiographs, computed tomography scans of the ear structure, ophthalmology consultation, and management and intervention as needed.

Treatment of Structural Malformations

Phase I: Early Intervention for Jaw Asymmetries Our rationale for early treatment is that some of the unfavorable secondary adaptations to the deficient growth of the mandible can be prevented, and where condylar and coronoid structures exist (types I and IIA), additional bone apposition can be achieved by providing a substitute for the normal advancing mechanisms.[30–33] A functional appliance of the activator type, with or without a buccal shield, is used routinely in our HFM patients in the initial treatment phase. Generally, this treatment is started at the time of the eruption of the 6-year molars (Fig. 2–7).

Phase II: Mandibular Surgery The second treatment phase is surgical lengthening or reconstruction of the affected mandibular ramus. If this is done during the mixed dentition stage, it is often possible to avoid a surgical procedure on the maxilla by minimizing the secondary growth inhibition on the affected side.[26, 31, 34] The exceptions are situations in which the maxillary dental midline is severely deviated from the facial midline and orthodontic correction of the dental midline discrepancy is impossible. It it generally not possible to correct a severely canted maxillary occlusal plane until an open bite has been created by surgical

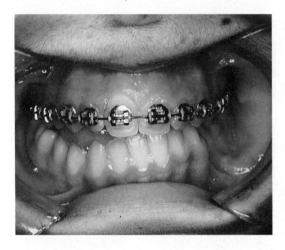

FIGURE 2–7. Open bite on the contralateral side and a level occlusal plane in the maxilla as a result of functional appliance treatment.

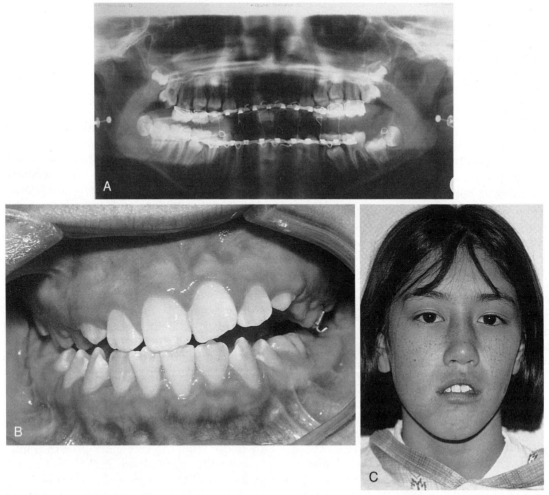

FIGURE 2–8. *A,* Open bite created by mandibular ramus lengthening (same individual as in Figure 2–2). *B,* Maxillary left molar has been extruded to contact with mandibular teeth. The maxillary teeth are canted to the left, while in the mandible the dental midline has been overcorrected. *C,* Facial view of the same patient. The chin position has been corrected by lengthening the left side of the mandible.

repositioning of the mandible. If maxillary surgery is anticipated, both jaw procedures can be postponed until most of the child's growth is completed. The more general growth remaining in a youngster, the higher the probability that the asymmetry will redevelop owing to less growth on the reconstructed side than on the contralateral side of the mandible. A transplanted costochondral graft may also grow excessively, thereby creating an asymmetry.

Lengthening of the affected mandibular ramus by distraction has become popular.[35–37] This technique has both advantages and disadvantages, and cases should be selected carefully. When distraction osteogenesis can be applied in such a way that significant muscle lengthening is achieved, this approach has a major advantage over other lengthening procedures in selected cases.

Following the mandibular surgery, the position of the mandible relative to the maxilla is secured by a bite registration splint and interarch fixation wires. Depending on the type of mandibular surgical procedure, the length of the fixation may vary from 2 weeks, if rigid or semirigid fixation was achieved, to 6 weeks, if the entire mandibular ramus was reconstructed. Following removal of the interarch fixation wires, the splint is attached to the maxilla with elastics to allow removal for cleaning. Light guiding elastics are placed to the mandible to ensure precise and controlled mandibular movements into the splint.[8] This is a period for reattachment of muscles and ligaments, retraining of the neuromuscular system to a new position of the mandible, and new bone formation as the bone graft is gradually replaced and remodeled. This important adjustment period should last for several weeks. The progression of new bone formation and remodeling is monitored by panoramic radiographs. Continued growth of the reconstructed ramus-condyle unit is still unpredictable, and many factors play a role.[38]

Phase III: Closure of Open Bite on the Affected Side The postsurgical treatment phase blends into the next phase if it is expected that the unilateral maxillary underdevelopment can be corrected without a surgical procedure. The open bite created by lengthening of the affected mandibular ramus is protected by a maxillary bite plate.

Auxiliary springs are placed on this plate for active extrusion of the maxillary teeth on the affected side (Fig. 2–8).

Phase IV: Orthodontic Treatment Full orthodontic treatment is started after eruption of the permanent teeth and after most of the jaw growth is completed. Standards for treatment outcome for these patients are the same as those for any other orthodontic patient. It is important not to resort to interarch elastic mechanics, which may contribute to redevelopment of jaw asymmetry. It should be recognized that it may be very difficult, if not impossible, to completely correct unfavorable dentoalveolar adaptations. This is a particular challenge in the presence of an asymmetric palate and tongue (Fig. 2–9).

Additional Surgical Procedures Reconstruction of a malformed or missing ear usually requires three surgical procedures, which are generally started when the patient is about 6 years old. Additional surgical procedures are often necessary to correct bony chin asymmetry, nasal septal deviation, and soft tissue deficiency. The asymmetric genioplasty and nasal septal reconstruction are done simultaneously. As the last procedure, soft tissue augmentation may be indicated. If the soft tissue asymmetry is mild, the transferred tissue may be a double dermis graft obtained from the buttock.[25] However, if more tissue bulk is needed, a muscle flap transfer by microvascular procedures may be the choice[38] (Fig. 2–10).

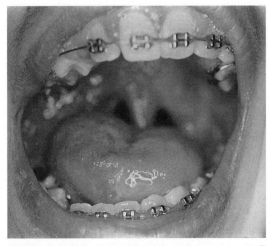

FIGURE 2–9. Asymmetry of palate and tongue typically seen in hemifacial microsomia.

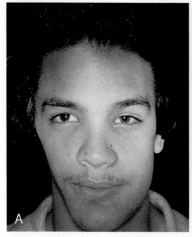 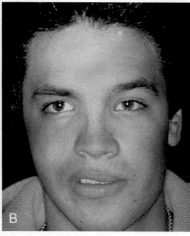

FIGURE 2–10. *A,* After skeletal correction, the soft tissue and contour differences may become even more marked than before correction. *B,* After microvascular transfer of muscle tissue.

Mandibulofacial Dysostosis (Treacher Collins Syndrome)

An English ophthalmologist, Treacher Collins, described features of this syndrome in 1900.[39] The same syndrome was also described by Franceschetti and Klein in 1949.[40] They used the term *mandibulofacial dysostosis* (MFD), which is now the more commonly used name for this constellation of structural and functional abnormalities. MFD has an autosomal dominant inheritance pattern, and the responsible gene has been located on the long arm of chromosome 5. This gene has now been cloned, and 10 mutations within the coding sequence have been identified.[2]

The incidence of MFD is not known, although it is recognized as a rare syndrome. The family history is negative for 60% of individuals with MFD. Consequently, only a few family studies have been done. It has been established that the gene mutations can be present without clinical signs of the condition.[41] This fact further complicates genetic counseling for parents of an affected child when neither of them exhibits clinical signs of the syndrome.

Structural Characteristics

The clinical findings include malar hypoplasia with discontinuity of the zygomatic arch, downslanted palpebral fissures, missing eyelashes on the lower eyelid, malformed and/or prominent ears with varying degrees of hearing loss, high nasal bridge with lateral buildup, narrow forehead and skull, and narrow and steep cranial base.[42–46] The mandible and the TMJ structures are usually severely affected in MFD[47–49] (Fig. 2–11). The mandibular condyles are usually present but small. The coronoid processes are present but vary in size. The mandibular plane is usually steep, with a marked antegonial notch. Mandibular ramus height is short, as is the length of the body of the mandible; the chin is therefore retruded and low. The distance from the chin to the hyoid bone is short, and maximal jaw opening is often reduced owing to this short distance. Posterior face height is short, and the inclination of the maxillary as well as the mandibular plane is steep. As a result, one may see a class I molar relationship and even an anterior crossbite in the presence of a very small mandible (see Fig. 2–11*D*). Often there is an anterior open bite, presumably owing to lack of bone proliferation at the condylar cartilage–bone interface. The suprahyoid muscles are short in this syndrome, which may contribute to the shape and growth pattern of the lower jaw. There is also a rather high incidence of choanal atresia, which interferes with nasal breathing. Clefting of the secondary palate has been reported in 30% to 35% of patients, and other types of velar problems such as short soft palate and inadequate palate elevation have been reported in another 30% to 40%.[49–51]

Functional Impairments

Respiration may be a serious problem for newborns as well as for older individuals with MFD. Several factors contribute to the airway problems, including choanal atresia, steep cranial base with anterior positioning of the posterior pharyngeal wall, short vertical dimensions in the posterior maxilla and nasopharynx, narrow cranial base with reduced distance between the pterygoid plates, and posteriorly positioned tongue due to a small and retruded mandible. It is not unusual for a tracheotomy to be required.[44, 45, 51, 52] Feeding difficulties are often seen and may be associated with respiratory problems or with a velopharyngeal problem such as an overt cleft, submucous cleft, or inadequate velopharyngeal function. Stenosis or atresia of the ear canals has been reported in approximately 50% of studied individuals.[43, 46] Reports also indicate a malformation of ossicles in nearly all individuals with MFD.[46, 53] Owing to the very high incidence of auditory problems, speech and language delay is a common finding, particularly if adequate measures to provide hearing within an acceptable range have not been taken from infancy.

Facial and Jaw Growth

In general, the structural abnormalities and disproportions seen at birth or in early infancy tend to become more marked as growth progresses. The midline structure with the nose and anterior maxilla continues to grow at a near normal rate while the lateral facial structures, primarily the zygomatic arch, remain hypoplastic or missing and the mandible continues its abnormal growth pattern with increasing disproportions between posterior and anterior face height.[47]

Overall Management

The overall team management for an infant with MFD includes immediate atten-

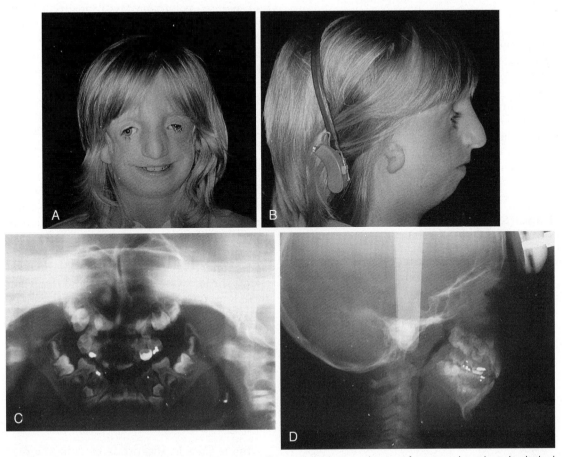

FIGURE 2–11. *A,* Mandibulofacial dysostosis (Treacher Collins syndrome). Note absence of zygoma, downslanted palpebral fissures, and broad, prominent nasal bridge *B,* Note absence of auricle, ear canal, and profile characteristics. *C,* Panoramic radiograph demonstrating bilateral mandibular malformations. *D,* Note marked antegonial notch, steep mandibular plane, and end-to-end incisor relationship despite the very small mandible.

tion to respiration, feeding, and hearing. Examination for choanal atresia is needed, and the condition of the ear structures should be assessed as early as possible. Spinal radiographs and renal sonograms should be obtained, and any eye problems should be ruled out. Speech and language development and psychosocial issues should be monitored closely. Speech therapy is often indicated, particularly for those in whom the velopharyngeal system is structurally defective. Uninterrupted wearing of hearing aids is essential when augmentation is required.

Treatment of Structural Malformations

Several surgical interventions are usually required in individuals who express a moderate to severe phenotype of MFD. These include, but are not limited to, choanal atresia repair, repair of cleft palate, placement of pressure equalization tubes, external ear reconstruction, mandibular ramus lengthening with or without joint reconstruction, lengthening of the posterior maxilla, zygomatic arch augmentation, rhinoplasty, and genioplasty. The surgical specialists must work closely with the rest of the team members. It is essential that the orthodontist is closely involved and is an active participant in the long-term planning and treatment. Extensive and long-term orthodontic treatment is always indicated for individuals with MFD.

Nager Syndrome (Nager Acrofacial Dysostosis)

Several of the malformations seen in this syndrome are similar to those seen in MFD. The term *acrofacial dysostosis* brings attention to the extremities (acral). The preaxial limb abnormalities that characterize Nager syndrome are diagnostic and differentiate this syndrome from MFD. This is a very rare syndrome with only 35 cases published.[54] Most cases are sporadic occurrences, but there is some evidence that an autosomal recessive inheritance pattern must be considered.

Structural Characteristics

Although craniofacial features in Nager syndrome and MFD are very similar, Nager individuals often have more extensive mandibular and temporomandibular involvement, often with extremely restricted jaw movements. In our center we have been caring for 15 children with Nager syndrome. In addition to the limb abnormalities, skeletal abnormalities including spinal and mandibular malformations (including missing joint structures and severe restrictions in movement), zygomatic arch discontinuity, and ear abnormalities with bilateral hearing loss, there is congenital absence of most of the soft palate[55] (Fig. 2–12).

Functional Impairments

Respiration and feeding problems are primarily due to the retruded mandible and tongue and severely restricted jaw opening. The bilateral hearing loss varies according to the severity of the ear abnormalities. There may be speech problems due to the impaired hearing, but in the absence of a soft palate, velopharyngeal closure cannot be achieved, and the speech is very hypernasal. In those individuals with very restricted jaw opening, chewing is not possible; oral hygiene is a major problem for the same reason. Severe dental decay without the option to treat adequately is often the case. Owing to the hand and limb abnormalities, manipulating implements may be difficult, and self-care may not be possible.

Facial and Jaw Growth

Overall poor growth and short stature are expected in Nager syndrome. Owing to the missing TMJ structures, the ankylosis, and the overall mandibular, zygomatic, temporal bone, and masticatory muscle involvement, there is very little growth of the lower face. The nose and anterior position of the maxilla appear prominent in relation to the deficient zygomatic areas and the extremely retruded mandible and chin. There is extreme crowding of teeth. Often the posterior teeth decay because of poor oral hygiene and poor access for treatment.

Overall Management

Team care is essential for this complex entity. The immediate concerns are with breathing and feeding, which often require placement of both a tracheostomy tube and

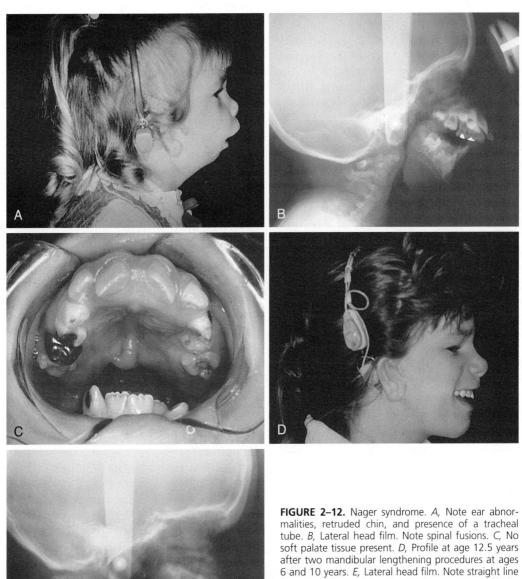

FIGURE 2–12. Nager syndrome. *A,* Note ear abnormalities, retruded chin, and presence of a tracheal tube. *B,* Lateral head film. Note spinal fusions. *C,* No soft palate tissue present. *D,* Profile at age 12.5 years after two mandibular lengthening procedures at ages 6 and 10 years. *E,* Lateral head film. Note straight line from the chin to the abnormal temporomandibular articulation.

a gastrostomy tube. Tube feeding may be necessary for a long time if jaw restrictions are severe.

Treatment Protocol

Following is a summary of our treatment protocol.

Immediate Intervention Tracheostomy and gastrostomy tubes should be placed to facilitate respiration and feeding.

Later, but as Early as Possible Stimulation to oral feeding, placement of hearing aids, speech and language stimulation, and sign language should be instituted.

Management of Jaws and Dentition Fluoride treatment and low sugar intake should be initiated to minimize tooth decay. At 3 to 4 years of age, release of mandibular ankylosis, followed by splint or functional appliance therapy, should be undertaken. A spring-loaded stretching device may be used as well. At age 6 or 7 or later, depending on several factors, lengthening of the mandibular rami should be started. Depending on the characteristics of the case, this can be done using bone grafts or distraction techniques. This treatment should be followed by splint and functional appliance therapy until orthodontic appliances can be placed after eruptions of permanent teeth. Additional surgical procedures may be indicated for the mandible. The maxilla and zygomatic arches may need reconstruction as well. Severe scoliosis is a frequent finding, and physical and occupational therapy are usually indicated. The hypernasal speech remains a problem, as little can be done surgically because of the absence of a soft palate, and obturation is usually not possible because of the poor condition of the dentition (see Fig. 2–12C).

Rare Syndromes with Temporomandibular Involvement

Miller and Reynolds syndromes have clinical craniofacial findings that are similar to those in Nager syndrome, but the limb abnormalities are postaxial rather than preaxial. The expectations for growth and the treatment are the same as for Nager syndrome. Cerebrocostomandibular syndrome also presents with similar TMJ restrictions and growth inhibition of the mandible (Fig.

2–13). Various syndromes may have a component of arthrogryposis. This may result in severe restriction of jaw movements with significantly impaired growth. The treatment procedures for the joint ankylosis and for lengthening of the mandibular rami are similar to those described earlier.

Overgrowth Disorders

ETIOLOGIC FACTORS

Most conditions of hemihyperplasia have unknown causes. Unilateral condylar hyperplasia may be associated with asymmetric size and growth of other structures, such as extremities, but is generally not apparent at birth. Theories for the pathogenesis of hemihyperplasia include vascular abnormalities, altered neurotrophic influence, endocrine abnormalities, and hyperplasia of neural crest cells.[56–61] As an example of congenital hemihyperplasia, a child with Klippel-Trénaunay-Weber syndrome is presented (Fig. 2–14). Absent any generalized unilateral tissue enlargement, unilateral condylar hyperplasia may develop subsequent to trauma. More commonly, although still rare, condylar hyperplasia may occur in a growing teenager without known cause.

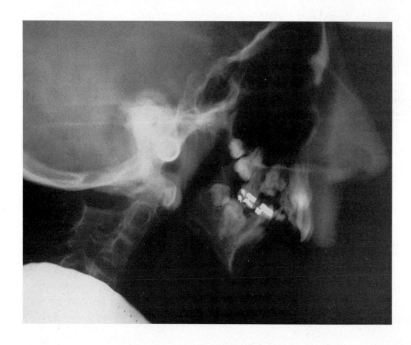

FIGURE 2–13. Cerebrocostomandibular syndrome. Note mandibular malformations, maxillary overdevelopment, long and prominent nasal bone, and spinal fusions.

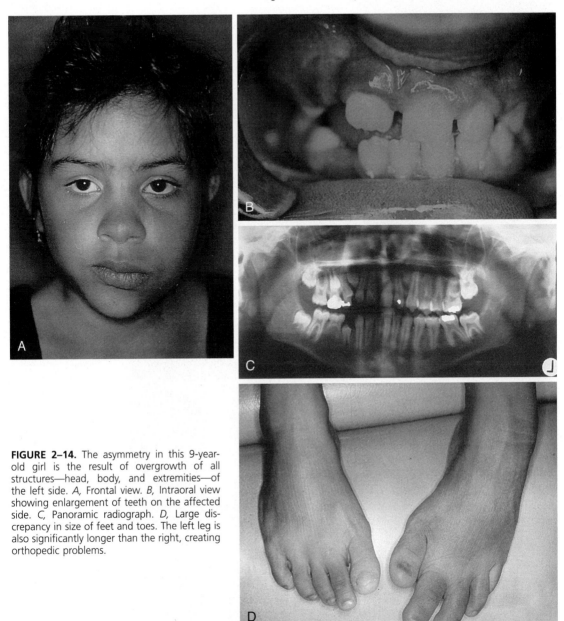

FIGURE 2–14. The asymmetry in this 9-year-old girl is the result of overgrowth of all structures—head, body, and extremities—of the left side. *A,* Frontal view. *B,* Intraoral view showing enlargement of teeth on the affected side. *C,* Panoramic radiograph. *D,* Large discrepancy in size of feet and toes. The left leg is also significantly longer than the right, creating orthopedic problems.

DEVELOPMENTAL CONDYLAR HYPERPLASIA

Idiopathic condylar overgrowth is usually unilateral and presents as a developing mandibular asymmetry. The outset may be at the start of pubertal growth but may also become manifest later, as growth on one side continues after the other side has stopped growing. Two distinct patterns of overgrowth are observed.[62] The condyle itself may become enlarged; this is generally associated with a lengthening of the ramus and may lead to an open bite on the affected side if the process proceeds fast and the maxillary teeth and alveolar process do not compensate with overdevelopment (Fig. 2–15). The deviation of the chin is generally less marked than the asymmetry in the level of the mandibular plane. The other pattern of overgrowth is characterized by a condyle of normal size and shape with excessive growth at the cartilage-bone interface. This generally results in an elongated condylar neck, a marked shift of the mandibular midline to the contralateral side, and crossbite. This pattern may or may not result in increased vertical growth in addi-

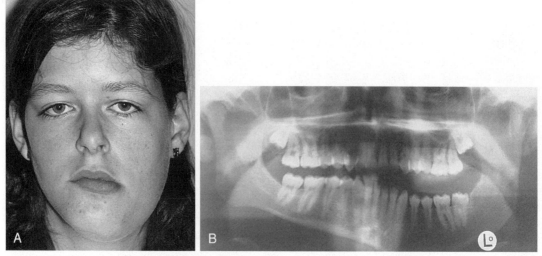

FIGURE 2–15. *A, B,* Overgrowth of the left side of the mandible, vertical type. Note lateral open bite, minimal midline shift.

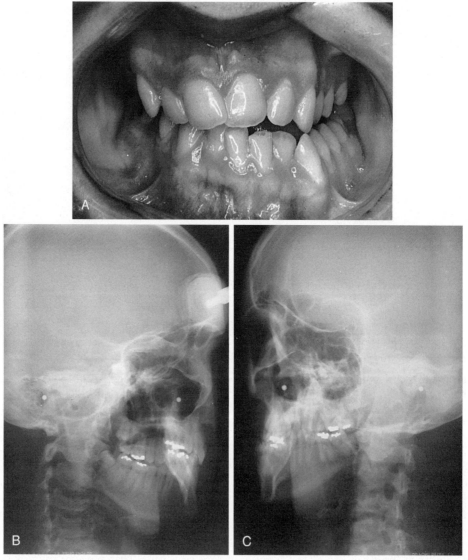

FIGURE 2–16. Overgrowth of the right side of the mandible, horizontal type. *A,* Note lower dental midline shift to the left and dental compensations. *B,* Left oblique head film. Note class I molar relationship. *C,* Right oblique head film demonstrating class III molar relationship. There is no increase in vertical development.

tion to the excessive horizontal growth component (Fig. 2–16). Neither type is generally associated with discomfort or pain. The condition of condylar hemihyperplasia is usually diagnosed after it is noted that the chin has shifted away from the midline or that there have been changes in the occlusion.

Overall Management

Standard multiview cephalometric films, tomograms, computed tomography, and magnetic resonance imaging allow for descriptions and measurements of asymmetry, but only longitudinal studies provide information on growth changes and velocity. To assess whether active growth is occurring at a given time, bone scans are now routinely used.[60, 63–65]

Interceptive Treatment and Correction of Asymmetries

Adaptive maxillary changes in response to the developing mandibular asymmetry should be counteracted or prevented if possible. For example, a unilateral bite block would prevent excessive vertical development on the affected side. Depending on the diagnostic work-up, a decision to remove or reconstruct the affected condyle may also be made.[65–67] It is interesting to note that condylar cartilage may develop on a reconstructed condyle if the disk and other joint structures are present.[68]

If, at the time of diagnosis, the maxilla is affected, two-jaw surgery may be necessary. If the condylar growth activity has subsided, as determined by bone scans and by radiographs at follow-up examinations, the surgical approach may be shortening of the mandibular ramus or body combined with a LeFort I procedure. The orthodontic treatment should focus on reduction of undesirable dentoalveolar adaptations and on arch coordination. This is challenging treatment, as the adaptations occur in all three planes of space. The orthodontic treatment should precede and follow the surgical treatment of the end-stage corrections.

REFERENCES

1. Poswillo D: The aetiology and pathogenesis of craniofacial deformity. Development 1988;103(suppl 207):103–111.

2. Gladvin AJ, Dixon J, Lofthus SK, et al: Treacher Collins syndrome may result from insertions, deletions or splicing mutations, which introduce a termination codon into the gene. Hum Mol Genet 1996;5:1533–1538.

3. Johnston MC, Bronsky PT: Prenatal craniofacial development: New insights on normal and abnormal mechanisms. Crit Rev Oral Biol Med 1995;6:25–79.

4. Cousley RRJ, Wilson DJ: Hemifacial microsomia: Developmental consequence of perturbation of the auriculofacial cartilage model. Am J Med Genet 1992;42:461–466.

5. Naora H, Kimura M, Otani H, et al: Transgenic mouse models of hemifacial microsomia: Cloning and characterization of insertional mutation region on chromosome 10. Genomics 1994;23:515–519.

6. Cohen MM Jr, Rollnick BR, Kaye CI: Oculoauriculovertebral spectrum: An updated critique. Cleft Palate J 1989;26:276–286.

7. Gorlin RJ, Pindborg J, Cohen MM Jr: Syndromes of the Head and Neck, ed 2. New York, McGraw-Hill, 1976, pp 546–552.

8. Peterson-Falzone S: An introduction to complex craniofacial disorders. In Berkowitz S (ed): Cleft Lip and Palate, vol 2. San Diego, Singular Publishing Group, 1996, p 209.

9. Grabb WC: The first and second branchial arch syndrome. Plast Reconstr Surg 1965;36:485–508.

10. Rollnick BR, Kaye CI, Nagatoshi K, et al: Oculoauriculovertebral dysplasia and variants: Phenotypic characteristics of 294 patients. Am J Med Genet 1987;26:361–375.

11. Tenconi R, Hall BC: Hemifacial microsomia: Phenotypic classification, clinical implications and genetic aspects. In Harvold EP (ed): Treatment of Hemifacial Microsomia. New York, Alan R. Liss, 1983, pp 39–49.

12. Grix A Jr: Malformations in infants of diabetic mothers. Am J Med Genet 1982;13:131–137.

13. Johnson JP, Fineman RM: Branchial arch malformation in infants of diabetic mothers: Two case reports and a review. Am J Med Genet 1982;13:125–130.

14. Peterson-Falzone SJ, Seto S, Golabi M: Hemifacial microsomia in children of diabetic mothers. SENTAL annual meeting and personal communication, 1989.

15. Avon SW, Shiveley JL: Orthopaedic manifestations of Goldenhar syndrome. J Pediatr Orthop 1988;8:683–686.

16. Figueroa AA, Friede H: Craniovertebral malformations in hemifacial microsomia. J Craniofac Genet Dev Biol 1985;11(suppl):167–178.

17. Gosain AK, McCarthy JG, Pinto RS: Cervicovertebral anomalies and basilar impressions in Goldenhar syndrome. Plast Reconstr Surg 1994;93:498–506.

18. Gibson JNA, Sillence DO, Taylor TKF: Abnormalities of the spine in Goldenhar syndrome. J Pediatr Orthop 1996;16:344–349.

19. Vento AR, La Brie RA, Mulliken JB: The O.M.E.N.S. classification of hemifacial microsomia. Cleft Palate Craniofac J 1991;28:68–76.

20. Horgan JE, Padwa BL, La Brie RA, Mulliken JB: O.M.E.N.S.-Plus: Analysis of craniofacial and extracraniofacial anomalies in hemifacial microsomia. Cleft Palate Craniofac J 1995;32:405–412.

21. Cousley RR: A comparison of two classification systems for hemifacial microsomia. Br J Oral Maxillofac Surg 1993;31:78–82.

22. David DJ, Mahatumarat C, Cooter RD: Hemifacial microsomia: A multisystem classification. Plast Reconstr Surg 1987;80:525–535.

23. Pruzansky S: Not all dwarfed mandibles are alike. Birth Defects 1969;1:120.

24. Kaban LB, Mulliken JB, Murray JE: Three-dimentional approach to analysis and treatment of hemifacial microsomia. Cleft Palate J 1981;18:90.

25. Harvold EP, Vargervik K, Chierici G (eds): Treatment of Hemifacial Microsomia. New York, Alan R. Liss, 1983.

26. Vargervik K, Kaban LB: Hemifacial microsomia—diagnosis and management. In Bell (ed): Modern Practice in Orthognathic and Reconstructive Surgery. Philadelphia, WB Saunders, 1992, pp 1533–1559.

27. Chierici G, Miller AJ: Experimental study of muscle reattachment following surgical detachment. J Oral Maxillofac Surg 1984;42:485.

28. Storey A: Temporomandibular joint receptors. In Anderson OJ, Matthews B (eds): Mastication. Bristol, England, John Wright and Sons, 1976, p 50.

29. Petrovic A, Stutzman J, Oudet C: Control processes in postnatal growth of condylar cartilage of the mandible. In McNamara JAJ (ed): Monograph No. 4. Craniofacial Growth Series. Ann Arbor, University of Michigan, 1975, p 100.

30. Melsen B, Bjerregaard J, Bundgaard M: The effect of treatment with functional appliances on a pathologic growth pattern of the condyle. Am J Orthod 1986;90:503–512.

31. Vargervik K, Ousterhout DK: Factors affecting longterm results in hemifacial microsomia. Cleft Palate J 1986;23(suppl):53–68.

32. Silvestry A, Natali G, Iannetti G: Functional therapy in hemifacial microsomia: Therapeutic protocol for growing children. J Oral Maxillofac Surg 1996;54:278.

33. Kaplan RG: Induced condylar growth in a patient with hemifacial microsomia. Angle Orthod 1987;59:85.

34. Kaban LB, Moses ML, Mulliken JB: Correction of hemifacial microsomia in the growing child. Cleft Palate J 1986;23(suppl):50–52.

35. McCarthy JG, Schreiber J, Karp N, et al: Lengthening of the human mandible by gradual distraction. Plast Reconstr Surg 1992;89:1–8.

36. Molina F: Mandibular distraction in hemifacial microsomia, technique and results in 56 patients [abstract]. Cambridge, Craniofacial Society of Great Britain, 1994.

37. Chin M, Toth BA: Distraction osteogenesis in maxillofacial surgery using internal devices: Review of five cases. J Oral Maxillofac Surg 1996;54:45–53.

38. Vargervik K, Hoffman WY, Kaban LB: Comprehensive surgical and orthodontic management of hemifacial microsomia. In Turvey TA, Vig KWL, Fonseca RJ (eds): Facial Clefts and Craniosynostosis: Principles and Management. Philadelphia, WB Saunders, 1996, p 537.

39. Treacher Collins E: Case with symmetrical congenital notches in the outer part of each lower lid and defective development of the malar bone. Trans Ophthalmol Soc UK 1900;20:190–192.

40. Franceschetti A, Klein D: Mandibulo-facial dysostosis: New hereditary syndrome. Acta Ophthalmol 1949;27:143–224.

41. Marres HA, Cremers CW, Dixon MJ, et al: The Treacher Collins syndrome: A clinical, radiological, and genetic linkage study on two pedigrees. Arch Otolaryngol Head Neck Surg 1995;121:509.

42. Kolar JC, Munro IR, Farkas LG: Anthropometric evaluation of dysmorphology in craniofacial anomalies: Treacher Collins syndrome. Am J Phys Anthropol 1987;74:441–451.

43. Marsh JL, Celin SE, Vannier MW, Gado M: The skeletal anatomy of mandibulofacial dysostosis (Treacher Collins syndrome). Plast Reconstr Surg 1986;78:460–468.

44. Arvystas M, Shprintzen RJ: Craniofacial morphology in Treacher Collins syndrome. Cleft Palate Craniofac J 1989;26:14–22.

45. Peterson-Falzone SJ, Figueroa AA: Longitudinal changes in cranial base angulation in mandibulofacial dysostosis. Cleft Palate J 1986;26:14–22.

46. Pron G, Galloway C, Armstrong D, Posnick J: Ear malformation and hearing loss in patients with Treacher Collins syndrome. Cleft Palate Craniofac J 1993;30:97–103.

47. Herring SW, Rowlatt UF, Pruzansky S: Anatomical abnormalites in mandibulofacial dysostosis. Am J Med Genet 1979;3:225–229.

48. Goldberg J, Enlow D, Whitaker L, et al: Some anatomical characteristics in several craniofacial syndromes. J Oral Surg 1981;39:489–498.

49. Roberts F, Pruzansky S, Aduss H: An x-radiocephalometric study of mandibulofacial dysostosis in man. Arch Oral Biol 1975;20:265–281.

50. Peterson-Falzone SJ, Pruzansky S: Cleft palate and congenital palatopharyngeal incompetency in mandibulofacial dysostosis: Frequency and problems in treatment. Cleft Palate J 1976;13:354–360.

51. Johnston C, Taussig LM, Koopmann C, et al: Obstructive sleep apnea in Treacher Collins syndrome. Cleft Palate J 1981;18:39–44.

52. Shprintzen RJ, Croft C, Berkman MD, Rakoff S: Pharyngeal hypoplasia in Treacher Collins syndrome. Arch Otolaryngol 1979;105:127–131.

53. Kay ED, Kay CN: Dysmorphogenesis of the mandible, zygoma, and middle ear ossicles in hemifacial microsomia and mandibulofacial dysostosis. Am J Med Genet 1989;32:27–31.

54. Chemke J, Mogilner BM, Ben-Litzhak I, et al: Autosomal recessive inheritance of Nager acrofacial dysostosis. J Med Genet 1988;25:230–232.

55. Jackson IT, Bauer B, Saleh J, et al: A significant feature of Nager's syndrome: Palatal agenesis. Plast Reconstr Surg 1989;84:219–226.

56. Cohen MM Jr: A comprehensive and critical assessment of overgrowth and overgrowth syndromes. Adv Hum Genet 1989;18:181–303.

57. Cohen MM: Wiedemann-Beckwith syndrome, imprinting, IGF2 and H19: Implications for hemihyperplasia, associated neoplasms, and overgrowth. Am J Med Genet 1994;51:233–234.

58. Chen Y-R, Bendor-Samuel RL, Huang CH: Hemimandibular hyperplasia. Plast Reconstr Surg 1996;97:730–737.

59. Slootweg PJ, Miller H: Condylar hyperplasia: A clinico-pathological analysis of 22 cases. J Maxillofac Surg 1986;14:209–214.

60. Gray RJ, Sloan P, Quayle AA, Carter DH: Histopathological and scintigraphic features of condylar hyperplasia. Int J Oral Maxillofac Surg 1990;19:65–71.

61. Norman JE, Painter DM: Hyperplasia of the mandibular condyle: A historical review of important early cases with a presentation and analysis of twelve patients. J Maxillofac Surg 1980;8:161–175.

62. Obwegeser HL, Makek MS: Hemimandibular hyperplasia–hemimandibular elongation. J Maxillofac Surg 1986;14:183–208.

63. Cisneros GJ, Kaban LB: Computerized skeletal scintigraphy for assessment of mandibular asymmetry. J Oral Maxillofac Surg 1984;42:513–520.

64. Pogrel MA: Quantitative assessment of isotope activity in the temporomandibular joint regions as a means of assessing unilateral condylar hypertrophy. Oral Surg Oral Med Oral Pathol 1985;60:15–17.

65. Robinson PD, Harris K, Coghlan KC, Altman K: Bone scans and the timing of treatment for condylar hyperplasia. Int J Oral Maxillofac Surg 1990;19:243–246.

66. Kaban LB: Congenital and acquired growth abnormalities of the temporomandibular joint. In Keith DA (ed): Surgery of the Temporomandibular Joint. London, Blackwell Scientific, 1988, pp 67–75.

67. Lineaweaver W, Vargervik K, Tomer BS, Ousterhout DK: Posttraumatic condylar hyperplasia. Am Plast Surg 1989;22:163–171.

68. Perrott DH, Vargervik K, Kaban LB: Costochondral reconstruction of mandibular condyles in nongrowing primates. J Craniofac Surg 1995;6:227–237.

CHAPTER

3

Masticatory Myalgias

Christian S. Stohler

The masticatory myalgias form a subset of the larger diagnostic entity of temporomandibular disorders (TMDs). This subset was proposed because of the belief that etiologic, prognostic, and therapeutic differences justify the distinction.

About half of all cases of TMDs are classified as masticatory myalgias or painful masticatory muscle disorders.[1, 2] As for the other subsets of TMDs, a broad range of clinical presentations is found with respect to severity, comorbidity, and impact. The milder forms are comparable to an episodic headache; the most serious presentations change the lives of affected persons in major ways.

In their search for cures, patients with persistent facial pain consult a large number of providers and are offered many types of treatment.[3, 4] Consequently, it is highly likely that patients with persistent facial pain find their way to an oral surgeon because of desperation and the belief that nothing short of surgery will provide lasting relief. With this perspective in mind, this chapter provides oral surgeons with the current understanding of the masticatory myalgias, emphasizing issues relevant to their practice.

Clinical Presentations

Patients' complaints are dominated by reports of pain that varies in intensity and spatial distribution both interindividually and intraindividually over time. As far as the masticatory myalgias are concerned, pain is usually the greatest clinical challenge that clinicians and patients face. In most cases, the dysfunction is a secondary issue.

Pain descriptors that are most frequently chosen by patients with persistent facial pain include *aching* (chosen by 53%), *tight* (46%), *throbbing* (44%), *tender* (43%), *exhausting* (37%), *nagging* (36%), *sharp* (36%), *tiring* (35%), and *shooting* (30%). More than 20% of facial pain patients select words such as *radiating* and *pressing*, but these pain descriptors are less likely to be chosen by patients suffering from other chronic pain conditions. The words *torturing* and *terrifying* are chosen by 54% and 38%, respectively, of cancer patients, but they are used by only 10% and 6% of facial pain patients in the description of their pain experience.[5]

With only 18% of patients reporting pain limited to the head and face, pain in locations other than the trigeminal dermatomes represents a common finding among patients with persistent facial pain (Fig. 3–1). Between 50% and 60% of patients report the painful involvement of the upper cervical dermatomes (C2–6). The percentage of patients with pain distributions involving the thoracic (T1–12), lumbar (L1–5), and sacral (S1–4) dermatomes ranges, depending on the specific dermatome, from 16% to 34%, 23% to 26%, and 2% to 20%, respectively.[6] Although jaw muscle pain represents the main attribute, pain involvement beyond the head-face region appears to influence the clinical picture to a significant degree as far as functional abilities and mood are concerned. If pain exists in locations other than the trigeminal (V1–3) and upper cervi-

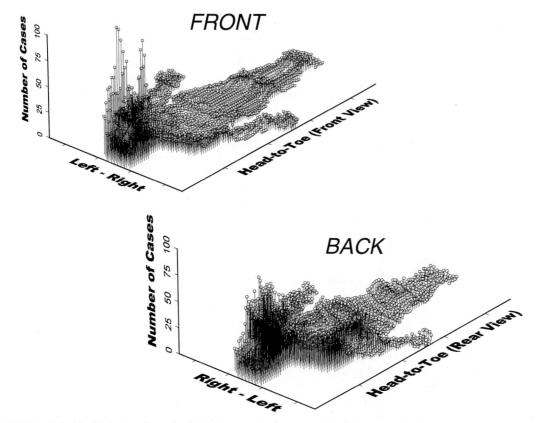

FIGURE 3–1. Bodily distribution (front, back) of the reporting frequency of pain in a sample of 200 patients with persistent facial pain. (Adapted from Turp JC, Kowalski CJ, O'Leary TJ, Stohler CS: Pain maps from facial pain patients indicate a broad pain geography. J Dent Res 1998;77:1465–1472.)

cal dermatomes (C2–4), it is associated with significantly increased pain-related disability and depressive preoccupation.[7]

Other symptoms that are often reported include the inability to open the mouth fully and the disturbing perception of bite shifts or teeth not coming together properly. Perceived changes in the bite are amplified by the exquisite sensibility of the tooth-supporting tissues, which allows the detection of very small changes in the dental occlusion during conscious biting.[8] The limited range of mandibular motion and the altered mandibular posture and bite represent motor symptoms that are viewed by some as the dysfunction responsible for pain. Others consider these symptoms to be the direct consequence of pain (see later).

Infrequent pain of low or even high intensity is more likely perceived as a nuisance when compared with the experience of lasting pain of an even lesser intensity. Persistent pain can disrupt the lifestyle of the affected person in a major way, causing significant functional limitations and restric-

tions in daily activities to varying degrees.[7, 9–12] Changes in mood such as anger, frustration, fear, and sadness are characteristic features that accompany persistent pain. Tension, worry, and irritability are also prevalent mood types in those with persistent pain. Differences among patients can also be expected in terms of medication usage, patient autonomy, disability-related expenditures, and productivity loss.[13–16] Furthermore, there is evidence that pain has negative consequences on the sufferer's memory. A comparison of young women when they were experiencing at least moderately severe menstrual pain and when they were pain free made it clear that pain impedes access to memories of pleasant personal experiences.[17]

Classification and Diagnostic Criteria

Is the diagnosis of the masticatory myalgias any more advanced than it was a decade ago? This is a question frequently asked by patients, particularly those who experience unsatisfactory treatment outcomes.

The masticatory myalgias are recognized by the presence of symptoms and signs that are far from being distinctive. The identifying features include the report of pain of muscle orign and tenderness to the palpation of the muscles of mastication. A painful response to palpation has to occur in at least 3 of 20 jaw muscle sites, with at least one of these sites being located on the same side as the complaint of pain. The presence of limited mouth opening is not a mandatory feature for the masticatory myalgias according to the research diagnostic criteria for TMDs (RDC/TMD).[18]

Categorical classification systems, such as the RDC/TMD or the classification system of the American Academy of Orofacial Pain,[19] have tremendous appeal to practitioners. They facilitate communication with other providers, patients, and insurance carriers. Although a categorical diagnostic system works well if distinct clinical features are available, limitations become apparent when dealing with symptoms and signs that recur in more than one class. Because there are no clear boundaries between the subsets of TMDs, case assignment is probabilistic rather than absolute, raising the question of whether categorical classification schemes will ever work satisfactorily. However, in the absence of valid biomarkers, it is clear that the development of improved classification systems will have to wait.

With the introduction of a second axis in the RDC/TMD,[18] scoring pain intensity, affect, and pain-related disability became a controversial issue for patients. However, it is a fact that patients with persistent pain experience significant changes in their lives, and it is not surprising that these changes induce emotional reactions that must be considered. Interactions with health providers, insurance carriers, and family members who understand little of the patient's situation or the suffering it causes may compound the problem. Such additional information can at least educate the profession and the public about the seriousness of the condition and trigger an appropriate level of compassion and understanding. It may also prevent unsuccessfully managed patients from receiving treatments applicable to acute pain that have little chance of success and may entrench the already existing pain problem.[20]

Additional shortcomings of the available taxonomies for the TMDs are becoming increasingly recognized. Masticatory myalgias are rarely limited to a single topographic domain.[6, 21–25] Boundaries between related muscle conditions are rather soft with respect to tension-type headache and regional myofascial pain involving the upper cervical spine (Fig. 3–2). Furthermore, the frequent overlap of the symptoms and signs of the masticatory myalgias with broad-based myofascial pains or the widespread pain distributions found in fibromyalgia represents another concern. Because patients with TMDs and widespread pain are least tolerant of experimentally induced pain over the masseter muscles,[23] differences in central neural processing have to be assumed. Because widespread pains have usually existed for longer durations than conditions involving local and regional pain at a patient's first presentation to a tertiary care setting, different prognostic properties among these conditions should be assumed.[4] The choice of treatment target, such as local versus systemic, is another issue that has a bearing on the type of treatment rendered to patients (see later).

Finally, the insurance coverage depends on the diagnostic assignment. The controversy over whether a patient's problem is a medical or a dental condition is often left to the patient to resolve, in the absence of any evidence in support of one view or the other. However, there is no question that a patient with chronic disabling pain should never have to fight for a particular diagnosis in order to get reimbursement for *necessary* diagnostic and therapeutic procedures.

Etiology and Pathogenesis

The traditional thinking on the etiology of the masticatory myalgias rests on the hypothesis that abnormal skeletal or dental alignment and the associated muscular dysfunction are the causes of pain and its persistence. Structural abnormalities, such as certain types of occlusal interferences, dental malocclusions, malpositions of the condyle in the glenoid fossa, or malalignment

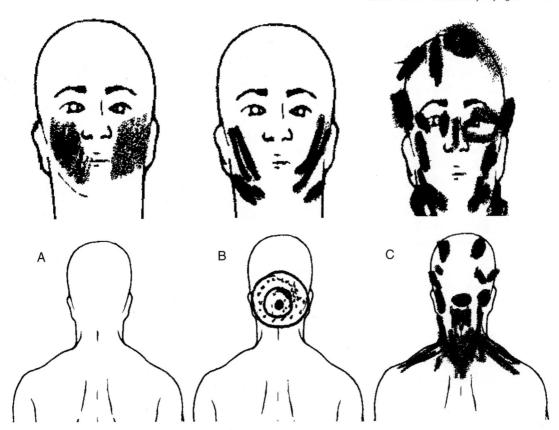

FIGURE 3–2. Examples of head, face, and neck pain maps of patients classified as having masticatory myalgias according to the research diagnostic criteria for temporomandibular disorders. Note the differences in pain distributions among cases A, B, and C.

of the disk and condyle, are believed to produce and maintain pain and the mandibular dysfunction.

Because muscles are believed to have to work harder in the presence of structural abnormality, the key assumption is that malalignment initiates muscle hyperactivity. Besides structural factors, mental stress was later added to the list of conditions that can cause muscle hyperactivity, because reasons were needed to explain pain in the absence of structural abnormality or the persistence of symptoms following structural correction. A vicious circle that is based on the mutually reinforcing relationship between pain and muscle hyperactivity is assumed to account for the progressive pathophysiologic processes. Specifically, muscle hyperactivity is supposed to cause pain, which in turn reinforces abnormal muscle function.[26] Reports of symptom relief following structural correction have been used as proof of the hyperactivity–vicious circle theory. However, experimental evidence in support of this theory is lacking. It

is also important to note that the goal of breaking the vicious circle is often used to justify aggressive treatment.

Epidemiologic data challenge the idea of a vicious circle and assumptions of the progressive nature of the TMDs and the masticatory myalgias. Rather than being progressive in nature, there is evidence that, with few exceptions, symptoms tend to be non-progressive, self-limited, or fluctuating over time.[27] The masticatory myalgias do not represent a temporally stable disease entity. Fifty percent, 63%, and 57% of patients with masticatory myalgias reported being free of pain at the 1-, 3-, and 5-year follow-up examinations, respectively; the majority of the remaining cases were diagnosed as TM arthritides or disk conditions. Only 23%, 13%, and 7%, of cases were reassigned as masticatory myalgias at the 1-, 3-, and 5-year follow-up examinations.[28]

The clinical literature also challenges the key assumption of the hyperactivity–vicious circle theory. Analytic reviews of the original literature concluded that muscle hyperactivity is not a unifying feature of patients with persistent pain, putting into question the hyperactivity–vicious circle theory and the rationale for treatments that are aimed at reducing nonexisting muscle hyperactivity.[29-31]

Although complaints of difficulty with mouth opening and perceived changes in the maxillomandibular relationship can be viewed as a form of motor dysfunction, there is little evidence that they cause pain. Alternatively, there is good evidence that changes in the jaw relationship can be caused by pain (Fig. 3–3).[32] Pain-related changes in motor function that are traditionally referred to as being the dysfunction do not appear to represent a maladaptive behavior. On the contrary, the altered motor behavior in pain is believed to serve adaptive-protective purposes. Unlike the hyperactivity–vicious circle theory to explain the development of pain and dysfunction, the pain-adaptation model predicts the adaptive response to functioning in pain.[29-31] With the demise of the hyperactivity–vicious circle theory, the prevailing etiologic thinking is no longer supported. Other etiologic factors need to be considered.

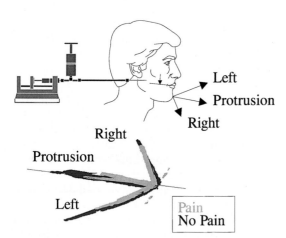

FIGURE 3–3. Example of pain-induced changes in mandibular range of motion and jaw relationship. Upper panel shows the stimulus delivery system for producing tonic experimental jaw muscle pain. Subject was instructed to perform maximal left, right, and protrusive movements in the presence and absence of pain. The lower panel shows the gothic arch tracing in the presence and absence of pain. Note the reduction in the range of motion, as shown by the limitation of the lateroexcursive and protrusive movements in the situation of pain and the position of the tip of the gothic arch, which is located more anteriorly in the situation of pain. (Adapted from Obrez A, Stohler CS: Jaw muscle pain and its effect on gothic arch tracings. J Prosthet Dent 1996;75:393–398.)

As far as TMDs are concerned, initial onset in both males and females is more likely to occur before age 50 than later in life, although this does not mean that severe symptoms cannot occur in old age.[33, 34] The preponderance of women in clinical populations is a striking observation in need of an explanation. The problem also seems to be more severe for female patients both physically and emotionally.[35] One popular explanation assumed that differences in care-seeking behaviors between the sexes accounted for the large number of women in clinic populations. However, gender differences in health services use and symptom perception are insufficient to explain the greater involvement of women.[36]

Evidence is emerging in support of a biologic explanation for this difference. Because the chances of seeking treatment increases by 77% with the use of supplemental estrogen in the postmenopausal years, or by 19% in subjects on oral contraceptives,[37] female hormones have been implicated in the modulation of pain. Another clue that may light on the etiology of the masticatory myalgias comes from a phase I clinical trial in which subjects were injected with recombinant human nerve growth factor (rhNGF). Subjects reported pain in the bulbar and jaw musculature that tended to worsen with chewing. Pain was also noted with swallowing, and abdominal and limb muscles were occasionally perceived as painful as well. Both sexes were affected, but women were more susceptible to rhNGF than men.[38] Furthermore, evidence from basic research supports the formulation of a link between NGF and estrogen that may be relevant in the masticatory myalgias. Unlike previous hypotheses, the NGF-estrogen link is consistent with the fluctuating course of the masticatory myalgias, the fact that the condition is more frequent in women of reproductive age than in any other group, and the fact that the condition is more serious in women than in men.[39]

In summary, it is clear that the scientific advances in recent years support the abandonment of the hypothetical model of etiology that stifles progress and drives therapists to search for structural abnormalities that are probably variations of normality in a large number of cases or even the direct consequence of pain.

Management Issues

In their search for cures, 22% of patients with persistent facial pain seek treatment from an oral and maxillofacial surgeon. The only health professionals more likely to be consulted by patients with persistent facial pain are general dentists (54% of cases), family physicians (27%), and physical therapists (24%). With oral surgeons ranked in the fourth place among a list of 44 different care providers consulted by 206 consecutive patients before their referral to a tertiary care clinic, the oral surgeon assumes an important place.[4]

Because the dentist–oral surgeon's practice is limited to treating the head and face, the patient's history understandably emphasizes orofacial complaints over similarly disturbing symptoms in other parts of the body. It is therefore not surprising that close matches between patients' chief pain complaints and whole body pain drawings occur only in those patients whose pain is restricted to the head-face region. If concomitant pain occurs outside the head and face area, the additional pain sites in the neck, shoulder, arm, chest, abdomen, back, and leg are rarely acknowledged in the chief complaint. In fact, the strength of agreement beyond chance between the verbal report of pain and the pain drawing is only slight for neck, shoulder, arm, abdomen, back, and leg and poor for chest.[40] Thus the dentist–oral surgeon's attention is aimed at the region of the primary disciplinary focus. This can be a problem in clinical decison-making when diagnostic or therapeutic services are initiated without knowledge of disease involvement beyond the head and face.

In clinical decision-making, a narrow disease focus places substantial weight on local symptoms and signs. Interventions for diseases with a broader involvement tend to be more medical than surgical in nature. With only 18% of persistent orofacial pain patients exhibiting pain that is limited to the trigeminal system,[6] the potential exists for 82% of such patients to receive insufficient consideration of their concomitant conditions in other parts of the body. A strong focus on the masticatory system can prevent the clinician from launching treatments that emphasize a systemic rather than local target. Because a high percentage of subjects with masticatory myalgias fulfill the diagnostic criteria of conditions such as tension-type headache, regional myofascial pain, and fibromyalgia, the question of treatment focus must have a bearing on the choice of treatment.

At first impression, this does not appear to be an issue for the oral surgeon, because muscle conditions, in contrast to conditions involving the temporomandibular joints (TMJs), are not likely to be treated by means of surgery. However, the differentiation of muscle and joint conditions is often a problem, with false-positive joint involvement being a real possibility. Problems with differentiating muscle and joint conditions become obvious when considering that large numbers of neurons located in the subnucleus caudalis receive input from the TMJ and masseter muscle and respond to nociceptive input from both structures.[41-43] This raises questions regarding the validity of the choice of the TMJ as the treatment target, because nociceptive input from muscle could elicit similar central effects.

Clinical decisions are further complicated by the fact that more than one subset of TMDs can be present in one subject or even on one side of the face. Should the treatment focus on the muscles of mastication or the TMJ? Which of the two conditions shapes the overall clinical presentation in a major way? Alternatively, are changes in central neural processing responsible for the present state, thus diminishing the chance of success of any peripheral intervention, irrespective of its peripheral target? The presence of comorbidity may be troublesome as well. What benefit can be expected from TMJ surgery in the case of concomitant neck-shoulder myofascial pain or even fibromyalgia? With about 30% of healthy and pain-free volunteers showing evidence of disk displacement, what measures are in place to ensure that this structural variation does not become the focus of treatment in a case of disabling myofascial pain involving the jaw, neck, and shoulders? Clearly, the issue is the validity of diagnostic assignment, which ultimately determines the patient's fate.

The oral surgeon is also confronted with another problem. Because patients with widespread pain conditions are generally in pain for longer times before referral to a specialty clinic than those with involvement of only the head, face, and upper neck,[6] there is a greater likelihood of more serious and treatment-resistant presentations. Besides these cases involving greater complexity and persistence, these patients are also likely more desperate and will consider treatments with even questionable outcomes because nothing else seems to work. This is captured in the words of a patient: "What is there to lose?" In an attempt to help a desperate patient, experimental treatments may be offered that later prove to be flawed.[44]

Finally, a change in viewpoint is indicated. Rather than being impressed by the success rates of 70% to 90% reported for masticatory myalgias using an array of treatments,[45-54] the 10% to 30% of cases that do not respond to available treatments should receive serious consideration. Twenty-eight percent of patients with persistent pain are dissatisfied or very dissatisfied with the care that they received.[4] This suggests that quoting figures of high success rates in discussions with patients who have experienced multiple treatment failures may not represent a true or likely scenario.

ACKNOWLEDGMENT: The writing of this chapter was partly supported by NIH RO1 DE8606-09, "Pain-Modulated Jaw Motor Function" (CSS), and NIH RO1 DE12059-02, "Pathogenesis of TMD Myalgia Symptoms" (CSS).

REFERENCES

1. Marbach JJ, Lipton JA: Treatment of patients with temporomandibular joint and other facial pain by otolaryngologists. Arch Otolaryngol 1982;108:102–107.
2. List T, Dworkin SF: Comparing TMD diagnoses and clinical findings at Swedish and US TMD centers using research diagnostic criteria for temporomandibular disorders. J Orofac Pain 1996;10:240–253.
3. Glaros AG, Glass EG, Hayden WJ: History of treatment received by patients with TMD: A preliminary investigation. J Orofac Pain 1995;9:147–151.
4. Turp JC, Kowalski CJ, Stohler CS: Treatment-seeking patterns of facial pain patients: Many possibilities, limited satisfaction. J Orofac Pain 1998;12:61–66.
5. Turp JC, Kowalski CJ, Stohler CS: Pain descriptors characteristic of persitent facial pain. J Orofac Pain 1997;11:285–290.
6. Turp JC, Kowalski CJ, O'Leary, TJ, Stohler CS: Pain maps from facial pain patients indicate a broad pain geography. J Dent Res 1998;77:1465–1472.
7. Turp JC, Kowalski CJ, Stohler CS: Greater disability with increased pain involvement, pain intensity and depressive preoccupation. Eur J Pain 1997;1:271–277.
8. Owall B, Moller E: Oral tactile sensibility during biting and chewing. Odontol Rev. 1974;25:327–346.
9. Hawley DJ, Wolfe F: Pain, disability, and pain/disability relationships in seven rheumatic disorders: A study of 1,522 patients. J Rheumatol 1991;18:1552–1557.
10. Von Korff M, Ormel J, Katon W, Lin EH: Disability and depression among high utilizers of health care: A longitudinal analysis. Arch Gen Psychiatry 1992;49:91–100.
11. Hazard RG, Haugh LD, Green PA, Jones PL: Chronic low back pain: The relationship between patient satisfaction and pain, impairment, and disability outcomes. Spine 1994;19:881–887.
12. Tesio L, Granger CV, Fiedler RC: A unidimensional pain/disability measure for low-back pain syndromes. Pain 1997;69:269–278.
13. Dworkin SF: Behavioral, emotional, and social aspects of orofacial pain. In Stohler CS, Carlson DS (eds): Craniofacial Growth Series, vol 29, Biological and Psychological Aspects of Orofacial Pain. Ann Arbor, Center for Human Growth and Development, University of Michigan, 1994, pp 93–112.
14. Dworkin SF: Somatization, distress and chronic pain. Qual Life Res 1994;3(suppl 1): S77–S83.
15. Wilson L, Dworkin SF, Whitney C, LeResche L: Somatization and pain dispersion in chronic temporomandibular disorder pain. Pain 1994;57:55–61.
16. Okeson JP: Management of Temporomandibular Disorders and Occlusion. St. Louis, Mosby–Year Book, 1993, pp 349–350.
17. Eich E, Rachman S, Lopatka C: Affect, pain, and autobiographical memory. J Abnorm Psychol 1990;99:174–178.
18. Dworkin SF, LeResche L: Research diagnostic criteria for temporomandibular disorders: Review, criteria, examinations and specifications, critique. J Craniomandib Disord 1992;6:301–355.
19. McNeill C: Temporomandibular Disorders: Guidelines for Classification, Assessment, and Management. Chicago, Quintessence, 1993, pp 1–141.
20. Foreman PA, Harold PL, Hay KD: An evaluation of the diagnosis, treatment, and outcome of patients with chronic orofacial pain. N Z Dent J 1994;90:44–48.
21. Blasberg B, Chalmers A: Temporomandibular pain and dysfunction syndrome associated with generalized musculoskeletal pain: A retrospective study. J Rheumatol Suppl 1989;19:87–90.
22. Krause SJ, Tait RC, Margolis RB: Pain distribution, intensity, and duration in patients with chronic pain. J Pain Symptom Manage 1989;4:67–71.
23. Hagberg C: General musculoskeletal complaints in a group of patients with craniomandibular disorders (CMD): A case control study. Swed Dent J 1991;15:179–185.
24. Allerbring M, Haegerstam G: Characteristics of patients with chronic idiopathic orofacial pain: A retrospective study. Acta Odontol Scand 1993;51:53–58.
25. Hagberg C, Hagberg M, Kopp S: Musculoskeletal symptoms and psychosocial factors among patients with craniomandibular disorders. Acta Odontol Scand 1994;52: 170–177.
26. Travell JG, Rinzler S, Herman M: Pain and disability of the shoulder and arm: Treatment by intramuscular infiltration with procaine hydrochloride. JAMA 1942;120:417–422.
27. Randolph CS, Greene CS, Moretti R, et al: Conser-

vative management of temporomandibular disorders: A posttreatment comparison between patients from a university clinic and from private practice. Am J Orthod Dentofacial Orthop 1990; 98:77–82.

28. Huggins KH, Dworkin SF, Saunders K, et al: Five-year course for temporomandibular disorders using RDC/TMD [abstract]. J Dent Res 1996;75:352.

29. Lund JP, Donga R, Widmer CG, Stohler CS: The pain-adaptation model: A discussion of the relationship between chronic musculoskeletal pain and motor activity. Can J Physiol Pharmacol 1991;69:683–694.

30. Lund JP, Stohler CS, Widmer CG: The relationship between pain and muscle activity in fibromyalgia and similar conditions. In Voeroy H, Merskey H (eds): Progress in Fibromyalgia and Myofascial Pain. Amsterdam, Elsevier, 1993, pp 311–327.

31. Lund JP, Stohler CS: Effect of pain on muscular activity in temporomandibular disorders and related conditions. In Stohler CS, Carlson DS (eds): Craniofacial Growth Series, vol 29, Biological and Psychological Aspects of Orofacial Pain. Ann Arbor, Center for Human Growth and Development, University of Michigan, 1994, pp 75–91.

32. Obrez A, Stohler CS: Jaw muscle pain and its effect on gothic arch tracings. J Prosthet Dent 1996;75:393–398.

33. Salonen L, Hellden L, Carlsson GE: Oral health status in an adult Swedish population: Prevalence of signs and symptoms of dysfunction in the masticatory system. Swed Dent J Suppl 1990;70:1–22.

34. Hiltunen K, Schmidt-Kaunisaho K, Nevalainen J, et al: Prevalence of signs of temporomandibular disorders among elderly inhabitants of Helsinki, Finland. Acta Odontol Scand 1995;53:20–23.

35. Lundeen TF, Levitt SR, McKinney MW: Discriminative ability of the TMJ scale: Age and gender differences. J Prosthet Dent 1986;56:84–92.

36. Von Korff M, Wagner EH, Dworkin SF, Saunders KW: Chronic pain and use of ambulatory health care. Psychosom Med 1991;53:61–79.

37. LeResche L, Saunders K, Von KM, et al: Use of exogenous hormones and risk of temporomandibular disorder pain. Pain 1997;69:153–160.

38. Petty BG, Cornblath DR, Adornato BT, et al: The effect of systemically administered recombinant human nerve growth factor in healthy human subjects. Ann Neurol 1994;36:244–246.

39. Stohler CS: Masticatory myalgias: Emphasis on the nerve growth factor–estrogen link. Pain Forum 1997;6:176–180.

40. Turp JC, Kowalski CJ, Stohler CS: Temporomandibular disorders—pain outside the head and face is rarely acknowledged in the chief complaint. J Prosthet Dent 1997;78:592–595.

41. Sessle BJ, Hu JW, Amano N, Zhong G: Convergence of cutaneous, tooth pulp, visceral, neck and muscle afferents onto nociceptive and non-nociceptive neurones in trigeminal subnucleus caudalis (medullary dorsal horn) and its implications for referred pain. Pain 1986;27:219–235.

42. Kojima Y: Convergence patterns of afferent information from the temporomandibular joint and masseter muscle in the trigeminal subnucleus caudalis. Brain Res Bull 1990;24:609–616.

43. Dalle R, Raboisson P, Woda A, Sessle BJ: Properties of nociceptive and non-nociceptive neurons in trigeminal subnucleus oralis of the rat. Brain Res 1990;521:95–106.

44. Spagnoli D, Kent JN: Multicenter evaluation of temporomandibular joint Proplast-Teflon disk implant. Oral Surg Oral Med Oral Pathol 1992; 74:411–421.

45. Greene CS, Laskin DM: Long-term evaluation of conservative treatment for myofascial pain-dysfunction syndrome. J Am Dent Assoc 1974; 89:1365–1368.

46. Greene CS, Laskin DM: Long-term evaluation of treatment for myofascial pain-dysfunction syndrome: A comparative analysis. J Am Dent Assoc 1983;107:235–238.

47. Carraro JJ, Caffesse RG: Effect of occlusal splints on TMJ symptomatology. J Prosthet Dent 1978;40:563–566.

48. Cohen SR: Follow-up evaluation of 105 patients with myofascial pain-dysfunction syndrome. J Am Dent Assoc 1978;97:825–828.

49. Dao TT, Lavigne GJ, Charbonneau A, et al: The efficacy of oral splints in the treatment of myofascial pain of the jaw muscles: A controlled clinical trial. Pain 1994;56:85–94.

50. Nel H: Myofascial pain-dysfunction syndrome. J Prosthet Dent 1978;40:438–441.

51. Okeson JP, Hayes DK: Long-term results of treatment for temporomandibular disorders: An evaluation by patients. J Am Dent Assoc 1986;112: 473–478.

52. Magnusson T, Carlsson GE: A 2 1/2 year follow-up of changes in headache and mandibular dysfunction after stomatognathic treatment. J Prosthet Dent 1983;49:398–402.

53. Strychalski ID, Mohl ND, McCall, WD Jr, Uthman AA: Three year follow-up TMJ patients: Success rates and silent periods. J Oral Rehabil 1984;11:71–78.

54. Wessberg GA, Carroll WL, Dinham R, Wolford LM: Transcutaneous electrical stimulation as an adjunct in the management of myofascial pain-dysfunction syndrome. J Prosthet Dent 1981;45:307–314.

Pathophysiology of Articular Disk Displacements of the Temporomandibular Joint

Stephen B. Milam

Displacement of the articular disk of the temporomandibular joint (TMJ) from its normal position was recognized as a clinical problem over 100 years ago.[1] Subsequently, surgical repositioning of the disk[1] or its removal[2, 3] was suggested as a remedy for the condition. Since these early reports, several others have associated joint pain, limited mandibular movement, and joint sounds with displacement of the articular disk of the TMJ.[4-13]

The incidence of articular disk displacement is unknown. Based on human cadaver studies, the incidence is estimated at approximately 2% to 67% of the general population.[14-22] Radiographic studies suggest that up to 70% of patients seeking treatment for a suspected TMJ disorder have articular disk displacement.[23]

The structure and biochemical composition of contacting surfaces of the TMJ may be altered by articular disk displacements. Disk deformation and/or perforation, atypical cellular architecture, osteophyte formation, subchondral bone resorption, disruption of the physical continuity of the articular surface of the mandibular condyle, and adhesion formation have all been observed in studies of human cadaver TMJs with articular disk displacement.[14, 19, 24-28] These anomalies have been described as degenerative changes. The implication of a disease process has had an impact on the clinical management of patients with signs

of articular disk displacement for the past four decades. However, there is still considerable debate concerning the mechanisms involved in articular disk displacement and the significance of this phenomenon relative to the pathogenesis of degenerative TMJ disease.

Definition of Disease

According to *Stedman's Medical Dictionary, disease* is "an interruption or perversion of function."[29] One may argue that this definition is too broad in scope and inadequate. For example, an acute injury could produce an interruption or perversion of the function of an affected tissue or organ. However, an acute injury is frequently self-limited and reversible with healing. Few would classify such a self-limited process as a disease, although an interruption or perversion of function could be shown. Clearly, the definition should reflect the notion of progression. Perhaps, a more complete definition of *disease* would be a process resulting in an interruption or perversion of function that is not self-limited.

If this definition of disease is accepted, one can argue that all diseases require intervention. This argument is valid because a disease, by definition, results in loss of function and is not self-limited. A derangement that results in a temporary loss of function may not require therapeutic intervention. Indeed, it could be argued that some "therapeutic" interventions may actually be deleterious. Anyone who has studied biologic systems appreciates the complex interactions of molecules involved in cell signaling and tissue matrix repair following injury. Misdirected "therapeutic" intervention could impair biologic processes that are involved in the restoration of function. In a worst-case scenario, interferences with these normal biologic processes by either pharmacologic or nonpharmacologic means could lead to a progressive dysfunctional state (i.e., disease). Therefore, it is important for us to study molecular events that underlie both adaptive and disease processes affecting the TMJ.

Adaptation versus Disease

Does an articular disk displacement inevitably progress to advanced degenerative TMJ disease? The notion that articular disk displacement results in an unfavorable biochemical situation that ultimately culminates in a progressive degenerative joint disease was revitalized by Farrar in the 1970s[23, 30] and summarized in a classification scheme developed by Wilkes.[31] The view that the natural progression of this disorder culminates in advanced degenerative TMJ disease is supported by animal studies that have revealed significant biochemical and histologic changes in the mandibular condyle and temporal bone following diskectomy.[32–34] Similar changes in humans were suggested by radiologic studies of patients who had undergone diskectomy[35–37] and in cadaver studies.[14, 24] Thus, the model proposed by Wilkes has been generally accepted by the clinical community. Both surgical and nonsurgical approaches to "reposition" the displaced articular disk have been carried out with the belief that a successful long-term repositioning of the articular disk was possible and would, if successful, abort the inevitable progression to advanced degenerative joint disease. General acceptance of the model has been so strong that many surgeons believe that if the articular disk cannot be salvaged owing to excessive deformity or lost structural

integrity, it should be replaced with either an autologous graft or an alloplastic implant.

It would appear that articular disk displacements do culminate in degenerative TMJ disease from the preceding discussion. However, several studies have provided evidence of a remarkable adaptive capacity of the TMJ.[33, 38–43] Marked and rapidly occurring (i.e., <4 weeks) adaptive responses can be evoked in the rhesus monkey TMJ by the alteration of occlusal patterns.[44, 45] Similar adaptive changes of the articular surfaces of the TMJ have been documented in response to forced protrusion[46–49] or forced retrusion[50, 51] of the mandible. It is argued that articular tissues affected in this fashion may be better adapted to accommodate new mechanical stresses imposed on the TMJ by mandibular growth and changing dentition.[52, 53]

It is possible that many changes observed in the structure of the TMJ following articular disk displacement do not represent a disease state. In previous animal studies investigating the effects of diskectomy on the articular tissues of the mandibular condyle and temporal bone, no effort was made to assess the animals for signs of TMJ dysfunction. We attempted to document functional derangement in the masticatory function of rabbits following diskectomy using video recordings of jaw movements while feeding. In these preliminary studies, we were unable to differentiate operated animals from unoperated controls (Milam and associates, unpublished observations, 1987).

In many instances, it is likely that the articular tissues of the human TMJ adapt or remodel in response to articular disk displacement. One must assume, however, that the adaptive capacity of the TMJ is not infinite. Histologic and arthroscopic studies of human TMJs have identified structural defects believed to represent failure in the adaptive mechanisms of the TMJ.[14–22, 54] In addition, there are instances in which individuals appear to sustain a progressive functional derangement of the TMJ. Therefore, some individuals are apparently capable of mounting an adaptive response to an articular disk displacement; other individuals may not adapt to these structural derangements, and a progressive degenerative joint disease may result. What accounts for the apparent variability in the physiologic response to articular disk displacement?

Several factors may directly or indirectly influence the adaptive capacity of the TMJ. These include age, sex, psychological stress, systemic illness, and the nature and existence of previous TMJ injury.[55–58] Theoretically, these factors may compromise the adaptive capacity of the TMJ, leading to a disease state. In the pathologic state, it is assumed that the delicate balance between catabolic and anabolic responses of affected articular tissue is perturbed, and adaptation yields to disease.[52]

Intraarticular Forces and Degenerative TMJ Disease

It is the consensus of researchers in the field that degenerative TMJ disease is the result of maladaptation to increased joint loading.[6, 7, 21, 25, 59–63] However, little is known about the actual forces transmitted to the articular surfaces of the human TMJ during function. Mathematical modeling and limited animal data indicate that several factors may influence loading of the TMJ during function.[64–71] These include the status of the dentition, the total bite force, ipsilateral and contralateral muscle force ratios, and the mechanical properties of food eaten.[72] In addition, studies of human TMJs suggest that the articular structures may be differentially loaded. This is suggested by asymmetric remodeling of the articular surfaces of both the mandibular condyle and the temporal bone.[21]

There have been a few attempts to measure intracapsular pressures of the TMJ during function. Lower joint space forces up to 17.7 kg have been recorded in an adult monkey using an implanted piezoelectric foil.[73] During masticatory function, superior joint space pressures up to 20 mm Hg (0.39 pounds/square inch) were recorded in weanling pigs.[74] More recently, intracapsular pressures ranging from slightly subatmospheric to 200 mm Hg (3.9 pounds/square inch) were recorded in symptomatic human TMJs during function.[75] However, these measurements reflect global hydrostatic pressures within the superior joint space and not contact stresses. Chen and Liangfeng attempted to estimate contact stresses

in the human TMJ using finite element modeling (FEM).[76] Estimates provided by these studies greatly exceed those contact stresses previously thought to exist in the TMJ. In fact, FEM predictions indicate that the contact stresses generated within the TMJ with function can approach, in magnitude, those stresses generated in knee and hip joints with functional loading (i.e., up to 1650 pounds/square inch).[76] It should be noted that FEM estimates are based on certain unproven assumptions about intraarticular movements and material properties. Therefore, these estimates may not be accurate. However, recent studies of the articular tissues of the pig TMJ revealed mechanical properties that are typical for tissues subjected to heavy vertical stresses.[77] These observations indicate that the articulating structures of the TMJ are loaded during function, although the characteristics of contact stresses produced in the human TMJ are currently unknown. Furthermore, it is currently unknown whether articular disk displacements adversely affect joint loads or joint-loading patterns.

Articular Disk Displacement and Degenerative Joint Disease: Cause or Effect?

As previously mentioned, "degenerative changes" of the mandibular condyle and temporal bone have been observed in animals following diskectomy, disk perforation, or disk displacement.[33, 34, 59, 60, 78, 79] In addition, studies of human TMJs provided evidence that articular disk displacement is associated with an increased incidence of degenerative joint disease or osteoarthrosis.[21, 80] These observations provide evidence that the articular disk affords some protection against excessive loading. These data also support the popular notion that articular disk displacements may contribute to degenerative joint disease by increasing functional demands on articular fibrocartilages of the TMJ.

However, de Bont and colleagues argued that degenerative joint disease may precede articular disk displacement.[80] Histologic studies of 22 human TMJs were conducted, revealing "osteoarthritic changes" affecting the articular surfaces of the TMJ in 50% of joints (i.e., four of eight) with normal disk-condyle relationships.[80] Degenerative changes were also observed in 79% of joints (i.e., 11 of 14) that had articular disk displacements.[80] These investigators suggested that the sliding properties of affected articulating surfaces of the joint are adversely affected by molecular events that precede articular disk displacement. Subsequently, joint stiffness and friction increase, leading to articular disk displacement. If this model is accurate, one could argue that articular disk displacement is a sign of degenerative joint disease and not its cause.

Extracellular Matrix Degradation and Degenerative TMJ Disease

The TMJ is formed from a complex organization of extracellular matrix molecules and cells. A variety of extracellular matrix molecules have been identified in articular structures of the TMJ. These include collagens,[81–85] cartilage proteoglycans,[84–88] and glycoproteins.[83–85, 89, 90] Collagens and proteoglycans have received considerable attention because of their relative abundance and their contribution to the biomechanical properties of articular cartilage. However, other matrical constituents may also contribute in a significant way to the continued health of these specialized articular tissues.

Loss of the cartilaginous matrix in degenerative joint disease involves the destruction of specific extracellular matrix molecules. The destructive processes probably involve specific enzymes[91–97] but may also involve nonenzymatic processes.[98–101] However, it should be reemphasized that these degradative events may not necessarily signal a disease process. As for all connective tissues, these degradative events are a necessary component of normal tissue remodeling. As previously discussed, the principal difference between a disease state and normal remodeling apparently lies with the uncoupling of catabolic and anabolic tissue responses. In disease, the mechanisms that hold the degradative processes in check may be lost or severely curtailed.[102–104] In addition, the synthetic responses of specialized cell populations in diseased tissue may be restricted.[104, 105] Thus, the rate of degradation exceeds the rate of synthesis, resulting in an insufficient replacement of tissue in a disease state.

A consistently observed change in the extracellular matrix of articular cartilage obtained from degenerative joints is the disruption of the collagenous matrix and a loss of proteoglycans.[34, 102, 104–109] It is generally believed that collagens found in the articular fibrocartilage of the temporal bone and mandibular condyle and in the articular disk function to provide form and tensile strength to the tissue.[108] Animal studies have provided evidence that an early physical effect related to collagen degradation is an increase in the hydration of the articular cartilage of the TMJ.[34, 79] This phenomenon is commonly described in other joints after similar experimental manipulations.[103]

Cartilage is composed primarily of water. In fact, water accounts for 78% of the weight of the fibrocartilage of the rabbit mandibular condyle.[79] Water is attracted to this specialized tissue primarily by the presence of large aggregating cartilage proteoglycans (Fig. 4–1). These enormous aggregate molecules (up to 200 million daltons) are composed of proteins and repeating disaccharide molecules known as glycosaminoglycans (therefore the term *proteoglycans*). The predominant glycosaminoglycans found in the articular fibrocartilage of the TMJ are keratan sulfate, chondroitin 6-sulfate, and chondroitin 4-sulfate.[85] These glycosaminoglycans are covalently linked to core proteins to form proteoglycan monomers called aggrecans.[110, 111] Aggrecans are, in turn, noncovalently associated with hyaluronic acid. This association is stabilized by link proteins.[112, 113] Large aggregating cartilage proteoglycans are formed in this way. They carry a significant negative charge by virtue of the large number of carboxyl and sulfate moieties contributed primarily by the glycosaminoglycans.[112] The net negative charge of these macromolecules attracts extracellular water molecules and ions.[114]

Tissues composed of proteoglycans are typically resilient to compressive loading because of their structured water content.[115] The loss of these molecules from articular cartilage is believed to eventually lead to structural failure with loading. It is interesting to note that one of the earliest observed changes in osteoarthritic joints is the loss of large aggregating cartilage proteoglycans from affected articular tissues. On the

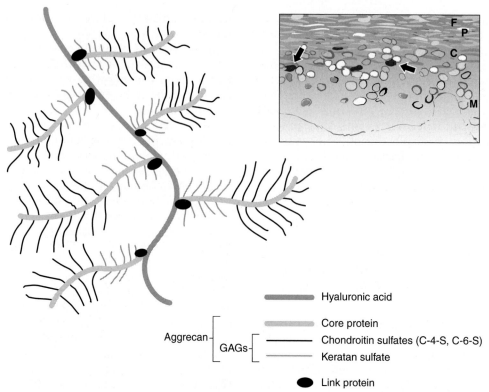

FIGURE 4–1. Large aggregating cartilage proteoglycans in the temporomandibular joint (TMJ). Fibrocartilages of the TMJ are composed of large aggregating proteoglycan molecules. The inset photomicrograph depicts the immunolocalization of keratan sulfate, a component glycosaminoglycan (GAG) molecule, in fibrocartilage of the mandibular condyle. These feather-like molecules are composed of GAGs (chondroitin sulfates and keratan sulfate) that are covalently linked to core protein(s). This structure is called a proteoglycan monomer or aggrecan. Aggrecan molecules are noncovalently associated with a single, centrally located hyaluronic acid molecule. The interaction between hyaluronic acid and aggrecan is stabilized by link protein. Large aggregating proteoglycan molecules can reach molecular weights exceeding 100 million daltons. These enormous molecules carry a vast negative charge owing to the large number of sulfate and carboxyl groups contained in the GAG component. Cations and water are attracted to proteoglycan molecules. It is believed that large aggregating proteoglycan molecules contribute to the resiliency of articular tissues of the TMJ by attracting and structuring extracellular water. C, chondroblastic layer; F, fibrous layer; M, mineralization zone; P, prechondroblastic layer.

basis of these observations, one would predict a net loss of water from the affected tissues. However, as previously noted, studies have demonstrated an increase in the water content of these tissues in the initial phases of degenerative joint disease. What is the explanation for this apparent discrepancy?

Large aggregating cartilage proteoglycan molecules are normally intertwined among collagen molecules found in the articular fibrocartilage of the TMJ (Fig. 4–2). It is believed that collagen molecules physically restrain these proteoglycan molecules, much like string wrapped around a sponge physically restrains the sponge. It appears that as the collagenous matrix of an articular fibrocartilage becomes increasingly degraded, its restraining influence on large

aggregating cartilage proteoglycans is lost.[103] These negatively charged proteoglycan macromolecules expand, like sponges, increasing water absorption. Thus, the initial effect of collagen degradation in articular tissues is an increase in their water content.

As large aggregating cartilage proteoglycan molecules expand and attract more water, they become increasingly vulnerable to enzymatic and nonenzymatic degradation.[116] Eventually these molecules are lost from affected articular tissues.[103, 104, 108] Israel and colleagues[117] measured degradation products of cartilage proteoglycan molecules in lavage fluid obtained during TMJ arthroscopy. These investigators found a significant correlation between the presence of these proteoglycan degradative products and degenerative joint disease, as assessed visually by arthroscopic examination. Thus an early and key event in degenerative joint disease is loss of the integrity of the collagenous matrix of articulating structures, followed by loss of proteoglycans.

Collagens may also have other important functions in articular tissues of the TMJ. Cells may communicate with one another over relatively long distances by applying tension or "sensing" tension through the extracellular matrix.[118] This form of intercellu-

lar communication is mediated by specific transmembrane receptors, termed *integrins*.[119–121] Previous studies provided evidence that this form of intercellular communication may influence the metabolic activities of resident cell populations. For example, cells in muscle tendons subjected to tensile forces synthesize type I collagen and fibronectin.[122] However, the same cell population subjected to compressive loads is induced to make type II collagen and proteoglycans.[122] Similar cellular responses have

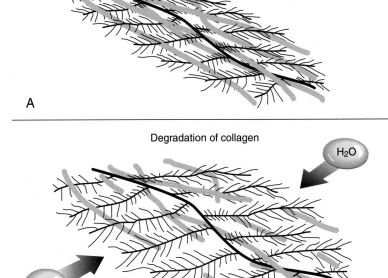

A

Degradation of collagen

B

FIGURE 4–2. Degradation of large aggregating cartilage proteoglycans (PGs). Large aggregating proteoglycan molecules are embedded in a collagenous matrix in articular tissues of the temporomandibular joint. It is currently believed that the collagenous matrix confines the larger aggregating proteoglycan molecules to a restricted space, much like string wrapped around a sponge confines the shape of the sponge (A). As the collagenous matrix of diseased articular tissue is degraded by enzymatic and nonenzymatic processes, previously confined large aggregating proteoglycan molecules expand and attract more water to the affected tissue (B). However, with expansion, proteoglycan molecules are more susceptible to degradation and are eventually lost from diseased articular tissue. As proteoglycan molecules are degraded, water is lost from these tissues (C). Articular tissues affected in this manner lose their resiliency to compressive loading. As a result, diseased articular tissues are increasingly vulnerable to injury by mechanical stress.

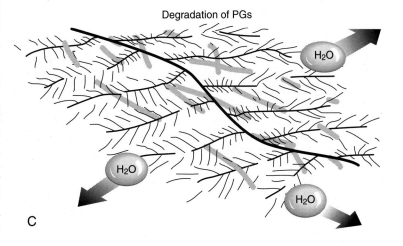

Degradation of PGs

C

been observed in supporting tissues of the articular disk of the TMJ that are loaded following articular disk displacement.[123] Disk perforation, in addition to signaling excessive loading forces, may disrupt the transmission of tensile forces required to maintain cells in the region in a "fibroblast" phenotype. The combination of disruption of this signaling mechanism and compressive loading apparently favors a chondrogenic phenotype in affected areas of the TMJ disk.[43, 123] Thus, disruption of the collagenous component of articular tissues could have a significant impact on the metabolic activities of cells found in this specialized tissue.

Dermatan sulfate, a glycosaminoglycan normally associated with a 37-kD core protein to form the small proteoglycan known as decorin, is also found in the articular disk of the TMJ.[124–127] Decorin belongs to a family of small proteoglycans that includes fibromodulin and biglycan. Decorin binds to both type I and type II collagen. In vitro, these interactions can inhibit collagen fibrillogenesis. In addition, decorin can bind and inhibit transforming growth factor beta (TGF-β).[128]

TGF-βs are dimeric peptides (approximately 25 kD) that are synthesized by cells in the TMJ and exert a variety of biologic effects, including an increase in the synthesis of extracellular matrix molecules, the inhibition of matrix-degrading enzymes, and the suppression of immune cell function.[129–134] TGF-β effects are probably fundamental in normal healing responses in the TMJ. Decorin can influence these important effects by binding to and inhibiting the TGF-βs.[128] Therefore, changes in the relative abundance of decorin in an articular tissue, such as the articular disk, of the TMJ could significantly influence many important biochemical events. It is important to realize that a modification of the molecular composition of the extracellular matrix of an articular tissue can strongly influence both the mechanical properties and the cellular and biochemical activities of the affected tissue. In fact, the nature of these extracellular matrix modifications could be the primary determinant of the tissue response to the evoking injury. Furthermore, these modifications could ultimately dictate whether the response leads to remodeling or disease.

Mechanisms of Tissue Degradation in the TMJ

Both enzymatic and nonenzymatic processes are likely to contribute to extracellular matrix degradation in the TMJ. The enzymatic agents that are most likely involved in the degradative processes are proteinases, particularly metalloproteinases.[104, 135, 136] Oxygen-derived free radicals constitute the principal nonenzymatic agents that could be involved in the degradation of the articular structures of the TMJ.[98, 100, 101, 137–139]

ENZYMATIC DEGRADATION

Several proteinases have been implicated in the degradation of cartilaginous matrices in degenerative joint diseases. These include various members of the metalloproteinase family,[91, 140] serine proteases of the plasminogen-plasmin cascade,[141] and cysteine proteinases such as calpain and lysosomal cathepsins.[142–144] These proteinases are produced by a variety of cells that populate articular tissues. Chondrocytes synthesize metalloproteinases, including collagenase (MMP-1) and stromelysin (MMP-3).[92, 145–148] Chondrocytes also synthesize lysosomal proteinases, including cathepsins D, B, and L.[95, 149–157] Synoviocytes can synthesize collagenase (MMP-1), 72-kD gelatinase (MMP-2), and stromelysin (MMP-3).[158–161] Polymorphonuclear leukocytes may also contribute elastase, collagenase (MMP-8), 92-kD gelatinase (MMP-9), and cathepsin G.[104, 135, 136] Articular disk cells from the rabbit TMJ are capable of synthesizing 92-kD gelatinase (MMP-9), 72-kD gelatinase (MMP-2), collagenase (MMP-1), and stromelysin (MMP-3).[162, 163] In addition, several plasma proteinases, including plasmin, thrombin, and kallikrein, may be present in sufficient concentrations to contribute to the degradative process under certain conditions.[136]

Zardeneta and associates recently characterized proteinases recovered from symptomatic human TMJs with articular disk displacement by arthrocentesis.[164] Ten consecutive 2-mL fractions were collected and analyzed for proteinase activity using sensitive colorimetric and fluorimetric bioassays.

Fractions displaying proteinase activity were further studied using substrate-specific zymography and characterized with respect to sensitivity to known proteinase inhibitors. This study identified both active and latent metalloproteinases in these lavage samples. Three interesting observations were made during this study. First, proteinases were found to exist in both active and latent forms. Latent forms of the enzymes are not biologically active but can be made active by enzymatic, and perhaps nonenzymatic, modification. Therefore, latent proteinases are proenzymes that can be "recruited" into service if the environment permits their activation.

Second, specific proteinases were eluted by arthrocentesis of the superior joint space at different outflow volumes. Some proteinases were recovered in early fractions (i.e., at outflow volumes of 2 to 6 mL), and others were recovered in late fractions (i.e., at outflow volumes of 16 to 20 mL). This observation is consistent with the view that these proteinases are differentially distributed in synovial fluid and articular tissues of the TMJ. Furthermore, the data suggest that arthrocentesis is effective at removing (or diluting) these enzymes from the various fluid and tissue compartments within the TMJ, assuming sufficient volumes are used in the lavage procedure.

Finally, no correlation was observed between TMJ pain, as assessed by the difference in pain visual analogue scores obtained before and after an intracapsular injection of local anesthetic, and total proteinase activity. Coleman and Weisengreen histologically examined TMJs obtained from 45 cadavers.[165] These investigators observed signs of articular disk displacement with degenerative changes in 22.2% of the joints examined. However, none of the individuals with signs of degenerative joint disease had a history of TMJ problems before death. This study was one of the first to question the assumed relationship between degenerative joint disease and symptoms. Other studies have provided evidence that symptoms, particularly joint pain, and signs of degenerative joint disease are not strongly correlated.[166] Likewise, Zardeneta and associates did not observe a correlation between proteinase activity and TMJ pain.[164]

Endogenous Mechanisms to Control Proteinase Activities

Under normal circumstances, these degradative enzymes are controlled by failsafe mechanisms that limit their destructive activities. For example, an intact cartilaginous matrix limits access for proteinases that are not deposited directly into the cartilage matrix (i.e., by chondrocytes). In addition, some matrix-degrading enzymes are inhibited by other proteins found in the extracellular matrix. These include the tissue inhibitors of metalloproteinases (TIMP-1 and TIMP-2)[158, 167] and alpha-1-antitrypsin.[168] Both TIMP-1 and TIMP-2 are produced by resident cells in the TMJ.[162, 163] Alpha-1-antitrypsin inhibits several enzymes, including collagenase (MMP-1), 72-kD gelatinase (MMP-2), stromelysin (MMP-3), elastase, and cathepsin B.[168] Finally, cytokines that appear to suppress catabolic activities in articular cartilage, such as the TGF-βs, downregulate the synthesis of matrix-degrading enzymes and stimulate the synthesis of inhibitory molecules (i.e., TIMPs).[147, 169-174] Several isoforms of TGF-β have been identified in the articular fibrocartilage of the porcine mandibular condyle.[56] These isoforms may be secreted into the extracellular matrix of this tissue in an inactive form. As the matrix is degraded, these TGF-β isoforms may be released from the matrix and activated so that they can inhibit further degradation of the cartilaginous matrix. The activated TGF-β isoforms may also stimulate chondrogenesis in the articular fibrocartilage, effectively coupling anabolic responses with catabolic responses.[174, 175]

Assuming that proteinases are involved in the pathogenesis of degenerative joint disease, one can envision that disease may result from the overproduction of these enzymes. Disease may also result if the endogenous mechanisms that normally function to suppress the activities of proteinases are impaired. In this instance, a degradative event could prevail even in the absence of an unusual production of active proteinases. Future research will undoubtedly focus on endogenous proteinase inhibitory pathways and their role in the pathogenesis of degenerative TMJ disease.

NONENZYMATIC DEGRADATION

Free radicals are molecules or ions that contain an odd number of electrons (i.e., unpaired electrons). The presence of one or more unpaired electrons makes these molecules highly reactive. When two free radicals react with each other, the unpaired electrons from each molecule pair to form a stable molecule. In this instance, both free radicals are eliminated. However, free radicals often react with nonradical molecules, and the free radical acquires an electron from the nonradical molecule. The products generated from these reactions are themselves free radicals, because they now contain unpaired electrons. In this fashion, free radicals can generate chain reactions that can destroy molecules, inhibit molecular activities, and/or stimulate molecular activities.

Blake and colleagues postulated a mechanism that may be involved in free radical generation in articular joints.[176] The mechanism is based on a model of hypoxia-reperfusion injury.[177–179] With unfavorable joint loading, intraarticular pressures may exceed capillary perfusion pressure in vascularized tissues of a joint. A brief period of hypoxia may result during the loading phase of a joint movement. Blake and colleagues provided evidence that such a mechanism is possible in human joints.[176] They observed a 33% reduction in synovial fluid Po_2 (from 61 to 41 mm Hg) in arthritic human knee joints with isometric quadriceps contraction.[176] An 87% reduction in synovial capillary perfusion was concurrently observed in knee joints during this exercise.[176]

Intraarticular pressures have been recorded in human TMJs during function that exceeded estimated capillary perfusion pressures for the vascularized tissues of the joint.[75, 180, 181] It is reasonable to speculate that, under abnormal conditions (e.g., articular disk displacement), contact stresses on vascular tissues of the TMJ could greatly exceed in magnitude the end capillary perfusion pressures of these tissues. Therefore, the hypoxia-reperfusion model cannot be refuted on the basis of inadequate intraarticular pressures. Interestingly, the placement of an occlusal splint prevented the elevation of hydrostatic pressures in the superior joint space of these TMJs during clenching.[181] Splint therapy may therefore be an effective intervention to protect the TMJ against a hypoxia-reperfusion injury.

Mechanism of Hypoxia-Reperfusion Injury

Adenosine triphosphate is converted to hypoxanthine in tissues affected by increasing hypoxia. In addition, xanthine dehydrogenase is converted to xanthine oxidase by a calcium-calmodulin–activated protease.[177, 179] This protease becomes active when energy-starved cells fail to maintain low cytosolic calcium levels. Xanthine oxidase generates a superoxide radical by univalent reduction of oxygen (O_2) instead of the reduced form of nicotinamide adenine dinucleotide (NADH).[177] Therefore, when the joint is relaxed and articular tissues are reperfused, xanthine oxidase may react with accumulated hypoxanthine or xanthine in the presence of oxygen to form the superoxide radical (O_2^-). In support of this model, McCord and Fridovich observed a rapid increase in knee synovial fluid Po_2 and free radical production with cessation of exercise.[177] The superoxide radical may then react with hydrogen peroxide to form the extremely reactive hydroxyl anion (OH•).[182] This hypoxia-reperfusion model can account, in part, for free radical generation in TMJs exposed to loads that may produce intraarticular pressures that exceed the capillary perfusion pressure of vascularized tissues in the joint.

There are other mechanisms by which free radicals may be generated in articular joints. Free radicals may be produced from molecular damage by excessive mechanical forces. For example, fingernail cutting generates a high yield of sulfur-centered free radicals.[183] The lubrication of articular surfaces by synovial fluid normally protects these surfaces from excessive frictional forces during joint movement. It is speculated that the articular disk of the TMJ further reduces mechanical stress by distributing contact forces over broad areas and by providing four lubricated surfaces. However, if these protective mechanisms are impaired (by changes in the physical properties of synovial fluid and/or displacement or perforation of the articular disk), mechanical forces generated with joint movement could be sufficient to damage tissue, yielding free radicals in the process. Theoretically, these free radicals could cause additional damage to affected tissue.

Oxygen-derived free radicals may also be formed during arachidonic acid metabolism. The hydroperoxidase-catalyzed conversion of prostaglandin G_2 to prostaglandin H_2 (cyclooxygenase pathway) and the transformation of 5-hydroperoxyeicosatetraenoic acid (5-HPETE) to 5-hydroxyeicosatetraenoic acid (5-HETE) (lipoxygenase pathway) both yield free radicals.[184, 185] Prostaglandin E_2 and leukotriene B_4 are products of these pathways. These arachidonic acid metabolites have been identified in physiologic concentrations in TMJ synovial fluid obtained from patients with articular disk displacements.[54] Furthermore, the levels of these arachidonic acid metabolites correlated with the severity of synovitis as graded during arthroscopic examination,[54] but did not correlate with joint pain (Zardeneta and associates, unpublished observations, 1995).

The role of free radicals in degenerative arthritides is unknown. Superoxide and hydroxyl radicals degrade hyaluronic acid from synovial fluid, reducing its viscosity.[182] A variety of synovial fluid proteins and extracellular matrix proteins may be degraded or significantly modified by free radicals. For example, the hydroxyl radical is capable of degrading collagens, fibronectins, elastin, laminins, fibrinogen, and immunoglobulins in vitro.[186–189] Free radicals may damage cartilage matrix by direct and indirect actions.[188]

Free radicals may also adversely affect cellular function in articular tissues. For example, oxygen-derived radicals generated from the hypoxanthine-xanthine oxidase system transiently inhibit transcription of the mitochondrial genes for 12S rRNA and the NADH dehydrogenase subunit 4 (ND4) in rabbit articular chondrocytes.[190] Free radicals may also influence gene expression by regulating activities of the transcription factor known as nuclear factor kappa β (NF kappa β).[191, 192] NF kappa β is a transcription factor that may activate gene transcription in several resident cell populations in the joint.[193] Collectively, these findings suggest that oxygen-derived free radicals may contribute to degenerative processes in affected joints by (1) degrading important molecules in articular tissues and synovial fluid and (2) influencing the synthetic func-

tions of resident cell populations in the joint. However, it is currently unknown whether free radicals are a major cause of the disease or a consequence of tissue damage. In fact, little is known of the role that these extremely reactive molecules may play in adaptive or degenerative responses of the TMJ to articular disk displacement.

Nitric Oxide and Degenerative Joint Disease

Nitric oxide (NO) is a free radical that may be involved in a variety of important biologic processes. For example, NO regulates vascular tone by activating guanylate cyclase in smooth muscle cells of vessels. This elevates cyclic guanosine monophosphate levels in these cells, resulting in relaxation and vasodilatation.[194] NO has a short half-life in the presence of oxygen (i.e., 6 to 10 seconds), limiting it to autocrine or paracrine functions.[195] It is produced by a variety of cell types, including endothelial cells, infiltrating leukocytes, synoviocytes, and chondrocytes.[195, 196] NO has a high affinity for iron atoms and may activate certain enzymes that contain a heme group.[197] This mechanism is apparently involved in the activation of guanylate cyclase[194] and cyclooxygenase[198] by NO. Other enzymes important in mitochondrial respiration and DNA synthesis may be inhibited by NO.[199] NO may also react with the superoxide radical to form the extremely reactive hydroxyl radical via a peroxynitrite pathway.

NO synthesis is increased in arthritic joints.[200] In an antigen-induced arthritic model, synovial inflammation and tissue destruction were markedly suppressed by N^G-monomethyl-L-arginine, an inhibitor of NO production.[201] These studies suggest a role of NO in the pathogenesis of inflammatory arthritides. It is likely that NO modulates vascular tone in the vascularized tissues of the TMJ. It is also possible that NO regulates prostaglandin synthesis in affected tissues of the TMJ by controlling the activation of cyclooxygenase-2.

Hemoglobin and Oxidative Stress in the TMJ

Perhaps the most damaging of all free radicals produced in living tissues is the hydroxyl radical (OH).[189, 202–207] Tissue damage following radiotherapy has been attributed, at least in part, to the formation of the hydroxyl radical in response to ionizing radiation.[203, 208] Previous investigators provided evidence that this free radical is capable of damaging molecules that are components of synovial fluid and implicated these extremely reactive molecules in the pathogenesis of degenerative joint disease.[204, 206] Hydroxyl radicals may be generated by several mechanisms, including the hypoxia-reperfusion mechanism proposed as a model of degenerative TMJ disease. Hydroxyl radicals are formed by the so-called Fenton and Haber-Weiss reactions (see later).[202, 209] Ferrous iron (Fe II) is required for the Fenton reaction.

Haber-Weiss cycle

$$O_2^- + Fe^{3+} \rightarrow Fe^{2+} + O_2$$

$$2\,O_2^- + 2H^+ \rightarrow H_2O_2 + O_2$$

Fenton reaction

$$H_2O_2 + Fe^{2+} \rightarrow \bullet OH + OH^- + Fe^{3+}$$

Recently, we reported that the α chain of hemoglobin (αHb) was recovered from cell-free lavage fluid obtained by arthrocentesis of the superior joint space of symptomatic human TMJs with articular disk displacements.[210] The presence of this protein was not due to gross contamination of lavage by red blood cells. αHb was found to elute in the first 4 mL of outflow volume collected by arthrocentesis. A second protein peak, eluting at 12 to 20 mL of outflow volume, contained a relatively high amount of αHb. We provided evidence that the majority (up to 89%) of αHb recovered from symptomatic human TMJs by arthrocentesis existed in a denatured state. Previous studies provided evidence that hemoglobin in a denatured, but not native, conformation can contribute iron for the Fenton reaction, leading to the production of hydroxyl radicals.[211]

Hemoglobin is a potent inflammatory agent. Hemoglobin deposited into articular joints elicits an intense inflammatory response that can lead to bone and cartilage destruction.[212] This phenomenon is particularly evident in extreme cases of repeated hemarthrosis associated with coagulopathies such as hemophilia.[213]

As hemoglobin decomposes following its deposition into a tissue, it provides a reactive heme group that can function as a Fenton reagent.[211] In other words, hemogobin-derived iron can catalyze the formation of the extremely reactive hydroxyl radical. As previously mentioned, hydroxyl radicals are capable of destroying molecules of the extracellular matrices of affected articular tissues. Free radical–mediated damage to collagens, fibronectins, elastin, laminins, hyaluronic acid, and proteoglycans has been documented in vitro.[187, 214] Because the biomechanical properties of articular tissues of the TMJ are determined to a large extent by the molecular composition of their extracellular matrices, loss of specific extracellular matrix molecules due to free radical damage could contribute to unfavorable joint biomechanics that could perpetuate joint injury. Indeed, such a mechanism could be involved in the weakening of supporting tissues of the articular disk, eventually leading to its displacement.

In summary, the presence of denatured hemoglobin in the TMJ may account for progression of degenerative TMJ disease because it has been shown that (1) hemoglobin prolongs and intensifies inflammation in synovial tissue, (2) heme iron may lead to the formation of hydroxyl radicals via the Fenton reaction, and (3) hydroxyl radicals may damage vital extracellular matrix molecules and cells, culminating in degenerative joint disease.

Free Radical Defense Mechanisms

The biologic activities of free radicals generated during function are tightly regulated to reduce damage in normal joints. For example, NO is rapidly oxidized to inactive nitrite and nitrate in the presence of oxygen. Furthermore, hemoglobin binds NO and in doing so inhibits its activity.[199] Also, synovial fluid hyaluronic acid may offer some protection against free radical injury.[215]

Oxygen-derived free radicals may be inhibited or converted to innocuous molecular species in articular tissues. Superoxide anion is converted to hydrogen peroxide by superoxide dismutases found in articular tissues.[216–220] Hydrogen peroxide is, in turn, converted to water by the enzyme catalase.[179, 182] Adjuvant-induced arthritis is reduced by superoxide dismutase.[219, 220] In a similar fashion, bone resorption, initiated either by interleukin-1 or by oxygen-derived free radicals generated from the hypoxanthine-xanthine oxidase system, can be inhibited by superoxide dismutase in vitro.[221] It is interesting to note that beneficial effects of superoxide dismutase have been reported in a preliminary study of its use to treat patients with persistent TMJ pain and dysfunction.[222]

The extracellular matrices of all tissues contain low-molecular-weight species, such as vitamin C, vitamin E, and glutathione, that serve as free radical scavengers.[101, 136] These and other so-called antioxidants have been marketed as a remedy for a variety of maladies, including aging. However, there is some concern that the overzealous use of these agents may have detrimental effects in some instances. For example, vitamin C may exacerbate free radical–mediated events that are driven by the Fenton reaction. When ferrous iron (Fe II) reduces hydrogen peroxide to generate the hydroxyl radical (OH) in the Fenton reaction, it becomes ferric iron (Fe III). Vitamin C (reduced ascorbate) converts Fe III back to Fe II, allowing for another cycle of hydroxyl radical generation via the Fenton reaction.[223–225] In situations of localized iron overload (e.g., bleeding into articular tissues, iron overload disease), a constant dietary source of reduced ascorbate (e.g., excessive vitamin supplementation) could convert the hydroxyl radical generation process from a one-cycle event to an ascorbate-driven repetitive cycle. Vitamin C does have antioxidant properties. However, it is becoming increasingly evident that local factors (e.g., local iron loads, tissue concentrations of reduced ascorbate) determine to a large extent whether vitamin C will exert pro-oxidant or antioxidant effects. This concern may not be trivial, because it is now known that in patients with iron overload diseases, such as hemochromatosis, vitamin C may exert lethal effects.[225]

Alterations in the Synthetic Capacity of Cells

In degenerative TMJ disease, we assume that the degradative processes are allowed to continue in an unchecked fashion. As previously noted, it is likely that these degradative processes involve an increased synthesis of matrix-degrading enzymes, the generation of free radicals, and a reduction in the efficacy of fail-safe mechanisms that exist to limit both proteolytic and nonproteolytic destruction of affected articular tissues. Failure of the structural integrity of affected articular surfaces may also be attributed, in part, to reduced synthetic function of local cell populations.

Chondroblasts are normally highly responsive to changes in their extracellular matrix. For example, embryonic chondroblasts can resynthesize a cartilage matrix depleted by enzymatic digestion in vitro in only a few days.[226] Under certain conditions, articular chondroblasts of the TMJ may initially increase their synthesis of proteoglycans in response to increased functional loads.[79] The responsiveness of chondroblasts to changing functional demands significantly contributes to the adaptive capacity of articular tissues in the TMJ. However, the chondroblast's capacity for repair may be limited. With continued and/or excessive loads, the chondroblast may fail. Haskin and colleagues provided evidence that chondroblast failure with excessive loading may be associated with disruption of specific cytoskeletal elements, F-actin and tubulin.[227] The integrity of the cytoskeleton is required for various cell functions, including gene regulation and protein synthesis.[228] Heat shock protein induction has also been observed in cells subjected to a 20-minute continuous compressive force.[227] It is believed that heat shock proteins function primarily to preserve only vital cellular functions during stress in an attempt to conserve energy.[229] These observations indicate that an important element in the pathogenesis of TMJ disease associated with articular disk displacement involves impairment of vital cellular functions in affected articular tissues. Under such conditions, anabolic events likely will not keep pace with the catabolic events mentioned earlier. The obvious net result of this imbalance would be tissue loss.

Changes in the molecular composition of articular tissues associated with the pathogenesis of degenerative joint disease can have a profound impact on local cellular activities. There is a mounting body of evidence that changes in the molecular composition of the extracellular matrix may profoundly affect phenotypic gene expression of resident cell populations. For example, prechondroblasts are thought to be pluripotential cells that can be committed to either a chondroblast phenotype or a fibroblast phenotype. These pluripotential cells may receive "signals" from specific extracellular matrix molecules by way of transmembrane receptors (i.e., integrins).[85, 119, 120] Werb and coworkers provided evidence that inhibition of the interaction between fibronectin and its integrin receptor (α5β1 integrin) can alter gene expression in rabbit synovial fibroblasts.[230] Fibronectins are extracellular matrix glycoproteins that promote cell adhesion and facilitate cell migration.[119, 231] In this study, treatment of attached and spread synovial fibroblasts with a monoclonal antibody directed against the α5β1 integrin or with synthetic peptides that inhibited the binding of fibronectin to the integrin receptor induced expression of collagenase (MMP-1) and stromelysin (MMP-3). Thus, cell interactions with molecules of the extracellular matrix can strongly influence gene expression.

Interestingly, a commonly observed change in the extracellular matrix of osteoarthrotic cartilage is an accumulation of fibronectins (up to a 10-fold increase).[232-234] In vitro studies provided evidence that accumulated fibronectin may inhibit chondrogenesis by providing "signals" to prechondroblasts that "instruct" them to become fibroblast-like cells at the expense of forming cartilage-producing cells (i.e., chondroblasts).[235, 236] Fibronectins may also regulate proliferation of these cells. For example, mandibular chondrocytes proliferate in a serum-enriched growth medium in vitro.[237] This proliferative response can be significantly inhibited, in a reversible fashion, with a monospecific antibody directed against the α5 subunit of the α5β1 integrin (i.e., the fibronectin receptor).[237] Collectively, these studies indicate that fibronectin stimulates a proliferative response by prechondroblasts and inhibits the expression of a chondroblast phenotype. These observations could explain the fibrotic changes observed in articular fibrocartilage of degenerate TMJs.

In summary, the extracellular matrix affords structural integrity to a tissue and determines the biomechanical properties of that tissue. The extracellular matrix also profoundly affects specific cellular activities, including gene expression. Disruption of the normal integrity of the extracellular matrix, as occurs with degenerative TMJ disease, can have a profound affect on *both* the biomechanical properties and the cellular activities of affected articular tissues. These secondary effects could be primary determinants of the progression of the disease. Articular tissues rendered increasingly vulnerable to the effects of mechanical stress by virtue of altered mechanical properties may not be able to adapt if chondrogenesis is inhibited by changing cell–extracellular matrix interactions.

Cytokines and Degenerative Joint Disease

The synthesis of matrix-degrading enzymes in the TMJ may be stimulated by proteins known as cytokines. Cytokines are peptide hormones that can evoke strong cellular responses. Cytokines are extremely potent molecules that typically exert biologic activity in 10^{-9} to 10^{-12} M concentrations. The cytokines that have been implicated in degenerative joint disease are interleukin-1 (IL-1),[238-246] tumor necrosis factor (TNF),[247-249] interleukin-6 (IL-6),[250] and interleukin-8 (IL-8).[251, 252] Of course, this is only a partial list of the more than 100 known cytokines. Conceivably, many more cytokines could be intimately involved in both adaptive and disease responses in the human TMJ. Of those cytokines currently believed to be involved in the pathogenesis of degenerative joint disease, IL-1 has received the most attention from researchers in the field.

CYTOKINE-MEDIATED AMPLIFICATION IN DEGENERATIVE JOINT DISEASE: THE IL-1 EXAMPLE

The term IL-1 refers to a group of three polypeptide hormones: IL-1α, IL-1β, and IL-1 receptor antagonist.[253] IL-1α and IL-1β are agonists for both types of IL-1 receptor described to date and evoke similar biologic responses. They generally differ on the basis of relative potencies (IL-1β > IL-1α) and by the fact that IL-1α is produced in an active form, whereas IL-1β is produced in an inactive precursor form.[254] The inactive precursor form of IL-1β is activated by a protease, termed IL-1 converting enzyme or convertase, that appears to be synthesized only by cells of the myelomonocytic lineage.[255]

Virtually all cells either have IL-1 receptors or synthesize these receptors when involved in an inflammatory process. Thus, IL-1 can evoke a multitude of cellular responses in an involved tissue. IL-1 induces the synthesis and release of several matrix-degrading enzymes by synoviocytes and chondrocytes. These include both fibroblast-type (MMP-1) and polymorphonuclear leukocyte–type collagenases (MMP-8), stromelysin (MMP-3), 72-kD (MMP-2) and 92-kD (MMP-9) gelatinases, and cathepsins.[249, 256] IL-1 is also capable of downregulating the expression of naturally occurring inhibitors of these enzymes.[158] Other cytokines may potentiate (basic fibroblast growth factor, platelet-derived growth factor-AB) or inhibit (TGF-β) IL-1 induction of matrix-degrading enzymes.[256] IL-1 upregulates the synthesis of other cytokines, including IL-6[245, 257–260] and IL-8,[251, 258, 261] which may be responsible for many of the biologic activities that have traditionally been attributed to IL-1. Collectively, these studies indicate that IL-1, and perhaps other cytokines, promote the net loss of cartilaginous matrix by increasing the synthesis of matrix-degrading enzymes and reducing the synthesis of molecules that function to restrict the activities of these enzymes.

IL-1 also regulates the synthesis of extracellular matrix molecules in articular fibrocartilage. IL-1 downregulates the synthesis of cartilage-specific type II collagens[243, 262] and increases the synthesis of type I collagen,[243, 262] fibronectin,[262] and several integrins, including the α5β1 integrin.[263–265] IL-1 may also activate heat shock proteins in chondrocytes, which could account, in part, for the inhibitory effect this cytokine has on glycosaminoglycan synthesis by chondrocytes.[266]

IL-1 stimulates arachidonic acid metabolism by increasing phospholipase activity in chondrocytes[239] and synoviocytes.[267] IL-1 increases prostaglandin E_2 production by chondrocytes obtained from primate mandibular condyles in femtomolar concentra-tions.[237] As previously mentioned, prostaglandin E_2 and leukotriene B_4 have been specifically implicated in the pathogenesis of degenerative TMJ disease.[54]

NO may be produced by target cells in response to IL-1.[268–270] IL-1 may also contribute to the production of oxygen-derived free radicals by stimulating arachidonic acid metabolism.[239] It is interesting to note that free radicals generated by hypoxia and reoxygenation stimulate IL-1 and IL-6 synthesis by cultured endothelial cells.[271] The synthesis of these cytokines under these experimental conditions is significantly inhibited in the presence of free radical scavengers (superoxide dismutase or glutathione peroxidase).[271] Therefore, it appears that both free radical production and inflammatory cytokine synthesis are involved in positive feedback mechanisms that perpetuate these signaling mechanisms. However, there may be a negative regulatory mechanism involved in the interrelationship between free radical production and cytokine expression. For example, both IL-1 and TNF upregulate the expression of manganous superoxide dismutase (MnSOD) in pancreatic islets.[272] MnSOD is a free radical scavenger that catalyzes a dismutation reaction between two superoxide anions and two hydrogen ions, forming oxygen and hydrogen peroxide. Therefore, an upregulated expression of this enzyme would be expected to offer some protection against superoxide anion–mediated toxicity.

CYTOKINES AND TMJ REMODELING AND DISEASE

Cytokines are likely involved in both remodeling and degenerative processes affecting the TMJ. TNF and IL-1 have been detected in human TMJ lavage fluid.[273–276] In a preliminary study, the levels of TNF in synovial fluid correlated with symptoms associated with disk displacement.[274] In addition, primary cultures of chondrocytes obtained from primate mandibular condyles respond to physiologic concentrations of IL-1 in vitro.[237] Future studies will be required to delineate the relative contributions of specific cytokines to both remodeling and degenerative processes in the TMJ.

Neurogenic Inflammation and Degenerative TMJ Disease

Neuropeptides (i.e., substance P, calcitonin gene–related peptide [CGRP] have been identified that can produce inflammation when released or injected into tissue.[277–285] Substance P, a neuropeptide found principally in small-diameter neurons believed to be involved in nociception, evokes a strong inflammatory response when injected into joints.[286, 287] Furthermore, substance P can be released into joints following antidromic stimulation of a sensory nerve providing innervation to the affected joint.[288] Substance P released in this fashion produces inflammation in the joint. Substance P is not the only neuropeptide found in these neurons, and there is evidence that other neuropeptides may also modulate immune function.[285, 289]

Substance P– and CGRP-containing nerve terminals have been identified in the TMJ.[290–292] In the rat, a dense network of substance P–containing nerve terminals is located in the anterior capsule and supporting tissues of the disk near its anterior margin.[290, 292] An abundant network is also found in the retrodiskal tissues of the joint.[291] It is conceivable that traction or compression of these nerve-rich structures could evoke the release of these neuropeptides into affected regions of the joint, which would initiate an inflammatory response.

Several studies have provided a substantial body of evidence that neuropeptides involved in neurogenic inflammation increase both IL-1[278, 280, 293] and TNF[280] synthesis. Interestingly, IL-1 upregulates the expression of substance P, in what appears to be a positive response loop.[294–297] The effect of IL-1 on substance P synthesis by affected neurons may be mediated by leukemia inhibitory factor.[298] Leukemia inhibitory factor is produced by synoviocytes,[299] chondrocytes,[300] and sympathetic neurons[298, 301] in response to IL-1 or TNF. In this regard, O'Byrne and colleagues observed a dose-dependent increase in synovial fluid substance P levels following injection of IL-1 into the rabbit knee joint.[302] Therefore, cytokines and neuropeptides may self-perpetuate molecular events that could eventually lead to degenerative changes in tissues of affected joints.

Factors that May Influence the Adaptive Capacity of the TMJ

SEX HORMONES

Several epidemiologic studies have provided evidence of a female predilection for temporomandibular dysfunction. In general, females tend to report more pain and exhibit a higher incidence of joint noise and mandibular deflection with movement than do male counterparts. Histologic studies of human cadaver TMJs also indicate that females have a higher incidence of articular disk displacement.[20]

Functional estrogen receptors have been identified in the female TMJ[303, 304] but not in the male TMJ.[55] High-affinity (kD = 5 × 10^{-10} M) estrogen receptors have been identified in macrophage-like synoviocytes.[305] In a model of osteoarthritis involving the rabbit knee joint (partial medial meniscectomy), systemically administered estradiol significantly reduced ^{35}S-incorporation into affected cartilage compared with operated controls.[306] Furthermore, the authors noted that articular cartilage from estradiol-treated animals was more friable than cartilage obtained from control animals. However, in these studies, safranin O staining of affected articular tissue was not appreciably different between experimental groups. Safranin O is a cationic dye that binds to anionic molecules such as glycosaminoglycans. These data indicate that estrogen may inhibit glycosaminoglycan degradation and synthesis.

Estrogen may also promote degenerative changes in the TMJ by increasing the synthesis of specific cytokines. Estradiol enhances the synthesis of IL-1 and IL-6 by peripheral blood mononuclear cells.[307] In contrast, testosterone may inhibit the release of these cytokines from stimulated monocytes.[307] In addition, prolactin, released from the pituitary in response to estrogen, exacerbates collagen-induced arthritis in mice.[308] Prolactin also stimulates cytokine production by lymphocytes and macrophages. Bromocriptine, a dopaminergic agonist that inhibits prolactin release from the pituitary, markedly (50%) suppresses the severity of collagen-induced arthritis in postpartum (i.e., hyperprolactinemic) mice.[308] Sex hormone regulation of cytokine production is complex and may be dependent on other coexisting factors. It is likely that sex hormones profoundly influence local cellular activities that may be associated with remodeling or degenerative processes in the TMJ.

Estrogens may mediate systemic effects that could inhibit their suspected local effects. Estrogens stimulate cortisol production, which could inhibit local inflammatory processes associated with a TMJ disorder. Therefore, the role of estrogens in the pathogenesis of degenerative TMJ disease is not clear at present. It is likely that the cumulative effects of sex hormones are dependent on several host factors, including genetic factors, age, preexisting disease, the integrity of the pituitary-adrenal axis, and possibly environmental factors.

AGE

With aging, it appears that the regenerative capacity of the articular tissues of the TMJ declines. Cell density in the prechondroblastic region decreases steadily with aging.[309] Prechondroblasts are the sole source of daughter cells in the fibrocartilage of the mandibular condyle and temporal bone.[310] With aging, there is also a progressive loss of cartilaginous matrix from this fibrocartilage. The cartilaginous matrix is gradually replaced with fibrous tissue that is sparsely populated with cells. Degenerative changes that occur with increasing frequency with age probably reflect the reduced synthetic capacity of these aged tissues.

OTHER FACTORS

Levine and colleagues suggested that sympathetic innervation may influence neurogenically mediated inflammatory responses.[311] These investigators provided evidence that conditions that reduce sympathetic tone can significantly decrease the severity of experimentally induced arthritis. It is conceivable from this model that heightened sympathetic tone (e.g., pain, psychological stress) could contribute to advancing degenerative joint disease. Cigarette smoking could also affect this process. Nicotine exacerbates certain arthritides, apparently by affecting sympathetic tone.[312] Other factors that may influence the adaptive capacity of the TMJ include diet, previous joint trauma (including surgical), and systemic illness (e.g., collagen vascular diseases, diabetes).

Model of Degenerative TMJ Disease

The etiology of articular disk displacement in the TMJ is unknown. A consensus among investigators in the field is that excessive loading of the TMJ leads to articular disk displacement. It is not clear at the present time whether articular disk displacement is the cause or the result of degenerative joint disease. However, articular disk displacement or articular disk perforation is associated with "degenerative" changes observed in articular tissues of the joint. In general, these changes become increasingly more pronounced as the articular disk becomes more displaced and eventually deforms against functional loading imposed by translational movements of the mandibular condyle.

How are mechanical forces transduced to biochemical reactions in the TMJ? As discussed earlier, mechanical forces can lead to the generation of destructive free radicals by at least three mechanisms: direct mechanical trauma (homolytic fission), hypoxia-reperfusion injury, and neurogenic inflammation (Fig. 4–3). Free radicals, particularly those formed in iron catalyzed reactions, are sufficiently reactive to destroy or sufficiently modify molecules in affected articular tissues. Under normal circumstances, these free radical–mediated reactions are tightly regulated and contained by endogenous scavenging mechanisms. Damage evoked by these reactions is confined, allowing for a healing or adaptive response. In susceptible individuals, genetic, dietary, environmental, hormonal, and/or local tissue factors may lead to an imbalance between the production of damaging free radicals and the free radical scavenging capacities of affected articular tissues. In addition, in discrete regions of vascularized articular tissues subjected to mechanical stress, bleeding could occur, resulting in a focal deposit of hemoglobin. As the depos-

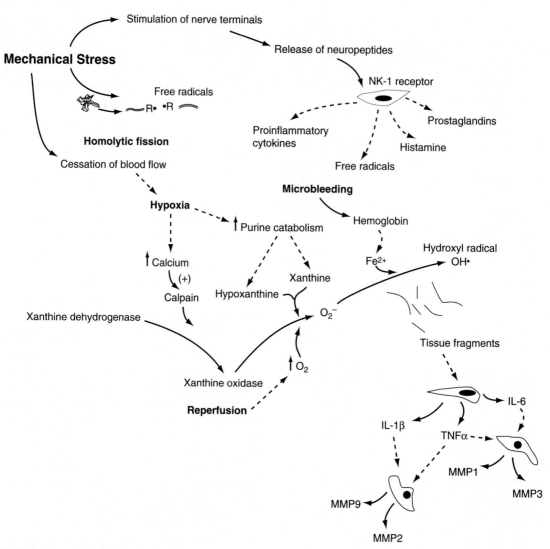

FIGURE 4–3. Model of the molecular biology of degenerative temporomandibular joint (TMJ) diseases. Mechanical stress can initiate molecular events that may culminate in degenerative joint disease in susceptible individuals. Traction or compression of nerve-rich structures of the TMJ (e.g., retrodiskal tissues, capsular ligament) can evoke the release of proinflammatory neuropeptides, such as substance P, calcitonin gene–related peptide (CGRP), and substance Y. Proinflammatory neuropeptides may stimulate resident cell populations to produce cytokines, free radicals, histamine, and prostaglandins that amplify the inflammatory response. Mechanical stress can also disrupt the physical integrity of molecules in articular tissues and generate highly reactive molecular species (free radicals) by a process known as homolytic fission. Finally, mechanical stress can lead to a hypoxia-reperfusion injury (see text). Free radical–mediated injury can be intensified by the presence of hemoglobin-derived iron that may be deposited into tissue by microbleeding (e.g., disruption of blood vessels with focal bleeding or from extravasation of erythrocytes in inflamed tissue). Tissue fragments generated by enzymatic or nonenzymatic (i.e., free radical) degradation can stimulate cells (synoviocytes, fibroblasts, chondrocytes) to produce proinflammatory cytokines and matrix-degrading enzymes. In this way, the sphere of injury may be expanded. IL, interleukin; MMP-1, collagenase; MMP-2, 72-kD gelatinase; MMP-3, stromelysin; MMP-9, 92-kD gelatinase; TNF, tumor necrosis factor.

ited hemoglobin decomposes, a reactive iron source is made available in the local tissue environment. Iron from partially decomposed, but not fresh, hemoglobin is sufficient to catalyze the production of the hydroxyl radical. The hydroxyl radical is a very reactive free radical that can destroy or significantly modify a variety of extracel-lular matrix and cellular molecules. Thus, it is possible that tissue destruction first occurs in joint regions subjected to unusual mechanical stresses, particularly in discrete areas where hemoglobin might accumulate in articular tissues (e.g., retrodiskal tissues) from bleeding.

Fragments of extracellular matrix molecules are rapidly generated by free radicals, particularly the hydroxyl radical. For example, fibronectin is markedly degraded in less than 1 minute by free radicals created in vitro under conditions believed to exist in the human TMJ. Some fragments of fibronectin, and probably fragments of many other extracellular matrix molecules, are chemotactic for proinflammatory cells, such as monocytes and macrophages. Also, these fragments may stimulate resident cell populations (synoviocytes) to produce proinflammatory cytokines (IL-1, IL-6, TNF), free radicals, and matrix-degrading enzymes. Both cytokines and matrix-degrading enzymes have been recovered from symptomatic human TMJs. Proinflammatory cytokines, as previously discussed, can evoke a cascade of molecular events, including arachidonic acid catabolism and the production and activation of matrix-degrading enzymes. Therefore, proinflammatory cytokines may be viewed as an amplification system that normally functions to initiate and orchestrate molecular events involved in inflammation and healing. In the proposed model of degenerative joint disease, cytokines and matrix-degrading enzymes could be mechanisms involved in the amplification of a tissue derangement originally produced by free radicals. In retrodiskal tissues, for example, this process could increase the sphere of damage produced by free radicals to the extent that the tensile strength of this tissue was significantly weakened. This could ultimately lead to loss in the posterior support of the articular disk, culminating in a typical anterior displacement.

The capsular ligament and retrodiskal tissues of the TMJ are richly innervated by substance P–, vasoactive intestinal polypeptide–, and CGRP-containing neurons. Stimulation of these nerve terminals by traction or compression could evoke a release of these neuropeptides into the surrounding tissue. Studies conducted by Holmlund and associates provided evidence that is consistent with this hypothesis.[313] They detected these neuropeptides in TMJ synovial fluid obtained from patients with articular disk displacements.[313] In fact, compared with neuropeptide levels detected in the knee joint, significantly higher concentrations of substance P, CGRP, and neuropeptide Y were found in the TMJ.[313] These neuropeptides can evoke an inflammatory response

when injected into articular joints.[277] Joint inflammation produced in experimental models of inflammatory arthritides can be significantly obtunded by manipulations that inhibit neuropeptide release.

Substance P and CGRP upregulate IL-1 synthesis by various cell populations in articular joints. IL-1, in turn, may increase the synthesis of these neuropeptides by neurons supplying the affected joint. Thus, a positive feedback loop may exist that perpetuates these signaling processes. This signaling mechanism may be further amplified by the presence of kinins and free radicals. These substances may lower the response thresholds of nerve terminals in affected tissues, resulting in the release of these neuropeptides with lower-intensity stimuli. Therefore, mechanical stresses impacting nerve-rich structures of the TMJ could trigger a molecular cascade leading to inflammation via a process known as neurogenic inflammation.

Changes in the molecular composition of the extracellular matrices of articulating tissues of the TMJ may therefore result from three basic mechanisms: direct mechanical trauma (homolytic fission), hypoxia-reperfusion injury, and neurogenic inflammation. These changes ultimately affect both the mechanical properties of the tissue and the cellular responses to the changing environment. Sometimes, articular disk displacements could result from a progressive weakening of the supporting tissues of the disk. Articular disk displacement could contribute to a progression of the disorder by creating an additional mechanical disadvantage or by promoting a direct impingement of articulating structures on nerve- or vessel-rich tissues in the affected joint. Nevertheless, it is apparent from clinical experience that, even in the face of these gross structural changes, many individuals do not sustain a lasting derangement of joint function.

Summary

The molecular events that underlie TMJ remodeling and degenerative diseases are complex and poorly understood. Structural changes associated with articular disk displacement in the TMJ are believed to be the result of a series of cascading molecular events that include free radical generation, cytokine synthesis and activation, neuropeptide synthesis and release, increased arachidonic acid metabolism, activation of matrix-degrading enzymes, and inhibition and/or reduction of protease inhibitor synthesis. These events ultimately alter the structural and molecular composition of the affected articular tissues. In some instances, articular disk displacement could result from these processes. In addition, these biologic processes can probably be modulated by other factors, including sex hormones, age, and physiologic responses to psychological stress. For these reasons, some individuals may experience a severe degenerative change in the face of physical stress imposed on the TMJ (i.e., articular disk displacement); other individuals, given a similar insult, can apparently mount an adaptive response and not exhibit signs of significant TMJ disease.

REFERENCES

1. Annandale T: On displacement of the interarticular cartilage of the lower jaw and its treatment by operation. Lancet 1887;1:411.
2. Lanz W: Discitis mandibularis. Zentralbl Chir 1909;36:289.
3. Pringle JH: Displacement of the mandibular meniscus and its treatment. Br J Surg 1918;6:385.
4. Isberg A, Widmalm SE, Ivarsson R: Clinical, radiographic, and electromyographic study of patients with internal derangement of the temporomandibular joint. Am J Orthod 1985;88:453.
5. Isacsson G, Isberg A, Persson A: Loss of directional orientation control of lower jaw movements in persons with internal derangement of the temporomandibular joint. Oral Surg Oral Med Oral Pathol 1988;66:8.
6. Stegenga B, de Bont L, van Loon J, et al: Classification of temporomandibular joint osteoarthrosis and internal derangement. 1. Diagnostic significance of clinical and radiographic symptoms and signs. Craniomandib Pract 1992;10:96.
7. Stegenga B, de Bont L, Boering G: Osteoarthrosis as the cause of craniomandibular pain and dysfunction: A unifying concept. J Oral Maxillofac Surg 1989;47:249.
8. Schellhas KP, Wilkes CH, Baker CC: Facial pain, headache, and temporomandibular joint inflammation. Headache 1989;29:229.
9. Montgomery MT, Van SJ, Harms SE: Success of temporomandibular joint arthroscopy in disk displacement with and without reduction. Oral Surg Oral Med Oral Pathol 1991;71:651.
10. Westesson PL, Brooks SL: Temporomandibular joint: Relationship between MR evidence of effusion and the presence of pain and disk displacement. AJR Am J Roentgenol 1992;159:559.
11. Widmalm SE, Westesson PL, Brooks SL, et al: Temporomandibular joint sounds: Correlation to joint structure in fresh autopsy specimens. Am J Orthod Dentofacial Orthop 1992;101:60.
12. Rohlin M, Westesson PL, Eriksson L: The correlation of temporomandibular joint sounds with joint morphology in fifty-five autopsy specimens. J Oral Maxillofac Surg 1985;43:194.
13. Gay T, Bertolami CN, Donoff RB, et al: The acoustical characteristics of the normal and abnormal temporomandibular joint. J Oral Maxillofac Surg 1987;45:397.
14. Castelli WA, Nasjleti CE, Diaz PR, et al: Histopathologic findings in temporomandibular joints of aged individuals. J Prosthet Dent 1985;53:415.
15. Davant TT, Greene CS, Perry HT, et al: A quantitative computer-assisted analysis of disc displacement in patients with internal derangement using sagittal view magnetic resonance imaging. J Oral Maxillofac Surg 1993;51:974.
16. Dijkgraaf LC, de Bont L, Otten E, et al: Three-dimensional visualization of the temporomandibular joint: A computerized multisectional autopsy study of disc position and configuration. J Oral Maxillofac Surg 1992;50:2.
17. Liedberg J, Westesson PL: Sideways position of the temporomandibular joint disk: Coronal cryosectioning of fresh autopsy specimens. Oral Surg Oral Med Oral Pathol 1988;66:644.
18. Liedberg J, Westesson PL, Kurita K: Sideways and rotational displacement of the temporomandibular joint disk: Diagnosis by arthrography and correlation to cryosectional morphology. Oral Surg Oral Med Oral Pathol 1990;69:757.
19. Nannmark U, Sennerby L, Haraldson T: Macroscopic, microscopic and radiologic assessment of the condylar part of the TMJ in elderly subjects: An autopsy study. Swed Dent J 1990;14:163.
20. Solberg WK, Hansson TL, Nordstrom B: The temporomandibular joint in young adults at autopsy: A morphologic classification and evaluation. J Oral Rehabil 1985;12:303.
21. Westesson PL, Rohlin M: Internal derangement related to osteoarthrosis in temporomandibular joint autopsy specimens. Oral Surg Oral Med Oral Pathol 1984;57:17.
22. Westesson PL, Bronstein SL, Liedberg J: Internal derangement of the temporomandibular joint: Morphologic description with correlation to joint function. Oral Surg Oral Med Oral Pathol 1985;59:323.
23. Farrar WB, McCarty WJ: Inferior joint space arthrography and characteristics of condylar paths in internal derangements of the TMJ. J Prosthet Dent 1979;41:548.
24. Helmy ES, Bays RA, Sharawy MM: Histopathological study of human TMJ perforated discs with emphasis on synovial membrane response. J Oral Maxillofac Surg 1989;47:1048.
25. Axelsson S, Fitins D, Hellsing G, et al: Arthrotic changes and deviation in form of the temporomandibular joint—an autopsy study. Swed Dent J 1987;11:195.
26. Brand JW, Whinery JJ, Anderson QN, et al: The effects of temporomandibular joint internal derangement and degenerative joint disease on tomographic and arthrotomographic images. Oral Surg Oral Med Oral Pathol 1989;67:220.
27. Kurita K, Bronstein SL, Westesson PL, et al: Arthroscopic diagnosis of perforation and adhesions of the temporomandibular joint: Correlation with postmortem morphology. Oral Surg Oral Med Oral Pathol 1989;68:130.

28. Blackwood HJJ: Cellular remodeling in articular tissue. J Dent Res 1966;45:480.
29. Stedman's Medical Dictionary. Baltimore, Williams & Wilkins, 1997, p 1966.
30. Farrar WB: Disk derangement and dental occlusion: Changing concepts. Int J Perio Res Dent 1985;5:34.
31. Wilkes CH: Internal derangements of the temporomandibular joint. Arch Otolaryngol Head Neck Surg 1989;115:469.
32. Yaillen DM, Shapiro PA, Luschei ES, et al: Temporomandibular joint meniscectomy—effects on joint structure and masticatory function in *Macaca fascicularis*. J Maxillofac Surg 1979;7:255.
33. Block MS, Bouvier M: Adaptive remodeling of the rabbit temporomandibular joint following discectomy and dietary variations. J Oral Maxillofac Surg 1990;48:482.
34. Hinton RJ: Alterations in rat condylar cartilage following discectomy. J Dent Res 1992;71:1292.
35. Brown WA: Internal derangement of the temporomandibular joint: Review of 214 patients following meniscectomy. Can J Surg 1980;23:30.
36. Eriksson L, Westesson PL: Long-term evaluation of meniscectomy of the temporomandibular joint. J Oral Maxillofac Surg 1985;43:263.
37. Tolvanen M, Oikarinen VJ, Wolf J: A 30-year follow-up study of temporomandibular joint meniscectomies: A report on five patients. Br J Oral Maxillofac Surg 1988;26:311.
38. Ghafari J, Heeley JD: Condylar adaptation to muscle alteration in the rat. Angle Orthod 1982;52:26.
39. Hinton RJ: Effect of condylotomy on DNA synthesis in cells of the mandibular condylar cartilage in the rat. Arch Oral Biol 1987;32:865.
40. Copray JC, Dibbets JM, Kantomaa T: The role of condylar cartilage in the development of the temporomandibular joint. Angle Orthod 1988;58:369.
41. Hinton RJ: Effect of condylotomy on matrix synthesis and mineralization in the rat mandibular condylar cartilage. Arch Oral Biol 1989;34:1003.
42. Hinton RJ: Jaw protruder muscles and condylar cartilage growth in the rat. Am J Orthod Dentofacial Orthop 1991;100:436.
43. Scapino RP: The posterior attachment: Its structure, function, and appearance in TMJ imaging studies. Part 1. J Craniomand Dis 1991;5:83.
44. Breitner C: Bone changes resulting from experimental orthodontic treatment. Am J Orthod 1940;26:521.
45. Breitner C: Further investigations of bone changes resulting from experimental orthodontic treatment. Am J Orthod 1941;27:605.
46. Charlier J-P, Petrovic A, Hermann-Stuzmann J: Effects of mandibular hyperpropulsion on the prechondroblastic zone of young rat condyle. Am J Orthod 1969;55:71.
47. Petrovic A: Mechanisms and regulation of mandibular condylar growth. Acta Morph Neerl Scand 1972;10:25.
48. Carlson DS, McNamara JA, Jaul DH: Histological analysis of the growth of the mandibular condyle in the rhesus monkey (*Macaca mulatta*). Am J Anat 1978;151:103.
49. McNamara JJ, Carlson DS: Quantitative analysis of temporomandibular joint adaptations to protrusive function. Am J Orthod 1979;76:593.
50. Adams CD, Meikle MC, Norwick KW, et al: Dentofacial remodeling produced by intermaxillary forces in *Macaca mulatta*. Arch Oral Biol 1972;17:1519.
51. Joho J-P: The effects of extraoral low-pull traction to the mandibular dentition of *Macaca mulatta*. Am J Orthod 1973;64:555.
52. Moffett BC, Johnson LC, McCabe JB, et al: Articular remodeling in the adult human temporomandibular joint. Am J Anat 1964;115:119.
53. Meikle MC: Remodeling. In Sarnat BG, Laskin DM (eds): The Temporomandibular Joint: A Biological Basis for Clinical Practice. Philadelphia, WB Saunders, 1992, p 93.
54. Quinn JH: Pain mediators and chondromalacia in internally deranged temporomandibular joints. In Bell W (ed): Modern Practice in Orthognathic and Reconstructive Surgery. Philadelphia, WB Saunders, 1992, p 471.
55. Milam SB, Aufdemorte TB, Sheridan PJ, et al: Sexual dimorphism in the distribution of estrogen receptors in the temporomandibular joint complex of the baboon. Oral Surg Oral Med Oral Pathol 1987;64:527.
56. Moroco JR, Hinton R, Buschang P, et al: Age-related changes of TGFβs in mandibular condylar cartilage. J Dent Res 1995;74:214.
57. Milam SB, Schmitz JP: Molecular biology of degenerative temporomandibular joint disease: Proposed mechanisms of disease. J Oral Maxillofac Surg 1995;53:1448.
58. Milam SB: Articular disk displacements and degenerative temporomandibular joint disease. In Sessle BJ, Bryant PB, Dionne RA (eds): Temporomandibular Disorders and Related Pain Conditions. Seattle, IASP Press, 1995, p 89.
59. Axelsson S, Holmlund A, Hjerpe A: An experimental model of osteoarthrosis in the temporomandibular joint of the rabbit. Acta Odontol Scand 1992;50:273.
60. Axelsson S: Human and experimental osteoarthrosis of the temporomandibular joint: Morphological and biochemical studies. Swed Dent J Suppl 1993;92:1.
61. De Bont LGM, Stegenga B: Pathology of temporomandibular joint internal derangement and osteoarthrosis. Int J Oral Maxillofac Surg 1993;22:71.
62. Stegenga B, Dijkstra PU, de Bont L, et al: Temporomandibular joint osteoarthrosis and internal derangement. Part II. Additional treatment options. Int Dent J 1990;40:347.
63. Stegenga B, de Bont L, Boering G, et al: Tissue responses to degenerative changes in the temporomandibular joint: A review. J Oral Maxillofac Surg 1991;49:1079.
64. Iwata T, Watase J, Kuroda T, et al: Studies of mechanical effects of occlusal force on mandible and temporomandibular joint. J Osaka Univ Dent Sch 1981;21:207.
65. Haskell B, Day M, Tetz J: Computer-aided modeling in the assessment of the biomechanical determinants of diverse skeletal patterns. Am J Orthod 1986;89:363.
66. Hatcher DC, Faulkner MG, Hay A: Development of mechanical and mathematic models to study temporomandibular joint loading. J Prosthet Dent 1986;55:377.
67. Faulkner MG, Hatcher DC, Hay A: A three-dimensional investigation of temporomandibular joint loading. J Biomech 1987;20:997.
68. Van ET, Klok EM, Weijs WA, et al: Mechanical capabilities of the human jaw muscles studied

with a mathematical model. Arch Oral Biol 1988;33:819.

69. Throckmorton GS, Groshan GJ, Boyd SB: Muscle activity patterns and control of temporomandibular joint loads. J Prosthet Dent 1990;63:685.

70. dos Santos J, de Rijk WG: Occlusal contacts: Vectorial analysis of forces transmitted to temporomandibular joint and teeth. Craniomandib Pract 1993;11:118.

71. Tuominen M, Kantomaa T, Pirttiniemi P: Effect of food consistency on the shape of the articular eminence and the mandible: An experimental study on the rabbit. Acta Odontol Scand 1993;51:65.

72. Hylander WL: Functional anatomy. In Sarnat BG, Laskin DM (eds): The Temporomandibular Joint: A Biological Basis for Clinical Practice. Philadelphia, WB Saunders, 1992, p 60.

73. Boyd RL, Gibbs CH, Mahan PE, et al: Temporomandibular joint forces measured at the condyle of Macaca arctoides. Am J Orthod Dentofacial Orthop 1990;97:472.

74. Ward DM, Behrents RG, Goldberg JS: Temporomandibular synovial fluid pressure response to altered mandibular positions. Am J Orthod Dentofacial Orthop 1990;98:22.

75. Dolwick MF: Personal communication, February 22, 1994.

76. Chen J, Liangfeng X: A finite element analysis of the human temporomandibular joint. J Biomech Eng 1994;116:401.

77. Teng S, Herring SW: Anatomic and directional variation in the mechanical properties of the mandibular condyle in pigs. J Dent Res 1996;75:1842.

78. Kantomaa T: Effect of functional change on cell differentiation in the condylar cartilage. J Anat 1987;152:133.

79. Lang TC, Zimny ML, Vijayagopal P: Experimental temporomandibular joint disc perforation in the rabbit: A gross morphologic, biochemical, and ultrastructural analysis. J Oral Maxillofac Surg 1993;51:1115.

80. De Bont LGB, Boering G, Liem RSB, et al: Osteoarthritis and internal derangement of the temporomandibular joint: A light microscopic study. J Oral Maxillofac Surg 1986;44:634.

81. Silbermann M, Reddi AH, Hand AR, et al: Further characterisation of the extracellular matrix in the mandibular condyle in neonatal mice. J Anat 1987;151:169.

82. Silbermann M, von der Mark K, Heinegard D: An immunohistochemical study of the distribution of matrical proteins in the mandibular condyle of neonatal mice. I. Collagens. J Anat 1990;170:11.

83. Strauss PG, Closs EI, Schmidt J, et al: Gene expression during osteogenic differentiation in mandibular condyles in vitro. J Cell Biol 1990;110:1369.

84. Ben AY, von der Mark K, Franzen A, et al: Immunohistochemical studies in the extracellular matrix in the condylar cartilage of the human fetal mandible: Collagens and noncollagenous proteins. Am J Anat 1991;190:157.

85. Milam SB, Klebe RJ, Triplett RG, et al: Characterization of the extracellular matrix of the primate temporomandibular joint. J Oral Maxillofac Surg 1991;49:381.

86. Ben AY, Lewinson D, Silbermann M: Structural characterization of the mandibular condyle in human fetuses: Light and electron microscopic studies. Acta Anat 1992;145:79.

87. Silbermann M, Frommer J: Dynamic changes in acid mucopolysaccharides during mineralization of the mandibular condylar cartilage. Histochemie 1973;36:185.

88. Symons NB: A histochemical study of the secondary cartilage of the mandibular condyle in the rat. Arch Oral Biol 1965;10:579.

89. Silbermann M, von der Mark K, Heinegard D: An immunohistochemical study of the distribution of matrical proteins in the mandibular condyle of neonatal mice. II. Non-collagenous proteins. J Anat 1990;170:23.

90. Tajima Y, Yokose S, Takenoya M, et al: Immunocytochemical detection of S-100 protein in rat mandibular condylar cartilage. Arch Oral Biol 1991;36:875.

91. Dean DD, Martel-Pelletier J, Pelletier J-P, et al: Evidence for metalloproteinase and metalloproteinase inhibitor imbalance in human osteoarthritic cartilage. J Clin Invest 1989;84:678.

92. Hasty KA, Reife RA, Kang AH, et al: The role of stromelysin in the cartilage destruction that accompanies inflammatory arthritis. Arthritis Rheum 1990;33:388.

93. Gunja SZ, Nagase H, Woessner JJ: Purification of the neutral proteoglycan-degrading metalloproteinase from human articular cartilage tissue and its identification as stromelysin matrix metalloproteinase-3. Biochem J 1989;258:115.

94. Flannery CR, Lark MW, Sandy JD: Identification of a stromelysin cleavage site within the interglobular domain of human aggrecan: Evidence for proteolysis at this site in vivo in human articular cartilage. J Biol Chem 1992;267:1008.

95. Fosang AJ, Neame PJ, Last K, et al: The interglobular domain of cartilage aggrecan is cleaved by PUMP, gelatinases, and cathepsin B. J Biol Chem 1992;267:19470.

96. Fosang AJ, Last K, Knauper V, et al: Fibroblast and neutrophil collagenases cleave at two sites in the cartilage aggrecan interglobular domain. Biochem J 1993;295:273.

97. Wilhelm SM, Shao ZH, Housley TJ, et al: Matrix metalloproteinase-3 (stromelysin-1): Identification as the cartilage acid metalloprotease and effect of pH on catalytic properties and calcium affinity. J Biol Chem 1993;268:21906.

98. Kang Y: The effect of free radicals on the rabbit articular chondrocytes in monolayer culture. Chin J Pathol 1991;20:100.

99. Vincent F, Brun H, Clain E, et al: Effects of oxygen-free radicals on proliferation kinetics of cultured rabbit articular chondrocytes. J Cell Physiol 1989;141:262.

100. Vincent F, Corral M, Defer N, et al: Effects of oxygen free radicals on articular chondrocytes in culture: c-myc and c-Ha-ras messenger RNAs and proliferation kinetics. Exp Cell Res 1991;192:333.

101. Henrotin Y, Deby DG, Deby C, et al: Active oxygen species, articular inflammation and cartilage damage. EXS 1992;62:308.

102. Johnson LC: Kinetics of osteoarthritis. Lab Invest 1959;8:1223.

103. Hamerman D: The biology of osteoarthritis. N Engl J Med 1989;320:1322.

104. Poole AR, Rizkalla G, Ionescu M, et al: Osteoarthritis in the human knee: A dynamic process of cartilage matrix degradation, synthesis and reorganization. Agents Actions Suppl 1993;39:3.

105. Sandy JD, Barrach H-J, Flannery CR, et al: The biosynthetic response of the mature chondrocyte in early osteoarthritis. J Rheumatol 1987;14:16.

106. Bollet AJ, Nance JL: Biochemical findings in normal and osteoarthritic articular cartilage. II. Chondroitin sulfate concentration and chain length, water, and ash content. J Clin Invest 1966;45:1170.

107. Mankin HJ, Lippiello L: The glycosaminoglycans of normal and arthritic cartilage. J Clin Invest 1971;50:1712.

108. Brandt KD, Radin E: The physiology of articular stress: Osteoarthrosis. Hosp Pract J 1987;15:103.

109. Helmy E, Bays R, Sharawy M: Osteoarthrosis of the temporomandibular joint following experimental disc perforation in *Macaca fascicularis*. J Oral Maxillofac Surg 1988;46:979.

110. Chandrasekaran L, Tanzer ML: Molecular cloning of chicken aggrecan: Structural analyses. Biochem J 1992;288:903–910.

111. Upholt WB, Chandrasekaran L, Tanzer ML: Molecular cloning and analysis of the protein modules of aggrecans. Experientia 1993;49:384.

112. Neame PJ, Christner JE, Baker JR: Cartilage proteoglycan aggregates: The link protein and proteoglycan amino-terminal globular domains have similar structures. J Biol Chem 1987;262:17768.

113. Neame PJ, Barry FP: The link proteins. Experientia 1993;49:393.

114. Muir H, Maroudas A, Wingham J: The correlation of fixed negative charge with glycosaminoglycan content of human articular cartilage. Biochim Biophys Acta 1969;177:494.

115. Kempson GE, Muir H, Swanson SAV, et al: Correlations between the compressive stiffness and chemical constituents of human articular cartilage. Biochim Biophys Acta 1970;215:70.

116. Heinegard D, Hascall VC: Aggregation of cartilage proteoglycans. III. Characteristics of the proteins isolated from trypsin digests of aggregates. J Biol Chem 1974;249:4250.

117. Israel HA, Saed-Nejad F, Ratcliffe A: Early diagnosis of osteoarthrosis of the temporomandibular joint: Correlation between arthroscopic diagnosis and keratan sulfate levels in the synovial fluid. J Oral Maxillofac Surg 1991;49:708.

118. Klebe RJ, Caldwell HB, Milam SB: Cells transmit spatial information by orienting collagen fibers. Matrix 1989;9:451.

119. Milam SB, Haskin C, Zardeneta G, et al: Cell adhesion proteins in oral biology. Crit Rev Oral Biol Med 1991;2:451.

120. Ruoslahti E: Integrins. J Clin Invest 1991;87:1.

121. Bosman FT: Integrins: Cell adhesives and modulators of cell function. Histochem J 1993;25:469.

122. Vogel KG, Keller EJ, Lenhoff RJ, et al: Proteoglycan synthesis by fibroblast cultures initiated from regions of adult bovine tendon subjected to different mechanical forces. Eur J Cell Biol 1986;41:102.

123. Blaustein DI, Scapino RP: Remodeling of the temporomandibular joint disk and posterior attachment in disk displacement specimens in relation to glycosaminoglycans content. Plast Reconstr Surg 1986;78:756.

124. Kadokura A: Purification and partial characterization of proteoglycans of bovine articular disc. Kanagawa Shigaku 1990;25:77.

125. Nakano T, Scott PG: Proteoglycans of the articular disc of the bovine temporomandibular joint. I. High molecular weight chondroitin sulphate proteoglycan. Matrix 1989;9:277.

126. Nakano T, Scott PG: A quantitative chemical study of glycosaminoglycans in the articular disc of the bovine temporomandibular joint. Arch Oral Biol 1989;34:749.

127. Scott PG, Nakano T, Dodd CM, et al: Proteoglycans of the articular disc of the bovine temporomandibular joint. II. Low molecular weight dermatan sulphate proteoglycan. Matrix 1989;9:284.

128. Andres JL, Stanley K, Cheifetz S, et al: Membrane-anchored and soluble forms of betaglycan, a polymorphic proteoglycan that binds transforming growth factor-beta. J Cell Biol 1989;109:3137–3145.

129. Centrella M, Massague J, Canalis E: Human platelet derived transforming growth factor beta stimulates parameters of bone growth in fetal rat calvariae. Endocrinology 1986;119:2306.

130. Centrella M, McCarthy TL, Canalis E: Transforming growth factor beta is a bifunctional regulator of replication and collagen synthesis in osteoblast-enriched cell cultures from fetal rat bone. J Biol Chem 1987;262:2869.

131. Sporn MB, Roberts AB, Wakefield LM, et al: Some recent advances in the chemistry and biology of transforming growth factor-beta. J Cell Biol 1987;105:1039.

132. Hauschka PV, Chen TL, Mavrakos AE: Polypeptide growth factors in bone matrix. Ciba Found Symp 1988;136:207.

133. Rosen DM, Stempien SA, Thompson AY, et al: Transforming growth factor-beta modulates the expression of osteoblast and chondroblast phenotypes in vitro. J Cell Physiol 1988;134:337.

134. Termine JD: Non-collagen proteins in bone. Ciba Found Symp 1988;136:178.

135. Birkedal-Hansen H, Moore WGI, Bodden MK, et al: Matrix metalloproteinases: A review. Crit Rev Oral Biol Med 1993;4:197.

136. Roughley PJ, Nguyen Q, Mort JS, et al: Proteolytic degradation in human articular cartilage: Its relationship to stromelysin. Agents Actions 1993;3:149.

137. Das UN: Interaction(s) between essential fatty acids, eicosanoids, cytokines, growth factors and free radicals: Relevance to new therapeutic strategies in rheumatoid arthritis and other collagen vascular diseases. Prostaglandins Leukot Essent Fatty Acids 1991;44:201.

138. Wang K, Xu SJ, Zhang FH, et al: Free radicals–induced abnormal chondrocytes, matrix and mineralization: A new concept of Kaschin-Beck's disease. Chin Med J Peking 1991;104:307.

139. Wei XQ: Free radical damage to chondrocytes and protection by selenium, tocopherol and ascorbic acid using serum-free medium method. Chung Hua Wai Ko Tsa Chih 1992;30:176.

140. McCachren SS: Expression of metalloproteinases and metalloproteinase inhibitor in human arthritic synovium. Arthritis Rheum 1991;34:1085.

141. Campbell IK, Piccoli DS, Butler DM, et al: Recombinant human interleukin-1 stimulates human articular cartilage to undergo resorption and human chondrocytes to produce both tissue and urokinase-type plasminogen activator. Biochim Biophys Acta 1988;967:183.

142. Buttle DJ, Saklatvala J: Lysosomal cysteine endopeptidases mediate interleukin-1 stimulated cartilage proteoglycan degradation. Biochem J 1992;287:657.

143. Suzuki K, Shimizu K, Hamamoto T, et al: Biochemical demonstration of calpains and calpastatin in osteoarthritic synovial fluid. Arthritis Rheum 1990;33:728.

144. Suzuki K, Shimizu K, Hamamoto T, et al: Characterization of proteoglycan degradation by calpain. Biochem J 1992;285:857.

145. Harvey AK, Stack ST, Chandrasekhar S: Differential modulation of degradative and repair responses of interleukin-1-treated chondrocytes by platelet-derived growth factor. Biochem J 1993;292:129.

146. DiBattista JA, Martel PJ, Wosu LO, et al: Glucocorticoid receptor mediated inhibition of interleukin-1 stimulated neutral metalloprotease synthesis in normal human chondrocytes. J Clin Endocrinol Metab 1991;72:316.

147. Harvey AK, Hrubey PS, Chandrasekhar S: Transforming growth factor-beta inhibition of interleukin-1 activity involves down-regulation of interleukin-1 receptors on chondrocytes. Exp Cell Res 1991;195:376.

148. Ballock RT, Heydemann A, Wakefield LM, et al: TGF-beta 1 prevents hypertrophy of epiphyseal chondrocytes: Regulation of gene expression for cartilage matrix proteins and metalloproteases. Dev Biol 1993;158:414.

149. Baici A, Lang A, Horler D, et al: Cathepsin B as a marker of the dedifferentiated chondrocyte phenotype. Ann Rheum Dis 1988;47:684.

150. Baici A, Lang A: Cathepsin B secretion by rabbit articular chondrocytes: Modulation by cycloheximide and glycosaminoglycans. Cell Tissue Res 1990;259:567.

151. Jasin HE, Taurog JD: Mechanisms of disruption of the articular cartilage surface in inflammation: Neutrophil elastase increases availability of collagen type II epitopes for binding with antibody on the surface of articular cartilage. J Clin Invest 1991;87:1531.

152. Baici A, Lang A: Effect of interleukin-1 beta on the production of cathepsin B by rabbit articular chondrocytes. FEBS Lett 1990;277:93.

153. Maciewicz RA, Wardale RJ, Wotton SF, et al: Mode of activation of the precursor to cathepsin L: Implication for matrix degradation in arthritis. Biol Chem Hoppe Seyler 1990;371:223–228.

154. Kiyoshima T, Tsukuba T, Kido MA, et al: Immunohistochemical localization of cathepsins B and D in the synovial lining cells of the normal rat temporomandibular joint. Arch Oral Biol 1993;38:357.

155. Vittorio N, Crissman JD, Hopson CN, et al: Histologic assessment of cathepsin D in osteoarthritic cartilage. Clin Exp Rheumatol 1986;4:221.

156. Martel PJ, Cloutier JM, Pelletier JP: Cathepsin B and cysteine protease inhibitors in human osteoarthritis. J Orthop Res 1990;8:336.

157. Nguyen Q, Mort JS, Roughley PJ: Cartilage proteoglycan aggregate is degraded more extensively by cathepsin L than by cathepsin B. Biochem J 1990;266:569.

158. Firestein GS, Paine MM: Stromelysin and tissue inhibitor of metalloproteinases gene expression in rheumatoid arthritis synovium. Am J Pathol 1992;140:1309.

159. Hamilton JA, Leizer T, Piccoli DS, et al: Oncostatin M stimulates urokinase-type plasminogen activator activity in human synovial fibroblasts. Biochem Biophys Res Commun 1991;180:652.

160. Partsch G, Matucci-Cerinic M, Marabini S, et al: Collagenase synthesis of rheumatoid arthritis synoviocytes: Dose-dependent stimulation by substance P and capsaicin. Scand J Rheumatol 1991;20:98.

161. Cutolo M, Sulli A, Barone A, et al: Macrophages, synovial tissue and rheumatoid arthritis. Clin Exp Rheumatol 1993;11:331.

162. Kapila S, Lee C, Richards DW: Characterization and identification of proteinases and proteinase inhibitors synthesized by temporomandibular joint disc cells. J Dent Res 1995;74:1328.

163. Breckon JJ, Hembry RM, Reynolds JJ, et al: Identification of matrix metalloproteinases and their inhibitor in the articular disc of the craniomandibular joint of the rabbit. Arch Oral Biol 1996;41:315.

164. Zardeneta G, Schmitz JP, Milam SB: Latent proteases recovered from human TMJ lavage fluid. J Oral Maxillofac Surg 1996;54:86.

165. Coleman RD, Weisengreen HH: Degenerative changes in the articular disc in later maturity. J Dent Res 1955;34:679.

166. De Leeuw R, Boering G, Van der Kuijl B, et al: Hard and soft tissue imaging of the temporomandibular joint 30 years after diagnosis of osteoarthrosis and internal derangement. J Oral Maxillofac Surg 1996;54:1270.

167. Talhouk RS, Bissell MJ, Werb Z: Coordinated expression of extracellular matrix-degrading proteinases and their inhibitors regulates mammary epithelial function during involution. J Cell Biol 1992;118:1271.

168. Awbrey BJ, Kuong SJ, MacNeil KL, et al: The role of alpha-1-protease inhibitor (A1PI) in the inhibition of protease activity in human knee osteoarthritis. Agents Actions 1993;3:167.

169. Bassols A, Massagué J: Transforming growth factor beta regulates the expression and structure of extracellular matrix chondroitin/dermatan sulfate proteoglycans. J Biol Chem 1988;263:3039.

170. Berchuck A, MacDonald PC, Milewich L, et al: Transforming growth factor-beta inhibits prostaglandin production in amnion and A431 cells. Prostaglandins 1989;38:453.

171. Brandes ME, Allen JB, Ogawa Y, et al: Transforming growth factor beta 1 suppresses acute and chronic arthritis in experimental animals. J Clin Invest 1991;87:1108.

172. Chandrasekhar S, Harvey AK: Transforming growth factor-beta is a potent inhibitor of IL-1 induced protease activity and cartilage proteoglycan degradation. Biochem Biophys Res Commun 1988;157:1352.

173. Chantry D, Turner M, Abney E, et al: Modulation of cytokine production by transforming growth factor-beta. J Immunol 1989;142:4295.

174. Joyce ME, Roberts AB, Sporn MB, et al: Transforming growth factor-beta and the initiation of chondrogenesis and osteogenesis in the rat femur. J Cell Biol 1990;110:2195.

175. Leonard CM, Fuld HM, Frenz DA, et al: Role of transforming growth factor-beta in chondrogenic pattern formation in the embryonic limb: Stimulation of mesenchymal condensation and fibronectin gene expression by exogenenous TGF-beta and evidence for endogenous TGF-beta-like activity. Dev Biol 1991;145:99.

176. Blake DR, Unsworth J, Outhwaite JM, et al: Hypoxic-reperfusion injury in the inflamed human joint. Lancet 1989;1:288.

177. McCord JM, Fridovich I: The reduction of cytochrome c by milk xanthine oxidase. J Biol Chem 1968;243:5753.

178. Granger DN, Rutili G, McCord JM: Superoxide radicals in feline intestinal ischemia. Gastroenterology 1981;81:22.

179. McCord JM: Oxygen-derived free radicals in post-ischemic tissue injury. N Engl J Med 1985; 312:159.

180. Nitzan DW, Mahler Y, Simkin A: Intra-articular pressure measurements in patients with suddenly developing, severely limited mouth opening. J Oral Maxillofac Surg 1992;50:1038.

181. Nitzan DW: Intraarticular pressure in the functioning human temporomandibular joint and its alteration by uniform elevation of the occlusal plane. J Oral Maxillofac Surg 1994;52:671.

182. McCord JM: Free radicals and inflammation: Protection of synovial fluid by superoxide dismutase. Science 1974;185:529.

183. Chandra H, Symons MCR: Sulphur radicals formed by cutting a-keratin. Nature 1987; 328:833.

184. Lands WEM: The biosynthesis and metabolism of prostaglandins. Annu Rev Physiol 1979;41:633.

185. Yamamoto S, Ohki S, Ogino N, et al: Enzymes involved in the formation and further transformation of prostaglandin endoperoxides. Adv Prostaglandin Thomboxane Res 1980;6:27.

186. Auer DE, Ng JC, Seawright AA: Free radical oxidation products in plasma and synovial fluid of horses with synovial inflammation. Aust Vet J 1993;70:49.

187. Baker MS: Free radicals and connective tissue damage. In Rice-Evans CA, Burdon RH (eds): Free Radical Damage and Its Control. Amsterdam, Elsevier, 1994, p 301.

188. Burkhardt H, Schwingel M, Meninger H, et al: Oxygen radicals as effectors of cartilage destruction: Direct degradative effect on matrix components and indirect action via activation of latent collagenase from polymorphonuclear leukocytes. Arthritis Rheum 1986;29:379.

189. Curran SF, Amoruso MA, Goldstein BD, et al: Degradation of soluble collagen by ozone or hydroxyl radicals. FEBS Lett 1984;176:155.

190. Vincent F, Corral-Debrinski M, Adolphe M: Transient mitochondrial transcript level decay in oxidative stressed chondrocytes. J Cell Physiol 1994;158:128.

191. Schieven GL, Kirihara JM, Myers DE, et al: Reactive oxygen intermediates activate NF-kappa B in a tyrosine kinase-dependent mechanism and in combination with vanadate activate the p561ck and p59fyn tyrosine kinases in human lymphocytes. Blood 1993;82:1212.

192. Kwak HS, Yim HS, Chock PB, et al: Endogenous intracellular glutathionyl radicals are generated in neuroblastoma cells under hydrogen peroxide oxidative stress. Proc Natl Acad Sci U S A 1995;92:4582.

193. Latchman D: Eukaryotic Transcription Factors. London, Academic Press, 1995.

194. Ignarro LJ: Signal transduction mechanisms involving nitric oxide. Biochem Pharmacol 1991;41:485.

195. Stefanovic-Racic M, Stadler J, Evans CH: Nitric oxide and arthritis. Arthritis Rheum 1993;36:1036.

196. Stadler J, Stefanovic-Racic M, Billiar TR, et al: Articular chondrocytes synthesize nitric oxide in response to cytokines and lipopolysaccharide. J Immunol 1991;147:3915.

197. Lancaster JR, Hibbs JB: EPR demonstration of iron-nitrosyl complex formation by cytotoxic activated macrophages. Proc Natl Acad Sci U S A 1990;87:1223.

198. Salvemini D, Misko TP, Masferrer JL, et al: Nitric oxide activates cyclooxygenase enzymes. Proc Natl Acad Sci U S A 1993;90:7240.

199. Moncada S, Palmer RMJ, Higgs EA: Nitric oxide: Physiology, pathophysiology, and pharmacology. Pharmacol Rev 1991;43:109.

200. Farrell AJ, Blake DR, Palmer RM, et al: Elevated serum and synovial fluid nitrite suggests increased nitric oxide synthesis in rheumatic diseases. In Moncada S, Marletta MA, Hibbs JB (eds): Biology of Nitric Oxide. Colchester, UK, Portland Press, 1992, p 166.

201. McCartney-Francis N, Allen JB, Mizel DE, et al: Suppression of arthritis by an inhibitor of nitric oxide synthase. J Exp Med 1993;178:749.

202. Gutteridge JM: Iron and oxygen: A biologically damaging mixture. Acta Paediatr Scand Suppl 1989;361:78.

203. Gajewski E, Rao G, Nackerdien Z, et al: Modification of DNA bases in mammalian chromatin by radiation-generated free radicals. J Biochem 1990;29:7876.

204. Saari H, Sorsa T, Konttinen YT: Reactive oxygen species and hyaluronate in serum and synovial fluid in arthritis. Int J Tissue React 1990;12:81.

205. Tadolini B, Cabrini L: The influence of pH on OH: scavenger inhibition of damage to deoxyribose by Fenton reaction. Mol Cell Biochem 1990;94:97.

206. Greenwald RA: Oxygen radicals, inflammation, and arthritis: Pathophysiological considerations and implications for treatment. Semin Arthritis Rheum 1991;20:219.

207. Kondo H, Nishino K, Itokawa Y: Hydroxyl radical generation in skeletal muscle atrophied by immobilization. FEBS Lett 1994;349:169.

208. Pardo L, Osman R, Banfelder J, et al: Molecular mechanisms of radiation induced DNA damage: H-abstraction and beta-cleavage. Free Radic Res Comm 1991;2:461.

209. Stadtman ER, Berlett BS: Fenton chemistry: Amino acid oxidation. J Biol Chem 1991; 266:17201.

210. Zardeneta G, Milam SB, Schmitz JP: Presence of denatured hemoglobin in diseased temporomandibular joints. J Oral Maxillofac Surg 1997; 55:1242–1248.

211. Sadrzadeh SMH, Graf E, Panter SS, et al: Hemoglobin: A biologic Fenton reagent. J Biol Chem 1984;259:14354.

212. Key JA: Experimental arthritis: The reactions of joints to mild irritants. J Bone Joint Surg 1929;11:705.

213. Nishioka GJ, Van Sickels JE, Tilson HB: Hemophilic arthropathy of the temporomandibular joint: Review of the literature, a case report, and discussion. Oral Surg Oral Med Oral Pathol 1988;65:145.

214. Greenwald RA: Oxygen radicals, inflammation, and arthritis: Pathophysiological considerations and implications for treatment. Semin Arthritis Rheum 1991;20:219.

215. Sato H, Takahashi T, Ide H, et al: Antioxidant activity of synovial fluid, hyaluronic acid, and two subcomponents of hyaluronic acid. Arthritis Rheum 1988;31:63.

216. Cerchiari EL, Sclabassi RJ, Safar P, et al: Effects of combined superoxide dismutase and deferoxamine on recovery of brainstem auditory evoked potentials and EEG after asphyxial cardiac arrest in dogs. Resuscitation 1990;19:25.

217. Gutteridge JM, Maidt L, Poyer L: Superoxide dis-

mutase and Fenton chemistry: Reaction of ferric-EDTA complex and ferric-bipyridyl complex with hydrogen peroxide without the apparent formation of iron(II). Biochem J 1990;269:169.

218. Singh R, Pathak DN: Lipid peroxidation and glutathione peroxidase, glutathione reductase, superoxide dismutase, catalase, and glucose-6-phosphate dehydrogenase activities in FeCl3-induced epileptogenic foci in the rat brain. Epilepsia 1990;31:15.

219. Vaille A, Jadot G, Elizagaray A: Anti-inflammatory activity of various superoxide dismutases on polyarthritis in the Lewis rat. Biochem Pharmacol 1989;39:247.

220. Yoshikawa T, Tanaka H, Kondo M: The increase of lipid peroxidation in rat adjuvant arthritis and its inhibition by superoxide dismutase. Biochem Med 1985;33:320.

221. Garrett IR, Boyce BF, Oreffo RO, et al: Oxygen-derived free radicals stimulate osteoclastic bone resorption in rodent bone in vitro and in vivo. J Clin Invest 1990;85:632.

222. Lin Y, Pape HD, Friedrich R: Use of superoxide dismutase (SOD) in patients with temporomandibular joint dysfunction—a preliminary study. Int J Oral Maxillofac Surg 1994;23:428.

223. Aisen P, Cohen G, Kang JO: Iron toxicosis. Int Rev Exp Pathol 1990;31:1.

224. Herbert V, Shaw S, Jayatilleke E, et al: Most free radical injury is iron-related: It is promoted by iron, hemin, holoferritin, and vitamin C, and inhibited by desferrioxamine and apoferritin. Stem Cells 1994;12:289.

225. Herbert V, Shaw S, Jayatilleke E: Vitamin C–driven free radical generation from iron. J Nutr 1996;126:1213S.

226. Fritton Jackson S: Environmental control of macromolecular synthesis in cartilage and bone. Proc R Soc Lond B Biol Sci 1970;175:131.

227. Haskin CL, Athanasiou KA, Klebe R, et al: A heat-shock–like response with cytoskeletal disruption occurs following hydrostatic pressure in MG-63 osteosarcoma cells. Biochem Cell Biol 1993;71:361.

228. Bissell MJ, Hall HG, Parry G: How does the extracellular matrix direct gene expression? J Theor Biol 1982;99:31.

229. Georgopoulos C, Welch WJ: Role of the major heat shock proteins as molecular chaperones. Annu Rev Cell Biol 1993;9:601.

230. Werb Z, Tremble PM, Behrendtsen O, et al: Signal transduction through the fibronectin receptor induces collagenase and stromelysin gene expression. J Cell Biol 1989;109:877.

231. Glukhova MA, Thiery JP: Fibronectin and integrins in development. Semin Cancer Biol 1993;4:241.

232. Chevalier X: Fibronectin, cartilage, and osteoarthritis. Semin Arthritis Rheum 1993;22:307.

233. Brown RA, Jones KL: The synthesis and accumulation of fibronectin by human articular cartilage. J Rheumatol 1990;17:65.

234. Vilamitjana AJ, Harmand MF: Biochemical analysis of normal and osteoarthritic human cartilage. Clin Physiol Biochem 1990;8:221.

235. Pennypacker JP, Hassell JR, Yamada KM, et al: The influence of an adhesive cell surface protein on chondrogenic expression in vitro. Exp Cell Res 1979;121:411.

236. Pennypacker JP: Modulation of chondrogenic expression in cell culture by fibronectin. Vision Res 1981;21:65.

237. Milam SB: Cell–extracellular matrix interactions with special emphasis on the primate temporomandibular joint. Ph.D. dissertation, University of Texas, 1990.

238. Balblanc JC, Vignon E, Mathieu P, et al: Cytokines, prostaglandin E2, phospholipase A and metalloproteases in synovial fluid in osteoarthritis. Rev Rhumat Mala Osteo Articulaires 1991;58:343.

239. Chang J, Gilman SC, Lewis AJ: Interleukin 1 activates phospholipase A2 in rabbit chondrocytes: A possible signal for IL-1 action. J Immunol 1986;136:1283.

240. Chang JS, Quinn JM, Demaziere A, et al: Bone resorption by cells isolated from rheumatoid synovium. Ann Rheum Dis 1992;51:1223.

241. Davies ME, Horner A, Franz B, et al: Detection of cytokine activated chondrocytes in arthritic joints from pigs infected with *Erysipelothrix rhusiopathiae*. Ann Rheum Dis 1992;51:978.

242. Flescher E, Garrett IR, Mundy GR, et al: Induction of bone resorbing activity by normal and rheumatoid arthritis T cells. Clin Immunol Immunopathol 1990;56:210.

243. Goldring MB, Birkhead J, Sandell LJ, et al: Interleukin 1 suppresses expression of cartilage-specific types II and IX collagens and increases type I and III collagens in human chondrocytes. J Clin Invest 1988;82:2026.

244. Hardingham TE, Bayliss MT, Rayan V, et al: Effects of growth factors and cytokines on proteoglycan turnover in articular cartilage. Br J Rheumatol 1992;1:1.

245. Harigai M, Hara M, Kitani A, et al: Interleukin 1 and tumor necrosis factor-alpha synergistically increase the production of interleukin 6 in human synovial fibroblast. J Clin Lab Immunol 1991;34:107.

246. Verschure PJ, Van NC: The effects of interleukin-1 on articular cartilage destruction as observed in arthritic diseases, and its therapeutic control. Clin Exp Rheumatol 1990;8:303.

247. Campbell IK, Piccoli DS, Hamilton JA: Stimulation of human chondrocyte prostaglandin E2 production by recombinant human interleukin-1 and tumour necrosis factor. Biochim Biophys Acta 1990;1051:310.

248. Campbell IK, Piccoli DS, Roberts MJ, et al: Effects of tumor necrosis factor alpha and beta on resorption of human articular cartilage and production of plasminogen activator by human articular chondrocytes. Arthritis Rheum 1990;33:542.

249. Pickvance EA, Oegema TJ, Thompson RJ: Immunolocalization of selected cytokines and proteases in canine articular cartilage after transarticular loading. J Orthop Res 1993;11:313.

250. Bender S, Haubeck HD, Van de Leur E, et al: Interleukin-1 beta induces synthesis and secretion of interleukin-6 in human chondrocytes. FEBS Lett 1990;263:321.

251. DeMarco D, Kunkel SL, Strieter RM, et al: Interleukin-1 induced gene expression of neutrophil activating protein (interleukin-8) and monocyte chemotactic peptide in human synovial cells. Biochem Biophys Res Commun 1991;174:411.

252. Elford PR, Cooper PH: Induction of neutrophil-mediated cartilage degradation by interleukin-8. Arthritis Rheum 1991;34:325.

253. Aggarwal BB, Gutterman JU: Human Cytokines: Handbook for Basic and Clinical Research. Boston, Blackwell Scientific Publications, 1992.

254. Mosley B, Urdal DL, Pricket K: The IL-1 receptor binds the human interleukin-1a precursor but not the human IL-1B precursor. J Biol Chem 1987;262:2941.

255. Black RA, Kronheim SR, Sleath PR: Activation of IL-1B by a co-induced protease. FEBS Lett 1989;247:386.

256. Chandrasekhar S, Harvey AK, Stack ST: Degradative and repair responses of cartilage to cytokines and growth factors occur via distinct pathways. Agents Actions Suppl 1993;39:121.

257. De M, Sanford TR, Wood GW: Interleukin-1, interleukin-6, and tumor necrosis factor alpha are produced in the mouse uterus during the estrous cycle and are induced by estrogen and progesterone. Dev Biol 1992;151:297.

258. Chaudhary LR, Spelsberg TC, Riggs BL: Production of various cytokines by normal human osteoblast-like cells in response to interleukin-1 beta and tumor necrosis factor-alpha: Lack of regulation by 17 beta-estradiol. Endocrinology 1992;130:2528.

259. Dinarello CA: Interleukin-1 and interleukin-1 antagonism. Blood 1991;77:1627.

260. Shalaby MR, Waage A, Espevik T: Cytokine regulation of interleukin 6 production by human endothelial cells. Cell Immunol 1989;121:372.

261. Dinarello CA: Reduction of inflammation by decreasing production of interleukin-1 or by specific receptor antagonism. Int J Tissue React 1992;14:65.

262. Goldring MB, Sohbat E, Elwell JM, et al: Etodolac preserves cartilage-specific phenotype in human chondrocytes: Effects on type II collagen synthesis and associated mRNA levels. Eur J Rheumatol Inflamm 1990;10:10.

263. Dedhar S: Regulation of expression of the cell adhesion receptors, integrins, by recombinant human interleukin-1 beta in human osteosarcoma cells: Inhibition of cell proliferation and stimulation of alkaline phosphatase activity. J Cell Physiol 1989;138:291.

264. Dedhar S: Signal transduction via the beta 1 integrins is a required intermediate in interleukin-1 beta induction of alkaline phosphatase activity in human osteosarcoma cells. Exp Cell Res 1989;183:207.

265. Milam SB, Magnuson VL, Steffensen B, et al: IL-1 beta and prostaglandins regulate integrin mRNA expression. J Cell Physiol 1991;149:173.

266. Cruz TF, Kandel RA, Brown IR: Interleukin 1 induces the expression of a heat-shock gene in chondrocytes. Biochem J 1991;277:327–330.

267. Gilman SC, Chang J, Zeigler PR, et al: Interleukin-1 activates phospholipase A2 in human synovial cells. Arthritis Rheum 1988;31:126.

268. Beasley D: Interleukin 1 and endotoxin activate soluble guanylate cyclase in vascular smooth muscle. Am J Physiol 1990;259:R38–R44.

269. Corbett JA, Wang JL, Sweetland MA, et al: Interleukin 1 beta induces the formation of nitric oxide by beta-cells purified from rodent islets of Langerhans: Evidence for the beta-cell as a source and site of action of nitric oxide. J Clin Invest 1992;90:2384.

270. Corbett JA, Kwon G, Turk J, et al: IL-1 beta induces the coexpression of both nitric oxide synthase and cyclooxygenase by islets of Langerhans: Activation of cyclooxygenase by nitric oxide. J Biochem 1993;32:13767.

271. Ala Y, Palluy O, Favero J, et al: Hypoxia/reoxygenation stimulates endothelial cells to promote interleukin-1 and interleukin-6 production: Effects of free radical scavengers. Agents Actions 1992;37:134.

272. Borg LA, Cagliero E, Sandler S, et al: Interleukin-1 beta increases the activity of superoxide dismutase in rat pancreatic islets. Endocrinology 1992;130:2851.

273. Rossomando EF, White LB, Hadjimichael J, et al: Immunomagnetic separation of tumor necrosis factor alpha. I. Batch procedure for human temporomandibular fluid. J Chromatogr 1992;583:11.

274. Shafer D, Rossomando E, White L, et al: Clinical implications of TNF-alpha in synovial fluid from TMJs. J Dent Res 1992;71:621.

275. Shafer DM, Assael L, White LB, et al: Tumor necrosis factor-α as a biochemical marker of pain and outcome in temporomandibular joints with internal derangements. J Oral Maxillofac Surg 1994;52:786.

276. Kubota E, Imamura H, Kubota T, et al: Interleukin 1B and stromelysin (MMP3) activity of synovial fluid as possible markers of osteoarthritis in the temporomandibular joint. J Oral Maxillofac Surg 1997;55:20.

277. Kimball ES: Substance P, cytokines, and arthritis. Ann N Y Acad Sci 1990;594:293.

278. Kimball ES, Persico FJ, Vaught JL: Substance P, neurokinin A, and neurokinin B induce generation of IL-1-like activity in P388D1 cells: Possible relevance to arthritic disease. J Immunol 1988;141:3564.

279. O'Byrne EM, Goldberg RL, Doughty JR, et al: Interleukin-1–induced cartilage degradation is independent of substance P level in rabbit knees. Agents Actions 1991;34:232.

280. Lotz M, Vaughan JH, Carson DA: Effect of neuropeptides on production of inflammatory cytokines by human monocytes. Science 1988;241:1218.

281. Brain SD, Cambridge H, Hughes SR, et al: Evidence that calcitonin gene-related peptide contributes to inflammation in the skin and joint. Ann N Y Acad Sci 1992;657:412.

282. Buckley TL, Brain SD, Collins PD, et al: Inflammatory edema induced by interactions between IL-1 and the neuropeptide calcitonin gene-related peptide. J Immunol 1991;146:3424.

283. Cambridge H, Brain SD: Calcitonin gene-related peptide increases blood flow and potentiates plasma protein extravasation in the rat knee joint. Br J Pharmacol 1992;106:746.

284. De AK, Ghosh JJ: Inflammatory responses induced by substance P in rat paw. Indian J Exp Biol 1990;28:946.

285. Green PG, Basbaum AI, Levine JD: Sensory neuropeptide interactions in the production of plasma extravasation in the rat. Neuroscience 1992;50:745.

286. Lam FY, Ferrell WR: Mediators of substance P–induced inflammation in the rat knee joint. Agents Actions 1990;31:298.

287. Lam FY, Ferrell WR, Scott DT: Substance P–induced inflammation in the rat knee joint is mediated by neurokinin 1 (NK1) receptors. Regul Pept 1993;46:198.

288. Yaksh TL: Substance P release from knee joint afferent terminals: Modulation by opioids. Brain Res 1988;458:319.

289. Smith GD, Harmar AJ, McQueen DS, et al: Increase in substance P and CGRP, but not somatostatin content of innervating dorsal root ganglia

in adjuvant monoarthritis in the rat. Neurosci Lett 1992;137:257.

290. Johansson A-S, Isacson G, Isberg A, et al: Distribution of substance P–like immunoreactive nerve fibers in temporomandibular joint soft tissues of monkey. Scand J Dent Res 1986;94:225.

291. Ichikawa H, Wakisaka S, Matsuo S, et al: Peptidergic innervation of the temporomandibular disk in the rat. Experientia 1989;45:303.

292. Kido MA, Kiyoshima T, Kondo T, et al: Distribution of substance P and calcitonin gene-related peptide-like immunoreactive nerve fibers in the rat temporomandibular joint. J Dent Res 1993;72:592.

293. Laurenzi MA, Persson MA, Dalsgaard CJ, et al: The neuropeptide substance P stimulates production of interleukin 1 in human blood monocytes: Activated cells are preferentially influenced by the neuropeptide. Scand J Immunol 1990;31:529.

294. Hart RP, Shadiack AM, Jonakait GM: Substance P gene expression is regulated by interleukin-1 in cultured sympathetic ganglia. J Neurosci Res 1991;29:282.

295. Jonakait GM, Schotland S: Conditioned medium from activated splenocytes increases substance P in sympathetic ganglia. J Neurosci Res 1990;26:24.

296. Jonakait GM, Schotland S, Hart RP: Effects of lymphokines on substance P in injured ganglia of the peripheral nervous system. Ann N Y Acad Sci 1991;632:19.

297. Jonakait GM, Schotland S, Hart RP: Interleukin-1 specifically increases substance P in injured sympathetic ganglia. Ann N Y Acad Sci 1990;594:222.

298. Shadiack AM, Hart RP, Carlson CD, et al: Interleukin-1 induces substance P in sympathetic ganglia through the induction of leukemia inhibitory factor (LIF). J Neurosci 1993;13:2601.

299. Hamilton JA, Waring PM, Filonzi EL: Induction of leukemia inhibitory factor in human synovial fibroblasts by IL-1 and tumor necrosis factor-alpha. J Immunol 1993;150:1496.

300. Campbell IK, Waring P, Novak U, et al: Production of leukemia inhibitory factor by human articular chondrocytes and cartilage in response to interleukin-1 and tumor necrosis factor alpha. Arthritis Rheum 1993;36:790.

301. Freidin M, Kessler JA: Cytokine regulation of substance P expression in sympathetic neurons. Proc Natl Acad Sci U S A 1991;88:3200.

302. O'Byrne EM, Blancuzzi VJ, Wilson DE, et al: Increased intra-articular substance P and prosta-glandin E2 following injection of interleukin-1 in rabbits. Int J Tissue React 1990;12:11.

303. Aufdemorte TB, Van SJ, Dolwick MF, et al: Estrogen receptors in the temporomandibular joint of the baboon (*Papio cynocephalus*): An autoradiographic study. Oral Surg Oral Med Oral Pathol 1986;61:307.

304. Abubaker AO, Raslan WF, Sotereanos GC: Estrogen and progesterone receptors in temporomandibular joint discs of symptomatic and asymptomatic persons: A preliminary study. J Oral Maxillofac Surg 1993;51:1096.

305. Cutolo M, Accardo S, Villaggio B, et al: Presence of estrogen-binding sites on macrophage-like synoviocytes and CD8+, CD29+, CD45RO+ T lymphocytes in normal and rheumatoid synovium. Arthritis Rheum 1993;36:1087.

306. Rosner IA, Goldberg VM, Getzy L, et al: Effects of estrogen on cartilage and experimentally induced osteoarthritis. Arthritis Rheum 1979;22:52.

307. Li ZG, Danis VA, Brooks PM: Effect of gonadal steroids on the production of IL-1 and IL-6 by blood mononuclear cells in vitro. Clin Exp Rheumatol 1993;11:157.

308. Whyte A, Williams RO: Bromocriptine suppresses postpartum exacerbation of collagen-induced arthritis. Arthritis Rheum 1988;31:927.

309. Livne E, von der Mark K, Silbermann M: Morphological and cytological changes in maturing and osteoarthritic articular cartilage in the temporomandibular joint of mice. Arthritis Rheum 1985;28:1027.

310. Livne E, Weiss A, Silbermann M: Articular chondrocytes lose their proliferative activity with aging yet can be restimulated by PTH-(1-84), PGE1, and dexamethasone. J Bone Miner Res 1989;4:539.

311. Levine JD, Goetzl EJ, Basbaum AI: Contribution of the nervous system to the pathophysiology of rheumatoid arthritis and other polyarthritides. Rheum Dis Clin North Am 1987;13:369.

312. Miao FJ, Benowitz NL, Basbaum AI, et al: Sympathoadrenal contribution to nicotinic and muscarinic modulation of bradykinin-induced plasma extravasation in the knee joint of the rat. J Pharmacol Exp Ther 1992;262:889.

313. Holmlund A, Ekblom A, Hansson P, et al: Concentrations of neuropeptides, substance P, neurokinin A, calcitonin gene-related peptide, neuropeptide Y and vasoactive intestinal polypeptide in synovial fluid of the human temporomandibular joint: A correlation with symptoms, signs and arthroscopic findings. Int J Oral Maxillofac Surg 1991;20:228.

CHAPTER

5

Arthritis of the Temporomandibular Joint

Keith Silverstein

Temporomandibular joint (TMJ) disorders have numerous etiologic factors, including trauma, infection, osteoarthritis (OA), and immunologic, metabolic, and neoplastic processes. Symptoms arise from the synovium, cartilage, or surrounding structures such as the capsule, bursa, and tendons. Clinicians involved in caring for patients with arthritic diseases are faced with a difficult diagnostic challenge because many of the diseases have similar presentations. The TMJ can be clinically involved in 50% to 60% of patients with rheumatoid arthritis (RA), whereas in nearly 70% there are radiographic abnormalities.[1, 2] Thirty percent of patients with juvenile rheumatoid arthritis (JRA) may have TMJ involvement, which can lead to abnormalities in mandibular growth, function, and cosmesis.[3, 4] Ankylosing spondylitis (AS) patients suffer from TMJ involvement more often than patients with psoriatic arthritis (PA) but less frequently than those suffering from RA and JRA.[5] Wenneberg and colleagues noted radiographic changes in 66% of subjects in their RA group, 38% in the PA group, and 30% in the AS group, whereas a control group revealed only 12%.[5] Cortical erosion of the condyle was more frequent in women with RA when compared to men, whereas in AS the reverse was true.[5] RA and PA groups were negatively correlated for age, suggesting young subgroups with early-onset and severe disease. Subcortical cysts, which occur with severe joint damage, were noted only in the RA group. Pain, crepitus,

and limited opening were the most common clinical features in all groups.[6] Because of the overlap between presentations and outcomes, the work-up must be organized and thorough. Subdividing the causes of arthritis into groups can aid in the work-up and diagnostic process.

Successful management of arthritides depends on the recognition of specific signs and symptoms. Limiting the differential diagnosis with thorough history taking is critical. The work-up should include questions regarding swelling, redness, pain at rest, duration of symptoms, rate of onset, location of involved joints, pattern of joint involvement, preceding events such as trauma, and time of day when symptoms are worst. Medications influencing symptoms and a thorough review of systems should be included. Physical examination should not be limited to the involved joints, as the skin, heart, lungs, and mucous membranes are often affected by the same disease process. Involved joints are observed for deformity, symmetry, and proximity. Palpation of these areas should be noted for pain, temperature, and range of motion. This should lead to the appropriate diagnostic studies, including radiologic studies, laboratory tests, and synovial fluid analysis.[2]

Normal synovial fluid is clear or straw colored and viscous from hyaluronic acid. Viscosity is reduced in inflammatory arthritides, and the synovial fluid flows like water—unlike the stringing produced by normal synovial fluid. Evaluation of cell counts, clot formation, and differences between serum and synovial glucose levels can aid in the diagnosis and differentiate arthritic conditions. The presence of crystals and the evaluation of their size, shape, and compensation under polarized light can be useful in the diagnosis of metabolic arthritides. Once the data are interpreted and the diagnosis is made, a treatment plan is produced. A review of the pathophysiology, signs, symptoms, and treatment options for these conditions is given later in the chapter.[7, 8]

Proper diagnosis is imperative when considering the perioperative period. Consideration should be given to multiorgan system damage and to medication side effects. Perioperative evaluation of each organ system should be thorough owing to the extra-articular manifestations of connective tissue diseases, RA, and other inflammatory arthritides.

When the cervical spine, TMJ, and cricoarytenoid joints are involved, anesthetic risks should be evaluated.[9] When peripheral involvement is severe or cranial neuropathies are present, the patient should be evaluated with flexion-extension, odontoid views, and magnetic resonance imaging (MRI) of the cervical spine.

Pleuritic and pericardial effusions, although rare, can cause compromised function, necessitating pulmonary and cardiac function testing. Swelling of involved areas can also lead to neurologic manifestations from entrapment, as in carpal tunnel syndrome. Some patients with RA may complain of Sjögren's syndrome, characterized by dry eyes and mouth. These patients should have lubrication placed prior to taping the eyes to prevent corneal abrasions. Raynaud's phenomenon can also be noted in the operating room, as the room temperature falls. Anesthetic and surgical plans must often take into consideration that these patients frequently are hypertensive and have underlying renal disease. Surgery on these patients may also trigger flare-ups. Spondyloarthropathies such as AS, PA, arthritis associated with inflammatory bowel disease, and Reiter's syndrome are grouped because of their similar presentation and immunogenetics. Involvement of the spine and thorax can lead to decreased range of motion and resultant restrictive lung disease. AS patients also suffer from aortic in-

sufficiency secondary to fibrotic changes in the aortic valve. Ten percent of these patients suffer from arrhythmias caused by fibrosis of the conduction system, necessitating cardiac evaluation.[2, 7, 10]

The multisystem involvement of patients with connective tissue diseases presents many perioperative concerns. Elective procedures are best delayed until the patient's disease is in an inactive state or under medical control. Extraarticular and organ system involvement should be addressed prior to the perioperative period.

Drug Therapy

Pharmacologic agents used to treat arthritides frequently have systemic side effects that influence perioperative decisions. These agents fall into three major groups: nonsteroidal anti-inflammatory drugs (NSAIDs), corticosteroids, and remission drugs such as immunosuppressives. These drugs work by altering the immune system and preventing the formation of inflammatory mediators.

Phospholipids in cell walls are converted to arachidonic acid. Cyclooxygenase then converts these to prostaglandins and thromboxane. The primary action of NSAIDs is to block cyclooxygenase from converting arachidonic acid into metabolites. NSAIDs have many side effects that must be considered perioperatively.

Platelet aggregation is inhibited by most NSAIDs. Aspirin inhibits platelets for their life span, which is 10 days, and should be discontinued accordingly preoperatively. Nonacetylated salicylates have no effect on platelets and can be taken up to the time of surgery. Other NSAIDs cause reversible acetylation of platelets and exert their effect only as long as they are present in the bloodstream. Half-lives should be checked for each individual drug to determine the amount of time they will be present.

NSAIDs also have side effects on the stomach and kidney. Renal function can be evaluated with serum creatinine levels, and the stomach mucosa can be examined with endoscopy. In patients with compromised renal perfusion or insufficiency, the renal cortex relies on prostaglandin E (PGE) to maintain renal cortex perfusion. NSAIDs decrease the level of PGE, which leads to a rise in creatinine and blood urea nitrogen. Discontinuing these agents usually resolves the problem. In approximately one third of these patients gastrointestinal side effects also develop, and the drug is discontinued for this reason. If NSAIDs are discontinued and flare-ups occur, symptoms can be managed with corticosteroids during the interval.

Corticosteroids have many systemic effects, although few have surgical implications. Wound healing is delayed in patients on steroid therapy, and sutures may need to be retained longer. Hypothalamic-pituitary-adrenal axis suppression by the exogenous steroids is a concern and must be addressed perioperatively. Doses of prednisone greater than 10 mg/day for more than several weeks in the past year suppress the axis, and it may take a year for the return to baseline. The maximal amount of endogenous steroid produced in a stressful surgical situation is 300 mg of hydrocortisone or 60 mg of prednisone. Patients receiving comparable doses do not need supplemental steroids. Those taking lower doses should be managed with 100 mg three times daily of hydrocortisone or an equivalent.

Methotrexate is a folic acid analogue that interferes with thymidine synthesis, leading to inhibition of DNA synthesis. The development of cirrhosis remains a concern, although it occurs in less than 1 in 1000 over 5 years. Other significant side effects include lung toxicity, occurring in 8% of patients, and, for unclear reasons, methotrexate increases the incidence of perioperative infection. The discontinuation of therapy 3 weeks perioperatively (the week prior to surgery, the week of surgery, and the week after surgery) is recommended to aid in wound healing.[10, 11]

Osteoarthritis

OA is a chronic noninflammatory disease affecting the articular cartilage of joints. This is the most common skeletal disease of the human body and is related to loss of cartilage and hypertrophy of bone. Recent estimates are that 40 million Americans, including 85% of the population over age 70, have some degree of OA.[12] Often the disease is characterized by mild symptoms despite severe damage. Radiologic evidence does not necessarily correlate with clinical symptoms.[13] In younger patients, evidence of cartilage destruction and bone degeneration can occur secondary to infection, trauma, or congenital problems. The exact mechanisms of joint degeneration remain unknown, but stresses on subchondral bone and cartilage are suspect.[14] Treatment objectives include symptomatic relief, reduction of stresses, and corrective procedures to aid in joint function.

ETIOLOGY

Forces applied to joints are dissipated by redistribution over the capsule, cartilage, and subchondral bone. The cartilage is designed to compress under loads. This is possible because the cartilage is made up of collagen and proteoglycan. Collagen on articular surfaces is unique in that it is type 2 collagen, which contains three alpha helical chains.[15] Proteoglycan, consisting of a protein backbone and glycosaminoglycan chains with negative charges, is also present and incorporates water molecules. This water is released as cartilage is loaded and is regained when the force is removed. The loss of this compressibility and elasticity is a central feature of degenerative joint disease and is related to water loss from the cartilage.[13, 14, 16]

Adult cartilage no longer synthesizes collagen unless it is damaged. During the stress response to trauma, DNA synthesis begins and chondrocytes collect to form new structure. OA also alters the structure of proteoglycans and glycosaminoglycans by changing the balance between degradation and synthesis.[17] Proteases such as cathepsin D and hydrolases are increased as degeneration progresses. These findings of increased degradation associated with increased DNA activity are typical in OA.[14] As the disease progresses, synthesis lags behind the degradation and a net loss of cartilage ensues. Repair of the degenerative process becomes haphazard, and repaired cartilage is not as organized as the original articular cartilage. Repair of the degenerated articular surface results in type 1 collagen instead of the original type 2 collagen.[15] Bone remodeling is active during this phase, and subchondral bone becomes sclerosed while the margins hypertrophy and overgrow.[12]

The initiating events leading to OA are correlated with the amount of work and load the joint is stressed by. Continuous loading of the joint can lead to a decrease in elasticity and fracture of the subchondral bone when compared to unloaded or paralyzed joints. The cartilage is then called on to dissipate more of the load, resulting in more water loss and inelasticity. The release of proteases during this cycle causes cartilage destruction. Similar degeneration occurs in normally stressed joints that are deformed and unable to dissipate loads. This is common in congenitally deformed joints.[14, 16]

PATHOLOGY

The earliest degenerative changes are seen in articular cartilage, as proteoglycans are lost at the surface. Chondrocytes are then stimulated, and DNA synthesis increases. These activated chondrocytes can be found in clusters at the articular surface. Flaking of the cartilage follows along collagen fibers, parallel with the joint surface.[17] Radiographs depict this stage of the disease as narrowing of the joint space as the cartilage surface is lost. Growth of surrounding bone is stimulated, resulting in osteophyte formation. As the degeneration continues, the articular cartilage is lost and subchondral bone is exposed and eburnated. Subchondral pseudocysts become evident as synovial fluid passes through the cartilage and cortical bone to fill marrow cavities.[12]

CLINICAL FEATURES

Degenerative joint disease is divided into primary and secondary forms. Primary OA is defined as the form with no predisposing factors and with symptoms beginning after the fifth to sixth decade of life. Secondary OA is associated with known underlying abnormalities or injuries, and symptoms begin decades earlier than with the primary form. Underlying processes found to predispose to secondary OA include septic arthritis or inflammatory states such as RA and PA. Trauma of the articular cartilage, meniscus removal, and aseptic necrosis have also led to early OA. Certain systemic diseases, for unknown reasons, may also predispose one to early OA. Patients suffering from diabetes mellitus and acromegaly have been found to have earlier and more severe degenerative disease, affecting multiple joints. Other commonly accepted reasons for the early development of OA include anatomic abnormalities and congenital aberrations such as slipped epiphyseal plates and shallow fossae.[14]

The most common complaint of patients with OA is pain with function and load bearing. Stiffness after a period of rest is common, but it subsides shortly (minutes) after function begins, unlike in RA. Examination reveals joints with less range of motion, tenderness to palpation, bony enlargement, and effusions. If degeneration causes complete denuding of the cartilage, crepitus may also be appreciated.

Associated findings in advanced OA include Heberden's nodes and Bouchard's nodes.[18] These are nodules at the base of the distal interphalangeal (DIP) joints and at the proximal interphalangeal (PIP) joints. The development of these nodes is secondary to the enlargement of bone surrounding the joint. Metacarpophalangeal (MCP) joints, wrists, elbows, and shoulders are usually spared unless a specific traumatic event has occurred. Involvement of the spine, leading to decreased range of motion, pain, stiffness, and possibly nerve root involvement, is more common and can result in radicular pain, sensory disturbances, and muscle spasm. OA of the hip can be the most crippling form and lead to the loss of ambulation. Pain with weight bearing and motion should be addressed early to prevent hip contracture and permanent deformity. Knees follow a similar course, unless a sports injury, such as torn meniscus, leads to earlier degeneration.[7, 9]

TEMPOROMANDIBULAR JOINT INVOLVEMENT

OA is the most common disease affecting the TMJ. Symptoms can be present without other joint involvement, which is rare in other arthritides.[2] Referred pain to the head and neck is a common finding. Patients with OA beginning in the fifth decade generally have slow-onset disease with mild symptoms. Those patients in their second to fourth decade of life have a more severe, symptomatic course. In these patients the disease generally develops from myofascial pain and dysfunction or an intra-articular disk derangement. Usually one TMJ is involved, but bilateral involvement does occur. Even when bilateral disease is evident, symptoms are usually unilateral.[12] Radiographic evidence occurs in 44% of asymptomatic patients.[7] Histologic involvement occurs in 40% to 60% of patients,[17] but clinical symptoms occur in only 8% to 16% of the population. Women are more likely to be afflicted with TMJ involvement, and the frequency increases with age.

Patients with TMJ involvement rarely complain of morning stiffness, although pain and tenderness increase as load and function increase throughout the day.[10] When morning symptoms are present, they generally last 30 minutes or less. Osteophytes form and marginal bone thickens, leading to palpable masses over the preauricular region. Patients can progress to a state where opening is limited and joint noise increases until locking occurs. Special imaging of the TMJ, including MRI and arthrograms, can reveal disk perforations and dislocations. Plain films and computed tomographic (CT) scans can reveal flattening of the condylar head, cyst formation of the subchondral bone, joint narrowing, osteophyte formation, and subchondral sclerosis.

In contrast to RA and other arthritides, laboratory work-ups rarely provide diagnostic data. The sedimentation rate is normal or slightly elevated, and synovial fluid analysis reveals a slight elevation in white blood cells.[18] Recent articles have reported inflammatory mediators in the synovial fluid, such as elevated levels of keratan sulfate, leukotriene B, and prostaglandins, but these are not yet diagnostic.[19]

The TMJ is like other articular joints in the body in that it has cartilage, synovial lining, synovial fluid, and subchondral bone. It differs in that the articulating surface is covered with fibrocartilage, not hyaline cartilage as are other articular joints. Articular cartilage receives its nutrition from the synovial fluid, not the subchondral bone. After maturity of the epiphyseal plate, perforating vessels can no longer supply the cartilage with nutrients or remove waste

products. Changes in the synovial fluid therefore influence the metabolism of the cartilage.[16]

Many hypotheses regarding the initial event triggering OA have been postulated, including mechanical, inflammatory, and chemical insults that release collagenases and proteolytic enzymes, causing degradation of the cartilage. Abnormal and repetitive mechanical stresses may exceed the functional capacity of normal articular tissues. The result is a decreased collagen stiffness, leading to increased hydration of the proteoglycan-water gel.[16] Other hypotheses suggest that cartilage breakdown is the result of weakness of the subchondral bone secondary to microfractures from excessive loading. Inflammatory mediators and waste products are also likely causes of degeneration. Alterations of synovial fluid or reduced quantities, causing improper lubrication and nutrition of the cartilage, may also play a role. These phenomena lead to friction of the cartilage and collagen destruction.[19]

Early in OA and chondromalacia, which are indistinguishable, the water content of the cartilage matrix is increased from swelling and breakdown of the collagen fibrils.[13, 20] Proteoglycans are depleted, and chondrocytes cluster while proliferating in an attempt to repair. These histologic findings are manifested mostly in the deeper layers of cartilage, sparing the superficial layer until advanced disease states, which may take years to develop.[21] As the disease progresses, chondrocytes degenerate and synovial cells destruct, releasing proteolytic and collagenolytic enzymes; this results in more degradation. As the process advances, tissues lose integrity and the cartilage splits and fibrillation occurs. This leads to adhesions as the cartilage thins. The marrow contained within the subchondral bone then fibroses. Macroscopic changes identifiable on radiographs include osteophyte formation, sclerosis, surface erosions, subchondral cysts, and deformations. Extraarticular responses such as muscle pain and atrophy may be evident as the mandible length is altered and the occlusion changes.[14]

Although OA may develop without disk displacement, internal derangements are highly correlated with TMJ OA.[22, 23] Cartilage degradation, altering the sliding properties of the joint surfaces, and alterations of the synovial fluid, giving rise to increased friction and adhesive wear, impair disk movement.[5] Degradative products from the OA cartilage are then released into the synovial fluid. When it is produced in large quantities, it cannot be reabsorbed by the synovial membrane or cleared. Mediators of inflammation are also released in response, causing synovitis. The osteoarthrosis and synovitis is termed osteoarthritis. The synovial membrane is not innervated, but the mediators of inflammation produced by the synovium stimulate capsular nociceptors.[24] This leads to joint tightness and continued stretching and elongation of the attachments, causing anterior displacement. Limitation of the mandibular opening can then ensue from the malpositioned disk. The periligamentous tissues, such as ligaments and muscles, are also subject to alteration from the changes in the articular surface. As the posterior attachment elongates, the nociceptors within the tissue are stimulated, causing pain. As the ligaments are subjected to tensile forces from the altered frictional capacity and elongation, they extend beyond their span of elasticity and deform. As they elongate, the collagenous component of the ligament is disrupted and the tissue may rupture or lacerate. It is these ligamentous attachments of the disk that keep it anchored to the condylar head and resist displacement. As the functional limits of the ligament are exceeded, nociceptors are stimulated, causing sprains and pain.[14] Anteriorly displaced disks are also subject to compressive loads placed on their posterior attachment. Maladaption, inflammation, and perforation are then possible as the inflammatory process continues. However, these are not the only adaptive changes that occur. There can be decreased vascularity and elastin content as collagen increases and fibrosis occurs. This can act as a pseudodisk and withstand compressive loads. Autopsy studies revealed 50% of elderly patients had joint degeneration, although no disk problems were reported. Eighty percent of patients with displaced disks had similar findings.[25] This may suggest that displaced disks are a sign of OA, not a cause of OA.

Classification and findings of TMJ OA should include the stage of cartilage destruction and the grade of synovitis rather than the degree of internal derangement. As reported by Dijkgraaf and others,[19] TMJ cartilage degeneration can be separated into four stages. In the first stage of OA, the *initial repair stage,* an imbalance of synthesis and degradation of extracellular matrix by chondrocytes is encountered. Growth factors, including insulin-like growth factor I, become evident in this stage.[19] Electron microscopy reveals increased metabolic activity, with increased DNA synthesis evident in chondrocytes and increased synthesis of the extracellular matrix. In the second stage of OA, the *early stage,* extracellular matrix synthesis increases but is exceeded by degradation from the increased activity of proteases. Cartilage swelling, resulting in an irregular surface and a net loss of articular cartilage, ensues.[19, 22, 26] Characteristic clusters of chondrocytes with increased metabolic activity in the swollen areas are also seen. Chondrocyte and cartilage necrosis follows in all cell layers, leaving attempts at repair disorganized.[22] Synovial fluid analysis during this early stage reveals metabolic products of arachidonic acid, interleukin-1 (IL-1), IL-6, tissue necrosis factor, and other proteases. Arthroscopic examination reveals swelling, softening, and fibrillations. Common clinical complaints during this phase include pain and limited range of motion. In the third stage of OA, the *intermediate stage,* articular cartilage is lost as synthesis is exceeded by degradation. Histologic evaluation reveals thinning, vertical splitting, and fibrillations of the cartilage as clusters of chondrocytes continue to necrose. Staining of proteoglycan continues to be reduced, and the collagen network becomes more haphazard. Biochemical markers such as cytokines and fibronectin continue to fill the joint space. Arthroscopically, cartilage continues to thin and a displaced disk may be evident. Pain with limited range of motion continues and can now be accompanied by joint clicking. In the fourth stage of OA, the *late stage,* increased degradation exceeds synthesis or reduced degradation equals decreased synthesis. Histologically, fibrillations are extensive, bone becomes denuded, and proteoglycan staining is nearly lost. Extracellular matrix synthesis is reduced, whereas protease activity can be reduced or increased if residual OA is occurring. Arthroscopic evaluation is remarkable for severe fibrillations, exposed bone, disk displacement, and possibly angiogenesis.[19]

DIAGNOSIS

Laboratory tests rarely reveal abnormalities, and the erythrocyte sedimentation rate remains normal. When coupled with a thorough clinical examination, radiographs can be an important diagnostic tool. Narrowed joint spaces, bone spurs, and subchondral cysts are typical in OA, but the work-up should exclude similarities with other arthritides.

TREATMENT

Realistic goals must be given to patients with OA because the disease can continue to progress despite therapy. Initial intervention should limit excessive and recurrent trauma. Moderate exercises and physical therapy should be started to strengthen the musculature supporting the joint. NSAIDs are usually sufficient to reduce pain, but the patient should be counseled on what side effects to look for because of their potential for prolonged use. Mild cases may also benefit from thermal therapy using warm and cold packs. The change in blood flow can influence inflammatory mediators and nerve endings. In more severe cases, thermal therapy can be obtained with ultrasound and infrared heat, which can provide deeper changes in perfusion. Orthopedic procedures, including débridement of loose bodies, osteotomy, and prosthetic replacement, should be reserved for patients with intractable pain. When choosing a procedure, the risks of surgery must be weighed against the benefit of pain relief and joint function.

Rheumatoid Arthritis

RA is a chronic systemic inflammatory disease predominantly affecting diarthrodial joints and frequently a variety of other organs. The causes are unknown. To guarantee uniformity in investigational and epidemiologic studies, the American College of Rheumatology has developed classification criteria (see box).

Classification Criteria for Rheumatoid Arthritis

1. Morning stiffness (> 1 hour)
2. Swelling (soft tissue) of three or more joints
3. Swelling (soft tissue) of hand joints (PIP, MCP, or wrist)
4. Symmetric swelling (soft tissue)
5. Subcutaneous nodules
6. Serum rheumatoid factor
7. Erosion and/or periarticular osteopenia, in hand or wrist joints, seen on x-ray

---

Criteria 1 to 4 must be continuous for 6 weeks and observed by a physician. Diagnosis requires at least four criteria.

RA occurs worldwide and in all ethnic groups, with a prevalence of 0.3% to 1.5% in most populations. The peak onset is between the fourth and sixth decades, but it may begin in childhood (JRA) or later in life. Females are two to three times more likely to be afflicted than males.[27]

ETIOLOGY

Three causes of RA have been investigated, although the etiology remains unknown. Genetic susceptibility has been demonstrated in family and twin studies. Afflicted patients have also demonstrated increased HLA-DR4 (60% to 70% versus the general population). The presence of this antigen has been correlated with increased levels of rheumatoid factor and the severity of joint destruction on radiograph. HLA-DR1 is found in populations seronegative for HLA-DR4, such as Israelis and Asians.[27]

RA has an autoimmune component, with 80% of RA patients testing positive for an immunoglobulin (Ig) directed at the Fc region of IgG known as rheumatoid factor (RF). High titers of RF have been correlated with severe joint destruction and subcutaneous nodules. Testing for RF by latex agglutination or sensitized sheep cell agglutination detects IgM antibodies, although IgG, IgA, IgE, and IgD antibodies have been described. IgM antibodies have the ability of complexing with five IgG molecules and are believed to be the cause of synovial inflammation. Smaller molecules, such as IgG antibodies, are believed to participate in the systemic manifestations and vasculitis common to this disease. Despite the strong association of RF with RA, it is not found only in this disease state. Chronic antigen presentation, as seen in diseases such as bacterial endocarditis, tuberculosis, viral infections, and advanced age, has also resulted in the formation of RF. None of these states is associated with HLA-DR4, suggesting the etiology may result from a combination of RF with the genetic antigen.[23]

The infectious hypothesis is based on polyarthritis associated with many viral and bacterial infections. Rubella, Epstein-Barr, and parvovirus have been implicated, but to date no vector has been identified.

PATHOPHYSIOLOGY

The hallmark of RA is synovial membrane proliferation and outgrowth causing erosion of articular cartilage and subchondral bone. The pannus or proliferating inflammatory tissue can lead to intraarticular and periarticular joint destruction, leading to deformity and dysfunction.

The etiology of RA remains unknown, but the pathophysiology is clear. After microvascular injury, synovial cells proliferate and swell and are infiltrated by mononuclear cells and T-lymphocytes. As the disease progresses, the synovium is infiltrated by plasma cells, macrophages, and more lymphocytes. Proliferation continues until the synovium becomes villous and vascularized.

Cellular and humoral roles have been identified. Activation of T-lymphocytes by unknown mechanisms occurs, resulting in the release of numerous inflammatory mediators and further proliferation of the synovium. IL-1, released from activated T-lymphocytes and macrophages, activates collagenases and PGE_2 by the synoviocytes. The monokines promote the degradation of proteoglycan by chondrocytes and the resorption of calcium from bone.

Humoral influences include the production of RF in the synovium, the formation of IgM-IgG complexes, and activation of the classic complement cascade. This leads to vascular permeability and phagocytosis of immune complexes. These neutrophils, filled with immune complexes, are called "RA cells" or "ragocytes" in the synovial fluid. Complexes are also trapped in the cartilage, causing changes in the matrix macromolecules. The production of inflammatory mediators, which is stimulated by the RA cells, results in the production of proteinases and prostaglandins. The inflammatory response destroys the cartilage, bone, tendons, and ligaments and stimulates fibroblasts, resulting in fibrosis. Collagenases activated at the interface of the pannus and cartilage by plasmin are probably responsible for the typical erosions seen over the joint surface.[27]

CLINICAL FEATURES

The onset of RA is different among individuals. The onset of joint pain occurs over weeks to months. Malaise, fatigue, and occasional episodes of fever accompany the joint symptoms. The pattern of joint involvement is generally polyarticular and symmetric, involving the PIP, MCP, wrist, elbow, shoulder, knee, ankle, and metatarsophalangeal (MTP) joints. The DIP joints are generally spared. Morning joint pain and stiffness lasting more than 1 hour or after periods of inactivity are hallmarks.

The course of the disease varies, but most patients suffer from some degree of joint deformity and disability. Classifications assessing functional capacity are evaluated frequently. Class 1 patients suffer no restriction in their normal activities. Class 2 individuals have moderate restrictions but can perform most activities. Class 3 patients suffer marked restrictions in their daily activities as well as in their occupational duties. The most incapacitated patients, confined to bed or wheelchair, are classified as class 4.[9]

ARTICULAR MANIFESTATIONS

RA can affect any diarthrodial joint but most commonly affects the hands, wrists, knees, and feet. The PIP and MCP joints swell early in the disease process, giving a spindle shape to the fingers. The DIP joints are usually spared, unlike in OA and PA, but the soft tissue surrounding the joint becomes lax, leading to ulnar deviation at the MCP joints. Hyperextension at the PIP joints with flexion of the DIP joints leads to swan-neck deformity. Synovial proliferation and effusion are common in the weight-bearing joints—thus the knees are commonly involved. Similar processes lead to compression of the median nerve, causing carpal tunnel syndrome. Further progression leads to severe joint destruction in the elbows, shoulders, hips, and ankles. The TMJ and the cricoarytenoid are rarely involved, but spinal involvement of the cervical region can lead to atlantoaxial subluxation in up to 30% of patients—in contrast to the spondyloarthritides, which affect the lower spine.[28]

TEMPOROMANDIBULAR JOINT MANIFESTATIONS

In approximately 50% to 75% of patients seropositive for RA, TMJ involvement develops during the course of the disease. The TMJs are involved bilaterally 30% to 75% of the time and are found in cases that have systemic manifestations.[29] Preauricular joint pain is described as deep and dull and increases with joint function. Advanced disease leads to decreased range of motion, decreased bite force, muscle tenderness, and the eventual destruction of joint anatomy, leading to clicking and crepitus. Severe limited motion occurs as the bone is destroyed and the joint space is filled with scar tissue leading to fibrous ankylosis.[3] Bony ankylosis is not typical in these patients. In severe cases, progressive class II occlusion develops, resulting in retrognathia and apertognathia, which can result in the development of obstructive sleep apnea. This is due to the progressive loss of bone height on top of the condyle, which eventually occurs in up to 80% of patients with TMJ symptoms.[30] Because RA starts in soft tissues, radiographic evaluation rarely reveals early pathology, despite joint symptoms. As the process continues, MRI evaluation can reveal TMJ disk destruction, displacement, and joint effusions. Later in the process, bony destruction is evident on radiographs in 19% to 84% of cases.[1, 30] As with most forms of arthritis involving the TMJ, radiographs reveal loss of joint space, condylar flattening, osteophyte formation, and erosion of the glenoid fossa. Radiographs of advanced RA reveal shortening of the posterior ramus, premature posterior occlusal contacts, and antegonial notching.

Diagnosis of rheumatoid arthritic TMJ involvement is generally easy, because it occurs late in the disease process. TMJ symptoms in a patient seropositive and clinically positive for RA are diagnostic. A distinguishing feature of RA involving the TMJ is morning stiffness that improves during the day or with function. Common joint symptoms such as pain and decreased range of motion, seen with most arthritides, are distinguished by changes in occlusal relationships and a changing profile. Radiographically, the joint space is narrowed and the condyle and glenoid fossa are eroded in late disease states. Progressive loss of ramus height secondary to lytic enzymes and osteoclast activity results in apertognathia and retrognathia, with antegonial notching. The patient most likely has normal-sized masseters, as opposed to a patient with a clenching and bruxism habit that overloads the joint.

EXTRAARTICULAR MANIFESTATIONS

Extraarticular manifestations such as low-grade fever, malaise, fatigue, weakness, and lymphadenopathy are common in RA. Other complications associated with RA are found in seropositive patients and can affect many organ systems.

Skin can have subcutaneous nodules in 25% of patients. These patients are always seropositive for RF and have severe articular destruction. Nodules occur in periarticular surfaces subject to pressure. Palmar erythema, vasculitis, and easy bruisability are also manifestations affecting the skin to different degrees.

Forty percent of patients with RA may also have pericardial lesions. Death from these lesions is rare, but they can cause debilitating symptoms when present. A congestive physiology caused by cardiomyopathies, resulting in right heart enlargement and peripheral edema, can occur. Conduction abnormalities secondary to nodules in the myocardium, valvular disease, and vasculitis of the coronary arteries have also been reported.

Rheumatoid pleural disease is common but is asymptomatic unless effusions become large or interstitial fibrosis causes restriction. Pulmonary function testing in this patient group reveals noncompliant lung expansion. This complication may also occur in patients treated with gold and D-penicillamine to control the chronic manifestations of the disease. Malignancy work-ups are also common in these patients because pulmonary nodules associated with the RA mimic cancer.

Although the central nervous system is generally spared, peripheral neuropathies are common. These lesions are caused by swelling of periarticular tissues, resulting in entrapment of peripheral nerves. This is the usual course found in carpal tunnel syndrome associated with RA. Vasculitis affecting the blood supply to nerves can also limit conduction in peripheral nerves.

Sjögren's syndrome is also common in patients seropositive for RF. The patient's eyes become dry, leading to scleritis and conjunctivitis. Rampant caries and rapidly advancing periodontal disease are also seen as a result of the associated xerostomia.

Occasionally, the triad of neutropenia, RA, and splenomegaly is associated with lymphadenopathy. Known as Felty's syndrome, it arises after the polyarticular destruction in seropositive patients. Recurrent infections with gram-positive bacteria are common but do not correlate with the severity of neutropenia. The neutropenia seems to occur secondary to hypersplenism and immune-mediated destruction of neutrophils.[2, 3, 9, 23, 27, 31]

TREATMENT

Most patients function with few restrictions despite the long and uncertain course of RA. Therefore, therapy with corticosteroids or immunosuppressives should be reserved for the most severe cases. Objectives of therapy include relief of pain, reduction of inflammation, minimization of side effects, preservation of muscle strength and joint function, and a return to a normal lifestyle. The initial program centers on adequate rest, anti-inflammatory drugs, and physical therapy to maintain joint function. Patients are instructed in exercise programs, which are limited to range-of-motion exercises during acute flare-ups. Salicylates are inexpensive, tolerated by most patients, and effective in controlling the inflammation associated with RA, although the doses required for control are higher than those for most inflammatory conditions. The other classes of NSAIDs are also effective and can be substituted based on side effects and cost. If NSAIDs are ineffective, slower forms of therapy such as the disease-modifying antirheumatic drugs hydroxychloroquine, gold, or penicillamine or the cytotoxic agents methotrexate or cyclophosphamide are considered.[32] Side effects are unique for each drug and must be monitored. Long-term corticosteroid use is reserved for patients with unresponsive and aggressive joint disease when function is jeopardized. Surgical consideration is limited to the most severe cases that are progressive and unresponsive to other forms of therapy. Success has been obtained with arthroplasties and total joint reconstructions using alloplasts. Synovectomy has also proved to be helpful if medicinal agents fail.

An increasingly popular approach is to start multiple drug therapy as is done with chemotherapy. The hope is to induce remission early in the disease. The more toxic drugs are then dropped from the therapy as remission occurs, and remission is maintained with less toxic drugs. Experimental therapies using interferon, cytokines, and cytokine antagonists are also in trial.[32]

Juvenile Rheumatoid Arthritis

JRA (Still's disease) is generally separated into three subtypes: systemic onset, pauciarticular, and polyarticular. Systemic-onset JRA represents 25% of occurrences and affects boys more often than girls. Extraarticular manifestations associated with the arthritis characterize its presentation. Fever is common and can precede arthritic symptoms by several months. Maculopapular rashes covering the trunk are often associated with fever episodes. Adenopathy, hepatosplenomegaly, pericarditis, and pleuritis are common findings and are generally self-limiting. One fourth of patients experience severe destructive polyarthritis, with laboratory findings significant for anemia and leukocytosis and negative for RF or antinuclear antibodies (ANA).

Pauciarticular arthritis accounts for 30% of patients with JRA, predominantly girls. This has a milder course and a good prognosis despite the early age of onset (2 to 4 years). In 50% of these patients iridocyclitis develops, which can lead to blindness, necessitating an ophthalmologic evaluation. These patients test negative for RF, although 50% to 60% test positive for ANA.

Polyarticular arthritis also has a good prognosis. It predominantly affects girls at around 2 years of age. This type accounts for 25% of patients with JRA. Initially, hands and feet are affected, then the peripheral joints. Twenty-five percent test positive for ANA, although RF is generally not found.

In addition to the three main subgroups of JRA, 5% to 10% of those with polyarticular disease test positive for RF. These patients present with symptoms at around age 12 and respond similarly to patients with the adult form of the disease.[10]

TEMPOROMANDIBULAR JOINT INVOLVEMENT

JRA affects one-quarter million young children. TMJ involvement occurs only when the condition is severe and progressive. TMJ involvement in patients with JRA has been reported in 5% to 65% of studies.[33] Any of the subtypes of JRA can affect the TMJ; however, it is most commonly seen in the polyarticular variant. Clinically, the patient experiences pain, tenderness, crepitation, clicking, and loss of function.[34] As the process continues, a class II occlusal relationship and micrognathia can develop, resulting in the classic bird-beak deformity. This deformity is a result of hindered growth of the condyle and ramus. Scarring of the capsular soft tissues and ligaments contributes to the lack of development. This deformity occurs in only 0% to 38% of patients and is related to age at onset of joint destruction. Plain radiographs have revealed destruction of the TMJ in 28.9% to 55% of affected children. The most common CT scan findings of the TMJs were reduced joint space and condylar size, condylar erosions, and condylar surface flattening. The

majority of erosion was seen on the lateral aspect of the condyle. Despite the reduction of joint space and degeneration of the condylar head, mandibular length was not greatly reduced when age was corrected for. These TMJ lesions are more prevalent in the JRA subtypes that typically have systemic manifestations. Other authors report TMJ involvement in prolonged severe cases and in those cases testing seropositive for RF.[34] CT may diagnose TMJ involvement earlier than clinical correlation. This may account for the higher prevalence of TMJ lesions found on CT scan (60%) than clinically. Onset is commonly associated with fever and generalized arthralgia, making it necessary to rule out infectious causes.

TREATMENT

Treatment of JRA centers on early recognition of the disease to limit deformity. Treatment has several main elements, including the reduction of inflammation, suppression of joint activity to limit long-term erosive changes, and prevention of disability. These can be accomplished by anti-inflammatory drugs and active home exercises. Pharmacologic agents are separated into immediate- and slow-acting agents. Immediate responders work within days to weeks and include salicylates, NSAIDs, and corticosteroids. The intermediate group functions within weeks to months and includes agents such as gold compounds, antimalarials, and D-penicillamine. The intermediate drugs are usually given in conjunction with immediate-acting drugs. Once remission is obtained, the drug of choice for JRA patients is methotrexate.[35] These patients must be monitored with liver function tests. Immunosuppressives such as cyclophosphamide and azathioprine can be alternative remission agents if the patient responds poorly to methotrexate. In addition to pharmacologic treatment, the goals of therapy include maintenance of masticatory function, prevention of growth disturbances, and preservation of function. These are accomplished with daily exercises, occlusal appliances, and psychological support. Surgery is reserved for correction of complications, including ankylosis and micrognathia.

Close monitoring of these patients is critical given their systemic complications and polypharmacologic treatment. Serial laboratory tests to monitor the complete blood count, electrolytes, and erythrocyte sedimentation rate must be maintained. Radiographs are followed every 6 to 12 months to evaluate joint anatomy. Continued joint destruction suggests that further therapy is indicated.

Ankylosing Spondylitis

AS (Marie-Strümpell disease, rheumatoid spondylitis) is a chronic progressive inflammatory disease primarily involving the articulations of the spine and adjacent soft tissues. The sacroiliac joint is always involved, with fewer cases affecting peripheral joints such as the hip, shoulder, and TMJ. The disease predominantly affects men in the third decade of life. An association between AS and histocompatibility complex HLA-B27 has been made, with 88% to 96% of patients testing positive for the antigen.[36]

The disease is worldwide, with a prevalence of 0.5% to 4% in white men, 10 times the rate found in women. The influence of histocompatibility gene HLA-B27 is unknown, but it is believed to be a marker for an associated gene. An infectious agent is still a likely cause of the HLA-B27–associated arthritides, but it has not been identified to date.

Physical examination early in the disease reveals loss of lumbar lordosis and decreased inspiratory expansion. Bent-over posture and rigid spine are pathognomonic. Significant laboratory findings include an elevated erythrocyte sedimentation rate, mild anemia, and a negative test for RF. These findings in a young man positive for HLA-B27 are diagnostic.[10, 36]

PATHOLOGY

The earliest evidence of pathologic change is seen in the sacroiliac joint. The disease spreads peripherally from the spine, but the skipping of segments is known to occur. The synovial reaction is similar to that in RA, with the occurrence of hyperpla-sia and the accumulation of lymphocytes and plasma cells. As cartilage and bone are destroyed, fibrosis occurs and radiolucent cysts become evident. The early diagnosis may be confusing, and infectious etiologies should be ruled out. Inflammation affecting tendon and ligament insertions leads to bony erosions and new ossification centers. When the outer annulus of the spinal column is involved, it can have a bamboo-like appearance.[36–38]

MANIFESTATIONS

The disease primarily affects men between the ages of 15 and 40 years, rarely affecting patients over the age of 50. Most patients have associated constitutional symptoms, including fatigue, malaise, and weight loss. Initially, the most common complaints are of stiffness, lower back pain, and hip pain. These symptoms are exacerbated in the morning and are commonly confused with sciatica. Approximately 25% of patients develop peripheral arthritis in later stages of the disease, but generally after back pain has occurred. The hips are often the site of debilitation, which may lead to ankylosis. Chest pain and pleurisy are often confused with cardiac pain but are usually secondary to costosternal and costovertebral inflammation. Atlantoaxial degeneration has been reported, although less frequently than in RA. Work-up, excluding involvement at the atlantoaxial joint, should be done whenever the patient may be scheduled for an operative procedure. Acute anterior uveitis, which can be the presenting symptom in 20% to 30% of patients, necessitates an ophthalmologic evaluation. Restricted lung disease and uremia have also been reported secondary to amyloidosis associated with AS. In the most severe cases, cauda equina syndrome occurs, where inflammation of the lumbosacral nerve roots leads to muscle weakness and loss of bladder and anal sphincter tone. Involvement of the root of the aorta can lead to focal medial necrosis, resulting in dilatation of the aortic ring. Aortic cusps may become fibrosed and shortened, leading to valve incompetence. Fibrosis can also affect the cardiac septum, causing defects in the conduction pathways.[9, 36, 39, 40]

TEMPOROMANDIBULAR JOINT INVOLVEMENT

As with most forms of systemic arthritis, TMJ involvement occurs—in 4% to 50% of patients late in the course of the disease.[37] The most common complaint is one of pain, stiffness, decreased range of motion, and eventually ankylosis. Symptoms were found to be worse when the disease was in an acute phase. The degree of TMJ involvement was found usually to parallel the severity of spinal and peripheral joint involvement. Patients with TMJ symptoms usually have a history of severe AS, with periods of nonambulation and height loss.[37] Thirty percent of patients have radiographically evident AS on plain films of the TMJs. These findings include erosion of the condyle and fossa, osteophyte formation, and subchondral sclerosis. As the disease progresses, severe narrowing of the joint space becomes evident.[10, 30] Extraarticular manifestations such as iritis, uveitis, and cardiac symptoms are common in patients with TMJ involvement.[5, 40]

TREATMENT

Prevention of spinal and joint deformity is the main therapeutic goal. Exercise is vital, and patients are instructed to maintain erect posture while walking, standing, and sitting. Although drugs fail to limit disease progression, they provide pain relief for the maintenance of correct posture. NSAIDs have been found to reduce pain and stiffness while enabling exercise. Slow-release preparations have been proven to be more effective and can be given with a cytoprotective drug, limiting gastric irritation. Glucocorticoid use is limited because of side effects, but patients with severe iritis and uveitis should be treated with intraocular steroids.[8] Another second-line drug with proven efficacy is sulfasalazine (Azulfidine), which has been beneficial in patients with peripheral arthritis such as TMJ disease and inflammatory bowel disease. Other immunosuppressives have not been beneficial. Surgical intervention should be limited to those patients with severe crippling disease.[4] The goal of procedures is to release contractures and increase joint function.

Psoriatic Arthritis

Psoriasis occurs in 1% to 2% of the population as a dermatologic disease. The prevalence of PA in patients with psoriasis is higher than that found in the general population, with arthritis associated with the skin lesions developing in 5% to 7% of these patients. There is a higher incidence in women. The etiology remains unknown, although a greater incidence among first-degree relatives suggests a genetic component. Ninety percent of patients are also positive for HLA-B27.[8]

Although in 20% of patients joint pain is the primary complaint, the majority (80%) have psoriasis for months to years prior to joint symptoms. This arthritic condition is generally less severe than RA with respect to joint deformity and limitation of function. Typically, a few joints are involved and symptoms are mild and intermittent.[41]

CLINICAL FEATURES

The majority of patients present with monoarticular or asymmetric polyarticular arthritis, involving scattered small joints of the hands and feet. Sausage fingers are often present and result from swelling of interphalangeal joints and the flexor tendon sheath. Peripheral joints are warm, swollen, and tender and show synovial proliferation. Flexion contracture and ankylosis can occur but are rare. No correlation exists between joint involvement and psoriatic skin lesions, but a relationship does exist between nail lesions (onycholysis) and the development of arthritis.[8]

Despite the prevalence of PA in other joints, there is dispute over the incidence of involvement of the TMJ—although most agree it is rarely associated.[5, 41–43] All reported cases have occurred prior to the fourth decade and have involved a preceding traumatic event. TMJ involvement is described as episodic, sudden, and usually unilateral. TMJ symptoms are nondiagnostic, although the joint and muscle pain around the affected joint is the most common complaint.[42] Patients have reported morning stiffness, crepitus, and eventual loss of interincisal opening. If advanced disease is unmanaged, ankylosis can occur and has been reported.[41] Unlike in early RA and JRA, TMJ involvement in early PA is evident on radiographs in up to 82% of cases.[5] Early findings include erosion, flattening of the condylar head, osteoporosis, and joint space narrowing.

DIAGNOSIS

The diagnosis of PA is suggested by the presence of arthritis in a patient with psoriatic skin or nail lesions. Asymmetric joint involvement, negative testing for RF, and absence of rheumatoid nodules should differentiate PA from RA.[8, 10] PA can be associated with hyperuricemia in 20% of cases. This can be differentiated from gouty arthritis by synovial fluid analysis. Laboratory abnormalities include hypoproliferative anemia and elevated erythrocyte sedimentation rate. Characteristic radiographic findings include severe destruction of isolated joints, osteolysis, ankylosis, whittling of the tufts of the terminal phalanges, and pencil-cup deformity of the fingers and toes.[18]

TREATMENT

Immunosuppressive agents such as methotrexate have been used successfully but are reserved for severe cases resulting in joint destruction. Occasionally, the improvement of skin lesions may lead to improvement of involved joints.[8, 11]

Reiter's Syndrome

Reiter's syndrome is characterized by arthritis in association with one or more of the following: urethritis, cervicitis, bacillary dysentery, eye inflammation, and mucocutaneous lesions. The majority of patients are young males who are positive for HLA-B27. The causes of this syndrome are unknown but have been noted to follow bacillary dysentery and sexual exposures.[9] This has led to the hypothesis that an infectious agent is associated with the etiology. A genetic component is also likely because 80% of white patients are positive for HLA-B27. The risk for developing Reiter's syndrome is 20% in an HLA-B27–positive individual with nonspecific urethritis or bacillary dysentery.[9]

Histologically, the skin and mucosal lesions are similar, whereas the synovium is more like rheumatoid synovium. Skin lesions (keratoderma blennorrhagicum) are characterized by hyperkeratosis, parakeratosis, and acanthosis, and pustules and microabscesses develop in the epidermis. The dermis then becomes edematous, with infiltrating lymphocytes, plasma cells, and neutrophils. Mucosal lesions are similar but lack the keratinizing cells. Synovium is characterized by edema, extravasation of erythrocytes, and infiltration of neutrophils, lymphocytes, and plasma cells. After months of this type of inflammation, the synovium becomes villous, similarly to rheumatoid arthritic synovium, and pannus formation occurs over the articular surfaces.[33]

Symptoms commonly occur after exposure to infectious agents. Early complaints of mucopurulent urethritis following sexual exposure are common. Arthritis following 3 to 4 days later appears with mucocutaneous lesions and conjunctivitis. These symptoms of Reiter's syndrome have also been reported following bacillary dysentery.

Arthritis associated with Reiter's syndrome is described as acute in onset and involving two or more joints. Joints are characterized as warm, erythematous, and painful. Knees and ankles are primarily affected, whereas the hips and shoulders are usually spared. The distribution of joint involvement is asymmetric and variable. Symptoms peak at around 2 weeks, and arthritic pain lasts 2 to 4 months. Episodic recurrences are common for several years, necessitating periodic monitoring for contracture development and joint deformity.[29]

DIAGNOSIS

As in AS, cardiac conduction defects and aortic valvular lesions can develop but are infrequent. Laboratory testing reveals an elevated erythrocyte sedimentation rate and leukocytosis. RF is not identified, but HLA-B27 is found in the majority of patients. Radiologic examination often reveals new periosteal bone formation along the shaft of the involved joint.[9]

The differential diagnosis of Reiter's syndrome should rule out gonococcal arthritis early. Urethral culture and synovial fluid analysis can be used for diagnosis, because both processes have associated arthritis, urethritis, and cervicitis. If doubt still exists, a trial of penicillin can be given to the patient, who is monitored for response. If symptoms continue, Reiter's syndrome should be considered.

TMJ involvement is rare but may be underreported owing to nonspecific findings. Symptoms involving the TMJ are asymmetric and acute. Pain, tenderness, and a warm, erythematous joint are the usual findings.[29] Bony changes are rarely appreciated on radiographs until late-stage disease has occurred. Diagnosis is based on the triad of symptoms that is present in 70% of patients within the first 10 days of the disease.[44]

TREATMENT

Treatment consists of 10 to 14 days of tetracycline for the urethritis, which does not affect the arthritis.[10] Mucocutaneous lesions and conjunctivitis require no treatment, but iritis should be treated with intraocular glucocorticoids to limit scarring.[9] Symptomatic relief of arthritic pain can be obtained with indomethacin, phenylbutazone, and physical therapy. Although systemic glucocorticoids are rarely indicated, local injection into the joint can provide relief in resistant joint inflammation. Immunosuppressive agents are reserved for those severe cases resulting in joint deformity.

Lupus

Lupus is a disease in which the patient's immunologic system causes tissue injury. Hallmark is the presence of autoantibodies to nuclear components. The course of lupus is variable, with some cases going into spontaneous remission, some responding to corticosteroids, and some nonresponsive to any therapy. Although the etiology remains unknown, viral infection, genetic predisposition, and immunoregulatory abnormalities appear to play roles.[9]

ETIOLOGY

No clear etiologic factor has been recognized, although multiple hypotheses have been postulated. The belief that viral infection in genetically predisposed patients plays a role is supported by the fact that virus-like tubuloreticulum is found in the cytoplasm of affected cells. These structures are believed to be secondary to viral cell injury. Another hypothesis is abnormal regulation of the immune system—as humoral immunity increases, cell-mediated immunity becomes suppressed. A genetic role is supported by the predisposition of both monozygotic twins developing the disease. The chance of two monozygotic twins having the autoantibodies is greater than that seen in nontwin siblings.[9, 33]

CLINICAL FEATURES

Lupus is primarily a disease of women in their second to fifth decade of life. The prevalence is about 3 in 100,000 persons. Five-year survival remains about 77%, although the prevalence of renal and neural disease decreases survival. Death usually ensues from uremia, heart failure, hemorrhage, and bacterial infections.[33]

Patients suffering from systemic lupus erythematosus (SLE) present with multiple complaints varying in frequency. Arthritis and arthralgia are the most common complaints, occurring in 92% of patients. Most commonly, the pain occurs in the hands, feet, and large joints. Synovial effusion as well as pain, redness, and warmth are frequently encountered. Joint architecture is rarely affected by the arthritis, and destruction is uncommon. Synovial fluid analysis reveals a relatively low white blood cell count (around 3000/mm³) with frequently seen mononuclear cells.[33] More common than joint destruction is osteonecrosis from extended corticosteroid use and associated myositis around the joint.

Fever occurs in 84% of the population with lupus and recurs throughout the course. Malaise, fatigue, anorexia, and weight loss are also common. Skin lesions, as stated previously, occur in around 72% of cases and may present over the malar eminences of the face 40% of the time. These eruptions can occur anywhere but primarily in exposed areas. Ultraviolet injury is believed to be the etiology of these eruptions. Alopecia and facial vasculitis have also been reported.[9]

Renal involvement is the most serious outcome of the disease. Clinically evident renal involvement occurs in about 50% of cases, ranging from proteinuria and a few red blood cells to massive hematuria with renal failure. A similar percentage of patients are afflicted with cardiopulmonary manifestations. Pericarditis is the usual complaint, with the typical physical and electrocardiographic findings. Symptomatic pleural involvement also occurs in 50% of patients. Patchy, transient infiltrates can be seen, which lead to pneumonitis.

Neurologic manifestations, although less frequent, can be substantial and lead to abnormalities in mental function, cranial nerve abnormalities, and seizures. Testing of these patients reveals abnormal electroencephalograms and increased protein in the cerebrospinal fluid.[9]

PATHOGENESIS

Tissue injury results from autoantibody directed against unrecognized self-antigens. The antibodies are directed against DNA, RNA, histones, and other nuclear antigens. Collectively, these are termed antinuclear antibodies (ANA). Antibodies to clotting factors and cardiolipin and antibodies directed at lymphocytes have also been recognized.[33] The antibodies themselves are harmless, as they cannot pass through cell membranes to react with nuclear material. However, when cell lysis occurs, the antigen is exposed to the antibodies and antigen-antibody complex is accumulated. As the antibodies attach to the antigen, hematoxylin bodies form in the areas of inflammation. These hematoxylin bodies are believed to be degenerated nuclei that have interacted with antibody. The collection of the antibody-antigen complexes, as well as complement, gathers in the kidney's basement membranes. This accumulation of inflammatory cells leads to inflammation, hypercellularity, and thickening of the basement membrane. The result is glomerulonephritis. As the disease advances, glomeruli become thrombosed and sclerosed, compromising kidney function. Interstitial nephritis has also been reported and further complicates function.[33]

Widespread vasculitis is also evident in most organs, including the synovium of the joints. The heart is unique because it can develop nonbacterial vegetation on the chordae tendineae cordis and valves, which can lead to Libman-Sacks endocarditis. The spleen and central nervous system are also commonly affected.

Skin lesions vary with the stage and severity of the disease. An erythematous, maculopapular rash within the butterfly distribution of the face is most common but not diagnostic. Chronic lesions show erythema, extravasation of red cells with inflammation, hyperkeratosis, and atrophy. On immunofluorescence, the epidermal-dermal junction is delineated. IgG and C3 are also found in this layer.

LABORATORY TESTS

Multiple laboratory tests can lead to the diagnosis of lupus. A mild normochromic, normocytic anemia is seen in 50% of these patients, whereas they can also suffer from reduced white blood cell and platelet counts. Autoantibodies directed at these hematologic cells are believed to be a mechanism. Similar antibodies can also be formed against clotting factors, causing unwanted bleeding.

Patients' renal function should be evaluated by creatinine levels and testing for blood and protein in the urine. Markers of inflammation, such as the erythrocyte sedimentation rate and plasma electrophoresis, can be monitored to evaluate the amount and type of immunoglobulin present. Antibody that responds to antigens presented by nuclear components (ANA) in a patient with clinical findings of lupus is diagnostic.[9]

The diagnosis of SLE should be considered in women 20 to 50 years old with three to four of the clinical symptoms previously described.[33] The presence of glomerulonephritis, hemolytic anemia, leukopenia, and thrombocytopenia should raise suspicion. A positive ANA test is required for diagnosis but is not diagnostic by itself. Positive ANA tests can be identified in RA, Sjögren's syndrome, and scleroderma and with the ingestion of certain drugs.

TREATMENT

SLE has no cure, but life can be prolonged and acute flare-ups can be managed with the appropriate agents. Arthritic symptoms, fever, and myalgia respond to NSAIDs and rest. Antimalarials and the avoidance of ultraviolet light have been successful in relieving the symptoms associated with skin eruptions and in limiting their formation. More severe symptoms, such as central nervous system disease, renal failure, and diminishing red and white blood cells should be treated with corticosteroids.[23] Immunosuppressive therapy has been beneficial in controlling severe clinical symptoms but is limited owing to side effects. Plasmapheresis in conjunction with steroids and immunosuppressives is reserved for the most severe cases with the poorest prognosis.[23]

Metabolic Arthritis

Pseudogout (calcium pyrophosphate dihydrate deposition [CPPD] disease) and gout are two metabolic processes that involve the TMJ.[45] As crystals form in the synovial lining, inflammation develops and causes joint destruction. Although gout affects 5% of men over 65 years old and 2% of women in the same age group, only a few cases of TMJ involvement have been reported.[45] Gout has no definitive changes on radiograph; however, in late-stage disease, erosions and punched-out lesions can be found.

PSEUDOGOUT SYNDROME

Various forms of arthritis are associated with calcium deposits within the joint. Almost 30% of nursing home patients over age 80 have been found to have radiographic evidence of chondrocalcinosis, a descriptive term given to the radiographic appearance of joints with CPPD disease, revealing its prevalence.[33] Radiographs may not always reveal chondrocalcinosis or deposits in the surrounding soft tissues; therefore, synovial aspiration is often needed for definitive diagnosis.

The cause of pseudogout has not been established, but local overproduction of pyrophosphate related to excessive activity of nucleoside triphosphate pyrophosphohydrolase, deficiency of phosphatases, and local changes in proteoglycans are likely factors. This combination with an abnormal cartilage matrix may act as a nidus or trigger for crystal deposition.[33] Elevated levels of organic phosphate are also evident in involved joints. This process has a predilection for joints lined with fibrocartilage as opposed to those lined with hyaline cartilage, and the knees, wrists, and second and third MCP joints are the most common sites.[33] The presence of these crystals does not always lead to the arthritic condition, as some patients are found to have chondrocalcinosis but no symptoms. In any event, the disease is slowly progressive, but it may become severe enough to justify joint replacement.

TMJ involvement is rare, with only 14 reported cases, most occurring unilaterally after the age of 40 and only one patient presenting with bilateral complaints.[10, 46–48] The most common joint complaints include acute pain, joint effusion, swelling, and limited range of motion. Unlike the case in other processes, patients may complain of flulike symptoms.[10] Displaced disks and existing damage of the cartilaginous surfaces have been postulated as foci for crystal deposition, although this remains unproven.[46] Acute flare-ups are believed to be secondary to shedding of crystals from articular cartilage during trauma and inflammatory episodes. Radiographic evaluation has revealed condylar and fossa erosions with narrowed joint spaces, but this is a common feature in most arthritides. More helpful findings include calcification of the disk, and osseous tophi within the joint can aid in diagnosis.[10]

Diagnosis

The deposition of crystals should alarm the clinician to a variety of diseases. Systemic conditions associated with CPPD disease include RA, chronic arthritides, gout, hypomagnesemia, hypothyroidism, amyloidosis, hypophosphatasia, hyperparathyroidism, hemosiderosis, hemochromatosis, and familial hypocalciuric hypercalcemia. In addition, there is a correlation with aging, trauma, surgical intervention, and chronic steroid therapy.[33] Aspiration of the synovial fluid may provide crystals, but diagnosis may not be considered until neoplastic processes are eliminated.[46] The diagnosis is confirmed when rod- or rhomusshaped, weakly birefringent crystals with positive elongation are found in the synovial fluid or articular tissues. Synovial fluid also contains leukocyte counts in excess of 100,000, 80% to 90% of which may be neutrophils, during acute attacks. Common histologic features include nodular and gritty granulomatous tissue within and surrounding the joint space. Fibrocartilage manifests degeneration with foci of crystals and multinucleated giant cells that are evident despite a lack of inflammation.[33, 46]

Treatment

The treatment of pseudogout involves thorough aspiration of crystals from the synovial fluid and occasionally surgical débridement of the joint. Symptomatic relief is obtained with NSAIDs, aspirin, and, rarely, steroids. Refractory joint involvement can be treated with the injection of corticosteroids into the joint. Intravenous colchicine has been used during acute attacks that are resistant to treatment, but it is usually reserved for the prevention of acute attacks.[29, 33, 46]

GOUT

The literature suggests that gout causes 5% of all arthritides.[33] The most classic joint to be involved is the first MTP joint, but any joint can be involved. Chronic or recurrent acute attacks can be polyarticular and mimic RA. The manifestation of gout is caused by monosodium urate crystal deposition in joints and soft tissues (tophi). Primary gout is the result of hyperuricemia associated with hypoxanthine-guanine phosphoribosyltransferase deficiency and phosphoribosylpyrophosphate synthetase variants, which are the result of complex genetic, metabolic, and renal factors interacting. The genetics of gout reveal that 25% of patients have first-degree relatives with hyperuricemia. Protein intake, being male, increased surface area, obesity, alcohol intake, and social status are also correlated with hyperuricemia.[9]

In the absence of chronic renal insufficiency, primary gout affects middle-aged men and postmenopausal women. The risks increase with age and hyperuricemia level. Even in quiescent periods, urate levels remain elevated. Urate concentration is associated with purine absorption, destruction, and excretion. Exogenous consumption is critical and must be limited in susceptible patients. Compromised renal function becomes a factor because urate is not released by the kidneys. Diuretics, polycythemia vera, and chronic hemolysis have also been reported as causes of gout.

Pathophysiology

Urate crystal deposition is leukotactic and activates the complement cascade and inflammatory peptides. White blood cells and other components of the inflammatory cascade ingest the urate crystals, while the byproducts of inflammation contribute to the arthritic process. Crystals may also be coated with IgG, which amplifies the inflammatory response by stimulating the neutrophils. Phagocytosis of crystals causes a rapid release of peptidases and other proteolytic enzymes, leading to damage of the surrounding tissues. This process of chemotaxis leading to an exaggerated inflammatory response can be blocked with colchicine.[33]

Crystals associated with hyperuricemia are described as rods or needles that reveal bright birefringence with negative elongation when viewed under polarized light. During acute attacks, crystals can be found intracellularly and leukocyte counts can range from 10,000 to 50,000, with 80% to 90% being neutrophils. Crystals can be found between acute attacks and can severely destroy joints.

Clinical Features

When gout causes acute arthritis, it is usually incapacitating. In 75% to 90% of these attacks, one joint is involved.[9] The majority involve the MTP joint of the great toe. The heel is the second most likely joint to be involved, then the knee, wrist, fingers, and elbow. As the disease progresses, attacks become polyarticular and can involve the shoulder, hip, TMJs, and even the spine. The classic presentation is an acute attack occurring at night. Joints are reported as hot, dusky red, and painful. The attacks usually follow a precipitating event such as trauma, surgery, alcohol consumption, dietary overindulgence, and infection.[33] Initially, these attacks are self-limiting, but 62% of patients have another event within the first year.[33] If untreated, the attacks become more frequent and severe, leading to permanent disability.

Chronic gout is related to the level of hyperuricemia as urate disposal progressively worsens; this becomes evident as tophi develop. The time from first attack to visible tophi ranges from 3 to 42 years, with an average of 11 years.[33] Joint destruction occurs from degradation of cartilage and bone, which leads to cystic erosions and overhanging ledges of eroded bone. Radiographs reveal soft tissue swelling early in the disease. As the severity progresses, cystic erosions and overhanging bone can be seen. Soft tissue tophi are commonly found around joints, bursae, the extensor surfaces of the forearms, and occasionally the ear lobes.

Treatment

The treatment of acute gout attacks includes the use of NSAIDs, colchicine, adrenocorticotropic hormone (ACTH), or corticosteroids. Treatment with medications that cause systemic side effects, such as steroids and ACTH, are reserved for severe cases, as seen in patients with end-stage renal disease and liver disease. Single joint involvement has been successfully managed with joint injection, as long as infections are ruled out first.[45] Recurrent attacks are treated with low doses of NSAIDs or colchicine to suppress inflammation, but crystal accumulation continues.[9] Patients suffering from frequent attacks are also placed on uricosuric agents such as probenecid or allopurinol. Avoidance of foods containing purine metabolites and weight reduction over a prolonged period are also recommended. Rapid weight loss should be avoided because it has been found to precipitate attacks.[33]

REFERENCES

1. Akerman S, Kopp S, Nilner M, et al: Relationship between clinical and radiographic findings of the temporomandibular joint in rheumatoid arthritis. Oral Surg Oral Med Oral Pathol 1988;66:639.
2. Fries JF: Approach to the patient with musculoskeletal disease. In Wyngaarden JB, Smith LH Jr, Bennett JC (eds): Cecil Textbook of Medicine, ed 19. Philadelphia, WB Saunders, 1988, p 1488.
3. Carlsson GE, Kopp S, Oberg T: Arthritis and allied diseases of the temporomandibular joint. In Zarb GA, Carlsson GE (eds): Temporomandibular Joint. Function and Dysfunction. Copenhagen, Munksgaard, 1979, p 269.
4. Franks AST: Temporomandibular joint in adult rheumatoid arthritis. A comparative evaluation of 100 cases. Ann Rheum Dis 1969;28:139.
5. Wenneberg B, Kononen M, Kallenberg A: Radiographic changes in the temporomandibular joint of patients with rheumatoid arthritis, psoriatic arthritis, and ankylosing spondylitis. J Craniomand Disord Facial Oral Pain 1990;4:35.
6. Eyanson S, Hutton CE, Brandt KD: Erosive temporomandibular joint disease as a feature of the spondyloarthropathy of ulcerative colitis. J Oral Surg 1982;53:136.
7. Hansson TL: Pathological aspects of arthritides and derangements. In Sarnat BG, Laskin DM (eds): The Temporomandibular Joint: A Biological Basis for Clinical Practice, ed 4. Philadelphia, WB Saunders, 1992, pp 165–182.
8. Moll JM, Wright V: Psoriatic arthritis. Semin Arthritis Rheum 1973;3:55.
9. Cush JJ, Lipsky PE: Approach to articular and musculoskeletal disorders. In Wilson JE, Braunwald E, Isselbacher KJ, et al (eds): Harrison's Principles of Internal Medicine, ed 12. New York, McGraw-Hill, 1991.
10. Abubaker AO: Differential diagnosis of arthritis of the temporomandibular joint. Oral Maxillofac Surg Clin North Am 1995;7:1.
11. Abubaker AO, Laskin DM: Nonsurgical management of arthritis of the temporomandibular joint. Oral Maxillofac Surg Clin North Am 1995;7:51.
12. Zarb GA, Carlsson GE: Osteoarthrosis/osteoarthritis. In Zarb GA, Carlsson GE, Sessle BJ, Mohl ND (eds): Temporomandibular Joint and Masticatory Muscle Disorders, ed 2. Copenhagen, Mosby, 1995, p 298.
13. Stegenga B, DeBont LGM, Boering G: Osteoarthritis as the cause of craniomandibular pain and dysfunction: A unifying concept. J Oral Maxillofac Surg 1989;47:249.
14. Stegenga B, DeBont LGM, Boering G, Van Willigen JD: Tissue responses to degenerative changes in the temporomandibular joint: A review. J Oral Maxillofac Surg 1991;49:1079–1088.
15. Salo LA, Raustia AM: Type two and type three collagen in mandibular condylar cartilage of patients with temporomandibular joint pathology. J Oral Maxillofac Surg 1995;53:39.
16. DeBont LGM, Stegenga B: Pathology of the temporomandibular joint: Internal derangement and osteoarthrosis. Int J Oral Maxillofac Surg 1993; 22:71–74.
17. Bjornland T, Refsum SB: Histopathologic changes of the temporomandibular joint disk in patients with chronic arthritic disease: A comparison with internal derangement. Oral Surg Oral Med Oral Pathol 1994;77:572.

18. Calin A, Steinberg AD, Schumacher HR, et al: The spondylarthropathies. In Wyngaarden JB, Smith LH Jr, Bennett JC (eds): Cecil Textbook of Medicine, ed 19. Philadelphia, WB Saunders, 1992, pp 1515–1554.

19. Dijkgraaf LC, De Bont LGM, Boering G, Liem RSB: The structure, biochemistry and metabolism of osteoarthritic cartilage: A review of the literature. J Oral Maxillofac Surg 1995;53:1182.

20. Kleinman HZ, Ewbank RL: Gout of the temporomandibular joint: Report of three cases. Oral Surg Oral Med Oral Pathol 1969;281.

21. Mankin HJ, Brandt KD: Biochemistry and metabolism of cartilage in osteoarthritis. In Moskowitz RW, Howel DS, Golberg VM, et al (eds): Osteoarthritis, Diagnosis and Management. Philadelphia, WB Saunders, 1984, p 68.

22. DeBont LGM, Boering G, Liem RSB: Osteoarthrosis and internal derangement of the temporomandibular joint. A light microscopy study. J Oral Maxillofac Surg 1986;44:634.

23. Katz WA: Diagnosis and Management of Rheumatic Diseases, ed 2. Philadelphia, JB Lippincott, 1988.

24. Dieppe PA, Harkness JAL, Higgs ER: Osteoarthritis. In Wall PA, Melzack R (eds): Textbook of Pain, ed 2. Edinburgh, Churchill Livingstone, 1989, p 306.

25. Howell DS: Etiopathogenesis of osteoarthritis. In Moskowitz RW, Howel DS, Golberg VM, et al (eds): Osteoarthritis, Diagnosis and Management. Philadelphia, WB Saunders, 1984, p 129.

26. Mankin HJ, Brandt KD: Pathogenesis of osteoarthritis. In Kelley WN, Harris ED, Ruddy S, et al (eds): Textbook of Rheumatology, ed 3. Philadelphia, WB Saunders 1989, p 1469.

27. Arnett FC: Rheumatoid arthritis. In Wyngaarden JB, Smith LH Jr, Bennett JC (eds): Cecil Textbook of Medicine, ed 19. Philadelphia, WB Saunders, 1988, p 1508.

28. Kopp S: Rheumatoid arthritis. In Zarb GA, Carlsson GE, Sessle BJ, Mohl ND (eds): Temporomandibular Joint and Masticatory Muscle Disorders, ed 2. Copenhagen, Mosby, 1995, p 346.

29. Kaplan SA, Buchbinder D: Arthritis. In Kaplan SA, Assael CA (eds): Temporomandibular Disorders: Diagnosis and Treatment. Philadelphia, WB Saunders, 1991, p 165.

30. Sugahara T, Mori Y, Kawamoto T, et al: Obstructive sleep apnea associated with temporomandibular joint destruction by rheumatoid arthritis. Report of case. J Oral Maxillofac Surg 1994;52:876.

31. Zide MF, Carlton DM, Kent JN: Rheumatoid disease and related arthropathies. Oral Surg Oral Med Oral Pathol 1986;61:119.

32. Golbus J: Rheumatoid arthritis. In Rakel RE (ed): Conn's Current Therapy. Philadelphia, WB Saunders, 1997, pp 995–1000.

33. Wyngaarden JB, Smith LH Jr, Bennett JC (eds): Cecil Textbook of Medicine, ed 19. Philadelphia, WB Saunders, 1992.

34. Schneiderman ED: The temporomandibular joint in juvenile rheumatoid arthritis: Computed tomographic findings. Pediatr Dentistry 1995;17:46.

35. Moore TL: Juvenile rheumatoid arthritis. In Rakel RE (ed): Conn's Current Therapy. Philadelphia, WB Saunders, 1997, pp 1001–1004.

36. Boland EW: Ankylosing spondylitis. In Hollander JL (ed): Arthritis and Allied Conditions, ed 7. Philadelphia, Lea & Febiger, 1966, pp 633–655.

37. Crum RJ, Loiselle RJ: Temporomandibular joint symptoms and ankylosing spondylitis. J Am Dent Assoc 1971;83.

38. Dachowski MT, Dolan EA, Angelillo JC: Ankylosing spondylitis associated with temporomandibular joint ankylosis: Report of a case. J Craniomand Disord Facial Oral Pain 1990;4:52.

39. Thompson GT, Steinfield SM, Gall RM: Ankylosing spondylitis. In Rakel RE (ed): Conn's Current Therapy. Philadelphia, WB Saunders, 1996, p 945.

40. Syrjanen SM: The temporomandibular joint in rheumatoid arthritis. Acta Radiol 1985;26:235.

41. Sanders B, Halliday R: Psoriasis and rheumatoid arthritis: Their relationship in TMJ ankylosis. J Oral Med 1979;34:4.

42. Rasmussen OC, Bakke M: Psoriatic arthritis of the temporomandibular joint. J Oral Surg 1982;53:351.

43. Stimson CW, Leban SG: Recurrent ankylosis of the temporomandibular joint in a patient with chronic psoriasis. J Oral Maxillofac Surg 1982;40:678.

44. Bomalsky JS, Jiminez SA: Erosive arthritis of the temporomandibular joint in Reiter's syndrome. J Rheumatol 1984;11:400.

45. Gross BD, Williams RB, DiCosimo CJ, Williams SV: Gout and pseudogout of the temporomandibular joint. Oral Surg Oral Med Oral Pathol 1987;63:551.

46. Chuong R, Piper MA: Bilateral pseudogout of the temporomandibular joint: Report of case and review of the literature. J Oral Maxillofac Surg 1995;53:691.

47. DeVoa RAI, Brants J, Kusen GJ, et al: Calcium pyrophosphate dihydrate arthropathy of the temporomandibular joint. J Oral Maxillofac Surg 1981;51:497.

48. Magno WB, Lee SH, Schmidt J: Chondrocalcinosis of the temporomandibular joint: An external ear canal pseudotumor. Oral Surg Oral Med Oral Pathol 1992;73:262.

CHAPTER

6

Epidemiology of Temporomandibular Disorders

Thomas B. Dodson

Since the 1970s, the number of articles published related to temporomandibular disorders (TMDs) has increased dramatically (Fig. 6–1). Whether TMD is a significant public health problem or there has simply been an explosion of interest in the problem is not clear. The purpose of this chapter is to review the epidemiologic literature estimating prevalence and treatment needs of TMD. The chapter is divided into four sections. The first part reviews the definition and importance of epidemiology and introduces a working definition of TMD. The body of the chapter focuses on the important epidemiologic findings since 1950. The epidemiology of pediatric and geriatric populations is reviewed in the third part. In the final section, the findings are summarized and future research goals outlined. The review is not exhaustive. The papers selected for inclusion in this review were chosen on the basis of historical interest and/or the application of sound epidemiologic methods to investigate TMD.

Definitions of Epidemiology and Temporomandibular Disorders

DEFINITION AND VALUE OF EPIDEMIOLOGY

Epidemiology is the study of the determinants, distribution, and frequency (prevalence/incidence) of disease in a population. The epidemiologist's goals are to identify risk factors for a disease (determinants), determine who has the disease (distribution), estimate how many people currently have the disease (prevalence), and determine how many new cases develop each year (incidence). The epidemiologist provides a valuable service to the practitioner by acquiring and disseminating information as to which patients are at risk for disease, identifying etiologic agents, determining the natural history of treated (and untreated) disease, and elucidating causal relationships between cause and disease, thereby preventing disease.

WORKING DEFINITION OF TEMPOROMANDIBULAR DISORDERS

A precept of epidemiology is that in order to investigate a disease, one has to define the disease in unambiguous terms. The fundamental epidemiologic challenge to studying TMDs in nonpatient populations is definitional. Specifically, how much abnormal function (i.e., pain, joint noise, or limitation of jaw motion) must be present to classify an individual as having the "disease"? Those familiar with research and treatment of TMD immediately recognize this to be a considerable investigational handicap. The definitions of TMD are so diverse as to make the term functionally meaningless.

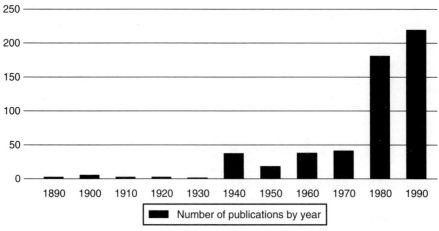

FIGURE 6–1. Number of TMD-related publications found in the American literature by year.

TMD is a heterogeneous collection of signs and symptoms that can be generally characterized by the presence of pain, TM joint noise, and limitation of jaw motion. TMDs can be broadly grouped as structural/organic (ankylosis, trauma, infection, neoplasia, or arthritis) or functional disorders (symptoms associated with function, i.e., pain, joint noise, or limitation of jaw motion). Epidemiologic research efforts have focused attention on functional TMDs, specifically myofascial pain dysfunction (MPD) and/or internal derangement (malrelationship of the condyle and articular disk). This chapter focuses on the major epidemiologic findings related to functional TMD.

Epidemiologic Findings of Importance to Temporomandibular Disorders

EPIDEMIOLOGIC STUDIES BEFORE 1950

Studies during the era before 1950 had several common features. First, the researchers were interested in functional lesions of the TM joint (arthrosis/arthritis), not myofascial pain. Second, the epidemiologic methods were unsophisticated. As will be seen with many future studies, these reports estimated disease prevalence by counting signs and symptoms of TMD. Finally, the study samples were derived from non-TMD patient populations.

Historically, Scandinavian researchers have made many significant contributions to the epidemiology of TMD. Their ready access to data may be due to having a stable, homogeneous population and a long history of socialized medicine. Not surprisingly, a Scandinavian published the first large-scale descriptive study of TMD. In 1947, Boman published an estimate of the frequency of TM joint symptoms in a non-TMD patient population.[1] In a sample of 1350 patients—hospital patients (n = 900), military personnel (n = 100), and children (n = 350)—Boman estimated the frequency of TM joint problems on the basis of eliciting positive findings on history (pain or joint noise) and clinical examination (joint noise or uncoordinated jaw movement). The prevalence of positive signs or symptoms was 31.6% in the hospital sample, 25% in the military sample, and 9.7% in the pediatric sample. Overall, females were more likely to have positive findings (32.4% versus 18.6%). The age range for positive findings was quite broad, with the peak frequencies at ages 20 to 40 and 60 to 70 in males and females, respectively. Pain had never been reported as severe and none of the study patients had sought treatment.

In 1949, Markowitz and Gerry attempted to estimate the prevalence of temporomandibular arthralgia using a cross-sectional study design and a sample composed of 700 unselected individuals examined at the U.S. Naval Hospital in Philadelphia.[2] Age, sex, and health status of the sample were not reported. A history of joint pain or the presence of articular signs was considered a positive finding, although articular signs were not well described. Overall, 28% of the sample had signs and symptoms of TM joint arthralgia and 6.4% of the subjects had sought treatment. Of patients with objective signs of TM joint arthralgia, 16.4% had no subjective complaints.

Summary of Pre-1950 Findings Despite significant flaws in study design, estimates of the prevalence of TMD in adults ranged from 25% to 31.6%. Other findings included gender differences, the broad age range of affected individuals, and the fact that the proportion of patients with clinical signs of TMD exceeded that of those subjects reporting symptoms. Despite methodologic flaws, these basic findings will be confirmed by future studies.

EPIDEMIOLOGIC STUDIES 1950 TO 1969

Epidemiologic studies conducted between 1950 and 1969 can be characterized by the use of a broader definition of TMD and sampling from TMD patient populations. In 1956, Dr. L. Laszlo Schwartz introduced the term *temporomandibular joint pain–dysfunction syndrome,* for a nonorganic disorder of the masticatory musculature.[3] By broadening the definition of TMD to include muscle as well as joint dysfunction, one would expect to see an increase in the prevalence estimates of TMD. The study samples during this era were based on TMD patient populations, and, therefore, we would predict demographic differences from the earlier studies, which were based on non-TMD patient populations.

In a 1956 British study, Hankey reported the demographic findings in a sample of 262 TMD patients.[4] The female-to-male ratio was 4:1, and 57% of the patients had symptoms before age 30, and 4% of the sample experienced symptoms after age 50. Schwartz and Cobin reported on 491 clinic patients evaluated for symptoms associated with the TM joint.[5] The female-to-male ratio was 4.3:1, and 77% of the patients were between the ages of 20 and 50 years. In another British study, Campbell reported a female-to-male ratio of 3.5:1 in a sample of 899 patients referred for treatment of TMD.[6]

In a sample of 100 patients treated for TMD, Thomson estimated the female-to-male ratio to be 3:1.[7] Females aged 18 to 30 composed 40% of the sample. He noted that

in terms of a population estimate from 1956, females aged 18 to 29 represented 7.06% of the population. Young females, therefore, were overrepresented in the patient sample when compared with the general population. Perry reported on a sample of 467 TMD patients.[8] The female-to-male ratio was 4:1. The peak age range was 21 to 50 years. This age range accounted for 83% of the sample with the 21 to 40 age range accounting for 44% of the sample.

Summary of Findings from 1950 to 1969 Studies during the 1950–1969 era focused on describing the demographics and symptoms of TMD patient samples. The demographic findings of TMD patient samples were quite different from those of previous non-TMD patient samples. The TMD patient samples were predominantly female (female-to-male ratios ranged from 3:1 to 4.5:1) and had a tighter age distribution (20 to 50 years). It was not clear, however, whether the demographic findings reflect fundamental differences between TMD patient and non-TMD patient samples or were a consequence of using a broader definition of TMD.

EPIDEMIOLOGIC STUDIES 1970 TO 1979

Prevalence Estimates of Temporomandibular Disorders and Treatment Needs

Recognizing methodologic weaknesses of earlier studies, reports published between 1970 and 1989 can be characterized by the introduction of sound epidemiologic methods to estimate the prevalence of the signs and symptoms of TMD in nonpatient populations (Fig. 6–2). In addition, there was a growing dissatisfaction with merely counting signs and symptoms of TMD to estimate prevalence and treatment needs. In the mid-1970s, we see the introduction and use of indices to measure TMD severity.

Scandinavian researchers pioneered population-based studies to estimate the prevalence of TMD. Agerberg and Carlsson used a cross-sectional study design and a random sample of individuals between 15 and 74 years of age to assess the frequency of TMD.[9] The authors assessed symptoms of TMD by using questionnaires. Of the questionnaires distributed, 91% were completed.

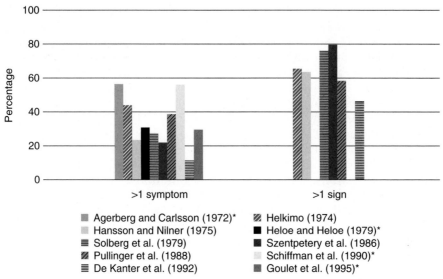

FIGURE 6–2. Estimated prevalence of TMD symptoms and signs, 1970–1995. *These studies reported the prevalence of symptoms only.

The final sample was composed of 1106 subjects (48% male). Overall, 57% of the sample reported at least one symptom of dysfunction. Although the distribution of symptoms by gender was more evenly divided than in studies based on TMD patient populations, women were more likely to report symptoms than men. For example, 44% of women and 34% of men ($P < .001$) reported TM joint noise. Age distribution of symptomatic subjects was less concentrated than the distribution reported in patient samples. Overall, 7% of the sample had sought treatment for TM disorders in the past. Women were more likely than men to have sought treatment (9% vs. 5%, $P < .05$). The authors concluded that "pain and symptoms of dysfunction of the masticatory system were thus relatively common in the populations examined and their sex and age distribution was clearly more even than in clinical series on record."

In 1974, Helkimo published a series of articles based on a dissertation investigating masticatory dysfunction.[10, 11] The study sample was composed of 321 Finnish Lapps (48.6% male) between the ages of 15 and 65. Symptoms of TMD were common (43%). On clinical examination, 45% of the sample had pain in response to TM joint palpation, 66% had pain on palpation of the muscles of mastication, and 48% had TM joint noise. With few exceptions, signs and symptoms of TMD varied little by age or sex. On the basis of

these findings, Helkimo concluded that in the study population, signs/symptoms of TM disorders were common, there were few significant differences between males and females, and disorders were well distributed across age groups. He also suggested that studies of functional disorders in TMD patient populations were not representative of TMD in the general population.

Using a sample of 1069 employed people ("healthy workers"), Hansson and Nilner conducted a cross-sectional study to estimate frequency and treatment needs of TM disorders.[12] The sample was predominantly male (92.3%) and ranged in age from 40 to 59 years of age. On the history, 23% of patients reported joint noise, 6% reported limitation of jaw motion, 3% reported pain with wide opening, and 7% reported preauricular pain. On clinical examination 65% of patients had joint noise in one or both joints, 37% reported pain in response to palpation of the muscles of mastication, and 10% reported TM joint pain. Overall, 79% of the patients had one or more signs and symptoms of TMD. The authors did not report on the demographic distribution or severity of signs/symptoms.

The researchers estimated that 25% to 30% of the sample was in need of some form of treatment. The authors' estimates of treatment need were much higher than those in any of the studies reported in this review. It is difficult to interpret this finding because the authors did not make explicit their parameters to determine treatment need. The authors recognized the limited value of measuring signs and symptoms of TMD and emphasized the point that more attention needs to be given to the epidemiologic study of the "diseases responsible for the symptoms."[12]

In 1979, Heloe and Heloe estimated the prevalence of TMD signs and symptoms in a population-based sample selected to represent the demographic and socioeconomic composition of the general Norwegian 25-year-old population.[13] The original sample size was 324, of whom 246 subjects completed the study. No comment was made on selection bias due to incomplete sampling of the study population. The sample was composed of 44.7% males. Data were collected regarding symptoms of TMD by using a structured questionnaire. Joint noise was reported by 31% of the patients (males = 21%, females = 38%), 8% reported pain with wide opening (male = 5%, female = 11%), and 5% reported TM joint pain (male = 6%, female = 4%). Four percent of the sample reported seeking treatment for TMD (male = 2%, female = 5%). Although the gender differences are not as marked in this sample as in TMD patient samples, in all but one category (TM joint pain), women consistently reported more symptoms than men and were 2.5 times more likely to have sought treatment in the past.

Solberg and colleagues reported on a non-TMD patient sample of young Americans (university students).[14] Using a cross-sectional study design, the authors estimated the prevalence of signs and symptoms of TMD by using questionnaires and clinical examinations. There were 739 individuals enrolled in the study (63% of the eligible population) with a mean age of 22.5 years, and 49.5% were male. In the sample, 25.9% reported a history of TMD symptoms. Except for headache ($P < .001$) the symptoms were evenly distributed between the sexes. On clinical examination, 76% of the sample had TMD signs. Overall, 76.3% of the sample had at least one positive sign or symptom (males = 68.5%, females = 84.2%). The authors estimated that less than 5% of the sample would require treatment. The gender differences were not as marked in this

sample as reported in the TMD patient sample studies; however, women reported a higher frequency of signs and symptoms. This study noted the discrepancy between the prevalence of reported TMD symptoms (26%) and signs of TMD documented by clinical examination (76%). The authors concluded that subclinical signs of TMD were common in this sample and awareness of symptoms was less common.

Development of Indices to Measure Temporomandibular Disorders

The development of indices to measure severity of TMD was an important research contribution. It was clear from the available studies that signs and symptoms of TMD were common. Despite the use of sound epidemiologic methods it was difficult to assess the severity and treatment needs of TMD. Counting signs and symptoms to assess the prevalence of TMD was of limited value because it did not discriminate by severity. Researchers, therefore, began to develop indices of TMD severity.

Using the sample previously described,[9] Agerberg and Carlsson developed an index of severity based on summing the number of symptoms.[15] They hypothesized a correlation of subjects who reported more symptoms with greater severity of symptoms. The index was of limited value because it was developed by using questionnaire data without the benefit of a physical examination. Also, no attempt was made to assess the validity or reliability of the index.

The Helkimo Index of TMD was developed by using data derived from patient history and physical examination.[16] The purpose of the index was to group individuals on the basis of the severity of their symptoms. The index has two components, based on the patients' reported symptoms (Anamnestic Index or A_i) and clinical examination (Dysfunction Index or D_i). The A_i scale ranges from A_i0 (having no symptoms) to $A_i III$ (the most severe symptoms such as locking or pain with opening). The Dysfunction Index is based on scoring the following clinical variables: range of motion, joint function, muscle pain, TM joint pain, and pain with jaw movement. The scores are summed and patients are grouped into one of four D_i categories ranging from D_i0 to D_iIII (no dysfunction to severe dysfunction).

Although the Helkimo Index may adequately group patients in terms of TMD severity, it provides little information on treatment need. Estimates of treatment need using the Helkimo Index were based on the assumption that increasing levels of the index were correlated with treatment need. In addition, the index provides no diagnostic or etiologic information. For example, patients with a fractured condyle, with severe symptoms of internal derangement or myofascial pain, or with TM joint ankylosis may all have the same D_i score.

The Craniomandibular Index (CMI), developed by Fricton and Schiffman, has been documented to be both reliable and valid.[17, 18] Like the Helkimo Dysfunction Index, the CMI is calculated on the basis of clinical findings of signs of TMD and is composed of two subindices, the Dysfunction Index (DI) and the Muscle Index (MI). The value of the two subindices is that they aid in grouping patients on the basis of primarily arthrogenous (DI) or myogenous (MI) clinical signs. The DI includes items related to range of motion, deviation, pain, and joint noise during movement, and TM joint tenderness. The MI includes items related to pain in response to palpation of the muscles of mastication and neck. Each item in the DI and MI is scored as 1 if positive. The DI is calculated by summing the total number of positive signs and dividing by 26 (range of DI = 0 to 1). The MI is computed by summing the total number of positive signs and dividing by 36 (range of MI = 0 to 1). The CMI is computed by averaging the sum of the DI and MI ([DI + MI]/2). The range of the CMI is 0 to 1.

The value of the CMI includes its ease of use after training/calibration; subindices to categorize clinical signs as primarily arthrogenous, myogenous, or both; and its documentation as being reliable and valid. One problem with the CMI is that clinical signs are not weighted on the basis of severity. For example, a patient who has a maximal incisal opening of 35 and a patient who opens 3 mm both receive a positive score of 1. The CMI shares the problem of other indices in that it provides no information regarding diagnosis or cause.

EPIDEMIOLOGIC STUDIES 1980 TO 1989

Earlier studies used cross-sectional data to estimate the point prevalence of TMD. Studies published in the 1980s began to collect data longitudinally. Longitudinal studies allow one to estimate the incidence (number of new cases per 100,000 population per year) of disease. (See the section on TM disorders in pediatric and geriatric populations for a review of studies using longitudinal designs.)

Using the Helkimo Index, Szentpetery and coworkers estimated the severity of TMD in a random sample of urban inhabitants.[19] The sample consisted of 600 people (45.7% male) with a mean age of 40.7 years (range 12 to 85). No TMD symptoms were reported by 79.3% of the sample (A_i0). Severe symptoms (A_iII) were reported by 5.3% of the sample. In contrast, 79.8% of the sample had objective clinical signs of TMD and 7.5% of the patients had moderate to severe signs (D_iII to D_iIII).

The most commonly encountered clinical sign was joint noise (46.5%). Women had joint noise more commonly than men, 57.1% to 34.7%, respectively ($P \leq .001$). Muscle tenderness was documented for 17.0% of the sample, again with women reporting a positive finding more commonly than men, 21.6% to 11.9%, respectively ($P \leq .01$). In the sample, 3.2% of the participants reported joint pain with palpation. Women reported it more commonly than men, 5.4% to 0.7%, respectively ($P \leq .01$).

To estimate the prevalence of TMD, Pullinger and associates reported on a nonpatient sample of young students (dental and dental hygiene students).[20] There were 253 eligible participants, of which 222 completed the study. The mean age of the sample was 23.9 years (19 to 40) and 54% were men. The authors chose this sample because young people have a higher risk for TMD and the data may be more representative of the population at risk.

Overall, 39% of the participants reported symptoms of TMD. Using the Helkimo Index, 41% of the sample had no clinical findings and 18% had moderate to severe clinical findings (D_iII to D_iIII). The most common clinical sign was joint noise (46.5%), and females outnumbered males, 57% to 35%, respectively ($P < .05$). Muscle tenderness to palpation was reported by 48% of the sample. Women had muscle tenderness more commonly than males, 68% to 33%, respectively ($P < .001$). Joint tenderness was elicited from 13.5% of the sample, and women were more commonly affected than men, 78% to 22% ($P < .001$).

Summary of Epidemiologic Findings 1980 to 1989 Although the actual numbers varied considerably, several trends were observed. Prevalence estimates suggest that TM disorders were common. Objective clinical signs were more common than patient report of symptoms. Signs and symptoms of TMD were common in the general population with the reported prevalence ranging from 21% to 57% for symptoms and 59% to 80% for signs. The demographic distribution of signs and symptoms in the general population was much different than in TMD patient samples. On average, females tended to have more signs and symptoms of TMD than men, but the differences are much smaller than in TMD patient samples. The introduction of TMD indices aided in grouping study participants by severity of TMD but failed to elucidate the underlying cause of the disorder. There was growing dissatisfaction with counting signs and symptoms to estimate the prevalence of TMD.

EPIDEMIOLOGIC FINDINGS SINCE 1990

The research in the 1990s can be characterized by the application of sound, sophisticated epidemiologic methods to estimate prevalence and treatment needs (see Figs. 6–2 and 6–3). As noted earlier, the indices used to assess the severity of TMD provided little information regarding disease states or cause. In the 1990s, attempts were made to estimate the prevalence of specific disease states: internal derangement (International Classification of Diseases, 9th revision [ICD-9] code 524.63) and structural bone changes of the mandibular condyle (ICD-9 codes 715.38, 716.98, 714.9, and 716.98).

Estimates of Prevalence and Treatments of Temporomandibular Disorders

Although the Scandinavians generated a large body of epidemiologic work on TMD,

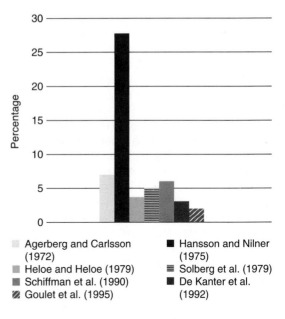

Agerberg and Carlsson (1972)
Heloe and Heloe (1979)
Schiffman et al. (1990)
Goulet et al. (1995)
Hansson and Nilner (1975)
Solberg et al. (1979)
De Kanter et al. (1992)

FIGURE 6–3. Estimated need for treatment of TMD.

it was not clear that it was appropriate to generalize their results to North American populations. In 1990, Dworkin and colleagues published the first large-scale epidemiologic study of TMD in the United States.[21] Using a sophisticated study design, the investigators compared randomly selected controls with symptomatic patients not seeking treatment and patients with symptoms of TMD seeking treatment. The study sample was composed of 210 community controls (COCO—random sample of individuals who reported no TMD symptoms in the previous 6 months prior to enrollment), 121 community cases (COCA—symptomatic patients not seeking treatment), and 261 clinic cases (CLCA—symptomatic patients seeking treatment). The authors assessed findings on the basis of history (symptoms: TM joint noise, limitation of jaw motion, and pain with function) and clinical examination (signs: range of motion, joint noise, pain on palpation of the TM joint and/ or muscles of mastication).

In terms of demographic findings, the mean age of the three groups was not different. The female-to-male ratio differed among the three groups (COCO, COCA, CLCA): 1.5:1, 3:1, and 5:1, respectively. For the self-reported symptoms, the frequency of joint noise in the three groups (COCO, COCA, CLCA) was 7%, 47%, and 75%, respectively and the frequency of pain with function was 8.5%, 21%, and 50%, respectively. In terms of clinical signs, the maximal incisal opening progressively decreased in the three groups from COCO to CLCA. Joint noise was commonly detected on physical examination in all three groups at rates generally higher than patient self-report. Thirty-two sites were palpated to assess pain on palpation of the TM joint and muscles of mastication. Clinic cases averaged 9.9 painful sites, community cases averaged 7.3 sites, and community controls averaged 3.1 sites ($P = .001$).

The principal study findings were as follows: (1) clinic cases and controls were distinguished most readily by report of pain with function, pain with palpation, and decrease in maximal incisal motion; (2) many clinical findings relevant to TMD were found with comparable prevalence in cases and controls; (3) clinical findings varied little by age; and (4) clinical findings of joint noise and other signs were more common than patient report of these problems. Using sophisticated epidemiologic methods, the authors confirmed many of the findings reported by the Scandinavian researchers, suggesting that these earlier studies may be used for comparative purposes.

Schiffman and associates estimated prevalence and treatment needs for TMD in a sample at risk: young (ages 22 to 24) predominantly female (nursing students) individuals.[22] The eligible population was 292 students. The Helkimo Anamnestic Dysfunction Index and the Symptom Severity Index were computed on the basis of 269 completed questionnaires. Clinical examinations were completed on 250 students and were used to calculate the Helkimo Clinical Dysfunction Index and the Craniomandibular Index (CMI).

On the basis of the questionnaire, 57% of the sample reported one or more symptoms of TM disorders. Joint noise was reported by 44% of the sample. Thirty-four percent reported severe symptoms (A_iII). On clinical examination, 45.7% of the study subjects had joint noise and 40% had pain on palpation. Overall, 26% of the sample had severe clinical dysfunction (D_iIII) and 33% had moderate clinical dysfunction (D_iII).

This study's value lies in the authors' attempts to discriminate among the various TMDs. The authors grouped the study sample on the basis of signs/symptoms consistent with a TM joint disorder, a muscle disorder, or both. TM joint dysfunction was grouped into internal derangement (ID) with reduction, ID without reduction (acute), and ID without reduction (chronic). Using the findings from the CMI or Helkimo Dysfunction Index, the authors estimated that 31% of the sample was free of TMD, 19% had primarily joint problems, 23% had primarily muscle problems, and 27% had both TM joint and muscle problems. Overall, the authors estimated that 6% of the sample had signs/symptoms of sufficient severity to warrant treatment. In the group with primarily muscle problems, 2% were candidates for treatment. Of patients with unilateral joint symptoms, 5% were candidates for treatment. Of patients with bilateral joint symptoms, however, 22% were candidates for treatment.

Spruijt and Hoogstraten published a methodologic review of TM joint noise.[23] The wide range of TM joint noise prevalence may be attributable to use of different study populations and measurement techniques. The most compelling methodologic issue, however, was discriminating joint noise due to disease from benign joint noise. Granted, TM joint noise may be an abnormal finding, but only a small fraction of the population with noise has pathologic noise. Consequently, when normal and abnormal cannot be discriminated, the prevalence of pathologic joint noise may be overestimated. Although other studies document a disparity between joint noise detected on examination and patient report of joint noise, in this study, there was concordance between joint noise reported by the subject and noise detected on clinical examination. This may reflect a definitional change in the clinical assessment of joint noise. For joint noise to be documented on clinical examination, it had to be reported by the patient and be palpable to the examiner. Commonly, joint noise may be assessed by using a stethoscope to magnify joint sounds. Consequently, joint noise assessed in this manner may be overrepresented and clinically normal joints were misclassified as being abnormal as a result of the presence of joint noise.

Utilizing data from a Dutch national dental survey, De Kanter and coworkers estimated the demand and need for treatment of TMD in adults.[24] A sample of 6577 persons was selected to be representative of the Dutch population aged 15 to 74 years. The final sample size was 3468. Assessment of TMD was based on questionnaires and clinical examinations. Severity of TMD was classified using the Helkimo Index. In terms of the questionnaire, 78.5% of the sample was free of symptoms and 4.9% had moderate to severe symptoms (A_iII). On clinical examination, 55.5% of the sample was free of signs of TM disorders and 2.8% had moderate to severe signs of disorder (D_iII and III). Despite the discrepancy in overall estimates of TMD based on symptoms (21.5%) and signs (44.5%), there was good concordance between patients who reported severe symptoms (4.9%) and those who reported moderate to severe clinical signs (2.8%). The authors estimated that 3.1% of the Dutch population needed treatment for TMD.

In a highly selected sample, Dibbets and van der Weele documented the prevalence of structural bony changes in the mandibular condyle.[25] A sample of subjects (n = 172) who had received orthodontic treatment and ranged in age from 7 to 17 years were followed longitudinally for a total of 15 years. In the initial sample (n = 163 radiographs to review), 1% of the sample had positive radiographic findings. By the completion of the study (n = 101 radiographs), 5% of the sample had evidence of structural bony changes of the condyle. The age at diagnosis of changes was between 12 and 16 years. All but one patient had one-sided changes. Notably, signs/symptoms identified with bony change did not assist in the differential diagnosis, nor did they show any obvious pattern.

Although the authors reported prevalence data, a conservative estimate of the incidence of new cases of bony changes in the mandibular condyle per year can be made. Assuming this sample is representative of patients undergoing orthodontic treatment and using a constant denominator of 172, the incidence of bony changes in the condyle was estimated to be 308 new cases/year per 100,000 orthodontic patients. Under no circumstances should this estimate of incidence be applied to the general population. As noted earlier, the sample on which the incidence estimate is based is highly selected (orthodontic patients) and may not be representative of the population of adolescents aged 7 to 17 years.

Lipton and colleagues estimated the prevalence and gender distribution of orofacial pain in the United States.[26] The estimates were based on data collected as part of the 1989 National Health Interview Survey (NHIS). The sample was composed of 45,711 households selected to be representative of the civilian, noninstitutionalized, nonmilitary population of the United States over the age of 18 years. Usable data were received from one person, age ≥ 18 years, per household for 42,370 of the 45,711 total interviewed households (response rate = 92.7%). Overall, 5.3% of the sample had reported jaw joint pain more than one time in the last 6 months. The female-to-male ratio was 2.1:1 (6.9% female, 3.5% male). In contrast, the female-to-male ratios for toothache, oral sores, and burning mouth were approximately 1:1.

Schiffman and associates attempted to ascertain the relationship between the severity of TM signs and symptoms and the stage of TM joint internal derangement.[27] Two clinicians examined 42 patients prior to bilateral TM joint arthrographic evaluation. The level of mandibular dysfunction was scored using the Helkimo Index and the Craniomandibular Index (CMI). Analysis revealed that the level of mandibular dysfunction as measured by the Helkimo Index and the CMI was not associated with TM joint internal derangement. This study confirmed previous speculation that indices provided information regarding the severity of mandibular dysfunction but provided no etiologic information.

Goulet and coworkers conducted a cross-sectional questionnaire study to estimate the jaw pain prevalence and treatment needs by using a randomized, stratified sample.[28] The study sample was designed to represent the general population in Quebec, Canada. The original sample size was 1675; the final sample size was 897, which represents a 53% response rate. Given this low response rate, the results should be interpreted with caution. Overall, 30% of those sampled reported a history of jaw pain. Only 7% of the sample, however, reported frequent jaw pain. Women were almost twice as likely as men (9% versus 5%) to report frequent jaw pain. In patients reporting jaw pain, 41% reported the pain severity as being moderate to severe. Overall, severe pain was reported by 1 of 7 women and 1 of 25 men, suggesting a relationship between pain severity and gender ($P < .01$). Joint noise was reported by 30% of the sample, and frequent episodes of joint noise were reported by 4%. Women were twice as likely to report joint noise as men ($P < .01$). In the 9 months prior to the interview, 2% of the sample reported seeking treatment for their symptoms. Overall, 3% of women and 1% of men reported seeking treatment ($P < .01$). Of patients seeking treatment, 70% were below the age of 45 years.

In a Swedish study published by Wanman and Wigren, the authors documented the need and demand for dental treatment in a stratified, randomly selected sample of three different age groups, 35-, 50-, and 65-year-olds.[29] The sample was selected to represent a Swedish community. Mandibular dysfunction was classified by using the Helkimo Index. By history, the proportion of symptom-free patients (A_i0) increased by age among the three age groups 57%, 59%, and 67%, respectively. On clinical examination, however, the proportion of patients free of signs of TMD (D_i0) decreased with age from 45% at 35 years and 46% at 50 years to 30% in the 65-year-olds. Most of the change was due to an increase in the proportion of patients with mild to moderate (D_iI or D_iII) severity scores. The proportion of patients with severe dysfunction index scores (D_iIII) was relatively unchanged among the three age groups.

There were significant discrepancies between professional assessment of treatment needs and actual treatment sought by patients in all three age groups. In the 35-year-old group, the professional assessment of treatment needs to manage TMD was 26%. Overall, 4% of the sample actually sought treatment. In patients seeking treatment, 66% received occlusal adjustment and 33% received splint therapy. In the 50-year-old group, the professional assessment of need for treatment was that 14% of the sample would benefit from treatment. Approximately 4.5% of the sample actually sought treatment. In the 65-year-old group, 7% of the sample was felt to benefit from treatment, but only 1.2% actually sought treatment.

In an attempt to estimate the prevalence of internal derangement of the TM joint, Katzberg and colleagues used radiographic imaging (magnetic resonance imaging [MRI]) to assess disk displacement in a group of asymptomatic volunteers and symptomatic patients.[30] The control group was composed of volunteers with a mean age of 28.3 years, and 49% were male. Overall, 33% of the control group had MRI evidence of at least one displaced disk. In the control group the distribution of men to women was almost one to one; however, the prevalence of MRI-diagnosed disk displacement for females was 39% versus 24% in males ($P = .12$). One should be cautious of generalizing the results of this study to other groups of populations. The authors did not describe well how volunteers were recruited so we have little information regarding potential selection biases in the study sample. The findings in this study regarding the prevalence of a potential disease state (internal derangement) in asymptomatic subjects, however, are comparable to those of other studies, in which the prevalence was estimated to be 32% and 21%.[31, 32] Given the high prevalence of disk displacement in otherwise asymptomatic subjects, one must consider the possibility that internal derangement represents a normal variant of disk position in adults.[33]

Summary Sound epidemiologic studies from the 1990s based on North American populations confirm many of the earlier findings reported by the Scandinavians. Specifically the signs and symptoms of TMD in the general population were common and clinical signs were detected more frequently than the number of subjects reporting symptoms would suggest. In addition, for many of the signs and symptoms in terms of both frequency and severity, females were more likely to have positive findings than males and more likely to seek treatment. Of interest, when examining subjects likely to seek treatment for their TMD in nonpatient samples, the age and gender distributions begin to approximate those seen in patient samples: predominantly female and young (below age 50). As suggested by earlier researchers, indices of TMD were documented to be nonspecific in terms of diagnoses. Some excellent work has been used to estimate treatment needs of TMD in the general population and the results are quite consistent: 3% to 6% of the population would benefit from treatment of TMD. The discrepancy between the professional need for treatment and actual treatment sought is of interest and would benefit from additional research. An important contribution of epidemiologic researchers in the 1990s was the effort to estimate the prevalence of specific disease states, and not simply to measure signs and symptoms of TMD. These studies addressing disease states use weaker methods so results should be interpreted cautiously. For those seeking additional information on the prevalence of TMD, De Kanter and associates have written an excellent review article.[34]

Temporomandibular Disorders in Pediatric and Geriatric Populations

The goals of epidemiologic research in pediatric and geriatric populations are similar in terms of assessing prevalence and treatment needs of TMD. In the pediatric population, however, the purpose of epidemiologic research was to assess potential preventative aspects of TM disorders. In the geriatric population, the epidemiologic research goal was to assess long-term consequences of TMD.

EPIDEMIOLOGY OF TEMPOROMANDIBULAR DISORDERS IN GERIATRIC POPULATIONS (Table 6–1)

In 1994, Schmidt-Kaunisaho and coworkers reported the results of an investigation to ascertain the prevalence of TMD in a sample of elderly residents of Helsinki, Finland.[35] The sample was composed of a randomly selected group of subjects born in 1904, 1909, and 1914 living in Helsinki in 1989 (population size of eligible subjects was 8035). The study sample was composed of 364 subjects of 600 selected subjects (response rate = 61%). Symptoms of TM disorders were scored by using the Helkimo Anamnestic Index (A_i). Overall, 34% of the sample reported some type of pain in the head and neck region. According to the Helkimo Index, 66% of all subjects were free of symptoms (A_i0), 14% had mild symptoms (A_iI), and 20% had severe symptoms (A_iII). Women reported symptoms more frequently than men ($P < .1$). Two percent of the sample reported their symptoms to be extremely severe. As the sample age increased, the proportion of subjects reporting symptoms decreased (37% at age 76, 32% at age 81, and 30% at age 86).

In a follow-up study, the authors reported the prevalence of signs of TMD in the same study sample, using the Helkimo Dysfunction Index (D_i).[36] The sample size was slightly smaller than in the other report (n = 342) and 29% were male. Overall, 20% of the sample were free of signs of TMD (D_i0). In the sample, 57% of subjects had mild signs (D_iI), 19% had moderate signs (D_iII), and 4% had severe signs (D_iIII) of TM dysfunction. Consistent with findings in samples of younger patients, clinical signs of dysfunction are documented more frequently than patient report of symptoms of dysfunction.

Soikkonen and colleagues reported the radiographic findings in the same study sample described.[37] The sample was composed of 124 edentulous subjects who had panoramic radiographic studies performed and evaluated. Of note, 17% were reported to have changes in condylar anatomic characteristics. The proportion of men and

TABLE 6–1.	Geriatric Samples—Estimates of TMD and Treatment Needs

Author	Design	Selection	Response Rate (%)	n	% Male	≥1 Symptom (%)	≥1 Sign (%)	Treatment Need (%)
Schmidt-Kaunisaho et al. (1994)	Cross-sectional	Randomly selected	61	364	28	34	—	—
Soikkonen et al. (1994)	Cross-sectional	Randomly selected	57	342	29	—	80	—
Bibb et al. (1995)	Cross-sectional	Eligible	50	429	42	12	35	<1

women having condylar abnormalities was 13% and 19%, respectively. Caution should be exercised in generalizing the findings from any of the studies described. Although the original sample may reflect the underlying study population, poor response rates of the samples undergoing evaluation of TMD may introduce selection bias that significantly affects the results in an unknown manner.

Bibb and associates estimated the prevalence of TMD signs and symptoms in a large elderly sample based in the United States.[38] The sample was composed of Medicare recipients, and the sample size was 429 subjects derived from an eligible sample of 866 subjects. The mean age of the sample was 74.4 years and 42% were male. Assessment of TM disorders was based on patient self-report and clinical examination. Overall, 12% of subjects reported a history of TMD and 6.5% reported pain with jaw function. Joint noise was documented in 35.2% of the sample, joint tenderness in 8.4%, muscle tenderness in 12.8%, and limitation of jaw motion in 22.4%. Overall, 1% of the sample had clinical findings or complaints that would warrant referral for evaluation and possible treatment. The authors assessed the relationship between TMD and health status measures. The lack of consistent relationship between TMD signs and symptoms and general health status suggests that TMDs are localized processes and not an extension of a general condition such as arthritis or depression, nor do they have a major impact on activities of daily living.

Summary The studies reviewed suggest that TMDs are not a major problem in the geriatric population. The implication of these findings is that intervention at a younger age to prevent problems in the future is not necessary. Treatment in the geriatric population should be focused on patients who demand treatment as a result of unacceptable symptoms of TMD, rather than attempting to screen and treat for TMD.[39]

EPIDEMIOLOGY OF TEMPOROMANDIBULAR DISORDERS IN PEDIATRIC POPULATIONS (Table 6–2)

Evaluation of TMD is of particular interest to pediatricians, pediatric dentists, and orthodontists because of the potential value of early detection and treatment in preventing problems in adulthood. It is not clear, however, that TMD is a significant problem in the pediatric population or that early detection and treatment play a role in preventing TMD-related problems in adulthood.

Unlike the cross-sectional studies seen commonly in the adult and geriatric populations, pediatric samples lend themselves to longitudinal studies. Magnusson and co-workers reported on a sample of 11- and 15-year-old subjects who had been examined for signs and symptoms of TMD 4 years earlier (ages 7 and 11).[40] The purpose of the study was to estimate the prevalence of TMD for each age group and to assess changes in the groups over time. The sam-

TABLE 6–2.	Pediatric Samples—Estimates of TMD and Treatment Needs							
Author	Design	Selection	Age Range (yr)	n	Male (%)	≥1 Symptom (%)	≥1 Sign (%)	Treatment Need (%)
Magnusson et al. (1985)	Longitudinal	Random	7–15	119	49	—	—	6.7
			7			35	32	
			11			61	55	
			15			66	66	
Wanman (1987)	Longitudinal	Eligible	17–19	258	51	—	—	—
			17			20.4	—	
			18			19.3	—	
			19			21.6	—	
Ohno et al. (1988)	Cross-sectional	Eligible	10–18	2198	49.8	11.5	—	—
Motegi et al. (1992)	Cross-sectional	Eligible	6–18	7337	44	12.2	—	0.2

ple was composed of 119 subjects (66 subjects in the 7- to 11-year age group and 53 subjects in the 11- to 15-year age group). The point prevalence of subjects reporting one or more symptoms of TMD increased with age (35% at age 7, 61% at age 11, and 66% at age 15). In terms of longitudinal changes, there was a significant increase between ages 7 and 11 in the frequency of children reporting one or more TMD symptoms (35% to 62%, $P < .01$). The changes between ages 11 and 15 were less dramatic. At age 11, 60% of the sample reported one or more TMD symptoms; 66% reported one or more symptoms at age 15.

Clinical function was assessed by using the Helkimo Dysfunction Index (D_i). The prevalence of TMD signs for each age group was 32% at age 7, 55% at age 11, and 66% at age 15. Only 2% of the sample had severe clinical signs (D_iIII). In terms of longitudinal changes in clinical signs, over the 4-year time periods, 52% of the sample had no change in the D_i score, 34% got worse, and 13% improved.

The findings of this study suggested that signs and symptoms of TMD were common in all age groups including children and that clinical signs increased with increasing age in children. It is important to stress that the clinical signs found in this investigation were mild and the need for treatment was small.

In research by Wanman published in 1987, the author performed a longitudinal study of TMD in adolescents (age 17).[41] The study purpose was to assess the prevalence of TMD at age 17 and follow the development (or remission) of TMD over the ensuing 2 years. The sample was composed of all 17-year-old residents of the Swedish town of Skelleftea. The original sample was composed of 285 subjects (100% of the eligible population) and a total of 258 subjects completed all three examinations at ages 17, 18, and 19. Males composed 51% of the sample. At age 17, 13 subjects (4.56%) of the sample were treated for TMD. At follow-up, another 6 subjects (2.2%) were treated and 7 subjects treated earlier were re-treated. Overall, 19 subjects (14 females and 5 males) were treated for TMD (6.67%).

Over time, there was little change in the proportion of subjects who reported one or more symptoms of TMD: age 17 to 20, 4%; age 18 to 19, 3%; and age 19 to 21, 6%. At

age 17 there was no significant difference in gender in the proportion of subjects reporting one or more symptoms. At ages 18 and 19, however, more females than males reported one or more symptoms ($P < .05$).

In terms of clinical signs (scored by using the Helkimo Dysfunction Index [D_i]), at age 17, 39% of males and 65% of females had clinical signs of TMD. At age 18, 45% of males and 60% of females had D_i scores greater than 0. At age 19, 43% of males and 57% of females had D_i scores greater than 0. Of the sample, at all ages examined, three subjects (all female at age 19) had severe D_i scores.

On the basis of the results of the study, the authors concluded (1) that signs and symptoms of TMD were common and mild in adolescents, (2) that females reported more signs and symptoms than males, and (3) that signs and symptoms fluctuated unpredictably over time. Given the frequency of signs and symptoms of TMD, the authors recommended that an examination of signs and symptoms of TMD was appropriate in this age group to document the frequency, intensity, and duration of signs and symptoms. The need and demand for treatment, however, were small.

In a large cross-sectional study of Japanese schoolchildren (age 10 to 18) the authors estimated the subjective recognition of TMD.[42] The sample size was 2198 and composed of 49.8% males. Overall, the subjective recognition of TM disorders was reported by 11.5% of the sample with no difference in the frequency by gender. Interestingly, the proportion of subjects reporting TMD decreased with age from 18.5% of primary school age children to 10.1% of senior high school age children. In the junior high school age group, 11.3% of the subjects reported TMD.

In another Japanese study, the authors reported the results of a large-scale cross-sectional study of subjects age 6 to 18 years.[43] Their findings were remarkably consistent with those of the Japanese study reported previously. The sample was composed of 7337 subjects, of whom 44% were male. TMD symptoms were reported by 12.2% of the sample with a slight female predominance (13% vs. 11.1%). When grouped by age, 5.7% of subjects aged 6 to 11 reported symptoms, 14.5% of subjects aged 12 to 14 reported symptoms, and

17.4% of subjects aged 15 to 17 reported symptoms. The increase in prevalence estimates of TMD with age was statistically significant ($P < .01$). Twelve subjects (0.2%) received treatment for TMD.

Summary Reportable signs and symptoms of TMD are common but generally mild in children. Treatment needs are few (range 0.2% to 6.6%). Although several authors report that examination and documentation of TMD are important,[28, 29] there is no evidence that early recognition and treatment play any role in preventing or alleviating future signs and symptoms of TMD. Given the dearth of information regarding treatment of TMD in the pediatric population, caution should be exercised in recommending and implementing treatment.

Summary of Findings and Directions for Future Research

Based on sound epidemiologic studies, TMDs do not represent a major public health problem. On the other hand, the studies suggest that between 3% and 6% of the nonpatient population may benefit from evaluation and management of signs and symptoms of TMD. In the United States, this represents a potential group of 7.5 to 15 million patients.

Epidemiologic research findings have treatment and management implications. Based on the studies in nonpatient populations, the clinical examination consistently detects more signs of TMD than does patient self-report. In fact, the clinical examination estimates the frequency of signs of TMD almost twice as often as the patient self-report of symptoms of TMD. Given these facts, in the absence of patient complaint, it is important to document signs of TMD but proceed cautiously with treatment recommendations. Treatment of the condition should not be worse than the condition itself.

Future research efforts should focus on a few key areas. For example, until we can explain the female/male discrepancy in patient samples, we cannot say we understand TM disorders. Future study samples should be derived from populations at risk for TM disorders. It is of little value to dilute the sample with low-risk individuals as doing

so may mask subtle risk factors. On the basis of current epidemiologic research, we have a good understanding of the distribution of TMD. We need to focus now on measuring the prevalence and treatment needs of specific disease entities that are included under the rubric of TMD. As such, there is little value in more studies of symptoms or severity of TMD. Based on current publications we have a good understanding of the distribution of signs, symptoms, and severity of TMD.

When reviewing articles related to TMD, one should keep in mind the following considerations because they have important ramifications in interpreting the results:

1. How was the study sample selected?
   a. Was it a random sample representative of a specific population, or was it a nonrandom convenience sample?
   b. Is the sample composed of TMD patients or non-TMD patients?
   c. What proportion of the eligible study sample actually enrolls in the study, and what effect might this have on the study results?
2. Does the author unambiguously define which TMDs are being investigated?
3. Finally, how is the disease state defined and measured? Much of the variability among the studies may be attributed to bias due to sample selection, disease definition and measurement, and response rates.

REFERENCES

1. Boman K: Temporomandibular joint arthrosis and its treatment by extirpation of the disk: A clinical study. Acta Chir Scand 1947;95:51–63.
2. Markowitz HA, Gerry RG: Temporomandibular joint disease. Oral Surg Oral Med Oral Pathol 1949;2:1309–1337.
3. Schwartz LL: A temporomandibular joint pain-dysfunction syndrome. J Chron Dis 1956;3:284–293.
4. Hankey GT: Affections of the temporomandibular joint. Proc R Soc Med 1956;49:983–999.
5. Schwartz LL, Cobin HP: Symptoms associated with the temporomandibular joint. Oral Surg Oral Med Oral Pathol 1957;10:339–344.
6. Campbell J: Distribution and treatment of pain in temporomandibular arthroses. Br Dent J 1958;105:393–402.
7. Thomson H: Mandibular joint pain: A survey of 100 treated cases. Br Dent J 1959;107:243–251.
8. Perry HT: The symptomatology of temporomandibular joint disturbance. J Prosthet Dent 1968;19:288–298.
9. Agerberg G, Carlsson GE: Functional disorders of the masticatory system. I. Distribution of symp-

toms according to age and sex as judged from investigation by questionnaire. Acta Odontol Scan 1972;30:597–613.

10. Helkimo M: Studies on function and dysfunction of the masticatory system. I. An epidemiological investigation of symptoms of dysfunction in Lapps in the north of Finland. Proc Finn Dent Soc 1974;70:37–49.

11. Helkimo M: Studies on function and dysfunction of the masticatory system. IV. Age and sex distribution of symptoms of dysfunction of the masticatory system in Lapps in the north of Finland. Acta Odontol Scand 1974;32:255–267.

12. Hansson T, Nilner M: A study of the occurrence of symptoms of diseases of the temporomandibular joint masticatory musculature and related structures. J Oral Rehabil 1975;2:313–324.

13. Heloe B, Heloe LA: Frequency and distribution of myofascial pain-dysfunction syndrome in a population of 25-year-olds. Community Dent Oral Epidemiol 1979;7:357–360.

14. Solberg WK, Woo MW, Hourston JB: Prevalence of mandibular dysfunction in young adults. J Am Dent Assoc 1979;98:25–34.

15. Agerberg G, Carlsson GE: Functional disorders of the masticatory system. II. Symptoms in relation to impaired mobility of the mandible as judged from investigation by questionnaire. Acta Odontol Scand 1973;31:335–347.

16. Helkimo M: Studies on function and dysfunction of the masticatory system. II. Index for the anamnestic and clinical dysfunction and occlusal state. Swed Dent J 1974;67:101.

17. Fricton JR, Schiffman EL: The craniomandibular index: Validity. J Prosthet Dent 1987;58:222–228.

18. Fricton JR, Schiffman EL: Reliability of a craniomandibular index. J Dent Res 1986;65:1359–1364.

19. Szentpetery A, Huhn E, Fazekas A: Prevalence of mandibular dysfunction in an urban population in Hungary. Community Dent Oral Epidemiol 1986;14:177–180.

20. Pullinger AG, Seligman DA, Solberg WK: Temporomandibular disorders. Part I. Functional status, dentomorphologic features, and sex differences in a nonpatient population. J Prosthet Dent 1988;59:228–235.

21. Dworkin SF, Huggins KH, LeResche L, Von Korff M, Howard J, Truelove E, Sommers E: Epidemiology of signs and symptoms in temporomandibular disorders: Clinical signs in cases and controls. J Am Dent Assoc 1990;120:273–281.

22. Schiffman EL, Fricton JR, Haley DP, Shapiro BL: The prevalence and treatment needs of subjects with temporomandibular disorders. J Am Dent Assoc 1990;120:295–303.

23. Spruijt RJ, Hoogstraten J: The research on temporomandibular joint clicking: A methodologic review. J Craniomandib Disord Facial Oral Pain 1991;5:45–50.

24. De Kanter RJ, Kayser AF, Battistuzzi PG, et al: Demand and need for treatment of craniomandibular dysfunction in the Dutch adult population [published erratum appears in J Dent Res 1993; 72(1):87]. J Dent Res 1992;71:1607–1612.

25. Dibbets JM, van der Weele LT: Prevalence of structural bony change in the mandibular condyle. J Craniomandib Disord Facial Oral Pain 1992; 6:254–259.

26. Lipton JA, Ship JA, Larach-Robinson D: Estimated prevalence and distribution of reported orofacial pain in the United States. J Am Dent Assoc 1993;124:115–121.

27. Schiffman EL, Anderson GC, Fricton JR, Lindgren BR: The relationship between level of mandibular pain and dysfunction and stage of temporomandibular joint internal derangement. J Dent Res 1992;71:1812–1815.

28. Goulet JP, Lavigne GJ, Lund JP: Jaw pain prevalence among French-speaking Canadians in Quebec and related symptoms of temporomandibular disorders. J Dent Res 1995;74:1738–1744.

29. Wanman A, Wigren L: Need and demand for dental treatment: A comparison between an evaluation based on an epidemiologic study of 35-, 50-, and 65-year-olds and performed dental treatment of matched age groups. Acta Odontol Scand 1995;53:318–324.

30. Katzberg RW, Westesson PL, Tallents RH, Drake CM: Anatomic disorders of the temporomandibular joint disc in asymptomatic subjects. J Oral Maxillofac Surgery 1996;54:147–155.

31. Kircos LT, Ortendahl DA, Mark AS: Magnetic resonance imaging of the TMJ disc in asymptomatic volunteers. J Oral Maxillofac Surg 1987;45:852.

32. Tasaki MM, Westesson P-L, Isberg AM: Classification and prevalence of temporomandibular joint disc displacement in patients and asymptomatic volunteers. Am J Orthod Dentofacial Orthop 1996;109:249–262.

33. de Bont LGM, Dijkgraaf LC, Stegenga B: Epidemiology and natural progression of articular temporomandibular disorders. Oral Surg Oral Med Oral Pathol Oral Radiol Endod 1997;83:72–76.

34. De Kanter RJ, Truin GJ, Burgersdijk RC, et al: Prevalence in the Dutch adult population and a meta-analysis of signs and symptoms of temporomandibular disorder. J Dent Res 1993;72:1509–1518.

35. Schmidt-Kaunisaho K, Hiltunen K, Ainamo A: Prevalence of symptoms of craniomandibular disorders in a population of elderly inhabitants in Helsinki, Finland. Acta Odontol Scand 1994; 52:135–139.

36. Hiltunen K, Schmidt-Kaunisaho K, Nevalainen J, et al: Prevalence of signs of temporomandibular disorders among elderly inhabitants of Helsinki, Finland. Acta Odontol Scand 1995;53:20–23.

37. Soikkonen K, Ainamo A, Wolf J, et al: Radiographic findings in the jaws of clinically edentulous old people living at home in Helsinki, Finland. Acta Odontol Scand 1994;52:229–233.

38. Bibb CA, Atchison KA, Pullinger AG, Bittar GT: Jaw function status in an elderly community sample. Community Dent Oral Epidemiology 1995; 23:303–308.

39. Greene CS: Temporomandibular disorders in the geriatric population. J Prosthet Dent 1994;72:507–509.

40. Magnusson T, Egermark-Eriksson I, Carlsson GE: Four-year longitudinal study of mandibular dysfunction in children. Community Dent Oral Epidemiol 1985;13:117–120.

41. Wanman A: Craniomandibular disorders in adolescents: A longitudinal study in an urban Swedish population. Swed Dent J Suppl 1987;44:1–61.

42. Ohno H, Morinushi T, Ohno K, Ogura T: Comparative subjective evaluation and prevalence study of TMJ dysfunction syndrome in Japanese adolescents based on clinical examination. Community Dent Oral Epidemiol 1988;16:122–126.

43. Motegi E, Miyazaki H, Ogura I, et al: An orthodontic study of temporomandibular joint disorders. I. Epidemiological research in Japanese 6–18 year olds. Angle Orthod 1992;62:249–255.

Clinical and Radiographic Diagnosis

CHAPTER

7

Clinical Evaluation for Temporomandibular Disorders and Orofacial Pain

James Fricton • Norman Mohl

Orofacial pain, including temporomandibular disorders (TMDs), is a common problem that, if misdiagnosed or inappropriately treated, may lead to chronic pain and a major personal crisis for the patient.[1–4] The potential complexity of these disorders can make traditional assessment and management of patients difficult. The variability of pain within and among individuals in terms of description, severity, location, and progression, which is frequently coupled with behavioral or psychosocial factors, may lead to diagnostic confusion in the clinician. Furthermore, symptoms such as nausea, tinnitus, paresthesias, and sensitive teeth, which are occasionally associated with orofacial pain, may suggest such diverse diagnoses as migraine headaches, otitis media, neuralgias, and tooth pulpitis. Thus, the frequently overlapping signs and symptoms exhibited by orofacial pain patients can be confusing, often resulting in multiple or vague diagnoses instead of a more specific differential diagnosis.

Several possible contributing factors, such as bruxism, postural habits, or emotional factors, may also complicate patient evaluation and, if neglected, can lead to inadequate or transient treatment outcomes.[5, 6] If orofacial pain continues without resolution, emotional and psychosocial problems such as depression, anxiety, sleep disturbances, task avoidance, and lifestyle disturbances may occur and further contribute to the problem.

Failure to consider each of these factors during the diagnostic process can lead to incorrect differential diagnoses, inadequate treatment regimens, and development of a chronic pain syndrome.

To address these issues in clinical practice and maximize patient outcomes, the complexity of orofacial pain disorders must be matched by the reliability, validity, and complexity of the diagnostic process. This chapter presents a protocol for enhancing diagnostic reliability and validity and thereby reducing the inherent uncertainty involved in evaluating patients with orofacial pain. It is hoped that this protocol will help clinicians understand each component of the diagnostic process and lead to more successful long-term management.

Problem List

The basis of this evaluation protocol is the establishment of a problem list, which, although patient-specific, is patterned after the problem-oriented medical record.[1–3, 7–9] The problem list includes specific definitions of chief complaints, historical information, physical examination findings, and contributing factors. This list is the essential component of the diagnostic "gold standard" for TMD and orofacial pain, which is based on the information gained from the chief complaint, history, physical examination, and, when indicated, consultations, imaging, or other diagnostic tests (Table 7–1).[10] The use of this information is also dependent on the existence of a diagnostic classification system that is based on valid, or at least acceptable, inclusion and exclusion diagnostic criteria. Thus, the definitions, criteria, classifications, and diagnostic processes and procedures used for any disorder should be able to differentiate that presumptive condition from normal structural or functional variability, from benign and subclinical conditions, and from other diseases or disorders with similar characteristics.[11] In addition, all contributing factors that may play a role in complicating the management of the disorder must, if at all possible, be identified. Comprehensive management then naturally follows by treating the diagnosed condition or conditions and reducing the contributing factors.

Establishing the patient's unique problem list depends on gathering as much accurate knowledge as possible about the patient as well as about his or her signs and symptoms.[12] To arrive at an accurate differential diagnosis in patients with orofacial pain, the techniques of history taking and physical evaluation must be well defined, reliable, and relevant. The physical examination should include an evaluation of the head and neck, the cranial nerves, and the masticatory and cervical musculoskeletal systems. Thus, the object is to develop a database for the patient that is sufficiently comprehensive, without being unwieldy, so that clinically useful information can be systematically obtained.[13] This chapter focuses on the techniques of history taking, physical examination, and additional diagnostic tests for orofacial pain with an emphasis on temporomandibular disorders.

The history of the problem often reveals information that points directly to a general diagnostic classification, if not to a specific

diagnosis (Tables 7–1 to 7–3). Physical examination of the patient should reinforce one's impression about the patient and provide more information in order to reduce uncertainty and ideally to lead to a more definitive diagnosis (see Table 7–2). Additional diagnostic studies, including blood studies, nerve blocks, pulp tests, radiographs, and psychometric testing, can, in some cases, help to rule out other disorders and provide information about possible contributing factors (see Table 7–3). These tests will rarely provide a definitive diagnosis in the absence of other clinical information. If, after completion of the diagnostic process, a high level of uncertainty about the diagno-

TABLE 7–2.	Standard Physical Examination for Temporomandibular Disorders and Orofacial Pain

General appearance
Mental status
Head and neck inspection
Cranial nerve function
Stomatognathic function
Muscle and joint palpation
Occlusal stability and function
Muscle strength and postural relationships

TABLE 7–3.	Diagnostic Studies for Temporomandibular Disorders and Other Orofacial Pain Disorders

Nerve blocks
    Peripheral nerve block
    Local infiltration
    Myofascial trigger point injection
    Sympathetic ganglion block
Radiographs
    TMJ arthrograms
    TMJ tomograms
    TMJ transcranials
    Panorex
    CT scan
    Individual films
    Angiogram
    Sialogram
Magnetic resonance imaging
Psychometric testing
Blood studies
Urinalysis
Radioisotope studies
Others

TABLE 7–1.	Components of an Evaluation for Patients with Orofacial Pain Disorders

History of presenting illness	Physical examination
Past medical history	Diagnostic studies
Personal history	Consultations

TABLE 7–4.	History of the Presenting Illness

Chief complaint and associated symptoms
Pain character
Pain severity
Temporal characteristics of the pain
Precipitating, aggravating, and alleviating factors
Onset date and events
Preexisting conditions
History of pain progression or persistence
Past and present medications
Past and present surgeries and other treatments
What led to referral

TABLE 7–6.	Review of Medical History

General health
Family history
Allergies
Past and present medication
Past surgeries
Previous hospitalizations
Past or present illnesses such as diabetes, heart
    disease, cancer
Last examination by a physician/dentist
Infectious diseases (hepatitis, human immunodeficiency
    virus, tuberculosis)
Bleeding disorders

sis persists or if a pathologic condition outside one's area of expertise exists, an appropriate consultation should be sought in order to gain an additional perspective on the patient's status.

HISTORY

In view of the fact that pain is a personal experience and can only be experienced and described by the patient, the history for pain problems in general is considered to be at least as important as the physical examination.[14] As Sir William Osler has succinctly described the importance of history, "Listen to the patient; he is giving you the diagnosis." The history should include defining each chief complaint and associated symptoms. This includes reviewing the character, severity, and temporal characteristics of the pain; precipitating, aggravating, and alleviating factors; onset and history of pain; past and present medications, surgeries, and other treatments; a personal history; a medical history; and a review of systems (Table 7–4). Clinicians must listen carefully, patiently, and nonjudgmentally as the patient describes each type of pain or complaint present, including the locations, character, severity, and duration of the symptoms. Chronic pain patients often have

multiple pain complaints with different descriptions, which may suggest that multiple conditions and diagnoses are involved in the problem. The manner in which the patient relates to the pain can also give important clues to the cause.[15]

The patient's chief complaint is a very important first step in the diagnostic process, especially since it may include varying qualitative or quantitative descriptors for pain. This can help the physician discern affective or sensory components of the pain and help him or her arrive at a differential diagnosis.[16, 17] Migraine headaches, for example, are typically described as throbbing pain, whereas tension-type headaches are usually of a constant and steady quality with a dull pressure sensation. In addition, the pain may vary in timing during the day, week, or year. Cluster headaches occur in clusters of weeks or months, and the patient is pain-free at other times. The pain from trigeminal neuralgia occurs for seconds to minutes with little pain in between pain attacks.

An adequate and relevant medical, dental, and personal history is also essential to the diagnostic process (Tables 7–5 to 7–8). An elaborate and lengthy illness history, for

TABLE 7–5.	Components of Personal History

Family	Social
Childhood	Relationships
Education	Health
Occupational	

TABLE 7–7.	Review of Systems

General health	Gastrointestinal
Dermatologic system	Genitourinary
Lymph nodes	Endocrine
Head, ear, eye, nose, throat	Obstetric-gynecologic
Dental	Neurologic
Hematopoietic	Muscle
Cardiovascular	Bones, joints
Respiratory	Psychiatric

TABLE 7–8.	General Appearance and Mental Status Evaluation
Color	Behavior
Gait	Appearance
Stability	Mood
Coordination	Affect
Ambulation	Language
Orientation	Nonverbal
Awareness	Memory

example, suggests a chronic pain problem and also gives clues as to what treatments to avoid. A medication history may reveal a chemical dependency problem or give clues to the physical aspects of the problem. For example, although the symptoms may be similar, carbamazepine usually improves a paroxysmal neuralgia but not an attack of acute muscle pain, thus helping to differentiate them. A personal history also allows the clinician to understand the patient and can uncover important contributing factors such as family stress, depression, or a familial predisposition. A medical history and review of systems are also critical to ruling out any medical or dental problem that may contribute to the symptoms as a primary or secondary diagnosis. Furthermore, questioning the patient about serious illnesses, hospitalizations, or previous medical care can reveal the presence of a related illness such as hypothyroidism, rheumatoid arthritis, labile hypertension, or Sjögren's syndrome that may contribute to orofacial pain. In summary, history taking for orofacial pain requires time, patience, ability to listen, and knowledge to ask the relevant follow-up questions. Without these available, the diagnosis and patient outcome may be compromised.

PRINCIPLES OF PHYSICAL EXAMINATION

A differential diagnosis may be established at any time, from the initial history to after several visits of diagnostic tests or trials. By the time a clinician is familiar with the patient's problem through a thorough history, the diagnosis or diagnostic group of most pain conditions should come into focus with an improved level of certainty. The physical examination for pain

may then be used to reduce uncertainty further by confirming thoughts about the history and refining the differential diagnosis. If the level of uncertainty at this stage is still too high, diagnostic tests such as temporomandibular joint (TMJ) imaging, consultations, or treatment trials may be necessary to secure a less uncertain differential diagnosis.

Physical examination for temporomandibular disorders and orofacial pain varies, depending on the location of the pain and the tentative impression or diagnosis. A physical examination may include inspection, palpation, percussion, auscultation, smell, and measurements to ascertain whether an abnormality or dysfunction that is related to the chief complaint is present. Inspection can reveal considerable information about the patient to the alert clinician. Slouching posture can point to depression; postural rigidity or clenching behavior can show excess muscle tension in the neck, shoulders, or jaws and may be associated with myofascial pain. Asymmetry, swelling, weakness, loss of function, dysfunction, skin changes, and other signs may lead to a finding of neoplastic disease or an infectious process. Inspection of the skin may reveal scars of past surgeries, skin trophic changes of causalgia, and color changes in local infection or systemic anemia. The patient's facial expression can reveal specific emotions, his or her relationship with the clinician or others in the room, or reactions to the specific questions being asked.

Palpation is the process of using touch to examine the body for signs of abnormalities. It can include finger palpation of the muscles for myofascial trigger points, the skin for hyperesthesia in causalgia, cold hands in migraine, lymph nodes for lymph adenopathy, joints for swelling and tenderness of arthritis, abdomen for organomegaly, and the rest of the head, face, neck, or body for a variety of possible conditions. Percussion of a part of the body can also be used in an attempt to detect clinical signs. For example, relative densities of parts of the body can be ascertained by listening to the sound produced by striking a finger against the opposite hand while it lies flat against the body part. Such a method is often used to reveal abnormalities in such organs as the lungs, liver, stomach, and urinary bladder. Percussion of teeth with the opposite end of a mirror can elicit problems with individual teeth.

Auscultation is the act of listening to body sounds through a stethoscope. Such conditions as the bruit of an arteriovenous fistula, aneurysms, murmurs of the heart and vessels, rales and friction rubs of lungs, crepitus in the joints, carotid, vertebral, and basivertebral insufficiency, and bowel sounds in a scrotal hernia can often be detected by this technique. Smell is also important in detecting abnormal odors in the breath, sputum, vomitus, feces, urine, or pus. Infections, diabetes, lung abscess, pancreatic disturbances, gas gangrene, and many other illnesses have distinctive odors. Thus, a clinician managing chronic pain patients should use all the senses and be aware of the possibility of a serious underlying disease that is causing the persistent pain.

A general appearance assessment includes factors such as ambulation, general malaise, postural imbalances, and general motor function (see Table 7–8). Motor function of the body includes three systems: the pyramidal or corticospinal system, the extrapyramidal system, and the cerebellar system.[18] Lesions of the pyramidal system can cause paralysis, weakness, muscle spasticity, and hyperactive deep tendon reflexes. Lesions of the extrapyramidal system cause postural instability and diminished muscle tone and function. Lesions of the cerebellar system affect coordination of movements of the trunk and extremities on the contralateral side. Central or peripheral lesions of the nervous system can also be uncovered by detecting sensory deficits in each nerve's distribution. Symptoms of numbness or tingling can be verified by accurate two-point discrimination testing, pin prick tests, and light touch tests. Disturbance of stereognosis, or inability to recognize size and shape of objects, reflects a parietal lobe lesion. Reflex testing of the deep tendon and superficial tendons can reveal upper or lower motor neuron disease, as in compression neuropathy or multiple sclerosis.

A mental status examination reveals the patient's state of awareness, general appearance, behavior, mood, affect, language function, nonverbal function, and memory (see Table 7–8). Abnormalities in the patient's mental status may point to a psychiatric condition or a higher cortical lesion such as intracranial neoplasm, cerebral vascular accidents, hematomas, edema, or arteriovenous malformations within or causing traction on the cortex. Clinicians should be aware of normal and abnormal characteristics of each aspect of mental status. Patients should be alert and aware of most activities occurring in the room. When a patient is dull or drowsy with attention that wanders, that state may indicate the presence of drug intoxication, depression, or an upper brain stem lesion. In general, most patients appear clean and well dressed. Grossly inappropriate dress may indicate secondary gain, counterproductive intentions, poor social environment, or alcoholism. The patient should respond to questions in a reasonable manner without unprovoked disruptive or unusual behavior. Inability to maintain a coherent line of thought may indicate a higher central nervous system (CNS) neuraxis lesion and memory disturbances. Patients should report accurately what they are feeling (mood), and their report should be consistent with the way the clinician views the patient's affect. Gross fluctuations or inconsistencies in mood and affect, either reported or observed, may indicate a central lesion or emotional disturbance. Language function is a patient's ability to comprehend language, acknowledge what is said, repeat words, name objects, write, and read. It can be affected by motor dysfunction and cognitive deficits. Nonverbal function is the ability to comprehend visual spatial relationships. It can be assessed by asking the patient to copy a three-dimensional-appearing cube from an example. Memory assessment includes immediate recall (recall five digits), ability to learn (name object and ask what it is later), and ability to retrieve old material (past presidents, address, names).

CRANIAL NERVE EXAMINATION

Assessment of cranial nerve function includes objective testing of each of the 12 cranial nerves (Table 7–9).[9] The olfactory nerve (I) can be tested by asking the patient to identify familiar odors such as tobacco, coffee, cloves, and peppermint. The nasal passages should be clear and each nostril tested with the eyes closed. The optic nerve (II) can be tested for visual acuity, the fundi

TABLE 7–9.	Cranial Nerves and Testing Their Function

Cranial Nerve	Function Test
I	Smell
II	Visual acuity
	Visual fields
	Pupils
	Size
	Shape
	Reaction
	Eye movement
III, IV, VI	Ptosis
	Diplopia
	Convergence
	Nystagmus
V	Facial sensation
	Sensory 1
	Sensory 2
	Sensory 3
	Motor of masticatory muscles
	Taste
	Corneal
VII	Motor of facial muscles
	Taste
VIII	Subjective hearing
	Rinne/Weber's test
IX	Swallow
	Cough
	Sensory
X	Gag reflex
	Speech
XI	Motor of neck muscles
XII	Motor of tongue muscles
Cervical	Motor
	Sensory

examined with an ophthalmoscope, and the visual fields examined with a confrontation approach. In the third technique, the patient is asked to cover one eye and fix his or her sight on the eye of the examiner about 40 inches (1 m) away. The examiner moves a flicking finger or pen light from the periphery to the center along a radius perpendicular to the interocular line until the target comes into the patient's vision. The examiner also observes the finger and compares the patient's visual field to the examiner's visual field to determine limitations in the patient's visual field. Any limitation may reflect blind spots caused by migraine, cataract, choroiditis, neuritis, retinitis, optic neuritis, optic atrophy, or tumors of the pituitary gland.

The oculomotor nerve (III) controls most eye movement and motion of the upper eyelid. Movement can be tested by asking the patient to follow the examiner's finger or pen light 20 inches away. The target should be moved right and left and then superiorly and inferiorly to determine limitations. The trochlear nerve (IV) innervates the superior oblique muscle, and, on contraction, causes the eye to rotate downward and outward. The abducens (VI) innervates the external rectus muscle and causes double vision if dysfunctional. This motor nerve is ordinarily the first one affected in such conditions as cavernous sinus thrombosis.

The trigeminal nerve (V) supplies sensation to the superficial and deep structures of the head and face and motor function to the muscles of mastication. Testing of the sensory division includes using a pin prick and the light touch of a cotton-tipped applicator to determine diminished or absent sensation compared to that of the contralateral side or another division. The ophthalmic, maxillary, and mandibular nerves need to be examined for sensation. The ophthalmic division (V1) supplies sensation to the conjunctiva, cornea, eyeball, upper eyelids, forehead, scalp, and nose. The maxillary division (V2) supplies sensation to the side of the nose, upper lips, cheeks, lower eyelids, lower temple, palate, and maxillary teeth and gingiva. The mandibular division (V3) supplies sensation to the jaw, cheeks, lower lip, tongue, floor of mouth, and mandibular teeth and gingiva. V3 also supplies the motor neurons to the temporalis, masseter, lateral pterygoid, and medial pterygoid muscles.

The facial nerve (VII) supplies taste to the anterior two thirds of the tongue and innervates all of the facial muscles, including the orbicularis oris, orbicularis oculi, frontalis, and buccinator muscles. Nerve VII can be tested by asking the patient to blow air in the cheeks, wrinkle the forehead, pucker the lips, smile, close eyes tight, and taste. The auditory nerve (VIII) supplies neural function for hearing and balance. Hearing can be tested using Weber's test or the Rinne test with a tuning fork. In testing hearing deficiencies with Weber's test, a middle ear obstruction is suspected if a resonating tuning fork on the middle forehead is heard more clearly on the affected side. A nerve dysfunction is suspected if it is heard better on the nonaffected side. In the Rinne test, a middle ear obstruction should be suspected if a tuning fork is heard better when placed on the mastoid than in front of the ear. An otoscope can also be used to determine patency of the tympanic membrane, rule out infections, and observe external ear obstructions.

The glossopharyngeal nerve (IX) supplies sensation to the upper pharynx and posterior part of the tongue and innervates the stylopharyngeus and pharyngeal constrictor muscles. Afflictions affecting these nerves are rare; however, when they occur they cause difficulty in swallowing or coughing and diminish the pharyngeal reflexes. Testing is done by asking the patient to swallow and cough. The vagus nerve (X) supplies sensory, motor, and autonomic function to the pharynx, larynx, lung, heart, and stomach. Afflictions eliminate the gag reflex and may cause deviation of the uvula, difficulties in swallowing and speech, as well as bradycardia. With recurrent laryngeal nerve damage, a nasal quality to speech is evident. Nerve IX can be tested by eliciting the gag reflex. The accessory nerve (XI) innervates the sternocleidomastoid and trapezius muscles. Afflictions affecting it decrease the ability to rotate the head and lift the shoulders. Testing can be done by repeating these movements against resistance. The hypoglossal nerve (XII) innervates the intrinsic and extrinsic tongue muscles and will typically result in asymmetric tongue function if afflicted. Nerve XII can be tested by asking the patient to stick out the tongue and move it left and right.

Disturbances of cranial nerve function result from a lesion of the cranial nerve ganglia or nuclei or efferent and afferent pathways associated with those nerves. Disturbances of the senses of smell, sight, sound, balance, taste, and touch of the face reflect a disorder affecting the cranial nerves. For example, meningitis can cause double vision, multiple sclerosis can cause optic atrophy and diminished vision, an acoustic neuroma can cause lack of sense of hearing. The motor function of the head and neck is mediated through the trigeminal (masticatory muscles), facial (facial expression), hypoglossal (tongue), and accessory (trapezius) cranial nerves. Paralysis, gross weakness, or spasticity of these muscles dictates further evaluation of these nerves through computed tomography (CT) scans,

magnetic resonance imaging, or neurosurgical evaluation. The important point is that pain may accompany any of these conditions as either a component of the problem or a coincidental event caused by other factors. The essence of differential diagnosis is to differentiate from among the several possibilities.

HEAD AND NECK INSPECTION

Inspection of the head and neck includes visual and manual inspection of each anatomic structure of the head and neck (Table 7–10). Clinicians should be aware of changes in symmetry, size, color, consistency, shape, or tenderness, the presence of which suggests an infectious, edematous, neoplastic, degenerative, obstructive, or dysfunctional process. Both diagnoses and contributing factors can be elicited during this assessment. Inspection of the hair and skin may reveal signs such as discoloration caused by hematoma, hemangioma, ulcers, or scarring due to herpes zoster. Abrasions may reveal recent trauma such as domestic abuse. Cranial asymmetry may reveal osteomas or old fractures. Lymph node enlargement may indicate tooth abscess, sinusitis, or serious cellulitis. Nasal asymmetry or septal deviation may indicate benign neoplasm, past trauma, or the source of nasal blockage and mouth breathing. The teeth and periodontium need to be examined clinically and radiographically for fractured teeth, pulpitis, caries, erosion due to abfraction, wear facets, excessive attrition, periodontal disease, or other oral abnormality. This includes testing for tooth mobility or fremitus. The salivary glands (sublingual, submandibular, and parotid) should be palpated for enlargement and inadequate,

TABLE 7–10.	Components of Head and Neck Inspection
Skull	Periodontium
Skin	Throat
Hair	Tonsils
Eyes	Vascularity
Ear	Nodes
Nose	Neck
Tongue	Salivary glands
Teeth	

cloudy salivary flow. Inspection of the eyes may reveal mydriasis (dilatation) due to neurasthenia or amphetamine ingestions or miosis (constriction) due to tabes dorsalis or narcotic ingestions. Wandering eyes and neck rigidity may reveal a meningitis condition. Inspection of the ear may reveal drainage, redness, or tenderness associated with an inner ear or auricle infection and the need for further tests and treatment. Facial symmetry can be assessed with inspection of the ears, eye level, facial size, nostrils, tip of nose, lips, and mentonian groove. It can be assessed intraorally with the frenula, palate, incisal position, and tongue. When the face is observed, particular attention should be paid to the lower third, from the base of the nose to the point of the chin.

The tongue warrants careful inspection because improper tongue position or chronic tongue habits can contribute to musculoskeletal pain. The presence of mucosal or tongue ridging indicates a tongue thrust habit against the teeth anteriorly, laterally, or both. The tongue often migrates to areas of lost teeth, also causing ridging or scalloping. Tongue volume should be examined for its ability to rest comfortably on the palate. Palatal shape could also be a factor if the tongue does not rest comfortably in its normal position. In correct tongue position the anterior third of the tongue lies on the rugae of the anterior palate. This can be determined by first observing whether the tongue position is between the dental arches as the lips are separated. If the tongue cannot be seen, it is probably in its palatal position. If it can be seen, an incorrect position probably exists. If the tongue position cannot be determined visually, the patient can simply be asked where the tongue is and asked to make a "cluck" sound. If this sound is done correctly, the tongue contacts the palate in its normal rest position, and a crisp, distinct cluck is produced. A patient can usually tell whether this sensation feels "usual" or not. If the tongue position is incorrect at rest, it most likely is incorrect during swallowing. Tongue position during speech may also create problems. Correct tongue position has two primary functions. First, the tongue's palatal position allows for optimal masticatory muscle relaxation, normal resting posture, and adequate freeway space. Second, it ensures that one's respiratory pattern is nasal rather than oral. Mouth breathing requires use of accessory anterior neck musculature and develops strained postural relationships because different air passages are involved. The tongue position influences breathing patterns. However, a clinician must not assume that every patient with a correct palatal tongue position has 100% nasal breathing.

Evaluation for a short upper lip should also be made. Poor lip closure can occur secondary to an anterior open bite, class II or class III malocclusions, mouth breathing, or prolonged childhood sucking habits. Each of these can add strain to the muscles and joints. For this evaluation, the patient is asked to curl the upper lip around the maxillary incisors. The upper vermilion border (red line where lip and upper lip tissue meet) should not be visible. If a patient has a short upper lip, complete lip closure at rest is difficult and these patients usually have up to half of their front teeth exposed when observed at rest.

Other hard and soft tissue indications of parafunctional habits should be evaluated. These signs include generalized tooth abrasion, localized wear facets, large buccinator or masseter muscles, tooth mobility or fremitus, and tongue or mucosal ridging. It is not unusual during an evaluation, particularly during the history, to notice masseter contraction caused by clenching. Childhood sucking habits that extend beyond the first few years of age, such as pacifier sucking or thumb sucking, can lead to increased use of the buccinator and neck muscles and anterior malocclusions or myofascial pain. Other habits such as nail biting, gum chewing, and tooth clenching and grinding can exert increased tension and forces on the masticatory muscles and teeth, which may lead to such conditions as myofascial pain, degenerative joint disease, excessive tooth wear, or tooth mobility.

ASSESSMENT OF CERVICAL FUNCTION

The cervical spine evaluation, if required, includes assessment of the posterior cervical spine, the upper thoracic spine, as well as the shoulders and upper extremities.[19] It should include active, passive, and resistive joint and muscle testing; muscle palpation;

TABLE 7–11.	**Components of Cervical Function Evaluation**
Cervical mobility	Cervical-thoracic junction
Pain in range of motion	Cervical lordosis
Noise in range of motion	Scoliosis
Radicular pain	Sleep position
Muscle strength	Distraction test
Forward head posture	Compression test
Lateral head tilt	Sensation upper extremity
Round shoulders	

neurologic evaluation of sensation; reflex testing; special cervical spine tests; and postural assessment (Table 7–11). Postural assessment includes observation of static and dynamic posture and questions regarding work positions, other daytime positions, and sleep positions. Static structural postural discrepancies can be elicited with specific radiologic studies, whereas functional postural problems, which are secondary to neuromuscular activity, must be assessed through observation of head position, spinal curves, and shoulder and pelvic levels. Assessment of overall spinal alignment begins cephalad and continues caudad to detect the presence of scoliosis, lordosis, or myalgia.

ASSESSMENT OF MASTICATORY SYSTEM FUNCTION

Assessment of the function of the masticatory system includes observations of the range of motion (ROM) of the mandible and the presence of pain and joint sounds during jaw movement (Tables 7–12 and 7–13). During the ROM assessment, the patient's max-

TABLE 7–12.	**Assessment of Masticatory Function**
Limits and pain in mandibular opening	Altered condylar movement including diminished translation or subluxation
Limits and pain in laterotrusion	Provocation tests including active resistance and sustained clenching
Pain in range of motion	
Deviation of opening (S curve or lateral)	Palpation of muscles
Joint noise in range of motion	Palpation of joint

imum opening from incisal edge to incisal edge should be measured with a millimeter rule and the opening pattern observed. The opening should then be stretched to determine whether pain exists and whether any limitation is fixed or flexible. The opening should be straight with no lateral deviations, S deviations, or jerkiness observed (Fig. 7–1). Maximum lateral excursive movements should also be measured, and any accompanying pain should be noted. Minimum normal jaw opening is considered to be two finger widths at the knuckles of the dominant hand or approximately 40 mm of incisal opening.[20, 21] Lateral motion should be 7 to 10 mm to both the right and left. Normal protrusive range is 7 to 10 mm. The lateral aspect of the TMJ should also be palpated while the jaw is closed and as it opens. The presence of subluxation or overt dislocation of one or both condyles can usually be determined by abnormal palpation during movement. If the range of motion is limited, the clinician must attempt to determine whether the limitation is due to contracture of one or more of the jaw closing muscles, a nonreducing anterior displacement of the articular disk (closed lock), coronoid process interference, a hematoma or infection, or some other condition, such as fibrous ankylosis or scleroderma, that will cause limitation.

In assessing sounds (clicking or crepitus) from the TMJ, palpation is generally sufficient because of the high prevalence and clinically insignificant nature of many TMJ sounds. Auscultation, e.g., use of a stethoscope, may be used if the palpation produces an equivocal result. The use of electronic devices to detect or record sounds from the TMJ is not recommended since such techniques produce a great many false-positive diagnoses.[22] Thus, the detection of sound from the TMJ is best done by direct palpation during repetitive opening, closing, and lateral movements (Fig. 7–2). It is also important to note that sounds in the TMJ do not imply abnormality or warrant treatment. Crepitus in the absence of pain may indicate the presence of osteoarthrosis, a noninflammatory degenerative process of the articular tissue that does not require specific therapeutic intervention. TMJ clicking is also exceedingly common in the population, may be caused by a variety of mechanisms, is usually not permanent, and does

TABLE 7–13.	**Problems in Mandibular Movement**
Maximum opening	Patient is asked to open as wide as possible and examiner measures the distance from incisal surface to incisal surface of maxillary and mandibular central incisors at the midline Positive result if 39 mm or less
Passive stretch opening	Gentle stretching by examiner beyond voluntary maximum opening and measure identical to maximum opening Positive result if 41 mm or less
Restriction	Positive result if maximum opening is less than 40 mm *or* subjective opinion of examiner that restriction exists for that individual
Pain on opening	Positive result if any pain, but not pressure or tightness, occurs with stretch *or* with maximum opening
Jerky opening	Positive result if not a smooth and/or continuous opening
S deviation on opening	An S curve deviation on opening or closing is positive result if >2 mm from midline
Lateral deviation on opening	A lateral deviation at full opening is positive result if >2 mm from midline
Protrusive	
Pain	Any pain, but not pressure or tightness, during or at maximum protrusion is positive result; teeth are slightly out of contact at end of range of motion
Limitation	Examiner measures the distance between labial surfaces of the maxillary incisors at maxillary midline when in centric occlusion and again at maximum voluntary protrusion; result is positive if the difference between the two values is less than 7 mm
Right and left laterotrusion	
a. Pain b. Limitation	Examiner marks the point on the mandibular incisors that matches the maxillary midline and measures the difference between this midline and the mandibular point after maximum laterotrusion; result is positive if <7 mm
Clinically can or is locked open	Voluntary or involuntary forward dislocation of the condylar head out of the glenoid fossa *combined* with fixation in that position (no time specified)
Clinically can or is locked closed	Voluntary or involuntary blocking of translation of the right and/or left condyle that is of short or permanent duration (fixation) as determined by manual palpation (condyle does not slide or translate anteriorly)
Rigidity of jaw	Resistance to manual rotation of jaw, voluntary or involuntary on manipulation suggests neuromuscular disorder

not necessarily imply that serious sequelae will follow.[10] If, however, these sounds are accompanied by joint pain, limitation in movement, and joint tenderness, therapeutic intervention is often indicated.

MUSCLE AND JOINT PALPATION

Tenderness of muscles is an essential criterion for diagnosing masticatory muscle disorders such as myofascial pain or myositis. In addition, tenderness on palpation of the TMJs strongly suggests the presence of synovitis or capsulitis of the joint. The diagnostic criteria for myofascial pain primarily involve

1. Localized tenderness to palpation at points in firm bands or skeletal muscle, tendons, or ligaments, often termed trigger points

2. Pain complaints that follow consistent patterns of referral from trigger points
3. Reproducible alteration or replication of the pain with specific palpation of the trigger point

Unfortunately, the intraexaminer and interexaminer reliability of muscle palpation is low, although prior calibration can improve its replicability.[23] The low reliability is due to several factors, such as the variability and cyclical nature of most orofacial pain, the patient's mood, and the patient's subjective perceptions based on previous experiences with pain. In addition, clinician-related variables such as the anatomic area palpated by the clinician and the amount of force applied can dramatically affect the patient's response to the palpation. Use of a pressure algometer for muscle palpation can reduce this latter variable and make palpa-

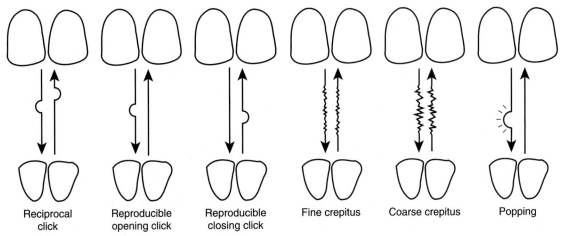

Reciprocal click | Reproducible opening click | Reproducible closing click | Fine crepitus | Coarse crepitus | Popping

FIGURE 7–1. Although many TMJs do not yield diagnostic information, some sounds are important. The TMJ noise must be audible to the patient and the corresponding dysfunction palpable by the examiner. **Reciprocal click:** Noise made on opening and closing from centric occlusion position that is reproducible on every opening and closing and can be eliminated with anterior repositioning of jaw suggests an early stage disk disorder. **Reproducible opening click:** Noise with *every* opening, no noise when closing, suggests deviation in form of disk or late stage disk disorder. **Reproducible closing click:** Noise with every closing, no noise when opening, suggests deviation in form of disk. **Crepitus (fine):** Fine grating noise on opening or closing suggestive of mild bone on bone contact, which may suggest surface defects on disk or a late stage disk disorder. **Crepitus (coarse):** Coarse grating noise on opening or closing suggestive of gross bone on bone contact and osteoarthritis or osteoarthrosis. **Popping:** Loud sound on opening that is audible to examiner at a distance without stethoscope suggests early stage disk disorder.

tion a more objective technique.[24] It is clear that all clinicians should make every effort to standardize their palpation techniques (location, size of surface palpated, pressure delivered, etc.) in order to improve the reliability of their assessments.

Muscle and joint palpation uses the technique and sites described in Figure 7–2. Muscle testing can also be accomplished in order to determine whether specific weakness exists. This weakness may be primarily due to muscle injury or secondary to a systematic muscular disease or neurologic disorder. Electromyography (EMG) cannot be used to diagnose muscle pain. The reliability, accuracy, sensitivity, and specificity of EMG are below the standards expected of a diagnostic test in diagnosing masticatory myofascial pain.[25]

OCCLUSAL EVALUATION

Examining the dentition and occlusion is an important part of the physical examination of a temporomandibular disorder (TMD) or orofacial pain patient. It may provide very useful information about the existence of bruxism or other oral habits and their possible effects on the dentition, periodontium, or other oral structures. Such an examination can also determine whether there has been a progressive change in occlusal relationships (midline shift, anterior open bite, unilateral posterior open bite, etc.) that may indicate the presence of such conditions as unilateral condylar hyperplasia, rheumatoid arthritis, or neoplasm. Noting the number of missing teeth, particularly loss of posterior occlusal support, is also important since this situation may predispose the TMJs to degenerative joint disease (osteoarthrosis), especially in the presence of bruxism.

Beyond these indications, the diagnostic validity of association of specific occlusal relationships with TMD is quite poor. Except for skeletal anterior open bites, overjets of greater than 6 to 7 mm, retruded contact position/intercuspal position slides greater than 4 mm, unilateral lingual crossbite, and five or more missing posterior teeth, occlusal factors have not been found to be correlated with TMD or orofacial pain.[26] Furthermore, some of these occlusal conditions may be the result of TMJ abnormality and not the converse.[26] It is for these reasons that several well respected organizations (The American Dental Association, National Institutes of Dental Research, American Academy of Orofacial Pain, and Royal College of Dental Surgeons of Ontario) have recom-

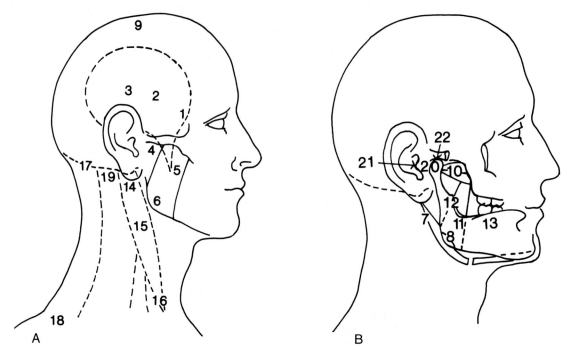

FIGURE 7–2. The muscle and joint sites for the masticatory system are used to develop a standardized technique for muscle palpation. The technique described here will assist the clinician in maintaining adequate reliability in assessing for tenderness. Palpation is performed by first locating the distinct band or part of joint and then using the sensitive spadelike pad at the end of the distal phalanx of the index finger to apply firm pressure at multiple sites in the area (approximately 0.5 to 1 pound per finger). The fingernail should be trimmed so that it does not cause false-positive findings. The patient is asked, "Does it hurt or is it just pressure?" The response is positive if palpation produces a clear reaction from the patient, i.e., palpebral response, or if the patient states that the palpation "hurts," indicating that the site is clearly more tender than surrounding structures or the contralateral structure. Any equivocal response by the patient is considered a negative response. Site 9 can be used as a reference site to demonstrate to the patient what "pressure" feels like. As a result of the poor accessibility of the lateral pterygoid site, the fifth finger should be used to palpate with the patient's jaw in laterotrusion to the ipsilateral side. Palpation of the lateral and superior aspects of the TMJ is accomplished with half mouth opening. Palpation of the posterior TMJ capsule is accomplished anterior to the tragus with the mouth open. The deep masseter is palpated immediately below the notch in the zygomatic arch with the mouth closed.

Palpation of extraoral muscle sites:
1. Anterior temporalis
2. Middle temporalis
3. Posterior temporalis
4. Superior masseter
5. Middle masseter
6. Inferior masseter
7. Posterior mandibular
8. Submandibular
9. Vertex or reference point

Palpation of intraoral muscle sites:
10. Lateral pterygoid site (open and move jaw laterally to palpate with posterior superior direction)
11. Medial pterygoid (sublingual palpation against ramus of mandible)
12. Temporalis insertion (run finger superior along the coronoid process)

Palpation of neck muscle sites:
13. Buccinator
14. Superior sternocleidomastoid
15. Inferior sternocleidomastoid
16. Middle sternocleidomastoid
17. Trapezius insertion
18. Upper trapezius
19. Splenius capitis

Palpation of temporomandibular joint sites:
20. Lateral aspect of joint site (slightly open jaw)
21. Posterior aspect of joint site (fully open jaw)
22. Superior aspect of joint site (slightly open jaw)

mended that, in most cases, TMD should be treated with conservative and reversible therapeutic modalities.

ADDITIONAL DIAGNOSTIC PROCEDURES, TESTS, AND STRATEGIES

It is quite clear that, if a high level of diagnostic uncertainty still exists after the history, physical examination, and clinical evaluations, consideration should be given to the use of additional diagnostic procedures, tests, or strategies. The use of such procedures, tests, or strategies must rest on the premise that they are reliable, are technically and diagnostically valid, are able to differentiate a disorder from among others with similar characteristics, and are cost-effective. Furthermore, a diagnostic procedure, test, or strategy, to have value, should be able to provide new information that is not already known to the clinician.[27] For example, there is no point in taking TMJ radiographs merely to determine whether the condyles translate during jaw opening since that information is already available from the physical examination. In addition, the less a diagnostic procedure, test, or strategy influences subsequent therapeutic decisions, the less relevance it has in differential diagnosis.[27] Thus, conducting a diagnostic test, the outcome of which will not alter the treatment options, is generally not indicated.

There are many diagnostic procedures, tests, and strategies that meet these standards and, therefore, are warranted in particular clinical situations. Among these are certain blood tests, urinalyses, biopsies, psychometric instruments, and imaging. With regard to the use of electronic instruments or devices, e.g., surface electromyography (EMG), thermography, sonography, electrovibrography (EVG), and mandibular kinesiology (jaw tracking), the evidence for their use in the differential diagnosis or monitoring of TMD and orofacial pain is not supportive.[28] In view of this, their use may present a risk of reaching either false-positive or false-negative diagnoses.[29–31] Thus, until scientific studies, using blinded evaluations to compare subgroups of TMD patients with matched controls and with individuals who have other orofacial pain conditions with

similar characteristics, demonstrate acceptable levels of reliability, validity, sensitivity, specificity, and predictive values, the use of electronic devices will continue to have questionable diagnostic utility and, therefore, will continue to be considered experimental. The conclusion is that the differential diagnosis of TMDs or other orofacial pain conditions is best accomplished by evaluation of the information obtained from the patient's history, clinical examination, and, when indicated, TMJ or other imaging.[32]

REFERENCES

1. Fricton JR: Behavioral and psychosocial factors in chronic craniofacial pain. Anesth Prog 1985; 32(1):7–12.
2. Fricton JR: Recent advances in temporomandibular disorders and orofacial pain (review). J Am Dent Assoc 1991;122(11):24–32.
3. Dworkin SF: Behavioral characteristics of chronic temporomandibular disorders: Diagnosis and assessment. In Sessle BJ, Bryant PS, Dionne RA (eds): Temporomandibular Disorders and Related Pain Conditions. Seattle, IASP Press, 1995, pp 175–192.
4. Rugh JD, Solberg WK: Psychological implications in temporomandibular pain and dysfunction (review). Oral Sci Rev 1976;7:3–30.
5. McCreary CP, Clark GT, Oakley ME, et al: Predicting response to treatment for temporomandibular disorders. J Craniomandibul Disord 1992;6(3):161–169.
6. Fricton JR, Olsen T: Predictors of outcome for treatment of temporomandibular disorders. J Orofac Pain 1996;10(1):54–65.
7. Aranda JM: The problem-oriented medical record: Experiences in a community military hospital. JAMA 1974;229(5):549–551.
8. DeGowin EL: Bedside diagnostic examination, ed 2. London, Macmillan, 1969, p 927.
9. Delp MH, Manning RP: Major's Physical Diagnosis: An Introduction to the Clinical Process, ed 9. Philadelphia, WB Saunders, 1981.
10. Mohl ND, Dixon DC: Current status of diagnostic procedures for temporomandibular disorders (review). J Am Dent Assoc 1994;125(1):56–64.
11. Mohl ND, Ohrbach R: Clinical decision-making. In Zarb GA, et al (eds): Temporomandibular Joint and Masticatory Muscle Disorders. Copenhagen, Munksgaard, 1994, pp 565–581.
12. Fricton JR, Kroening R: Practical differential diagnosis of chronic craniofacial pain. Oral Surg Oral Med Oral Pathol 1982;54(6):628–634.
13. Ohrbach R: Overview of patient evaluation. In Zarb GA, et al (eds): Temporomandibular Joint and Masticatory Muscle Disorders. Copenhagen, Munksgaard, 1994, pp 392–404.
14. Ohrbach R: History and clinical examination. In Zarb GA, et al (eds): Temporomandibular Joint and Masticatory Muscle Disorders. Copenhagen, Munksgaard, 1994, pp 407–432.
15. Swerdlow M: Problems in clinical evaluation of pain. In Payne JP, Burt RAP (eds): Pain: Basic

Principles, Pharmacology, Therapy. Baltimore, Williams & Wilkins, 1972.

16. Melzack R: The McGill Pain Questionnaire: Major properties and scoring methods. Pain 1975; 1(3):277–299.

17. Agnew DC, Merskey H: Words of chronic pain. Pain 1976;2(1):73–81.

18. Diamond S, Dalession DJ: The Practicing Physician's Approach to Headache, ed 2. Baltimore, Williams & Wilkins, 1978.

19. Clark GT: Examining temporomandibular disorder patients for cranio-cervical dysfunction. J Craniomandibul Pract 1983;2(1):55–63.

20. Fricton JR, Schiffman EL: The craniomandibular index: Validity. J Prosthet Dent 1987;58(2):222–228.

21. Schiffman EL, Fricton JR, Haley D, et al: The prevalence and treatment needs of subjects with temporomandibular disorders. J Am Dent Assoc 1990;120(3):295–303.

22. Widmer CG: Temporomandibular joint sounds: A critique of techniques for recording and analysis. J Craniomandibul Disord 1989;3(4):213–217.

23. Dworkin SF, LeResche L: Research diagnostic criteria for temporomandibular disorders: Review, criteria, examinations and specifications, critique (review). J Craniomandibul Disord 1992;6(4):301–355.

24. Schiffman E, Fricton J, Haley D, et al: A pressure algometer for MPS: Reliability and validity. Pain 1987;4(suppl):S291.

25. Lund JP, Widmer CG: Evaluation of the use of surface electromyography in the diagnosis, documentation, and treatment of dental patients (review). J Craniomandibul Disord 1989;3(3):125–137.

26. McNamara JA, Seligman DA, Okeson JP: Occlusion, orthodontic treatment, and temporomandibular disorders: A review. J Orofac Pain 1995;9(1):73–89.

27. Kassirer JP: Learning Clinical Reasoning. Baltimore, Williams & Wilkins, 1991, p 332.

28. Widmer CG, McCall WD, Lund JP: Adjunctive diagnostic tests. In Zarb GA, et al (eds): Temporomandibular Joint and Masticatory Muscle Disorders. Copenhagen, Munksgaard, 1994, pp 407–432.

29. Mohl ND, McCall WD, Lund JP, et al: Devices for the diagnosis and treatment of temporomandibular disorders. Part I. Introduction, scientific evidence, and jaw tracking (published erratum appears in J Prosthet Dent 1990;63(5):13A) (review). J Prosthet Dent 1990;63(2):198–201.

30. Mohl ND, McCall WD, Lund JP, et al: Devices for the diagnosis and treatment of temporomandibular disorders. Part III. Thermography, ultrasound, electrical stimulation, and electromyographic biofeedback (published erratum appears in J Prosthet Dent 1990;63[5]:13A) (review). J Prosthet Dent 1990;63(4):472–477.

31. Mohl ND, McCall WD, Lund JP, et al: Devices for the diagnosis and treatment of temporomandibular disorders. Part II. Electromyography and sonography (published erratum appears in J Prosthet Dent 1990;63[5]:13A) (review). J Prosthet Dent 1990;63(3):332–336.

32. Albino JEN: National Institutes of Health Technology Assessment Conference Statement: Management of Temporomandibular Disorders. 1996:NIH/NIDR.

CHAPTER

Temporomandibular Joint Imaging: Treatment Planning

Quentin N. Anderson

Medical imaging of the temporomandibular joint (TMJ) can be challenging. The TMJ lies within the skull base; has a concave, convex contour; and in lateral projection is overlapped by the skull base and opposite side. The TMJ is three-dimensional and inherently unstable (rotation-translation), and there is individual variability of approximately 20% between right and left sides.

Following Roentgen's discovery of x-rays in 1895, imaging studies have progressed from transcranial views to sophisticated computed tomography (CT) and magnetic resonance imaging (MRI) examinations. Transcranial views of the TMJ were refined between the 1930s and 1950s. CT examinations began in the late 1970s and 1980s, and MRI in the late 1980s and 1990s.

This chapter focuses on the availability and application of imaging devices, as well as their utility and value.

Transcranial Views

Early practitioners such as Costen, Lindbloom, and Grewcock[1] refined transcranial techniques, which have remained relatively stable since the 1950s. The design limitation of this technique is that only the lateral one third of the joint space can be visualized. The imaging technique is somewhat inflexible, and adaptation to anatomic variables is difficult (Fig. 8–1A).

Application This technique has limited application because it images only the lateral one third of the joint space.

Predictive Value Significant changes can be obscured, especially within the medial margins of the joint space. This technique has limited predictive value.

Cost/Benefit Ratio The cost/benefit ratio should be judged on a case-by-case basis.

Tomography

Tomography creates a two-dimensional picture of a three-dimensional structure. Objects in front of and behind the selected plane of imaging are blurred or obscured. This obviates superimposition of overlapping structures.

Mechanically, tomography is rather simplistic. The x-ray tube travels in one direction, with simultaneous x-ray film movement in the opposite direction. The result is a variable fulcrum point. Selected body sections can be obtained by mechanically moving the fulcrum point up or down. Optimal TMJ imaging studies are obtained with a wide arc of tube travel—30 to 40 degrees—and thin-section collimation—1- to 2-mm thick slices (Fig. 8–1B).

X-ray tube motion can be linear or complex (circular). In general, complex motion devices have been superseded by CT techniques. High-quality images using the suggested wide arc of tube travel and thin slices

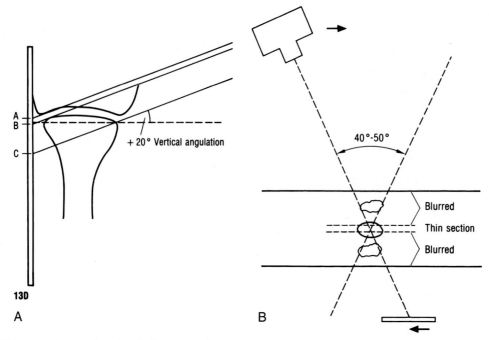

FIGURE 8–1. *A,* Diagram depicting the limitations of temporomandibular joint (TMJ) transcranial imaging. Only the lateral one third of the joint space can be visualized (A-B image projected onto the vertically oriented film). *B,* Overview of linear tomography. Thin-section images can be obtained without anatomic distortion. There is no limitation relative to the depth of focus. Complete images can be obtained along the transverse lateral-to-medial plane of the TMJ.

can routinely be obtained with linear tomography. Lateral corrected tomographic techniques using a localizing vertical submental view (VSM) for positioning have limited value. It is difficult to replicate exact VSM positioning, and right-to-left variability can be a challenge.

Sagittal tomographic studies from the outer lateral edge through the medial pole of the condyle in both closed and open positions are excellent for the detection of skeletal abnormalities. At our institution, we use a fluoroscope-assisted positioning technique—modified lateral correction. This technique facilitates through-put and replication on both initial and follow-up studies.

Coronal plane (anteroposterior) tomographic imaging of the TMJ can sometimes be helpful. In most cases, however, high-quality sagittal tomography is more than adequate to validate and classify osseous abnormalities.

UTILITY AND VALUE

Application Tomography is extremely useful for initial treatment planning and longitudinal follow-up studies.

Predictive Value Thin-section high-resolution lateral tomography in closed and open positions has significant predictive value.

Cost/Benefit Ratio Tomography has an excellent cost/benefit ratio for both initial and long-term follow-up examinations.

KEY FEATURES

Condylar Position

Sagittal tomographic techniques in both closed and open positions are an accurate means of assessing the condyle–glenoid fossa relationship. There is little if any anatomic distortion, as one would incur with transcranial views or Panorex images.

In general, the condyle–glenoid fossa relationship has little predictive value relative to disk cartilage position. Yang-Fangren's[2] and Pullinger's[3] studies documented a concentric condylar-glenoid relationship in only 58% to 65% of asymptomatic subjects. In our study groups, expected posterior condylar displacement with anterior disk cartilage position had little predictive value. In fact, our asymptomatic controls in other study groups were more likely to have a posterior condylar position.

Range of Condylar Motion

On full opening, the condyle should translate forward to the midhorizontal portion of the distal eminence. This correlates with an opening interincisal measurement between 40 and 50 mm.

Hypermobility and reduced range of motion are not predictive of disk cartilage position. The findings are nonspecific.

Degenerative Changes: Arthrosis

If excessive force or load is applied to any joint, this can lead to adaptive changes, or arthrosis.[4] Yale's condylar classification scheme depicts a rather uniform convex contour of the condyle. Adaptive changes (flattening of the articular contour, sclerosis and subarticular cystic change, and/or bone spur formation) often correlate with disk cartilage displacement. In our case studies, we found that the greater the number of documented adaptive changes within either the condyle or the glenoid fossa, the greater the chance of disk displacement or internal derangement.

Degenerative changes without internal derangement can occur but are seen in only a small number of cases—1% to 2%—and often in older populations ($\geq$35 years of age). The mean age of internal derangement in our study groups was the mid-20s.

Panorex Zonarc Studies

Panoramic studies portray the mandible as if it were split vertically down the midsagittal plane. The nose remains in the midline with the right and left jaw on either side of the film.

Simplistically, these studies are a special application of linear tomography. By adjusting the beam width wider or thinner, selected body sections can be obtained. Detailed discussions related to real images, ghost images, and double images are readily available in other textbooks and articles.[5]

In recent years, new technologies have been applied to panoramic principles for the imaging of other head and neck structures. Zonarc (Pallomex, Finland) panoramic equipment is designed such that selected images of the maxillofacial structures, temporal bone, and upper cervical spine can be obtained. Zonarc equipment orients the patient horizontally on a couch rather than in a seated, upright position. The horizontal position is useful for unstable patients, especially trauma cases (Fig. 8–2).

In general, Panorex views create distortion of the TMJ, off axis. Zonarc techniques, however, can be specifically programmed for the TMJ, with a significant reduction in distortion.

Application Routine mandibular studies that include the TMJ produce anatomically distorted images. This can be overcome by using specialized Zonarc studies.

Predictive Value Panorex Zonarc studies of the mandible and TMJ are a reasonable baseline for initial evaluation. By design, they are less optimal than thin-section tomography, and any skeletal discrepancies should be evaluated with tomography.

Cost/Benefit Ratio As an initial screening examination, Panorex Zonarc studies have an excellent cost/benefit ratio.

Computed Tomography

CT examinations of the TMJ began in the 1970s. The original CT scan times were approximately 1 to 2 minutes per slice and 1 to 5 minutes of computer reconstruction time per slice. Currently, dynamic spiral CT, which was introduced in the 1990s, is extremely fast; slice acquisition times are under 1 second, reducing motion artifact (Fig. 8–3). Another advantage of spiral CT is that the examination generates a volume data set rather than a simple slice thickness. Data from the spiral CT volume acquisition can be reformatted into multiple planes of imaging using computer techniques.

Other applications of spiral CT technology include three-dimensional imaging, CT angiography, and virtual reality imaging. Practitioners can visualize and formulate surgical approaches and new techniques through computer manipulation at the CT console.

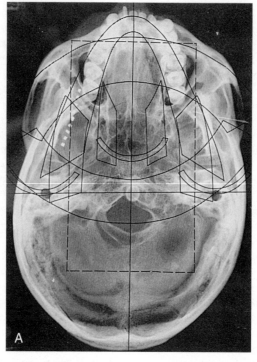

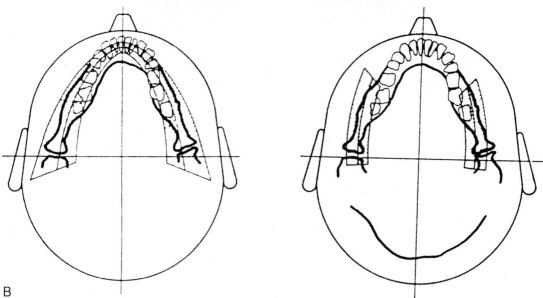

FIGURE 8–2. *A,* Diagram depicting the multiple imaging programs available with Zonarc, an advanced Panorex technology. *B,* Diagram depicting the specific Zonarc pathways for imaging the mandible and temporomandibular joint, with reduced distortion of the latter.

CT is extremely useful for revealing skeletal abnormalities of the TMJ but is of limited value in soft tissue evaluation. Anatomically, the disk cartilage is quite thin—a maximum of 3 mm thick—and its soft tissue CT characteristics are not unique. The surrounding joint capsule, tendon, and muscle have similar CT characteristics, making it difficult to isolate the disk cartilage. MRI studies, in contrast, have excellent soft tissue resolution and have superseded the initial enthusiasm for CT localization of the disk cartilage.

Application Skeletal abnormalities are optimally detected and classified using CT techniques.

Predictive Value Both spiral and fixed-slice CT techniques have excellent predictive value and should be used to evaluate skeletal abnormalities.

Cost/Benefit Ratio CT techniques, especially spiral CT, are very cost effective.

Magnetic Resonance Imaging

The basic principles of MRI evolved from biochemistry studies of the 1940s. In the late 1970s and early 1980s, these same principles were applied to whole body imaging. MRI equipment was designed with high- and low-strength magnetic field devices so that small tissue volumes within the body could be sampled for their unique resonant modulation patterns. Clinical MRI studies reflect the relative proton (H+) density within a given tissue volume. This is different from x-ray imaging, which depends on ionizing radiation and tissue absorption.

There are no significant biologic side effects of MRI, but there are precautions. Metallic clips, metallic foreign bodies, pacemakers, and some cardiovascular appliances can be affected and inadvertently displaced. TMJ joint prosthetic devices, dental fillings, and braces are not affected by the magnetic field.

MRI studies should be obtained in multiple planes of imaging—sagittal and coronal—using variable pulse sequences to create selected T1- and T2-weighted images. The studies should be further optimized by using a small field of view imaging coil. This enhances resolution of soft tissue and skeletal abnormalities.

The classification of disk position, or internal derangement, has not changed appreciably since the benchmark studies using arthrographic techniques. Arthrographic techniques require some sophisticated imaging equipment and operator skills.[6] MRI studies, in contrast, are universally available and, if appropriate techniques are followed, are just as precise as arthrographic examinations and less operator dependent.

Over the last 10 years, a significant amount has been written on abnormalities of the TMJ. There are three areas of concern: disk cartilage signal characteristics, joint effusions, and bone marrow signal patterns.

DISK CARTILAGE SIGNAL PATTERNS

The MRI signal pattern within the TMJ disk cartilage shows a low percentage of (H+) protons; it is a black, low-signal registration. Bright white signal patterns are usually indicative of inherent proteinaceous materials or water densities, such as edema patterns.

The knee fibrocartilage is comparable to the TMJ disk cartilage. Various signal patterns have been observed in the knee cartilage and the findings validated with arthroscopy and open surgery. The bright white signal pattern of knee cartilage has been graded from minimal involvement (grade I) to maximal involvement (grade III). In general, it is quite common to see an increase in signal pattern within the knee cartilage, but only when there is a break in contour of the fibrocartilage is it indicative of internal derangement or degeneration (grade III).

In similar fashion, we observed a relative increase in signal pattern within the TMJ disk cartilage. In our case studies, we failed to correlate a simple increase in signal in-

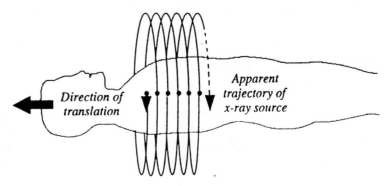

FIGURE 8–3. Diagram depicting the direction of patient motion, translation, and helical trajectory of spiral computed tomography (CT) imaging. Image data are collected continuously over a preprogrammed distance. Selected images at variable slice thicknesses and in multiple planar projections can be processed from the initial CT volume acquisition.

Direction of translation

Apparent trajectory of x-ray source

tensity with structural failure. We compared several groups, pre- and postoperatively, and found no positive correlation between disk cartilage failure and increased disk signal.

In addition to these anatomic findings, there is an inherent technical factor called the magic angle effect.[7] Any structure positioned at 55 degrees to the vector of the magnetic field can intrinsically undergo a signal conversion from black to white. The TMJ disk cartilage falls into this 55-degree relationship and is subjected to this conversion effect; that is, the black signal pattern is converted to a bright white signal.

Overall, we have concluded that an increase in signal intensity within the disk cartilage is most likely multifactorial. Signal alterations can be found in the normal TMJ disk cartilage, may be related to adaptive changes or aging, or may be caused by the magic angle effect.[8] We regard an increase in signal intensity as a nonspecific finding.

JOINT EFFUSIONS

Before the availability of MRI studies of the TMJ, it was difficult to document joint effusions. In our case studies, we found joint effusions to be quite common. They occurred in normal asymptomatic patients 15% to 20% of the time and in approximately 75% of patients with internal derangement. We found no significant correlation between the presence or amount of joint effusion and the patient's symptoms.

It is readily apparent that biochemical analysis of joint fluid will resolve this issue. The presence of biochemical mediators and protagonists, rather than the absolute presence of an effusion, is more predictive of TMJ dysfunction. The presence or absence of a joint effusion has little predictive value relative to classifying TMJ disorders.

INTENSITY OF BONE MARROW SIGNAL PATTERNS

An increase in bone marrow signal pattern (bright water density) has led some authors to propose that this is diagnostic of avascular necrosis (AVN). These findings are nonspecific and similar to those seen in transient osteoporosis (a self-limited disease), stress fractures, osteomyelitis, and nonspecific marrow infiltration.

Pathophysiologically, AVN is a failure of the microcirculation. AVN is multifactorial,[9] and in view of the multiple routes of collateral blood supply to the TMJ, there appears to be no valid correlation with vascular compression by a displaced disk. Extrinsic vascular compression has not been validated as an etiologic factor of AVN.

We found a minor increase in marrow signal pattern in 1% to 2% of study cases. Most often, these cases did not have any subarticular signal patterns typical of AVN, such as the crescent sign or double-line sign. Until these findings are validated with controlled longitudinal studies, there is little support for aggressive interventional therapy.[10]

Before the introduction of Proplast allograft materials, pre- and postsurgical planning was not affected by product failure or by recent Food and Drug Administration regulations. We are participating in an ongoing study to assess allografts using clinical imaging.

A new and ongoing area of interest at our trauma center is the evaluation of TMJ joint fractures.[11, 12] We have found that MRIs are not only useful in documenting fracture position but also predictive of concurrent disk cartilage and soft tissue injury. It seems logical that if surgical repair of skeletal deformities is undertaken, soft tissue injury should be considered. We believe that MRI examinations will be of benefit in the acute and long-term management of condylar fractures.

UTILITY AND VALUE

Application Except for the previously mentioned precautions, MRIs are an excellent means of evaluating soft tissue abnormalities of the TMJ.

Predictive Value MRI examinations of soft tissue abnormalities have a very high predictive value.

Cost/Benefit Ratio MRI is a cost-effective imaging study for initial treatment planning and long-term follow-up.

Summary

Multiple imaging avenues are available to evaluate TMJ disorders. Accurate assessment of skeletal and soft tissue abnormalities should be obtained before treatment planning. The cases depicted in Figures 8–4 to 8–18 illustrate the utility and value of various imaging pathways.

Text continued on page 142

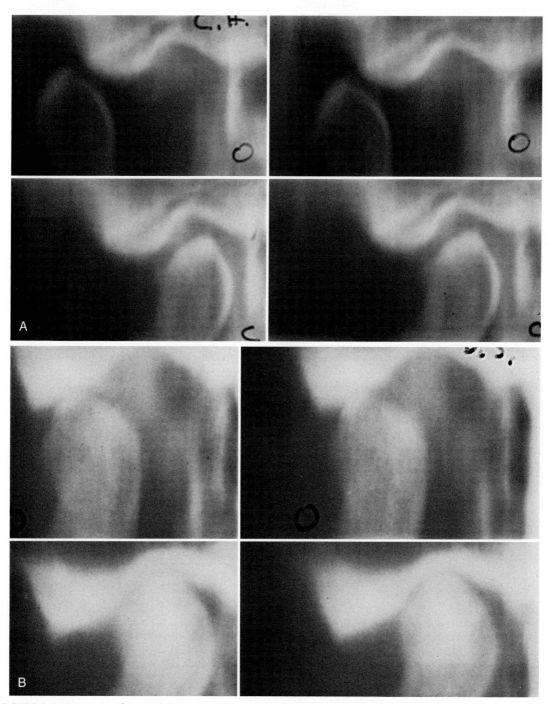

FIGURE 8–4. Two cases of internal derangement depicting adaptive degenerative findings. *A,* Closed and open position with mild grade I–II changes, a flat condyle, sclerosis, and small anteroposterior bone spur formation. *B,* Late-stage grade III changes, flat articular surfaces, severe sclerosis, and loss of joint space.

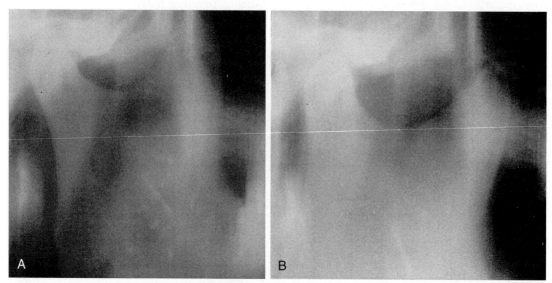

FIGURE 8–5. *A, B,* This case of coronoid process hypertrophy is well documented on both closed and open tomographic studies. The skeletal abnormality and the size and height of the coronoid relative to the temporomandibular joint are easily evaluated on a single study.

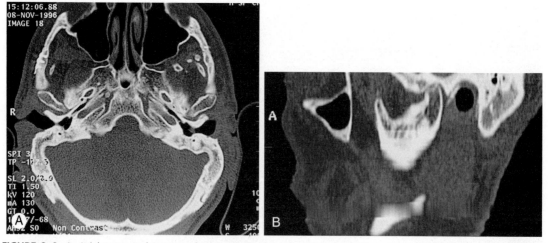

FIGURE 8–6. *A,* Axial computed tomography image of a postoperative coronoid resection. Residual bone fragments are identified in the temporal fossa and medial and lateral margins of the coronoid process. *B,* Computer-generated off-axis sagittal image that complements the axial study with an overview of the residual hypertrophy and deformity of the coronoid process.

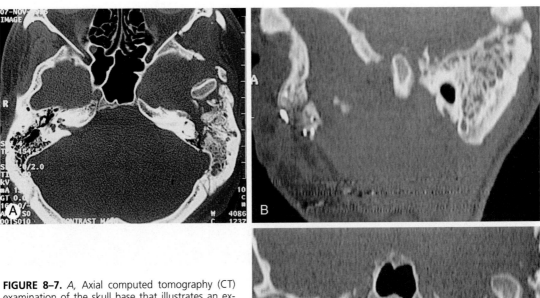

FIGURE 8–7. *A,* Axial computed tomography (CT) examination of the skull base that illustrates an extensive fracture deformity with extension into the glenoid fossa and disruption of the condylar-glenoid configuration. *B, C,* Off-axis computer-generated CT sagittal and coronal reconstructions depicting the extent of the fracture deformity within the glenoid fossa and the degree of condylar displacement into the middle cranial fossa.

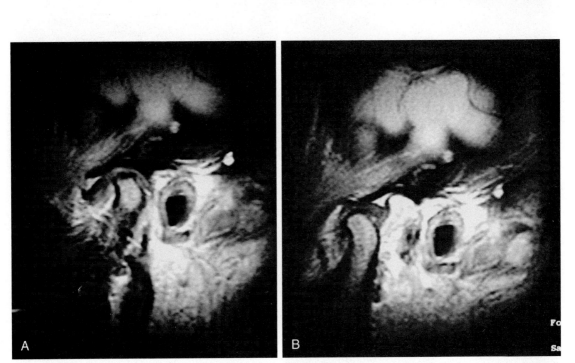

FIGURE 8–8. Two studies depicting a thickened, reducing disk cartilage. *A,* In the closed position, there is moderate hypertrophy throughout the disk cartilage, with a slight increase in signal intensity within the posterior attachment (bright white, nonspecific pattern). *B,* In the full open view, the disk is reduced, with hypertrophic thickening that extends into the posterior condylar attachment.

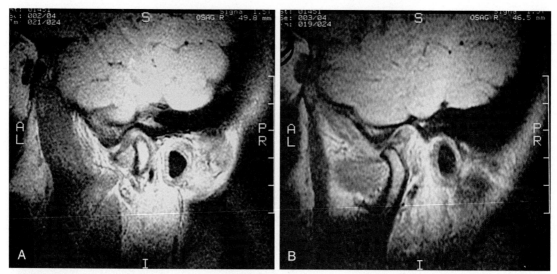

FIGURE 8–9. *A, B,* Two studies depicting a reducing hypertrophic disk cartilage, but with a more distinct focal area of increased signal pattern within the posterior one third of the disk. This finding of increased signal pattern is nonspecific and has no predictive value. Also note that the posterior condylar attachment is not appreciably thickened, as seen in Figure 8–8*B.*

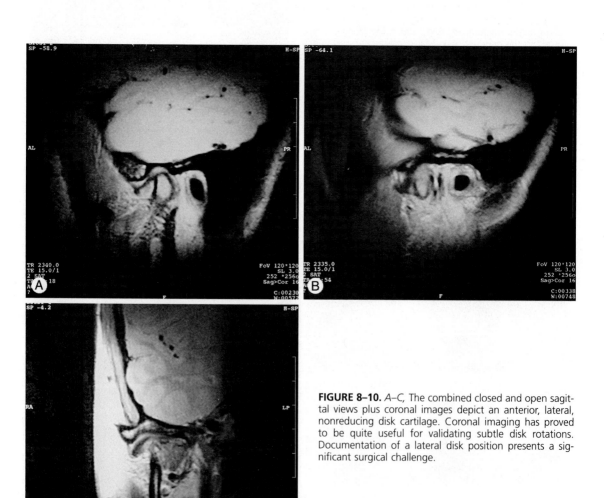

FIGURE 8–10. *A–C,* The combined closed and open sagittal views plus coronal images depict an anterior, lateral, nonreducing disk cartilage. Coronal imaging has proved to be quite useful for validating subtle disk rotations. Documentation of a lateral disk position presents a significant surgical challenge.

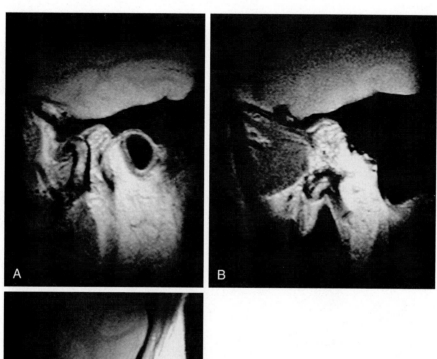

FIGURE 8–11. *A,* In the full open position, no identifiable disk cartilage can be clearly delineated. *B,* This more medial image in the same open position clearly outlines an incompletely reduced, medially displaced disk cartilage. *C,* The coronal image validates the medial rotation and documents additional degenerative findings. In the middle third of the condyle, there is a concave, black-bordered ring pattern. This degenerative process is quite interesting and could represent residual avascular necrosis or partial healing.

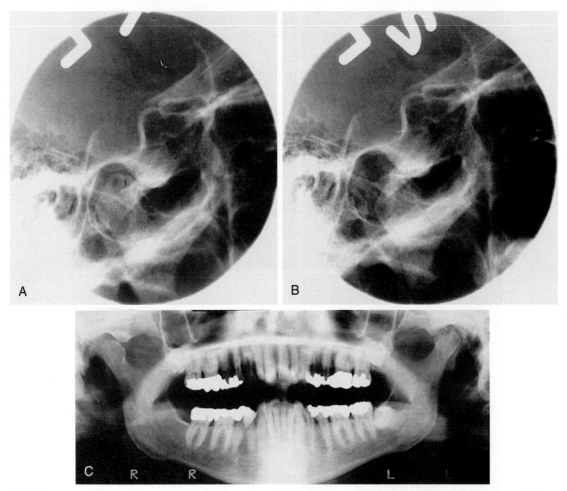

FIGURE 8–12. Summary of the principles of temporomandibular joint (TMJ) imaging. *A, B,* Closed-open transcranial views are of some value but do not clearly document significant skeletal abnormality of the condyle. *C,* Panorex study raises suspicion of skeletal abnormality within the left TMJ; there are subarticular cystic changes and possibly a flat articular contour.

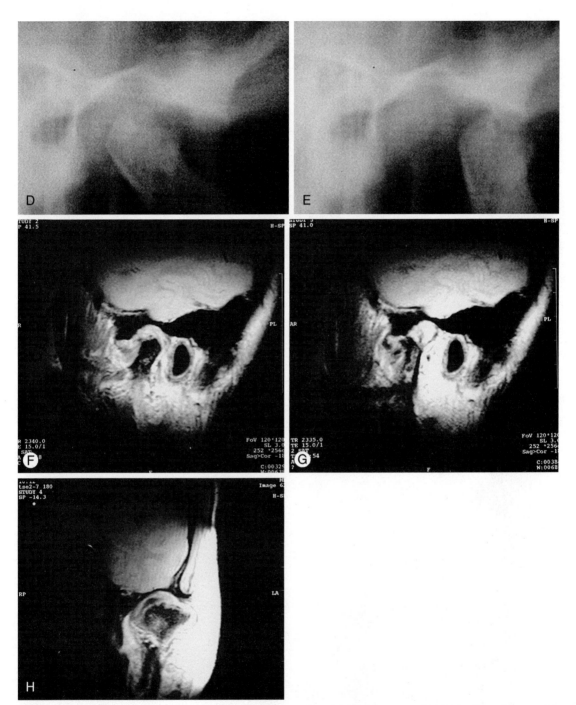

FIGURE 8–12 *Continued. D, E,* Closed and open tomographic studies clearly outline an eroded, flat contour of the condyle, with sclerosis in both the condyle and the distal eminence. These degenerative findings have a very high predictive value for internal derangement. *F–H,* This multiplanar magnetic resonance imaging (MRI) examination documents a nonreducing anteromedial displaced cartilage with degenerative condylar findings. There is decreased marrow signal pattern in the condyle, which simply correlates with the degenerative fibrotic changes within the marrow—a nonspecific finding. Black condyles have no predictive value relative to skeletal integrity. In addition, there are some very small filling defects (black signal pattern) within the joint effusion. These are residual loose joint bodies, secondary to the degenerative process, and fragments of bone and cartilage. Overall, this case illustrates that the Panorex examination is by far the best screening procedure, with follow-up documentation using tomography and MRI for classification of internal derangement.

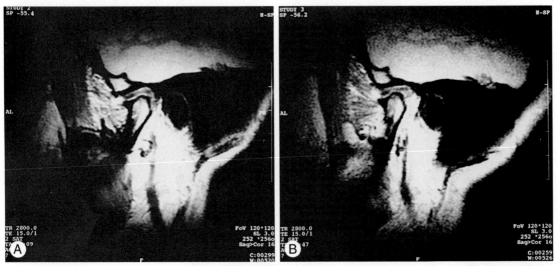

FIGURE 8–13. After meniscoplasty, the closed position (A) and open position (B) illustrate a relatively adherent disk cartilage, limited movement of the disk cartilage, and reduced range of condylar motion. This semifixated disk raises the potential of fibrosis, and residual adhesion. The degenerative black signal pattern within the bone marrow is simply fibrotic replacement.

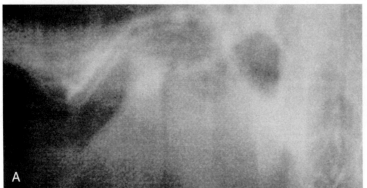

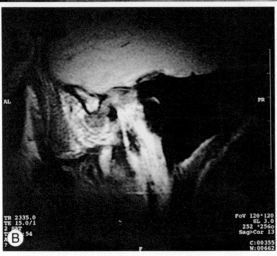

FIGURE 8–14. Allograft repair. A, Closed-position tomography illustrates a significantly deformed condyle, foreshortened with a flat sclerotic contour and a curvilinear calcification parallelling the inner border of the glenoid fossa, indicating a calcified allograft. B, Sagittal magnetic resonance imaging depicts the erosive soft tissue granuloma secondary to Proplast breakdown, with concave condylar erosion and concurrent degenerative change within the condyle (fibrotic black marrow pattern).

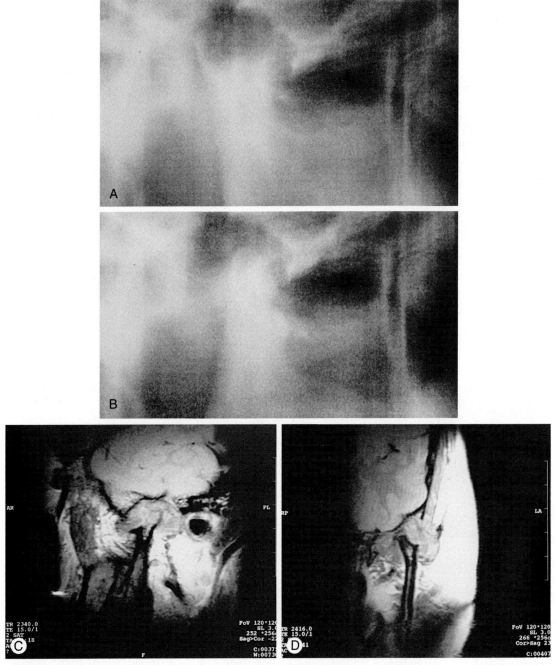

FIGURE 8–15. Allograft repair. *A, B,* Closed-open tomography illustrates more extensive erosive change within the condyle, plus irregular expansile erosion through the glenoid fossa. *C, D,* Sagittal and coronal magnetic resonance imaging documents extension of the Proplast granulomatous process through the glenoid fossa into the middle cranial fossa and over the anterolateral border of the joint space. The patient presented with a palpable left cheek mass.

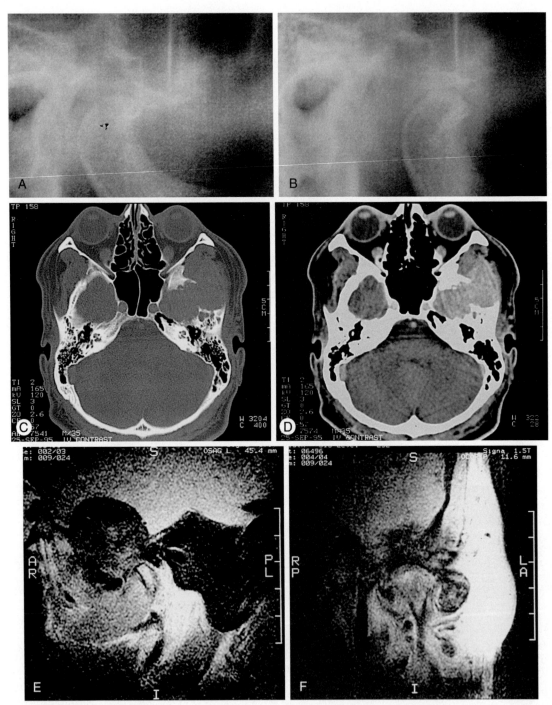

FIGURE 8–16. Primary temporomandibular joint (TMJ) tumor. The patient initially presented with pain and decreased range of motion—nonspecific TMJ findings. *A, B,* Closed and open tomography illustrates an extensive erosive process extending through the glenoid fossa. Similar involvement was seen in the allograft patient in Figure 8–15, but here there is a normal-appearing condyle. *C, D,* Axial computed tomography studies of the skull base demonstrate extensive bony erosion of the skull base, extending through the left middle cranial fossa. *D* was obtained after intravenous contrast enhancement and demonstrates a large, diffusely enhancing, bright white mass lesion engulfing the bony erosive process of the skull base and left glenoid fossa. *E, F,* Sagittal and coronal magnetic resonance imaging demonstrates that the mass has eroded through the glenoid into the middle cranial fossa, with expansion over the lateral border of the joint space. Note the low signal material within the joint effusion, similar to the case of loose joint bodies (see Fig. 8–12*F* and *G*). These low densities within the joint effusion are a significant feature of primary pigmented villonodular synovitis.

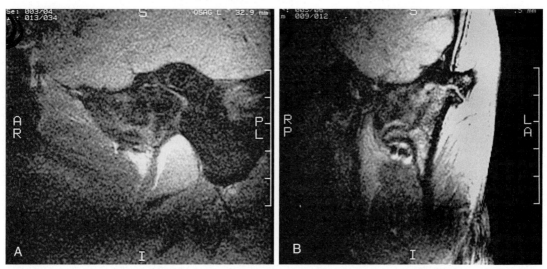

FIGURE 8–17. This patient presented with reduced range of motion with no known cause. After careful questioning, the patient related a history of facial injury. *A,* Sagittal magnetic resonance imaging (MRI) is nondiagnostic; there is no delineation of the glenoid fossa or condyle. *B,* Coronal MRI illustrates a healed medially depressed fracture of the condyle. The remaining disk elements have been displaced into the concave medial deformity of the healed fracture.

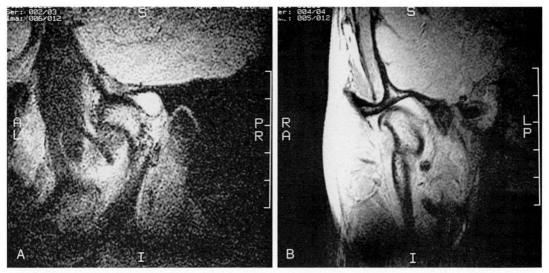

FIGURE 8–18. Acute condylar neck fracture, with images obtained in the closed position. *A,* Sagittal magnetic resonance imaging (MRI) clearly outlines the oblique condylar neck fracture (black linear signal pattern through the deformity). The displaced proximal segment of the condyle, with anteromedial rotation, is also well documented on the sagittal image. There is also a moderate joint effusion caused by hemorrhage. *B,* Coronal MRI not only validates the fracture deformity but also clearly outlines a laterally displaced disk cartilage and damage to the medial disk attachment. MRI of acute condylar fractures can be quite useful to document fracture deformities as well as assess concurrent soft tissue injury.

REFERENCES

1. Grewcock RJG: A simple technique for temporomandibular joint radiography. Br Dent J 1935;94:152–154.
2. Ren YF, et al: Condyle position in the TMJ. Oral Surg Oral Med Oral Pathol Oral Radiol Endod 1995;80:101–107.
3. Pullinger AG, Hollender L, Solberg WK, Petersson A: A tomographic study of mandibular condyle position in an asymptomatic population. J Prosthet Dent 1985;53:706–713.
4. Yale SH, Ceballos M, Resnoff CS, et al: Some observations on the classification of mandibular condyle types. Oral Surg Oral Med Oral Pathol 1963;16:572–577.
5. Langlais RP, et al: Diagnostic Imaging of the Jaws. Baltimore, Williams & Wilkins, 1994.
6. Katzberg RW, Dolwick MF, Helms CA, et al: Arthrotomography of the temporomandibular joint. AJR Am J Roentgenol 1980;134:995.
7. Ericsson SJ: The "magic angle" effect: Background physics and clinical relevance. Radiology 1993;188:23.
8. Scapino R: Histopathology associated with malposition of the human temporomandibular joint disc. Oral Surg Oral Med Oral Pathol 1983;55:382.
9. Takgi R: Angiography of the temporomandibular joint. Oral Surg Oral Med Oral Pathol 1944;78:539.
10. Colwell CW: The controversy of core decompression of the femoral head for osteonecrosis. Arthritis Rheum 1989;32:797.
11. Goss AN, Bosanquet AG: The arthroscopic appearance of acute temporomandibular joint trauma. J Oral Maxillofac Surg 1990;48:780.
12. Sullivan SM, Banghart PR, Anderson Q: Magnetic resonance imaging assessment of acute soft tissue injuries to the temporomandibular joint. J Oral Maxillofac Surg 1995;53:763.

Extrajoint Therapy

CHAPTER

Role of Splint Therapy in Treatment of Temporomandibular Disorders

Thomas Sollecito

History of Splint Therapy in Treatment of Temporomandibular Disorders

Splint therapy has been described in the literature as a treatment modality for temporomandibular disorders as early as 1877 as a means to effect a change in the temporomandibular joint complex. Through the years, intraoral splints have been advocated by many clinicians for varied purposes. The design of the splint has been modified for each specific purpose. In the 1940s through the 1960s Costen's concept of altering a patient's occlusion with a splint to restore vertical dimension, in hopes of relieving the signs and symptoms of temporomandibular disorders, was advocated by many practitioners. During that same period, Thompson was recognized as a proponent for mandibular repositioning with a splint, which was thought to afford the patient a suitable mandibular resting position. Other clinicians, at that time, advocated the use of splints to reposition the mandible, so as to allow a better seating of the condyle in the glenoid fossa. Still others were advocating the use of a pivotal splint to "unload" the joint. In the 1960s Ramfjord was credited with relating splint therapy to muscular function. In the 1970s and 1980s anterior repositioning appliances (splints), i.e., those that repositioned the mandible into a more

anterior position, re-emerged in popularity, and they are still used today. These appliances were used to treat internal disk disorders by advancing the condyle to force the repositioning of the disk over the condylar head mechanically.

From this brief historical perspective,[1] it is clear that clinicians over the years have used splints to treat and alleviate the signs and symptoms of acute and chronic, intracapsular and extracapsular, temporomandibular disorders.

Splint use in the treatment of TMD is still widely advocated today.[2] In general, an occlusal splint has therapeutic efficacy regardless of the type of splint being used.[3] In addition, the true mechanism by which splints are efficacious in reducing temporomandibular disorder symptoms is generally not well understood. Some clinicians elaborate on a mechanical or anatomic correction of the temporomandibular complex by a functional means.[4, 5] Other clinicians cite cognitive awareness of a parafunctional habit insofar as the occlusal splint reminds the patient of that habit.[6, 7] Still others claim a placebo effect of the occlusal guard[8] (Table 9–1).

In reviewing the use of splint therapy in the treatment of temporomandibular disorders, it is important to specify the diagnosis or diagnoses that the patient carries and is being treated for with regard to splint therapy. In this chapter, I review the use

TABLE 9–1.	Rationale for the Use of Splint Therapy in the Treatment of TMD

- Historically, splint therapy followed the presumed cause of TMD at the time.
- Splint therapy has been advocated to correct structural disharmony of both the TMJs and the occlusion.
- Splint therapy has been advocated to treat myofascial pain functionally.
- Splint therapy has been advocated as a device to aid in cognitive awareness.

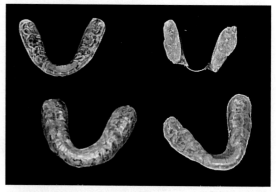

FIGURE 9–1. Various types of splints used for treatment of all types of temporomandibular disorders.

of splint therapy in myofascial pain disorders, in intracapsular disorders, and in surgery of the temporomandibular joint. I discuss the rationale for use as well as describe various types of splints used in each condition. In addition, I review the literature so as to draw some conclusions about the appropriateness of the splint treatment rationale and to discredit any myths involving the use of splint therapy in temporomandibular disorders.

Splint Therapy in Myofascial Pain

RATIONALE

In patients with myofascial pain, the presumed mechanism of action of an intraoral splint is via the relaxation of muscle, either by a mechanical change in the muscle itself[5] or by a change in the patient's function/parafunction when the teeth come together.[9] Many studies have corroborated that splint therapy decreases the symptoms of myalgia.[3, 10–12] Stabilization splint therapy has been shown to decrease the symptoms of

myofascial pain in 70% to 90% of the cases[3] (Table 9–2).

TYPES

There are various types of splints used to treat myofascial pain.[5] Included in this chapter are the most commonly used splints, since they are the most often cited in research of patients with myofascial pain (Fig. 9–1, Table 9–3). The most commonly used splint in the treatment of myofascial pain is known as the *stabilization splint*. It is a full-coverage maxillary or mandibular splint incorporating even posterior contact at the point of maximum closure (Fig. 9–2). The splint usually has anterior disocclusion in protrusive as well as canine guidance or group function in lateral excursions (Fig. 9–3). It is constructed in relation to the patient's centric occlusion or relation position.[5] Other names of this appliance are the *flat plane appliance*, the *University of Pennsylvania maxillary flat plane appliance*, the *Tanner mandibular appliance*, the *centric*

TABLE 9–2.	Rationale for the Use of Splint Therapy in the Treatment of Myofascial Pain

- Allows free mandibular movement
- Decreases muscular activity evidenced by EMG studies
- Does not allow full flexion of closing muscles
- Provides stable dental occlusion
- Aids in cognitive awareness
- Possible effect in bruxism
- Placebo effect

TABLE 9–3.	Types of Splints

- Stabilization splint
- Repositioning splint
- Mandibular orthopedic repositioning appliance or Gelb splint
- Pivot splint
- Soft splint
- Bite plane splint
- There are many variations of each basic category of splint. Each has a specific design thought to change jaw, muscle, or occlusal relationships structurally or functionally.

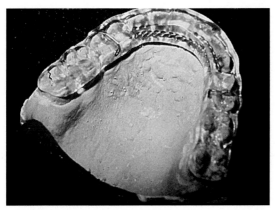

FIGURE 9–2. Stabilization splint.

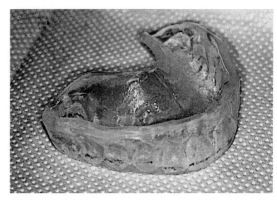

FIGURE 9–4. Soft splint.

relation splint, and the *muscle deprogramming splint.* Most often the appliance is made from a hard acrylic plastic resin.[5, 13]

Occasionally, the treatment of myofascial pain can include a resilient splint (soft splint) (Fig. 9–4). Usually this is a full-coverage "mouth guard" that can be used with good immediate results in patients suffering from myofascial pain. The advantage of a resilient splint is that it can be fabricated in the dental office and is less expensive.[5] A patient can also be referred to a local sporting goods store and make his or her own soft splint. Some clinical researchers feel that a hard splint is superior to a soft resilient one, if pain is related to bruxism.[14, 15]

Another splint is the bite plane splint, also known as the *Hawley bite plane,* which has been used to reduce muscle activity and treat patients with myofascial pain[5] (Figs. 9–5 and 9–6).

A variation of a conventional stabilization splint is the neuromuscular splint, which is constructed to conform to a three-dimensional mandibular representation of the jaw position when muscles are in a state of minimal electromyographic activity.[18, 19]

In addition to the overall styles of splints, many variations exist in the indexing of the opposing dentition on the occlusal surface of the splint, as well as slight modifications in the ultimate occlusal pattern of the patient's dentition in relation to the splint.[5]

Most often, in my practice of treating patients with myofascial pain, I use a conventional full-coverage maxillary splint with minimum to no indentations and anterior disocclusion in protrusive, and canine guidance in excursive, jaw movements. If I identify a patient who is clenching or grinding in the daytime and is unable to wear this type of splint, I prescribe a lower splint with no indentations that allows for free mandibular movement (Fig. 9–7).

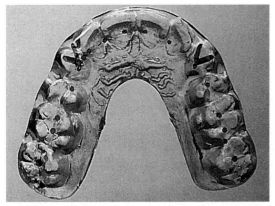

FIGURE 9–3. Occlusal scheme depicting centric occlusion, canine guidance, and anterior and posterior disocclusion in protrusive jaw movement.

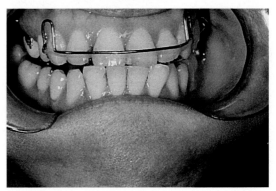

FIGURE 9–5. Hawley bite plate—note posterior disocclusion.

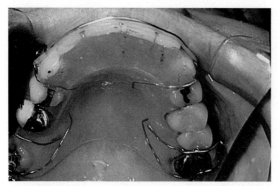

FIGURE 9–6. Occlusal view of Hawley bite plate.

REVIEW OF THE LITERATURE

A myriad of articles have been written concerning the use of splint therapy in treatment of temporomandibular disorders, specifically myofascial disorders.[20–24] Many of these studies evaluated surface electromyographs (EMGs) of the masseter and anterior temporalis muscles in various splint usages. As previously stated, stabilization splint therapy, in general, has been shown to decrease the symptoms of myofascial pain. Many investigators have tried to pinpoint the exact mechanism of the efficacious action that a splint offers in treating patients with this problem. In an article by Shi and Wang[16] an EMG analysis to record muscular activity in the masseter and anterior temporalis muscles of 60 patients noted an increase in the patient group during postural activity: i.e., those patients with myofascial pain had increased EMG findings at rest. This finding was noted to be reversed

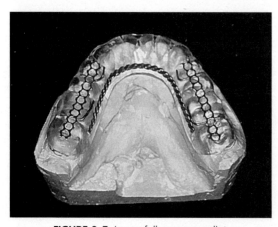

FIGURE 9–7. Lower full-coverage splint.

when a flat plane occlusal splint was used. After 3 months of occlusal therapy, the muscle activity according to the EMG returned to normal. This study suggested that the masseter and temporalis muscles, which are used in clenching, showed a significant decrease in hyperactivity. The authors concluded that the splint achieved a therapeutic result.[16] One counterargument cited against this study is that the signs and symptoms of temporomandibular disorders have traditionally been cyclic and that this was the natural course of the patient's myofascial disorder.[17]

One study evaluated the EMGs of patients who practice bruxism. Bruxism, the grinding of the teeth not during mastication, has been implicated as a cause and/or a perpetuating event in patients with myofascial pain. The EMG of nocturnal bruxers indicated less muscular (masseter and temporalis) activity after a patient was treated with a splint. Over time, however, the effect of splint therapy in treatment of patients with nocturnal bruxism became less certain.[25, 26] That is, the EMG results were less convincing that a continued decrease in muscular activity occurred. Another study found no significant decrease in bruxism with splint usage.[27]

Carlson and colleagues[19] compared muscle activity via EMG in conventional versus neuromuscular splints (discussed earlier). The purpose of this study was to investigate the effectiveness of and differences between these two appliances versus a placebo in which they used cotton rolls. No statistically significant difference was found between the centric relation conventional splint and a neuromuscular splint. There were, however, statistically significant differences found in the EMG values of the placebo versus the two treatment appliances. The study had a limited number of patients.

The results of another study, which showed that patients suffering from myofascial pain had a reduction in jaw pain with the use of an intraoral splint, also determined that these patients showed a decrease in depression and an increase in the use of planned action and rational thinking. In patients who were not treated with splints, these observations were not noted.[10] Assumptions of a cause-and-effect relationship can be made—since the patient's symptoms were alleviated, he or she experienced a decrease in depression. An opposing argument can be made, that the splint did nothing and the patient improved because he or she was less depressed.

In a study that compared acupuncture with splints in 61 patients with myofascial pain, it was noted that both yielded positive results, but acupuncture had more significant side effects.[28]

In investigating the difference between a soft splint (described earlier) and palliative treatment in myofascial patients, a soft splint was shown to be superior and more effective in relieving symptoms than palliative therapy only.[29] As discussed earlier, it is important to consider use of soft splints as an emergency measure in patients with acute myofascial pain.

In studies evaluating the change in efficacy of a splint that incorporated group function into its fabrication versus a splint that was fabricated by utilizing canine guidance,[30, 31] it was found that there was no significant advantage of one occlusal scheme over the other: that is, both occlusal schemes showed a decrease in muscle activity recorded via EMG. In this study, they used the same patient and changed the occlusal scheme on the intraoral guard.

In a study designed to determine whether the *continuous* use of a splint showed any additional benefit in relief of symptoms in patients with myofascial pain as opposed to the *intermittent* use of an intraoral splint, Wilkinson found that intermittent nocturnal use of a splint was better than continuous use of the splint.[32]

In an EMG study by Williamson and coworkers, the EMG of both the masseter and temporalis muscles in patients wearing an anterior repositioning appliance (Figs. 9–8 and 9–9) showed a decrease in muscular activity.[33] The 26 patients who were evaluated in this study all had anteriorly displaced disks with reduction and were being treated for such. Interestingly, the EMG results in these patients being treated with an anterior repositioning appliance revealed less muscular activity than in patients using a flat plane intraoral appliance. The significance of such a study is that it suggests that a patient who has an anteriorly as well as inferiorly displaced mandible has less muscular activity in the masseter and tem-

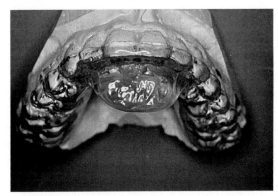

FIGURE 9–8. Maxillary anterior repositioning appliance. Note anterior flange.

poralis muscles than a patient who is in centric occlusion using a stabilization splint.

Many patients with myofascial pain in the muscles of mastication also suffer with myofascial pain in the cervical muscles. Some "trigger" points or "tender" points located in the neck muscles may refer pain to the patient's muscles of mastication, and vice versa.[34] A study[35] described by Manns recorded the electromyographic activity on the hyoid muscles, which are thought to stabilize the jaw during opening and closing. The hyoid group of muscles showed an *increase* in EMG activity while a patient utilized a stabilization splint.

The use of a stabilization splint did, however, show a *decrease* in sternocleidomastoid electromyographic activity when recorded during swallowing and tonic activity.[36] These patients all had cervical muscle spasms. In evaluation of the trapezius mus-

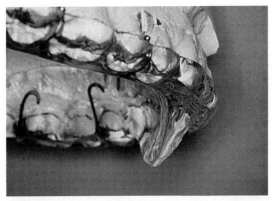

FIGURE 9–9. Lateral view of maxillary anterior repositioning appliance. Note that resting of lower incisors is anterior to this flange.

cle in the same study,[36] no significant improvements in EMG activity were observed with the use of an intraoral occlusal splint. One caveat to remember with these multiple electromyographic studies is that a change in pain in patients with temporomandibular disorders cannot be completely explained on the basis of the electromyographic evidence alone.[37]

In a parallel randomized, controlled, and blinded study performed by Dao and associates,[8] the therapeutic efficacy of splints was evaluated. Sixty-three subjects were evaluated and assigned into three groups. Group one was a passive control group who wore an occlusal splint 30 minutes at each appointment. Group two was an active control who wore a palatal splint (no occlusal coverage) 24 hours a day. Group three was the treatment group, who wore a full occlusal splint 24 hours a day. Over 10 weeks the subjects rated their pain intensity and unpleasant sensation after chewing. All pain ratings decreased significantly with time and quality of life improved for all groups. There were no significant differences between groups. The authors suggested that the gradual reduction in the intensity and unpleasantness of myofascial pain was not specific and not related to any type of treatment.[8] The findings in this study support the thoughts and ideas of Clark,[3] Greene and Laskin,[6] Rugh,[7] and Stohler,[58] who suggest that cognitive awareness and positive patient expectations may be more important than the structural value of an occlusal appliance in treatment of temporomandibular disorders.

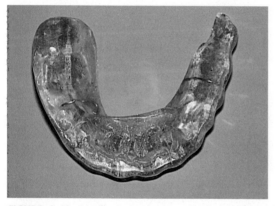

FIGURE 9–10. Maxillary anterior repositioning appliance worn unsupervised for 2 years.

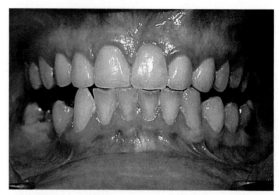

FIGURE 9–11. Patient's occlusion after 2 years unsupervised wear. Note open posterior malocclusion.

CONCLUSIONS AND MYTHS

Although there have been many theories presented and investigated to explain the effect of splint therapy in myofascial pain, it is apparent in the literature that no one theory has been validated. It appears that regardless of the type of splint utilized, patients usually respond positively in 70% to 90% of cases. The material of which a splint is made, the occlusal scheme that is incorporated into the bite surface of the splint, and the time in which a splint is worn seem to have minimal significance in the overall efficacy of treatment. The effect of splint therapy in treatment of myofascial pain certainly requires further investigation with randomized, controlled, and blinded studies in greater numbers of patients and for longer periods of time.

For the clinician who prescribes intraoral occlusal splint therapy for the treatment of myofascial pain, it is important to consider what has been proved and what is still equivocal. A conservative or reversible approach in treating patients is of utmost importance since long-term management of patients with some of the various types of intraoral appliances (Fig. 9–10) can have deleterious effects on the patients' occlusion (Fig. 9–11). On the basis of the published research that is currently available, it appears that occlusal splint therapy should be considered as a mode of therapy in patients with acute and chronic myofascial pain. This splint should have no deleterious effects on the patient's occlusion and should be monitored by the clinician at regular intervals.[38, 39]

Splint Therapy in Intracapsular Temporomandibular Disorders

RATIONALE

As in treatment of myofascial pain, splint therapy has been reported to be effective in pain management of those patients with intracapsular temporomandibular disorders including treatment of disc displacements and temporomandibular joint (TMJ) arthritis.[40, 41] How splints succeed in treating intracapsular disorders is also unknown at this time. Some theories have arisen regarding the use of splints in treatment of intracapsular disorders. Splints in the treatment of disk disorders, including anteriorly displaced disks with reduction and without reduction, are thought to recapture and reposition the disk physically to a corrected position above the condylar head.[4] Long-term outcomes of "repositioning" splint therapy are not as promising as once theorized. Studies have shown that the recapturing of a disk by use of a splint does not guarantee its correct position permanently, except in a very small percentage of patients.[42, 43] In other studies, the actual recapturing event is questioned.[44, 45] Clinicians have theorized that mechanically altering the position of the mandible can have two results: The first is that the condylar head being held in a more inferior, anterior position will mechanically persuade the disk to establish itself atop the condylar head in a more favorable position.[4] The second is that in wearing certain types of splints (i.e., pivotal splint, mandibular anterior repositioning appliance [ARA]) (Figs. 9–12 and 9–13) the condyle disk glenoid fossa relationship is "unloaded."[44, 46, 47] The theory hypothesizes that "unloading the joint" causes inflammation to decrease, range of motion to increase, and symptoms and signs of temporomandibular disorders to improve.

A similar theory holds true for patients who suffer with anteriorly displaced disks without reduction. Some clinicians use the term *disk dislocation* or *closed lock of the temporomandibular joint* to describe the condition of a meniscus that remains in an anterior position to the condyle and does not reduce on wide opening. Most clinicians further classify this subgroup of patients with intracapsular disorders into patients

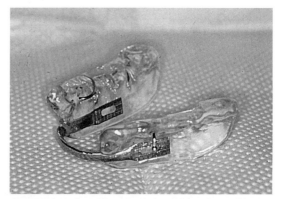

FIGURE 9–12. A pivot splint. Note that posterior acrylic blocks are thought to distract gently the condylar head when patient is in centric occlusion.

who have an acute closed locked situation and patients who have a chronic closed lock.[48] Patients with acute disk dislocation or acute closed lock (i.e., anteriorly displaced disks without reduction) are usually in severe pain, which increases when they try to open their jaw fully. Typically the jaw opens to approximately 22 to 30 mm and then firmly stops. Patients describe this condition as their jaw's feeling "stuck." Many of these patients also recall a history of joint clicking that preceded the limited opening, which ceases to exist once the disk does not reduce (i.e., lock). This results in limited opening. These patients are easily identified by the clinician since they have notable severely restricted condylar translation on opening as well as in lateral and protrusive jaw movements. Most clinicians, when faced with this patient population, try

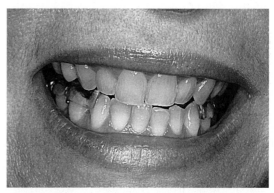

FIGURE 9–13. Mandibular anterior repositioning appliance (mandibular orthopedic repositioning appliance). Note occlusal index guides the mandible to a more anterior position, resulting in a class III occlusion. The condyle/disk relationship is reported to be "unloaded."

to manipulate the lower jaw and distract the condyle from the glenoid fossa to reduce the disk mechanically. If manipulation of the jaw is successful in reducing the disk, then splint therapy is indicated to continue to unload the joint and decrease inflammation while increasing range of motion.[49] A splint that may be used in this patient population is a maxillary anterior repositioning appliance (ARA) (see Figs. 9–8 and 9–9). An ARA used with careful monitoring in a very controlled time frame is helpful in holding the disk in a proper relationship to the condylar head. Many clinicians follow this ARA with a new stabilization splint or convert the existing ARA to a stabilization splint.[50]

Some patients with anteriorly displaced disks without reduction have chronic disk dislocations. These typically are the patients who experience limited jaw opening for a rather long period. Some of these patients possibly have an absence of significant pain, although their opening is significantly diminished. These patients many times are not able to be manipulated by the clinician to reduce the disk. They may also occasionally experience pain in the temporomandibular joint area if the jaw is stretched farther open or if there is impingement of retrodiscal tissue when moving the jaw into lateral excursive movements. Some of these patients in fact are very successful in adaptation.[51] The retrodiscal tissue itself may become moderately fibrosed such as to act as a pseudodisk. Use of a stabilization splint in these patients may be warranted during the early transition of fibrosis to decrease pain in the temporomandibular joint area.

Splints used in the treatment of arthritis of the temporomandibular joint are usually viewed as one particular mode of treatment in a multitherapy-based overall treatment plan. Generally, in treatment of patients with TMJ arthritis, the clinician tries to relieve the patient's pain, maintain and correct the patient's mobility and function, and prevent further deformation or degradation of the joint by suppressing the disease process. Appliance therapy in the management of temporomandibular joint arthritis should be only a *part* of the total management of the patient, which includes drug therapy, physical therapy, and possibly surgical therapy.[40, 52] The goals of splint therapy in the management of patients with temporomandibular arthritis are to minimize joint loading and provide the patient with a stable occlusion. These goals are thought ultimately to decrease jaw joint pain. Although there are multiple types of arthritis affecting the temporomandibular joint, splint therapy in each specific disorder is thought to have the same beneficial effect. Current controversy does exist concerning use of splint therapy in preventing the progression of arthritis in the temporomandibular joint.[53]

A study published by Boering and associates provided some of the first longitudinal data results regarding the natural progression of temporomandibular disorders. They and others concluded that temporomandibular intraarticular disorders follow a natural course independently of the treatment approach.[53–57] The clinician, therefore, should relate the treatment to the patient's pain and lack of functioning rather than trying to prevent some untoward temporomandibular disorder in the future. At this time, long-term follow-up of the use of splints in treating degenerative joint disease has not been done.[56] In addition, prevention of osteoarthritis or degenerative arthritis by use of an intraoral splint has not been proved.[55, 56]

TYPES OF SPLINTS

Once again, various types of splints have been used to treat intracapsular disorders. In addition, variations on basic designs of splints have also been used.[58] As noted, a stabilization splint has been used to treat joint pain, especially if this joint pain has been related to parafunctional habits.[51] In addition, a bite plane splint has been used to treat jaw joint pain. Various types of repositioning appliances have been used to alter condylar position at occlusal contact positions in an attempt to recapture a displaced disk (meniscus).[59] Repositioning appliances include the maxillary anterior repositioning appliance (ARA) (see Figs. 9–8 and 9–9), the ligated anterior repositioning splint (LARS), as well as various types of mandibular orthopedic appliances (MORAs) (see Fig. 9–13). These appliances are all designed with hard acrylic and cuspal indentations to guide the mandible to a predetermined position. The classic repositioning appliance is a full-coverage maxillary splint with an acrylic flange that rests lingual to the lower anterior teeth and has buccal and incisal indices of the lower cusp tips in its surface (see Figs. 9–8 and 9–9). This splint brings the mandible into a protrusive position. It is thought to be most effective at nighttime because it keeps the mandible forward during sleep, when it would otherwise tend to relax and retrude. This specific appliance has also been called the *pull forward appliance* as well as the *Farrar splint*. Other repositioning appliances are worn over the lower teeth and have deeper indices, which guide the mandible into an anterior position. Variations of this MORA are called the *Friedman, Gelb,* and *TMJ Blank appliances.*[5, 60, 61]

A pivotal type of appliance has also been used to "unload" the temporomandibular joint components and mildly stretch the joint[46] (see Fig. 9–12). These can be maxillary or mandibular appliances with occlusal contact only in the most posterior tooth. They can be designed to be either unilateral or bilateral, depending on the joint or joints involved in the disorder.

These active appliances, including the MORA as well as the pivotal appliance and TMJ Blank, can have adverse effects on the dentition when used to recapture the disk. The adverse occlusal effects many times are noted secondary to eruption changes in the dentition, or changes in jaw relations, or both (Figs. 9–14 to 9–16). This is an important consideration when prescribing these types of splints. It is therefore important to consider the patient's compliance when using any of these repositioning splints. An interruption in patient-doctor contact may result in drastic nonreversible occlusal changes with or without the reduc-

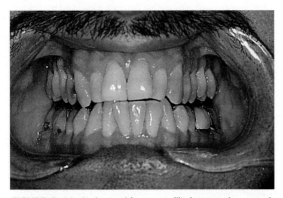

FIGURE 9–14. Patient with a mandibular anterior repositioning appliance.

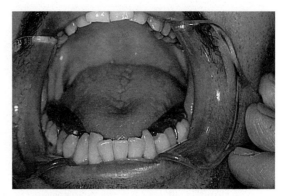

FIGURE 9–15. Patient with the appliance in place.

tion of pain in the temporomandibular joint area.[62, 63]

A REVIEW OF THE LITERATURE

In reviewing the literature concerning splint therapy used in intracapsular temporomandibular disorders, it is important to subcategorize the type of intracapsular disorder that is being treated. I will first discuss anteriorly displaced disks with reduction. Typically these patients describe to the clinician a painful clicking joint with signs and symptoms of capsulitis. These patients may also, in fact, have myofascial pain. In an article by Zamburlini and Austin, and another by LeBell and Kirveskari, the use of an anterior repositioning appliance (discussed earlier) versus a flat plane stabilization splint decreased jaw pain both in the muscles of mastication as well as in the preauricular area, the area associated with the joint.[42, 43] The anterior repositioning appliance, however, decreased joint tenderness better than the flat plane stabilization splint. In addition, when using the anterior positioning appliance, the patients noted a decrease in the amount of clicking. Even though clicking decreased in the short term, permanent long-term recapture of the articular disk was noted in about 10% to 30% of these patients.[42, 45]

In a study in the *Journal of Oral and Maxillofacial Surgery,* Kirk examined a total of 30 joints in 18 patients.[44] Twenty-seven of the 30 joints were treated with an anterior repositioning appliance (Sved type). The patients were treated until all of the joints were silent to auscultation. These patients were then evaluated with com-

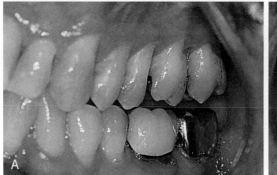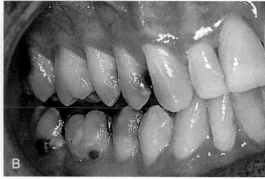

FIGURE 9–16. Note posterior disocclusion bilaterally, as a result of continual wearing of this appliance.

puted tomography (CT) scans as well as magnetic resonance imaging (MRI), while in both a centric occlusion position as well as an anterior repositioned position (i.e., with the Sved appliance in place). Comparisons were then made between the condyle and the disk. It was determined that there were some condylar positioning changes. The disk, however, appeared to be in the same position in all of the MRIs except three. Kirk concluded that the concept of disk recapture should be only a clinical term, not a true anatomic correction.[44] Moreover the joint noises were perhaps decreased as a result of increased joint space as opposed to any true recapturing of the disk. Chen in the *Australian Dental Journal* also refuted the concept of recapturing a displaced disk. It was also noted in this study that patients treated with an anterior repositioning appliance that moved the mandible into a more anterior position had a decrease in their symptoms of temporomandibular disorders.[45] In a study of 14 temporomandibular joints evaluated with MRI and treated with an anterior repositioning appliance, it was shown that recapture occurred in 30% of those cases. These patients were followed up for approximately 4 years, at which time 4 of the original 14 achieved stable repositioning.[64] This was confirmed with an MRI recording.

The significance of recapturing of the disk has also been controversial in assessment of patient recovery. In fact, whether the disk reduces may have little effect on overall symptoms.[17, 41] Cohen and MacAfee indicate that internal derangements of the temporomandibular joint can cause symptoms of temporomandibular disorders but also can lead to the more severe process of degenerative joint disease.[4] This, to date, has not been proved. In their article, Cohen and MacAfee state that maintenance of a proper anatomic meniscal condylar relationship is essential in preventing these degenerative joint changes and they advocate the use of anterior repositioning appliances to achieve proper meniscal position. In addition, Cohen noted that the use of magnetic resonance imaging to determine disk position in the management of internal derangements of the temporomandibular joint is an effective method of determining true discal position in the temporomandibular joint.[4]

Much has also been written on intrajoint pressures in the TMJ. In a review of the literature, it appears that intraarticular pressure has been recorded in an attempt to corroborate the theory of "joint unloading." In a study by dosSantos and deRiik in the *Journal of Oral Rehabilitation,* a proposed mechanical model to demonstrate the equilibrium of normal force vectors transmitted to the masticatory system with occlusal bite plane splints of different designs was introduced.[65] Occlusal contacts were imposed on the proposed models under the action of a masticatory force vector. This forced action created different responses within the joint and also at the level of the teeth. Intraoral appliances with smooth contacting surfaces or minor indentations (both with an increased vertical dimension) forced the mandible to assume a more anterior position, when compared with the intercuspal position in centric occlusion. This resulted in a concurrent increase in joint forces. It was noted that the bite splint that produced the least amount of increased joint force was the stabilization splint. This stabilization splint had a very minimal amount of increase in the occlusal vertical dimension.[65]

In an article in the *Journal of Prosthetic Dentistry,* Nitzan described the intraarticular pressure in the functioning human temporomandibular joint and its alteration by uniform elevation of the occlusal plane.[47] In his study, intraarticular pressure was measured at the posterior slope of the articular eminence in the upper compartment of the superior chamber of the temporomandibular joint. This intraarticular pressure was measured on 35 individuals, 28 of whom were females and 7 of whom were males. This was done under local anesthesia. The pressure measurements were recorded during rest position, maximum opening, and clenching. During maximum opening, the intraarticular pressure decreased, and, during clenching, the pressure always increased. One other notable finding was that females generated higher pressures in their joints than males, even though they had a lower bite force.[47] In 22 patients, the intraarticular pressure was also measured while they were clenching on an intraocclusal appliance. This appliance was designed so that it uniformly elevated the occlusal plane to reduce the force toward the temporomandibular joint. During clenching with the intraoral appliance in place, there was a decrease of 81.2%. It was suggested that an intraocclusal appliance was very effective in treatment of symptomatic temporomandibular joints in that it decreased the pressure in the upper joint space.[47] Most clinicians regard this as an appropriate guide to suggest that the use of an intraocclusal appliance during and after temporomandibular joint surgery is warranted. Another study, which further suggests that the use of splints may, in fact, decrease the "joint load," has shown that a fulcrum or pivotal splint located in the second molar area had a condylar lowering of about 1 to 3 mm in 90% of patients on repeated temporomandibular joint tomograms.[46] Thus, the use of splint therapy has been advocated in temporomandibular joint disorders consisting of anteriorly displaced disks with reduction.

Splint therapy has also been evaluated in anterior displaced disks without reduction. The literature supporting the efficacy of using splint therapies in anteriorly displaced disks without reduction seems to be less convincing. A small percentage of the patients who are treated "off the disk" with a stabilization splint may go through some posterior attachment changes in which the posterior tissue becomes more fibrous and acts as a pseudodisk. If a patient during the time of treatment is able to tolerate the decreased range of motion as well as pain, then eventually fibrous tissue replaces the heavily innervated and vascularized retrodiscal tissue, resulting in greater range of motion and less pain.[41, 49, 66] During this period of treatment "off the disk," both anterior repositioning splints as well as flat stabilization splints have been utilized and documented to decrease some of the pain and pressure in the joint itself.[41]

In contradiction, in a study by Lundh, 51 patients with temporomandibular joint pain associated with anteriorly displaced disks without reduction were placed in a 12-month clinical trial.[67] Half of the group was treated with the flat occlusal splint and the other half was untreated and left as a control group. Pain symptoms disappeared in about one third of the patients in each group. Another third of the patients in the control group also improved. Approximately 40% of those treated with the flat plane occlusal splint were noted to be worse at the end of treatment than in the beginning of the study. The author concluded that a statistically significant benefit of use of a flat occlusal splint over nontreatment in a control subject could not be identified and that in patients with painful disk displacements without reduction, the use of a flat occlusal splint should be reconsidered.[67] This article muddies the waters in suggesting that treatment of an acute closed lock for an anteriorly displaced disk without reduction should not include treatment with a flat plane occlusal splint. However, other case reports and studies[49] have suggested that manipulation of an acute closed lock by deflection of the mandible followed by continued stabilization splint therapy has had some success.[49, 68]

In addition, another study, described by Linde and colleagues, compared the 6-week treatment outcomes of patients with temporomandibular joint disk displacement without reduction.[50] In this study, they compared conventional splint therapy with transcutaneous electrical nerve stimulation (TENS) on symptomatic joints. Approximately half the patients treated with splints became pain-free or their temporomandibular joint pain improved at least 50% during rest and jaw function. Only 6% of the patients in the TENS-treated group improved. The conclusion was that flat occlusal splints in several respects were much better than TENS in treatment of symptoms associated with temporomandibular joint disk displacements without reduction.[50] One could infer from this study that at least 50% of the patients in this group did have good pain relief with flat occlusal splints.

As indicated, long-term follow-up regarding the use of a splint in treating degenerative joint disease has not been done. The study by Boering suggests that there is a natural progression or natural cessation of the temporomandibular disorder that is independent of the treatment used.[54, 55] However, it seems reasonable that if a patient is experiencing pain emanating from the temporomandibular joint area, use of a conservative splint may be beneficial in reducing some of the pain associated with arthritis.[40]

CONCLUSIONS AND MYTHS

It does appear, in reviewing the literature concerning splint therapy utilization in intracapsular disorders, that splint therapy many times can be efficacious in relieving signs and symptoms of temporomandibular disorders. The diminution of clicking, however, does not correlate well with patients' subjective symptoms. In addition, the theory of recapturing the disk by appliances seems unfounded or established in only a small percentage of patients. If, in fact, recapture does occur, the disk does not remain in the corrected position permanently, except in a small percentage of patients. Repositioning splint therapy may be superior, however, to flat splint therapy in reducing joint clicking and tenderness to palpation in the temporomandibular joint.[17, 42] It appears that repositioning appliances do offer short-term symptom reduction for acute pain associated with reciprocal clicking of the temporomandibular joint. This occurs especially when the pain is at the point of clicking and localized to the joint region or area when intermittent locking occurs.[17, 57]

The one problem, as previously discussed, with functional appliances, i.e., recapturing

appliances or repositioning appliances, is that, in an attempt to recapture the disk, the patient's dental occlusion may be adversely affected. In many patients with unsupervised wear of an anterior repositioning appliance a posterior open occlusion develops. This, on complete reduction of temporomandibular joint pain, may be corrected only by extensive prosthetic reconstruction or orthodontic treatment. It has been suggested that adverse effects as described can be prevented by the use of two splints, one worn to position the jaw and another one worn at night to maintain the teeth in their original alignment.[17]

The clinician who treats patients with temporomandibular disorders, especially those with intracapsular disorders, is faced with the decision as to the type of splint, i.e., stabilization versus a functional or repositioning splint, to utilize. At this time the literature is quite inconclusive in guiding the clinician as to which splint to use. If an anterior repositioning appliance or a functional splint is utilized, it is important to do frequent monitoring and frequent reevaluation to assess occlusal changes. This is absolutely required. If a patient is noncompliant or has a history of being lax in follow-up treatments, then an anterior repositioning appliance should *not* be considered. The majority of intracapsular disorders, including anteriorly displaced disks with reduction and without reduction, can be effectively treated with stabilization splints and other modalities. There are many articles to suggest that a flat stabilization splint reduces the symptoms of pain associated with those disorders. Because the nature of temporomandibular joint internal derangements and osteoarthrosis is nonprogressive in a majority of cases,[53] there is no true rationale for disk repositioning procedures via splint therapy. This makes the use of anterior repositioning appliances (which only in a minority of the cases reposition the disk) very limited in the way it should be prescribed.

Splint Therapy Utilization in Surgery of the Temporomandibular Joint

RATIONALE

Almost all patients with complaints of temporomandibular disorders, whether they are disorders related to the muscles of mastication or true intracapsular disorders, require a trial of conservative management. As a *part* of nonsurgical management of temporomandibular disorders, splint therapy should precede the decision to seek a surgical consultation. As stated earlier, the overall success rate for conservative management of temporomandibular disorder in general is anywhere from 70% to 90%. For those patients with intracapsular disorders unresponsive to conservative treatment, surgery may be required. The spectrum of surgical intervention that has been used to treat patients with temporomandibular disorders includes arthrocentesis, arthroscopy, arthrotomy, condylotomy, orthognathic surgery, and temporomandibular joint replacement.[48, 66, 69, 70] Various surgical interventions that are available for intracapsular temporomandibular disorders are detailed elsewhere in this volume.

Postoperative management of these surgical patients, i.e., those who require jaw joint surgery, requires adjunctive splint therapy in addition to physical therapy and medication therapy. Many open joint surgeries and occasionally temporomandibular joint arthroscopy procedures result in acute capsulitis. An occlusal splint, therefore, is thought gradually to reduce the pressure in the temporomandibular joint to allow for free movement of the mandible without dental intercuspation. A stabilization splint, therefore, is helpful for a period of 6 to 8 weeks after surgery to protect the jaw joint during healing. Splint therapy may have to be continued as the need for physical therapy and joint rehabilitation continues. Patients with intracapsular disorders that are treated with surgery may gradually (over a period of 6 months) be weaned off the splint. In general, postoperative splint therapy in this patient population must be monitored frequently because changes in pain, swelling, and muscle activity continue in the immediate postoperative weeks. In addition the patient's occlusion during the postoperative period may also change. If the splint is not adjusted frequently at this time, the muscles of mastication may become tender, causing jaw trismus, deviation on opening, or further muscle splinting. Some advocate that a stabilization splint be placed in the mouth the day after surgery and adjusted weekly for a period of 1 month.[48] Most patients achieve a stable occlusion post surgery in approximately 4 to 6 weeks. Adjustments may be necessary, however, for 3 to 4 months. Occlusal equilibration of the patient's natural dentition after that period may still be necessary to stabilize the patient's occlusion.

TYPES

Specific splint types that are used in the perioperative period for the TMD patient treated surgically include the stabilization splint, anterior repositioning splint, and LARS, which have been described earlier.

REVIEW OF THE LITERATURE

As noted, postoperative splint therapy does play an important role in the recovery from temporomandibular joint surgery. Although seemingly empirical, the indication for postoperative splint therapy at this time has not been adequately studied. In fact, much of the literature in this regard has been adapted from other studies involving splint therapy. Some of the studies have been mentioned, including those previously cited.

Splint therapy is thought to "unload" the jaw joint by putting less pressure on the joint itself.[47] This decrease in pressure is thought also to decrease postoperative inflammation as well as pain. In addition, a splint is thought to decrease any harmful effect from a patient's parafunctional habits, conscious as well as subconscious. In specific intracapsular disorders that are repaired surgically, including perforations of the disk that have been surgically plicated, as well as anteriorly displaced disks that are repositioned over the condylar head, many clinicians advocate the use of an anterior repositioning splint that moves the condyle slightly forward.[48] This is used for a period of approximately 2 months after surgery, thus allowing the best possibility of healing in the postdiscal attachment tissue. After 2 months of anterior repositioning, a stabilization splint is employed to allow for further unloading of the jaw joint as well as muscle relaxation.[48]

In patients who have osteotomies for treatment of the temporomandibular joints, splint therapy has only limited usage in the immediate postoperative phase.[48] Most of these patients do have or will have inter-maxillary fixation, and therefore the use of a removable splint is impossible. A ligated anterior repositioning splint (LARS) may be placed immediately postoperatively and surgically ligated into place to allow the jaw to change its position permanently.[48] After intermaxillary fixation in orthognathic surgeries, a stabilization splint may be used in stabilizing the patient's occlusion. This results in decreased muscular pain and improved joint function. In preoperative orthognathic surgery, a splint may also be used to relax the muscles of mastication to ensure proper condylar seating prior to permanently changing maxillomandibular relationships and to produce a more predictable postsurgical result, if in fact muscle splinting and/or guarding has altered the patient's maxillomandibular relationship.[48]

CONCLUSIONS AND MYTHS

Splint therapy plays many roles in surgery of the temporomandibular joint. Anterior repositioning splints, as earlier reported, can help maintain a surgically reduced disk. A stabilization splint can decrease jaw joint loading and thereby decrease inflammation in the postsurgical jaw joint. A stabilization splint may also decrease the negative forces to the jaw joint during parafunction postoperatively. A stabilization splint can also aid in the establishment of a proper occlusion in the postoperative patient. In addition the use of a stabilization splint is valuable in distinguishing muscular pain from true jaw joint pain. If the patient is placed on a stabilization splint and the pain ceases, temporomandibular joint surgery may not be necessary. True histologic benefits of postoperative temporomandibular joint splint therapy need to be substantiated in an animal model. Presently, much of the scientific literature that is available is that which has been adapted from other nonsurgical studies and used to support the role of splint therapy in surgery of the temporomandibular joint.

REFERENCES

1. McNeill C: History and evolution of TMD concepts. Oral Surg Oral Med Oral Pathol Oral Radiol Endod 1997;83:51–60.
2. Glass EG, Glaros AG, McGlynn FD: Myofascial pain dysfunction: Treatments used by ADA members. Cranio 1993;11(1):25–29.
3. Clark GP: A critical evaluation of orthopaedic interocclusal appliance therapy: Design theory and overall effectiveness. J Am Dent Assoc 1984; 108:359.
4. Cohen SG, MacAfee KA: The use of magnetic resonance imaging to determine splint position in the management of internal derangements of the temporomandibular joint. Cranio 1994;12(3):167–171.
5. Boero RP: The physiology of splint therapy: A literature review. Angle Orthod 1989;59(3):165–180.
6. Greene CS, Laskin VM: Splint therapy for the myofascial pain dysfunction syndrome: A comparative study. J Am Dent Assoc 1972;84:624–628.
7. Rugh JB: Home care and behavioral therapy. In McNeill C (ed): Current Controversies in Temporomandibular Disorders. Chicago, Quintessence, 1992, pp 142–152.
8. Dao TT, Lavigane GJ, Charmbonneau A, et al: The efficacy of oral splints in the treatment of myofascial pain of the jaw muscles: A controlled clinical trial. Pain 1994;56(1):85–94.
9. Clark GT, Beemsterboer PL, Solberg WK, et al: Nocturnal electromyographic evaluation of myofascial pain dysfunction in patients undergoing occlusal splint therapy. J Am Dent Assoc 1979; 99(4):607–611.
10. deLeeuw JR, Steenks MH, Ros WJ, et al: Assessment of treatment outcome in patients with craniomandibular dysfunction. J Oral Rehabil 1994; 21(6):655–666.
11. Turk DC, Zaki HS, Rudy TF: Effects of intraoral appliance and biofeedback/stress management alone and in combination in treating pain and depression in patients with temporomandibular disorders. J Prosthet Dent 1993;70(2):158–164.
12. Nemcovsky CF, Gazip F, Serfati V, et al: A comparative study of three therapeutic modalities in temporomandibular disorder population. Cranio 1992; 10(2):148–155.
13. Nelson SJ: Principles of stabilization bite splint therapy. Dent Clin North Am 1995;39(2):403–421.
14. Okeson JP: Management of Temporomandibular Disorders and Occlusion, ed 3. Philadelphia, WB Saunders, 1993, pp 402–448, 451–457.
15. Okeson JP: The effects of hard and soft occlusal splints on nocturnal bruxism. J Am Dent Assoc 1987;114:788–791.
16. Shi CS, Wang HY: Postural and maximum activity in elevators during mandible pre and post occlusal splint treatment of temporomandibular joint disturbance syndrome. J Oral Rehabil 1989;16:155–161.
17. Truelove E, Blasberg B: Orofacial pain review of the literature. In Millard HB, Mason DK (eds): Perspectives on the Second World Workshop on Oral Medicine. Ann Arbor, Michigan, University of Michigan Continuing Dental Education, School of Dentistry, 1995, pp 193–215.
18. Cooper BC, Cooper DL, Lucente FE: Electromyography of masticatory muscles and craniomandibular disorders. Laryngoscope 1991;101(2):150–157.
19. Carlson N, Moline B, Huber L, et al: Comparison of muscle activity between conventional and neuromuscular splints. J Prosthet Dent 1993;70(1):39–43.
20. Visser A, Naeige M, Hansson TL: The temporal/masseter co-contraction: An electromyographic and clinical evaluation of short-term stabilization

splint therapy in myogenous TMJ patients. J Rehabil 1995;22(5):387–389.

21. Long JH Jr: Interocclusal splint designed to reduce tenderness in lateral pterygoid and other muscles of mastication. J Prosthet Dent 1995;73(3):316–318.

22. Santander H, Miralles R, Jimenez A, et al: Influence of stabilization occlusal splint on cranial cervical relationships. Part II. Electromyographic analysis. Cranio 1994;12(4):227–233.

23. Moya H, Mirales R, Zuniga C, et al: Influence of stabilization occlusal splint on craniocervical relationships. Part I. Cephalometric analysis. Cranio 1994;12(1):47–51.

24. Attanasio R: Bite appliance therapy for myofascial pain and dysfunction. Oral Maxillofac Surg Clin North Am 1995;7(1):79–86.

25. Shan SC, Yun WH: Influence of occlusal splint on integrated electromyography of masseter muscle. J Oral Rehabil 1991;18:253–256.

26. Solberg WK, Clark GT, Rugh JD: Nocturnal electromyographic evaluation of bruxism patients undergoing short-term splint therapy. J Oral Rehabil 1975;2:215–223.

27. Holmgren K, Sheikholeslam A, Riise C: Effect of full arch maxillary occlusal splint on parafunctional activity during sleep in patients with nocturnal bruxism and signs and symptoms of craniomandibular disorders. J Maxillofac Surg 1994; 52(7):671–679.

28. List T, Helkimo M: Adverse effects of acupuncture and occlusal splint therapy in the treatment of craniomandibular disorders. Cranio 1992;10(4):318–324.

29. Wright E, Anderson G, Schulte J: A randomized clinical trial of intraoral soft splints and palliative treatment for masticatory muscle pain. J Orofac Pain 1995;9(2):192–199.

30. Borromeo GL, Suvinen TI, Reade PC: A comparison of the effects of group functioning and canine guidance in an interocclusal device on masseter muscle electromyographic activity in normal subjects. J Prosthet Dent 1995;94:174–180.

31. Rugh JV, Graham GS, Smith JC, et al: Effects of canine versus molar occlusal splint guidance on nocturnal bruxism and craniomandibular symptomatology. J Craniomandibul Disord Facial Oral Pain 1989;3:203–210.

32. Wilkinson T, Hansson TL, McNeill C, et al: A Comparison of the Success of 24 Hour Occlusal Splint Therapy versus Nocturnal Occlusal Splint Therapy in Reducing Craniomandibular Disorders. J Craniomandibul Disord Facial Oral Pain 1992;6:64–70.

33. Williamson EH, Navarro EZ, Zwemer JD: Comparison of electromyographic activity between anterior repositioning splint therapy and a centric relation splint. Cranio 1993;11(3):178–183.

34. Laskin DM: Diagnosis and etiology of myofascial pain and dysfunction. Oral Maxillofac Surg Clin North Am 1995;7(1):73–78.

35. Manns A, Velvivia L, Mirralles R, et al: The effect of different occlusal splints of the electromyographic activity of the elevator muscles. J Gnathol 1988;7:61–73.

36. Miralles R, Mendoza C, Santander H, et al: Influence of stabilization occlusal splints on sternocleidomastoid and masseter electromyographic activity. Cranio 1992;10(4):297–304.

37. Naeije M, Hansson TL: Short-term effect of the stabilization appliance in masticatory activity in myogenous craniomandibular disorder patients. J Craniomandibul Disord Facial Oral Pain 1991; 5:245–250.

38. NIH Technology Assessment Conference: Management of temporomandibular disorders. J Am Dent Assoc 1996;127:1595–1606.

39. National Institutes of Health Technology Assessment Conference Statement: Management of temporomandibular disorders, April 29-May 1, 1996. Oral Surg Oral Med Oral Pathol Oral Radiol Endod 1997;83:177–183.

40. Abubaker AO, Laskin DM: Non-surgical management of arthritis of the temporomandibular joint. Oral Maxillofac Surg Clin North Am 1995;7(1):51–61.

41. Okeson JP: Non-surgical treatments of internal derangement. Oral Maxillofac Surg Clin North Am 1995;7(1):63–71.

42. Zamburlini I, Austin D: Long-term results of appliance therapy using anterior disk displacement with reduction: A review of literature. Cranio 1991;9(4):361–368.

43. LeBell Y, Kirveskari P: Treatment of reciprocal clicking of the temporomandibular joint with a repositioning appliance and occlusal adjustment: Results after four and six years. Proc Finn Dent Soc 1990;86(1):15–21.

44. Kirk WS Jr: Magnetic resonance imaging on tomographic evaluation of occlusal appliance treatment for advanced internal derangement of the temporomandibular joint. J Oral Maxillofac Surg 1991; 49(1):9–12.

45. Chen CW, Boulton J, Gage JP: Splint therapy in temporomandibular joint dysfunction: A study using magnetic resonance imaging. Aust Dent J 1995;40(2):71–78.

46. Moncayo S: Biomechanics of pivoting appliances. J Orofac Pain 1994;8(2):190–198.

47. Nitzan DW: Intra-articular pressure in the functioning human temporomandibular joint and its alteration by uniform elevation of the occlusal plane. J Prosthet Dent 1993;69(3):293–297.

48. Bays RA: Arthrotomy and orthognathic surgery for temporomandibular disorders. In Kraus SL (ed): Temporomandibular Disorders, ed 2. New York, Churchill Livingstone, 1994, pp 237–276.

49. Chung SC, Kim HS: The effective stabilization splint on TMJ close lock. Cranio 1993;11(2):95–101.

50. Linde C, Isaacsson G, Jonsson RG: Outcome of eight week treatment with transcutaneous electric nerve stimulation compared with splint on symptomatic temporomandibular joint disk displacement without reduction. Acta Odontol Scand 1995;53(2):92–98.

51. Choi BH, Yoo JH, Lee WY: Comparison of magnetic resonance imaging before and after nonsurgical treatment of closed locks. Oral Surg Oral Med Oral Pathol 1994;78(3):301–305.

52. Mohamed SE: Non-surgical treatment of muscular disorders and TMJ disorders. Oral Maxillofac Surg Knowledge Update 1994;1:103–114.

53. deBont LGM, Dijkeraaf LC, Stegenga B: Epidemiology and natural progression of articular temporomandibular disorders. Oral Surg Oral Med Oral Pathol Oral Radiol Endod 1997;83:72–76.

54. Boering G: Temporomandibular Joint Osteoarthrosis: Analysis of 400 cases—A Clinical and Radiographic Investigation [thesis]. Groningen, The Netherlands, The Department of Oral and Maxillofacial Surgery, University of Groningen, 1966, pp 531–539. (Reprinted 1994.)

55. Boering G, Stegenga B, deBont LGM: Clinical signs of TMJ osteoarthrosis and internal derangement thirty years after non-surgical treatment. J Orofac Pain 1994;8:18–24.
56. deLeeuw R, Boering G, Stegenga B, et al: Symptoms of temporomandibular joint osteoarthrosis and internal derangement thirty years after non-surgical treatment. Cranio 1995;13(2):81–88.
57. Tallents RH, Katzberg RW, Macher DJ, et al: Use of protrusal splint therapy in anterior disk displacement of the temporomandibular joint: A one to three year follow-up. J Prosthet Dent 1990;63:336–341.
58. Stohler CS: Occlusal therapy in treatment of temporomandibular disorders. Oral Maxillofac Surg Clin North Am 1995;7(1):129–139.
59. Okeson J: Management of Temporomandibular Disorders and Occlusion, ed 2. St. Louis, CV Mosby, 1989, pp 413–439.
60. Orenstein ES: Anterior repositioning appliances when used for anterior disk displacement with reduction: A critical review. Cranio 1993;11(2):141–145.
61. Gelb ML, Gelb H: Gelb appliance: Mandibular orthopaedic repositioning therapy. Cranionclin Int 1991;1(2):81–98.
62. Owen AH: Orthopaedic/orthodontic therapy for anterior disk displacement: unexpected treatment findings. Cranio 1989;7:33–45.
63. Pertes RA, Attanosio R, Cinotti WR, et al: Occlusal splint therapy in myofascial pain disorders and internal derangements of the temporomandibular joint. Clin Prevent Dent 1989;11:26–33.
64. Bauer W, Augthun M, Wehrhein H, et al: Occlusal splint therapy in reciprocal TMJ clicking: A critical observation within a follow-up study. Fortschr Kieferorthop 1993;54(3):108–118.
65. dosSantos JD Jr., deRiik WG: Vectoral analysis of the equilibrium of forces transmitted to TMJ and occlusal biteplane splints. J Oral Rehabil 1995;22(4):301–310.
66. Sato S, Kawamura H, Motegi K: Management of non-reducing temporomandibular joint disk displacement: Evaluation of Three Treatments. Oral Surg Oral Med Oral Pathol Oral Radiol Endod 1995;80(4):384–388.
67. Lundh H, Westesson PL, Eriksson L, et al: Temporomandibular joint disk displacement without reduction: Treatment with occlusal splint versus no treatment. Oral Surg Oral Med Oral Pathol 1992;73:665–668.
68. Murakami K, Hosaka H, Moriya Y, et al: Short-term treatment outcome study for the management of temporomandibular joint closed lock: A comparison of arthrocentesis to nonsurgical therapy and arthroscopic lysis and lavage. Oral Surg Oral Med Oral Pathol Oral Radiol and Endod 1995;80(3):253–257.
69. Going R Jr: Arthroscopy in the conservative management of temporomandibular disorders. In Kraus SL (ed): Temporomandibular Disorders, ed 2. New York, Churchill Livingstone, 1994, pp 217–236.
70. Schwartz RB: Arthroscopy of the temporomandibular joint. Selected Readings Oral Maxillofac Surg 1996;4(4):1–45.

10

Physical Therapy Management of Temporomandibular Disorders

Steven L. Kraus

Nonsurgical treatment is the primary focus for patients experiencing symptoms and a limitation in function due to temporomandibular disorders (TMDs). Nonsurgical treatment options and the application and sequencing of the treatment options for TMD are controversial. Nonsurgical treatment options for TMD may include medication, mouth appliances, injections, stress management, and physical therapy. Physical therapy is both a conservative and a noninvasive form of management for TMD. This chapter has four objectives: first, to introduce clinical practice guidelines for physical therapy in the management of TMD; second, to familiarize the reader with physical therapy; third, to discuss TMD conditions that will best respond to physical therapy management; fourth, to give an overview of the cervical spine and its significance in head and neck pain management.

Clinical Practice Guidelines for Physical Therapy

An overview of clinical practice guidelines as they pertain to physical therapy intervention for TMD is important because current practice guidelines for physical therapy in TMD management are, at best, misleading. Clinical practice guidelines exist in all areas of medicine. Guidelines may be used as a means to understand the benefits of a certain intervention. The development of clinical practice guidelines is heralded by some experts as a prelude to a golden age of health care accountability and effectiveness.[1] Other experts, however, view the guidelines as a main element in a dangerous campaign to interpose governmental and health care managers between practitioners and patients—a campaign that could lead to diminished quality of care.[1] There are thousands of guidelines in existence. Many of these guidelines are proprietary, not based on science, or slanted toward a particular organization's or subspecialty's point of interest.[2]

Pertinent to this discussion are guidelines from the Agency for Health Care Policy and Research (AHCPR).[3] The AHCPR was created in 1989 as an extension of the U.S. Public Health Service to develop clinical practice guidelines in accordance with AHCPR regulations and procedures.[1] A majority of physical therapists and medical doctors are aware of the AHCPR recent guidelines, *Acute Low Back Problems in Adults*.[3] There have been many legitimate questions raised as to the agency's own guidelines used to acquire and review evidence for establishing these guidelines for acute low back pain.[1, 2] Weaknesses inherent in the AHCPR guideline development process would increase the likelihood of misinterpretation.[2, 4–6]

Dentists and dental organizations have become aware of the AHCPR guidelines on acute low back pain. Several task forces in dentistry refer to the AHCPR comments on modalities commonly used by physical therapists.[7, 8] Several task forces in dentistry also have conducted their own review of the literature pertinent to "physical therapy" management of TMD,[7–9] providing dentists or dental organizations the means to evaluate modalities commonly used by the physical therapist in the management of TMD.

A technical assessment conference (April 29–May 1, 1996) on TMD, sponsored by the National Institutes of Health (NIH), produced a Technology Assessment Statement.[7] Neither the conference planning committee, the expert panel, nor the conference itself included representation from the physical therapy profession.[10] The following is the final statement by the NIH on physical therapy:[7]

Physical Therapy: Physical therapy applications to TMD include a wide variety of evaluative techniques and treatment modalities that have been commonly used in other neurological and musculoskeletal disorders. These therapies generally are conservative and noninvasive. Benefits to TMD patients have been described, although few data are available to document these results.

A paper by Dr. Feine and colleagues[8] critiques the field of physical therapy on the basis of a Medline search of data from 1976 to 1996. Some modalities reviewed by Feine and coworkers[8] should have been excluded. For example, the use of diathermy is contraindicated for application to the temporomandibular joint (TMJ) area because the TMJ is located close to the eye. The U.S. Food and Drug Administration (FDA) has not yet approved laser treatment for use by a physical therapist, except in a research capacity. Transcutaneous electrical nerve stimulation is known to most physical therapists as an adjunctive modality and is considered only as a part of a comprehensive approach, not as a treatment unto itself.

The NIH position and Dr. Feine's paper on physical therapy are extremely narrow in perspective. They neither accurately nor adequately represent the profession of physical therapy and refer to physical therapy in the generic sense to mean a modality. This is a clear misrepresentation of the physical therapy profession. *Physical therapy,* as defined by the American Physical Therapy Association (APTA), is as follows:[11]

Physical therapy, which is the care and services provided by or under the direction and supervision of a physical therapist, includes:

1. *Examining patients with impairments, functional limitations, and disability or other health-related conditions in order to determine a diagnosis, prognosis, and intervention.*
2. *Alleviating impairments and functional limitations by designing, implementing, and modifying therapeutic interventions.*
3. *Preventing injury, impairments, functional limitations, and disability, including the promotion and maintenance of fitness, health, and quality of life in all age populations.*
4. *Engaging in consultation, education, and research.*

The APTA[12] advocates that

only physical therapists provide or direct the provision of physical therapy. Therefore the use of modalities, therapeutic techniques and exercises, unless provided by or under the direction of physical therapists, is not physical therapy. Other health care providers who use modalities and therapeutic techniques or exercises similar or identical to those used by physical therapists should be held to comparable educational and clinical standards.

The validity of research investigating physical therapy intervention for TMD should be seriously questioned when physical therapy is not defined and the credentials of the clinician are unclear. Conclusions based on research that investigates a single modality or therapeutic technique for single-tissue involvement also should be seriously questioned. Physical therapists seldom offer a singular treatment option for a patient who has myriad tissue and functional involvements. Physical therapists combine and sequence various treatment parameters, which may include modalities, therapeutic (manual) techniques, and exercise, as well as patient education and instructions in behavioral modifications.

Treatments offered are modified on the basis of the physical therapist's reassessment of the patient's signs and symptoms.

In summary, guidelines can appear to be beneficial to the public and the practicing clinician. Guidelines, however, can be incomplete and misleading.

Patient Accessibility to Physical Therapy

Patients have access to a physical therapist by way of self-referral or physician referral. Currently, more than 30 states have direct-access legislation. Patients in these states can consult physical therapists without a physician's referral. Patients can be assured that anyone who has a license in physical therapy must have graduated from an accredited program. Physical therapist education and training in the United States are uniform and standardized. Academic programs must meet the rigorous standards of an accreditation process. The Commission on Accreditation of Physical Therapy Education (CAPTE) is the independent accrediting agency for physical therapy education.

Though TMD patients can be seen directly by a physical therapist in those states that have direct access or by way of a medical referral to the physical therapist, the majority of patients with TMD are currently referred to a physical therapist by a dentist. Instead of consulting a medical doctor or physical therapist, patients often consult a dentist for TMD treatments for several reasons:

- Lay articles published in magazines and newspapers that describe in detail the reader's symptoms (e.g., headaches, facial, jaw, and neck pain); prospective patients conclude from these articles that the TMJ is the source of the patients' symptoms and help will be found by consulting a dentist.
- Word of mouth from neighbors or friends who received treatment from a dentist
- Patients' perception of the "cause" of their problems, i.e., teeth causing jaw pain
- TMD discovered during a routine dental visit

Once a dentist sees a patient, he or she may elect to initiate conservative and noninvasive care for the patient's TMD condition. Beyond this initial approach by the dentist, the patient can be referred to a physical therapist. When to refer to physical therapy is often a matter of clinical judgment. This author prefers physical therapy intervention before or during the nonsurgical dental care or before and then shortly after surgical intervention for the TMJ. The following guidelines can alert the dentist to those patients who should be referred to physical therapy at the earliest time possible:

- Chronic symptoms (more than 3 months in duration)
- Significant limitations with functional activities involving chewing, talking, and opening of the mouth
- Adjacent tissues to the TMJ, such as the muscles of mastication and cervical spine, that are involved are contributing to symptoms and limiting function of the jaw or neck
- Symptoms that have not responded to or are worsening after self-care management and/or the use of a mouth appliance and/or medication
- Patient demonstration of a lack of understanding and willingness to follow through with self-care management initiated by the dentist
- Postoperative arthroscopy or arthrotomy to the TMJ and postoperative orthognathic surgery
- "Significant" trauma received to the jaw, head, and/or neck

Management of TMD by a Physical Therapist

The widely used and accepted definition of TMD is as follows:

Temporomandibular disorders refer to a cluster of disorders characterized by the following main symptoms: pain and tenderness in the region of the muscles of mastication and the temporomandibular joint (TMJ), sounds during condylar movements, and limited or asymmetric mandibular movements.[9]

The term *TMD* evolved over time since previous terms were deemed too limiting, for example, "temporomandibular joint disturbances," "temporomandibular joint dysfunction," and "functional temporomandibular joint disturbances."[13] This definition includes not only problems related to the TMJs but also "all functional disturbances of the masticatory system."[13] Therefore, the term *TMD* implies a category of disorders, such as the TMJ and muscles of mastication, rather than a single diagnosis. There does exist a subclassification system for both the TMJ and muscles of mastication.[9]

For clinical and research purposes, three subgroups of TMD have been distinguished, according to the guidelines of the American Academy of Oral Facial Pain[9]:

- TMD with an arthrogenous component (TMD—A)
- TMD with an arthrogenous and myogenous component (TMD—A/M)
- TMD with a myogenous component (TMD—M)

Several studies have been completed, using these three subgroups of TMD.[14, 15] Physical therapy management of these three subgroups of TMD is covered in the next section.

Initially, TMD was thought to be caused by occlusal factors and therefore best treated by occlusal adjustments, prosthetic rehabilitation, and orthodontic treatment.[16] Occlusion is now considered to play a secondary role as an etiologic factor to TMD.[16–18] TMD is now thought to be a medical disorder in which diagnosis and treatment are based on principles used to treat other joints and muscles in the body.[19] Physical therapists treat nondiseased neuromuscular-skeletal conditions, which include the temporomandibular joint and associated muscles of mastication.

Other than doing nothing at all, treatment for any of the three subgroups of TMD should initially focus on instructing the patient in self-care management. This includes patient education, heat and/or cold application, awareness and control of oral habits, and, if necessary, a nonchew diet and over-the-counter nonsteroidal anti-inflammatory drugs (NSAIDs), such as aspirin and ibuprofen. Self-care management can be taught by the doctor or someone in the doctor's office who has proper training

and can respond appropriately to the patient's questions. Otherwise, the physical therapist can provide the home care instructions for TMD management. To understand the role of the physical therapist in TMD management is to go beyond the self-care treatment.

PHYSICAL THERAPY MANAGEMENT FOR TMD—A

A subclassification scheme for the patient population having TMD—A is the following[9]:

- Deviation in form
- Disk displacement
- Dislocation
- Inflammatory conditions
- Arthritides
- Ankylosis

Identifying the role for physical therapy intervention for the subclassifications of TMD—A listed is difficult. Identifying the role for physical therapy intervention for other medical diagnoses of the neuromuscular-skeletal system is also difficult. Physical therapists in the majority of cases do not treat medical diagnoses even though they may imply involvement of the neuromuscular-skeletal system.[20–24] For example, physical therapists do not treat degenerative disk disease of the spine, herniated nucleus pulposus, rheumatoid arthritis, and spondylosis. Likewise, physical therapists do not treat ankylosis, arthritides, or deviation in form of the TMJ. *Physical therapists treat impairments and functional limitations that are related to the disability of the patient, which may or may not have a correlation to the medical diagnosis.* An example is a loss of mouth opening (impairment). The patient's loss of mouth opening results in an inability to perform tasks involving talking (functional limitations). The patient's occupation demands extensive talking; thus the inability to open the mouth may prevent the patient from performing some aspects of his occupational duties (disability). The extent to which the patient perceives how the impairments and functional limitations affect his or her social roles will further impact the level of disability.[25] After physical therapy treatments, patients often have a return of function without symptoms, yet their medical or dental diagnosis—herniated disk, rheumatoid arthritis, spondylosis, or TMJ disk displacement/degenerative joint disease—still exists. *For research and outcome data to be meaningful, the diagnosis must match the skills of the clinician treating the diagnosis.*

The role of physical therapy in the treatment of TMD—A is to determine whether one or more of the following *physical therapy subclassification diagnoses* for TMD—A is present[26]:

- Inflammation
- Hypermobility
- Hypomobility

Inflammation

When a patient's primary complaint is "pain" of the TMJ, inflammation should be considered as one of the more probable sources of this complaint. TMJ tissues commonly inflamed are the posterior attachment (retrodiscal pad, superior and inferior stratums), collateral ligaments, and periarticular tissue (capsule/synovium and TMJ ligament). Generally speaking, tissues that are inflamed have varying degrees of vasodilatation (redness), swelling (exudate and bleeding from torn vessels), increase in blood flow and/or chemical and metabolic activity (heat), and irritation of nerve endings (pain). Inflammation can be acute, subacute, or chronic. Categorizing conditions in one of the three stages is difficult and is often subjective and is not considered here.

The cause of inflammation can be infection, disease, or trauma. Inflammation secondary to infection or disease requires dental and/or medical treatment. Infection or disease, e.g., various polyarthritides, are not common conditions of the TMJ. From the physical therapist's perspective, treatment for inflammation related to arthritides does not differ significantly from treatment offered for inflammation caused by trauma.

By far, the majority of inflammation of the posterior attachment and/or periarticular tissue is due to *either macrotrauma or microtrauma*. Macrotrauma to the TMJs may result from open joint surgery or a blow to the mandible. Microtrauma may occur when the TMJ tissues' physiologic range has been exceeded. An example would be opening wide during a dental procedure or by yawning. Duration, force, and repetition of opening would affect whether such an event would lead to inflammation. The TMJ is a load-bearing joint; however, microtrauma may result from TMD—M (masticatory muscle hyperactivity), which involves excessive or prolonged loading. TMD—M is covered later.

Inflammation is often accompanied by hypomobility (limited mouth opening) because the patient is unwilling to move his or her mouth in a functional range as a result of pain, associated muscle guarding, and/or joint effusion. However, inflammation of the periarticular tissue may lead to periarticular tissue tightness that also results in hypomobility. Acute inflammation of the periarticular tissue if left untreated progresses to the chronic stage, at which fibroblasts are formed, more collagen is produced, and periarticular tissue tightness develops.[27] Treatment of periarticular tissue tightness and a disk displacement without reduction, both of which result in hypomobility, are discussed later.

Diagnosis of Inflammation

A medical history focuses on events that may have caused macro- or microtrauma to the jaw. *Subjectively,* the patient reports having pain in the area of the TMJ with possible radiation into the temple, masseter, ear, and angle of the jaw. Patients often report that their pain is either increased or decreased by functional and/or parafunctional movements of the mandible. *Objective* confirmation of inflammation is made by the clinical examination, incorporating various palpation and selective loading procedures to the TMJs.[28, 29]

Treatment for Inflammation

Modalities

Modalities are used as part of a comprehensive treatment and not as a single approach. Primary goals for modalities are to lower pain and to enhance the healing process by reducing the effects of inflammation. Modalities discussed for the treatment of inflammation are moist or dry heat, ultrasound, cold, iontophoresis, and transcutaneous electrical nerve stimulation (TENS). These modalities are commonly used by this author. The duration and sequencing of modalities in conjunction with other procedures offered by the physical therapist are a matter of clinical judgment, experience of the clinician, and specific signs and symptoms of the patient. Before applying any modalities, the clinician must know specific indications and contraindications. More research is needed on the therapeutic effects of modalities on the TMJ. For now, research on other joint tissues is inferred to be applicable to the TMJ tissues. The following is only an overview; the reader is referred to the references for additional information.[30–32]

Thermal Agents

Moist/Dry Heat—Superficial Moist/dry heat is superficial heating. Changes in tissue temperature resulting from superficial heating depend on the intensity of the heat applied, time of heat exposure, and thermal medium (thickness of adipose tissue). When using tolerable superficial heat, temperature can be elevated up to 1°C at a depth of 3 cm. Superficial heating produces a therapeutic effect by elevating pain threshold, altering nerve conduction velocity, and decreasing muscle tension.

Superficial heating of the skin may produce a counterirritation effect to reduce pain. Superficial heating over a peripheral nerve (auriculotemporal nerve for primary TMJ innervation) can increase the threshold of sensory nerve conduction velocity, thus producing an analgesic effect. In both cases, superficial heating reduces the patient's perception of pain associated with inflammation.

Unrelated to inflammation but pertinent to the discussion of TMD—M are the effects of superficial heating on muscle. Heat decreases firing of the alpha motoneurons, thereby reducing tonic extrafusal fiber activity based on reflex mechanisms that are not totally understood. Muscle relaxation may also result from the analgesic effect of heating because the patient perceives less pain and as a result does less muscle guarding, which is a response to pain.

Increasing tissue temperature is usually associated with vasodilation, causing an increase in blood flow to the area. If the clinician suspects "significant" inflammation, superficial heat applied to the skin may be a relative contraindication. The clinician would have to weigh the benefits of the analgesic and neuromuscular effect in relation to the possible negative effects of vasodilatation of inflamed tissues of the TMJ.

Ultrasound—Deep Ultrasound has been used for more than 50 years in medicine. Ultrasound has similar effects to superficial heating of tissues. However, unlike in superficial heating, the biophysical effects result from the interaction of ultrasound with tissues at depths of 5 cm or more. Ultrasound has an anti-inflammatory effect. Ultrasound produces an increase in cell membrane and vascular wall permeability with enhanced blood flow to improve tissue repair and to reduce inflammation.[32] Physiologic effect is very dependent on the delivery parameters. For TMJ inflammation, pulsed ultrasound is applied. Pulsed ultrasound produces a nonthermal effect, therefore negating the effects that may be produced with continuous ultrasound in the presence of inflammation. Pulsed ultrasound is applied with a 5-cm or smaller sound head at a frequency of 3 MHz and low intensity of 0.5 to 0.8 W/cm^2 for 5 to 8 minutes.[32] Ultrasonic energy is frequency-dependent, so most absorption occurs at 1 to 2 cm below the skin surface at 3 MHz. This depth of ultrasound would be appropriate for the TMJ. Low-intensity continuous ultrasound may be used as inflammation decreases as determined by the reassessment of the patient's signs and symptoms.

Low-intensity continuous or pulsed ultrasound can be used in the treatment of acute and chronic wounds to enhance the reparative process.[33] Ultrasound applied within the first week may hinder the early stages of wound healing.[33] During the proliferation phase, which usually occurs in the second week, ultrasound would be beneficial. Ultrasound of higher intensity of 1.5 W/cm^2 is significant in the healing of traumatized soft tissue.[34] Timing and dosage of ultrasound are important considerations for facilitating the healing process after arthroscopy and arthrotomy.

When exercise was combined with ultrasound versus exercise alone, patients who had ultrasound reported a higher percentage of pain relief than those who received exercise only.[35] When appropriate, ultrasound should precede jaw exercises, when exercises are done to assist in the treatment of symptomatic periarticular tissue tightness or disk displacement without reduction.

Unrelated to inflammation but pertinent to the discussion of TMJ hypomobility are the biophysical effects of ultrasound on connective tissue and muscle. Elevation of tissue temperature by ultrasound preceding or during passive or active stretching has been postulated to alter the viscoelastic properties of collagen tissue and collagen molecular bonding, thus enhancing ease of stretch.[33] Unless sufficient intensity is used, the benefits of ultrasound are no greater than those of superficial heating. Ultrasound of 1.0 to 2.0 W/cm^2 was used on scar tissue secondary to lacerations, x-ray burns, and Dupuytren's contracture to reduce the size of keloids.[36] Ultrasound plays an important adjunctive role in the treatment of hypomobility secondary to capsular tightness and disk displacement without reduction by increasing collagen tissue extensibility.

Like superficial heating, ultrasound can decrease extrafusal fiber activity via a reflex mechanism. However, it may also affect the muscle spindle activity more directly because of its deeper penetration.[33] Ultrasound can elevate skeletal muscle temperature at the bone-muscle interface. Superficial or deep heating agents play an important adjunctive role in the treatment of TMD—M.

The following are general contraindications of superficial and deep heating:[30]

- Circulatory impairments that are prone to increased bleeding or hemorrhage (e.g., hemophilia)
- Post acute trauma with bleeding not controlled
- Potential capillary fragility in patients on long-term steroid therapy
- Elevation of tissues at the site of malignancy

Cold

Cryotherapy is used for reducing fever, controlling bleeding, decreasing muscle guarding, and, pertinent to this discussion, helping reduce inflammation and associated pain. Cold reduces bleeding by arteriolar vasoconstriction; decreases inflammation by decreasing metabolism and levels of vasoactive agents, e.g., histamine; and elevates the pain threshold by decreasing nerve-con-

duction velocity.[37] Cold to control inflammation can be applied to the TMJ by ice packs, ice cubes/cups for ice massage, or ice-soaked towels. During ice massage, the patient often experiences four distinct sensations: cold, burning, aching, then analgesia.

Unrelated to inflammation but pertinent to the discussion of TMJ—M are the biophysical effects of cold on muscle. Cold reduces muscle tension by decreasing pain and by decreasing the sensitivity of the muscle spindle afferent fiber discharge.[37] When applied by a vapocoolant to the affected muscle on passive stretch, cold is postulated to stimulate cutaneous afferents, producing a reflex decrease in gamma motoneuron firing and thus permitting more passive stretch of the muscle.[38]

Cold should be avoided in patients with cold-sensitivity conditions, including cold urticaria, cryoglobulinemia, cold intolerance, Raynaud's phenomenon, and paroxysmal cold hemoglobinurias.[37] Cold should not be applied over circulation-compromised areas (e.g., in peripheral vascular disease). Care should also be taken when the patient is hypertensive because cold can cause a transient increase in systolic and diastolic blood pressure.[37] Prolonged cold application for 1 hour or more over a superficial peripheral nerve can lead to neurapraxia or axonotmesis. Finally, the psychological response of the patient should be taken into account when applying cryotherapy.

There are certain clinical situations in which either heat or cold is clearly preferred. Often the choice is empirical. The following factors should be considered:[39]

1. Stage of injury
2. Area of body treated
3. Medical status
4. Patient preference

Iontophoresis

In iontophoresis a battery-powered system is used to deliver water-soluble ionizing drugs through the skin. The effects are dependent on the drugs used. Common drugs used for inflammation of the TMJ are dexamethasone sodium phosphate, methylprednisolone sodium succinate (Solu-Medrol), and lidocaine hydrochloride. Comparison of iontophoresis to systemic therapy and local injection showed that tissue concentration of the administered ion was higher for the iontophoresis than that obtained with systemic therapy but lower than that obtained by local injection.[40] Multiple treatments of iontophoresis would seem to be needed to be comparable to a single injection. However, the author is not aware of any research systematically comparing the ability of iontophoresis and joint injection to deliver medication to the TMJ. Therefore, it is not known whether these two treatment modalities are comparable.

Case reports, case series, and a clinical trial have shown patients who have been clinically diagnosed with capsulitis or tendonitis to have a decrease in signs and symptoms after the application of iontophoresis.[41-44] One study concluded that iontophoresis was no more effective than a saline placebo in providing pain relief or improvement in mandibular range of motion in patients with TMJ pain.[45] A recent double-blind randomized study investigated the effects of iontophoresis on limited mouth opening secondary to pain and a disk displacement without reduction.[46] All patients were asked to discontinue over-the-counter and prescribed medication for their condition. Use of intraoral appliances, jaw exercises, and self-administered heat or ice treatments was also discontinued. Results suggested that iontophoresis was effective in improving mandibular function, but not in reducing pain, in patients who had concurrent TMJ capsulitis and disk displacement without reduction. Iontophoresis is used by this author when the examination suggests localized inflammation of the periarticular tissue of the TMJ and/or masseter muscle.

Transcutaneous Electrical Nerve Stimulation

Transcutaneous electrical nerve stimulation (TENS) employs a small, portable, battery-operated unit. The unit has controls allowing the clinician to adjust the frequency, pulse width, and amplitude of an alternating current that is administered to the patient by electrodes of a variety of sizes and shapes. TENS has long been used as a means of pain control, largely on the basis of the "gait control theory" of Melzack and Wall. Gait control selectively activates large-diameter proprioceptive afferents to inhibit or balance small-diameter nociceptive input at the dorsal horn to block the patient's perception of "pain."[47] TENS has also been shown to produce reflex vasodilatation and decrease muscle guarding, thereby enhancing circulation and lymphatic drainage.[47] Optimal stimulation parameters for TMJ inflammation are a frequency of 1 Hz, pulse width of 75 to 100 μsec, and amplitude to the point of mild visible and rhythmic mandibular elevation without tooth or appliance contact.[32] Mannheimer states, "TENS performed in this manner is not designed to produce pain relief as its primary goal but to enhance the healing process by reducing the effects of inflammation."[32] Contraindications to TENS are epilepsy, transient ischemic attacks, and postcerebrovascular accidents.[47]

Hypermobility

The cause of hypermobility of the TMJ is unknown. Potential predisposing factors that have been suggested range from joint laxity to psychiatric disorders to skeletal abnormalities.[48] One study suggests that systemic hypermobility (ligament laxity) may be closely related to TMJ hypermobility.[49] Two studies on systemic hypermobility investigated whether a correlation exists between systemic hypermobility and disk displacements/osteoarthrosis of the TMJ.[50, 51] In one of the studies, the authors concluded that disk displacements of the TMJ are a sign of "joint hypermobility syndrome."[50] The other study showed that generalized joint hypermobility was not a predisposing factor to TMJ disk displacements and osteoarthrosis.[51] Regardless of the proposed etiologic factors for hypermobility, it is more often than not asymptomatic.

Diagnosis of Hypermobility

Hypermobility of the TMJ is identified when the condyle functions beyond the articular crest—an anatomic landmark on the temporal bone. The condyle moving past the articular crest is then functioning on the articular tubercle. A definitive diagnosis can only be made by a radiograph of the TMJ when the patient's mouth is fully opened. Hypermobility is such a benign condition that the expense and exposure to radiation do not justify radiographs for the sole purpose of identifying the condition. Often the clinical examination is sufficient to determine whether hypermobility is present.[26]

Subjectively, the patient often describes the jaw as "going out of place." This may be perceived as the patient touches the lateral poles of the TMJ. As the patient opens his or her mouth, the condyle(s) translates a significant distance anteriorly, causing the patient to interpret the sensation as the joint's "going out of place."

Objectively, the clinician palpates the lateral pole(s) of the TMJs to identify whether one or both of the following are present:

- Excessive anterior excursion of the lateral pole(s) during mandibular opening
- A "juddering" movement of the condyle(s) at the end of mandibular opening and at the beginning of mandibular closing, as a result of the condyle's going past the articular crest onto the articular tubercle during opening and closing movements of the mandible

This clinical examination for hypermobility has obvious flaws that contribute to false-positive or false-negative conclusions. Hypermobility, however, is one condition in which overdiagnosis or underdiagnosis is acceptable. The reason is that the condition is benign and the treatment is conservative, cost-effective, and reversible.

Treatment for Hypermobility

Only when hypermobility is accompanied by inflammation is treatment required, especially if pain occurs or is intensified at the end of full-mouth opening. Even if hypermobility were not present, avoiding or controlling the end range of joint movement would be therapeutic for the management of inflammation. Controlling asymptomatic hypermobility would only be necessary if the patient insisted that he or she did not want to experience the sensation of the jaw's "going out of place."

Primary treatment is simply telling the patient, "Do not open your mouth so wide" (conservative); if the patient applies this awareness exercise on a daily basis, only one treatment is needed (cost-effective). Patients only open wide if they eat a large sandwich, receive dental work, or have surgery requiring intubation. Because situations other than nonelective dental or surgi-

cal situations can be avoided, the only time a patient needs to open the mouth wide is in yawning. Yawning can be controlled by having the patient yawn with tongue pressed up against the palate of the mouth. Pressing the tongue up limits the patient's mouth opening to about 25 mm. The therapist can teach the patient additional cognitive awareness/neuromuscular exercises if necessary.[26]

Hypomobility

Hypomobility is limitation in functional movements of the mandible secondary to arthrogenous involvement. A review of the physiologic and neurophysiologic sequelae of hypomobility affecting the articular cartilage and mechanoreceptor activity of diarthrodial joints can be found in the reference section.[26] Functional movements affected by hypomobility include chewing food, opening the mouth to receive food, talking, and yawning.

There are various causes of TMD—A hypomobility. Ankylosis (bony or fibrous) results in complete restriction of movement. Hypomobility can be a result of fractures involving the TMJ or severe degenerative joint disease, neoplasia, aplasia, hypoplasia, and dysplasia of the bony components of the TMJ. If needed, treatment for these previous causes for hypomobility of TMD—A is rendered by the oral surgeon. Hypomobility may also stem from previous TMJ or orthognathic surgery. The more common causes of TMD—A hypomobility, which also respond best to physical therapy treatments, are *periarticular tissue tightness* and a *disk displacement without reduction.* Before a discussion of periarticular tissue tightness and disk displacement without reduction, the diagnosis of hypomobility is discussed.

Diagnosis of Hypomobility

Mandibular depression, protrusion, and lateral excursions are osteokinematic (movement of bone, e.g., mandible) movements frequently observed by the clinician to diagnose hypomobility. Mandibular hypomobility is present when any one or a combination of the following limited osteokinematic movements are present:

Mandibular depression: Actively, the patient is unable to achieve 36 mm of interincisal opening.

Functional interincisal opening is 36 mm and greater.

Mandibular protrusion: Actively, the patient is unable to achieve end-to-end position with the central incisors (this does not apply to class III patients).

Functional protrusion occurs when the lower central incisors can move past the upper central incisors.

Mandibular lateral excursions: Actively, during mandibular movement to the right, the patient is unable to achieve end-to-end position of the right bottom canine to the right upper canine; this also applies to the left canines when moving left.

Functional lateral excursion to the right occurs when the right bottom canine can move past the right upper canine; this also applies to the left canines during left lateral excursion.

Limitations and aberrant movements of the mandible are classically the same for periarticular tissue tightness and a disk displacement without reduction. The following is what the clinician typically sees in unilateral hypomobility of the TMJ:

Depression: Not functional, less than 25 mm of interincisal opening with the mandible deflecting to the side of the involved joint; deflection is movement of the mandible away from midline.

Protrusion: Not functional, with the mandible deflecting to the side of the involved joint.

Lateral excursion: Not functional to the opposite side of the involved joint with lateral excursion of the mandible to the same side functional.

Since limited mandibular dynamics are the same for periarticular tissue tightness and a disk displacement without reduction, history is the key to making the differential diagnosis. *Periarticular tissue tightness* is usually associated with a history of chronic inflammation resulting from trauma, long-term limited mobility, or strict immobiliza-

tion. *Disk displacement without reduction* usually has a sudden onset preceded by a history suggesting a disk displacement with reduction.

Limited opening can also be caused by a nonarthrogenous condition, such as TMD—M. Hypomobility of TMD—A origin and hypomobility of TMD—M origin can be differentiated by having the patient move the mandible into protrusion and lateral excursions. If protrusion and lateral excursions are normal, then TMD—M should be suspected. If it is limited, then TMD—A is suspected. Myogenous involvement typically does not restrict protrusive and lateral excursions as does arthrogenous involvement. A complete history and clinical examination confirm whether hypomobility is of an arthrogenous or myogenous origin.[26, 28] The treatment for hypomobility secondary to TMD—M is discussed later.

Periarticular Tissue Tightness

Periarticular tissue is the capsular-ligamentous tissue of joints. The entire lateral aspect of the TMJ capsule is thickened, forming the temporomandibular ligament. The TMJ ligament is regarded as part of and inseparable from the capsule. Here the terms *periarticular tissue* and *capsule* can be considered synonymous. Biomechanical and biochemical changes that occur with periarticular tissues of diarthrodial joints as a result of hypomobility have been well documented in the literature.[52–56]

Disk Displacement

Disk displacement is a very common condition affecting the TMJs. Experts disagree over the cause and treatment of disk displacements. The role of physical therapy in the treatment of disk displacement is based on the recognition and acceptance that the morbidity of the disk functioning off the condyle has not been demonstrated to be entirely pathologic and that patients can function in a pain-free state with minimal limitations in function with a disk displacement.[57–64] However, some researchers believe that the disk should not function off the condyle and that all efforts should be made to reposition the disk to its "normal" position on the condyle. Repositioning the disk to its normal position often requires various mouth appliances and/or arthrotomy and possible orthognathic surgical procedures. Long-term studies have shown that in a high number of patients who receive treatment to recapture the disk, the disk is often displaced again.[65-68]

I believe both treatment approaches are appropriate when based on rigid patient selection criteria. Criteria for making a decision to treat the disk off or on the condyle include the patient's age, traumatic or insidious onset, amount of time the disk has been displaced, symptomatic or asymptomatic, degree of functional limitations, and patient's response to previous treatment. Essentially, the decision to treat the disk on or off the condyle is based on the clinician's judgment and the patient's being well informed. *The patient needs to be well informed* of the pros and cons of all nonsurgical (no treatment, use of mouth appliance, and physical therapy) and surgical treatments (arthroscopy, arthrotomy, and orthognathic).

There are three well-defined stages of a disk displacement.[9] A discussion of the role of physical therapy for each stage follows.

Disk Displacement with Reduction—Stage I The diagnosis of a stage I disk displacement with reduction is classically made by the presence of joint noises, e.g., the reciprocal click. Additional clinical examination procedures can be found in the literature.[26, 28] The key to understanding the treatment of a stage I displacement is to know that it is functional. Patients can chew, talk, and yawn; they simply have joint noises as they perform these activities. Some patients with a stage I displacement may have a catch on opening related to the disk, or the opening becomes an effort because the "reduction" of the disk has become difficult. A treatment choice for this specific patient population may be progression to a disk displacement without reduction that is functional. Some patients with a stage I displacement may have inflammation and/or TMD−M. Patients with a stage I displacement and inflammation and/or TMD−M should be approached with treatment(s) as though the conditions simply coexist and are not related.

Patient Education The primary treatment offered by the physical therapist for a stage I displacement is education of the patient about the condition. If the decision to treat the disk off the condyle is made, patients need to be told that a stage I displacement and the associated joint noises do not mean that the joint is bad, diseased, or pathologic. The patient needs to know that he or she can function pain-free even with the disk(s) displaced. If the patient is consulting both a dentist and a physical therapist, it is important that the two professionals communicate as to what the emphasis should be on joint noises. Once agreement has been achieved, the two professionals can respond to the patient's questions in a consistent manner.

Inflammation If a stage I displacement is painful, pain results because inflammation is present. The initial approach that should be taken by the physical therapist is to assume that the stage I displacement and inflammation are independent and are simply coexisting. Treatment for inflammation has been covered. More often than not, as the inflammation is resolved, the patient returns to functioning in a pain-free state with joint noises. If the inflammation recurs or is not resolved to the patient's satisfaction, TMD−M is suspected.

TMD−M Treatment for TMD−M or masticatory muscle hyperactivity is covered later. TMD−M can be a source of the patient's symptoms, e.g., myofascial pain. As in the case of inflammation, a stage I displacement and TMD−M can also be independent of one another and simply coexisting. Often as TMD−M is treated, the patient states that the joint noises have lessened or have gone away. In such cases, the decrease in joint noises is assumed to be secondary to reduced joint loading because masticatory muscle hyperactivity has decreased.

Regardless of the inflammation and/or TMD−M that may be associated with a stage I displacement, resolution of the inflammation and/or TMD−M should occur in or around a 4- to 6-week period, with physical therapy intervention two to three times a week. If inflammation and/or TMD−M continues, a referral to a dentist for an appropriate mouth appliance to assist in controlling TMD−M is indicated. If the patient already has an appropriate mouth appliance and has undergone physical therapy treatments, he or she should be referred to an oral surgeon. In this situation, the stage I displacement is perpetuating the inflammation and/or TMD—M, and surgery may now be indicated.

Disk Displacement without Reduction—Stage II The diagnosis of a stage II disk displacement without reduction is made by history and altered mandibular dynamics. Patients often report having had joint noises prior to their limited function, suggesting a stage I displacement preceded the stage II displacement. Stage II displacement interferes with the patient's ability to perform functional activities. Objectively, altered mandibular dynamics associated with a unilateral stage II displacement are observed. The description of the altered mandibular dynamics seen with a stage II displacement is given in the section on hypomobility.

Physical therapists treating patients with a stage II displacement from a nondental referral are advised to have the patient consult a dentist who specializes in the treatment of TMD for a second opinion. For liability reasons, the patient should have a second opinion stating that physical therapy is a suitable option in the treatment of the stage II displacement. Treatment for a stage II displacement is covered later.

Disk Displacement with Osteoarthrosis—Stage III The diagnosis of a stage III disk displacement with osteoarthrosis is made by the presence of crepitus throughout the full range of opening and closing movements of the mandible. Stage III displacement, degenerative joint disease, and osteoarthrosis are considered synonymous in regard to the disk's being permanently displaced and undergoing significant changes. Though the integrity and mechanics of the TMJ are disturbed, the TMJ seems to adapt adequately to this altered disk position.[69] Patients who have a stage III displacement can have pain-free and near-normal mandibular dynamics.

Treatment—Stage III As in the treatment of a stage I displacement, physical therapy intervention centers on patient education and, if present, the treatment of inflammation and/or TMD—M.

Treatment for Periarticular Tissue Tightness and Stage II Displacement

The following therapeutic procedures and home exercises are used for either a capsular tightness or a stage II displacement. What is different in the application of the treatments for these two conditions is the degree of aggressiveness with which they are applied. For example, capsular tightness secondary to arthrotomy involving a repair to the disk warrants a less aggressive treatment approach than that used when diskectomy is performed. Though capsular tightness can be the result in both cases, the arthrotomy with the disk repair adds another variable to the postoperative rehabilitation. The disk repair often involves the "shortening" of disk attachments. Therefore, limitation in function may also be due to the surgical repair itself. This should not detract from the need to establish early mobility as long as the therapeutic procedures are applied in a controlled manner by the patient and physical therapist.[70] The time between the surgery and physical therapy would also dictate how aggressive the physical therapist would be in restoring functional movements of the mandible. Regarding stage II displacement, the only limitation in treatment is the patient's tolerance of the therapeutic procedures, which is discussed next.

Regardless of whether the patient has capsular tightness or a stage II displacement, an active interincisal opening of 25 mm should be expected.[26] Rotation of the condyle without any condylar translation allows up to 25 mm of opening. If the patient is unable to achieve 25 mm, this limitation is usually secondary to joint inflammation and/or TMD—M. Before therapeutic procedures are initiated for joint hypomobility, inflammation and/or TMD—M must be managed.

Modalities previously discussed can be used before, during, or after each therapeutic procedure. The choice and sequencing of modalities and therapeutic procedures as well as the degree of aggressiveness and length of time the therapeutic procedures are applied are determined by the patient's history and current signs and symptoms.

Finger Spread Stretch The patient rests supine with the cervical spine properly supported. The clinician stands at the head of the patient. Using the hand opposite the involved joint, the clinician places the thumb on the tip of the patient's lower central incisors and the index finger on the tip of the top central incisors. The patient is asked to open actively as the clinician follows with pressure of the fingertips on the patient's incisors. At the end of the available range, additional pressure is applied with the clinician's fingertips. While performing this exercise, the patient can be asked to extend the head to facilitate mouth opening.

An important modification to this manual exercise is performed at the time the patient can actively achieve opening to 25 to 30 mm. The patient is instructed to protrude the mandible forward and then open the mouth. Protruding the mandible translates the condyle to prevent forcing rotation beyond 25 mm. Valuable feedback from the therapist to the patient during the stretch helps the patient to understand what is expected when he or she does this exercise at home.

Joint Mobilization Techniques *Joint mobilization* is a general term that might be applied to any active or passive attempt to increase movement of a joint. Passive joint mobilization has been a popular treatment for the restoration of joint motion for many years. For better patient relaxation, the following techniques for the TMJ are best applied with the patient supine rather than sitting.

Distraction Distraction is a force applied parallel to the longitudinal axis of the bone—in this case, the neck of the condyle. Distraction is the first choice among intraoral techniques because of safety, ease, and effectiveness.

The patient is lying supine with appropriate support given to the cervical spine. The clinician stands on the opposite side of the involved joint. The clinician's thumb is placed on the patient's mandibular molars, on the side of the involved joint. If limitation of jaw opening prevents the placement of the thumb on top of the molars, the thumb may be positioned in the premolar area. The remaining fingers are wrapped around the chin comfortably. The clinician's other hand stabilizes the patient's cranium, with the middle or index finger palpating the lateral pole of the condyle for movement. While performing the distraction technique, the patient can actively open and close on command, using minimal muscle contraction. When the patient relaxes, additional distraction forces can be applied. Performing the distraction technique with active participation by the patient allows the patient to experience a less stressful, less painful movement of the joint. While performing

distraction, the patient can be asked to extend the head to facilitate mouth opening.

Translation The clinician's body position and hand placements are the same as in the distraction technique. The clinician's mobilizing hand translates the condyle in an anterior direction by passively pulling on the mandible. Translation is not performed only in the sagittal plane but also slightly across midline. Translation should be performed during varying degrees of distraction. Distraction simultaneous with translation helps the patient tolerate this technique better.

Lateral Glide The clinician's body position and the stabilizing hand are placed as in the distraction technique. The thumb contact of the mobilizing hand, however, is different. Thumb contact for this technique is on the top/inside of the molars. The rest of the fingers wrap around the mandible comfortably. Lateral glide is performed by pressing laterally with the thumb, while force is directed toward the table and patient's feet (final direction of the force generated by the thumb is as in following the slope of the patient's shoulder). This direction of force minimizes the discomfort on the contralateral side a patient would experience if a lateral force alone were applied.

Graded rhythmic oscillatory movements may be applied simultaneously with distraction, translation, and lateral glide joint mobilization techniques. Rhythmic oscillatory movements aid in pain inhibition and enhancement of joint mechanoreceptor activity.[26]

General rules to follow when applying joint mobilization techniques are as follows:

1. Patient and clinician must be properly positioned and relaxed.
2. Patient should be stabilized firmly.
3. Clinician must be willing to modify the technique on the basis of the tissue's response and patient's tolerance.
4. Clinician should use minimal force consistent with achieving the objective of the technique, which is to restore function.

Mobilization techniques when performed incorrectly or not indicated may result in the following:

1. Increase in pain
2. Increase in muscle guarding
3. Decrease in mobility

Static Tongue Blade Technique

Tongue blades are used to apply a low-load prolonged stretch (LLPS) to promote long-lasting elongation of the periarticular tissue. The effectiveness of LLPS has been well documented by laboratory studies.[71–73] The patient should be positioned supine for this procedure. The patient is instructed to place tongue blades on the side of the involved joint in the area of the molars. Using the tongue blades, the patient is told to "take up the slack and then some." If more than five tongue blades are used, try taping or gluing all but three of them together. The last tongue blade can be slid in or out between the remaining tongue blades. Actual duration of the LLPS is dependent on patient tolerance, but working up to a 10-minute stretch is adequate.

Studies have shown that raising the temperature of the stretched tissue and allowing the tissue to cool in a loaded position produce greater elongation of the treated tissue(s).[73–75] Ultrasound is used to enhance tissue extensibility with tongue blades in place.

Continuous Passive Motion

The importance of initiating early motion during the inflammatory phase, especially after surgical intervention, is widely accepted in the rehabilitation of other joints, such as the knee.[76] Use of passive motion on a continuous basis, as introduced by Salter and associates in 1970, has become an important area of study.[76] Salter has shown that continuous passive motion (CPM) applied in experimental animal studies is beneficial to soft tissue healing, bone and cartilage healing, swelling, hemarthrosis, and joint function.[76] It is reported that CPM in humans has resulted in positive effects on joint effusions, wound edema, pain, and reduction of capsular contractures and joint stiffness.[77, 78] Even though CPM has been used in a variety of orthopedic conditions, present indications and clinical studies for the use of CPM have largely focused on the rehabilitation of various knee disorders.

Though the potential benefit of CPM is known, there is insufficient clinical research to define the most appropriate device and protocol after arthroscopy or arthrotomy to the TMJ.[79] The term *CPM* may need to change because it indicates continuous motion. Motorized devices used on the TMJ are short term. Measurable outcomes in terms of therapeutic value and cost-effectiveness of CPM for TMD have not been fully researched. Timely physical therapy for TMD—A hypomobility produces therapeutic outcomes acceptable to the patient, surgeon, and insurance companies while avoiding the inconvenience and cost of CPM.

Home Exercise Program for Hypomobility

Tongue Up and Open/Close Patients having limited mobility with associated inflammation should be instructed to open and close the mouth with the tongue against the palate. Opening and closing with tongue up limit the condyle to rotation and prevent translation. This exercise creates controlled movement while increasing the patient's confidence that movement can occur without an increase in pain. This exercise can be performed numerous times throughout the day. Once inflammation is decreased, opening and closing can be performed with tongue down to allow opening beyond 25 mm.

Finger Spread Stretch and Static Tongue Blade Stretch After proper instructions to the patient, finger spread stretch and static tongue blade stretch therapeutic procedures can be continued at home. Patients do not have access to various modalities available in the physical therapist clinic. They can, however, apply heat and/or cold and, if available, a home TENS unit. Finger spread stretch can be applied with few repetitions many times a day, whereas static tongue blade exercise is applied for up to 10 minutes one to three times per day.

Dental Roll Distraction The dental roll distraction exercise is designed to distract the condyle. This is a *passive,* not an active exercise. The patient sits in a comfortable supported position. The patient places a dental roll ¼ inch in diameter between the back molars on the side to be distracted. The patient places the palm of the hand under the chin. The other hand is placed on the top of the head toward the forehead. Both hands are in front of the dental roll. With the patient relaxing the jaw, the chin hand applies a slight pressure superiorly as the other hand stabilizes the head. Hand pressure in the presence of relaxed jaw muscles creates a pivot over the dental roll, resulting in distraction of the condyle. The patient may elect to perform active protrusion several times while hand pressure is maintained. This procedure can be done 10 to 15 times each session, repeating 3 to 6 times per day.

Horizontal Tongue Blade Exercise The patient places seven tongue blades horizontally between the upper and lower central incisors. The patient does not bite on the tongue blades; rather the tongue blades are held in position by the patient's grasping the ends of the tongue blades. Seven tongue blades equals approximately 11 mm when placed between the central incisors. Translation normally begins at approximately 11 mm.[80] With tongue blades in place, the patient moves the mandible forward and backward repetitively 30 times per session, repeating 1 to 3 times per day. The forward and back motion of the mandible improves condylar translation. Should repetitive translation be performed with less than 11 mm of jaw opening, the patient usually feels pain or discomfort.

Capsule and Stage II Tissue Changes in Response to Treatment

Capsule Connective tissue responds to mechanical stress in a time-dependent or viscoelastic manner. The force/load applied needs to exceed the elastic range of a tissue; otherwise, the tissue returns to its original shape and prevents permanent elongation of the tissue.[81, 82] Beyond the elastic range or yield point is the plastic range of the tissue.[81, 82] Long-lasting elongation is dependent upon the intensity and duration of force applied.[83, 84] If loading is continued too far into the plastic range (fatigue point), tissue damage may result. The therapeutic procedures and home exercises previously discussed need to exceed the elastic range of the tight capsular tissue for permanent elongation to be achieved.

Stage II Displacement It is nearly impossible to predict whether a patient will regain function by going to a stage I displacement or progress to a stage III displacement. *Patients must be well informed and in agreement as to the possibilities.* If inflammation and/or TMD—M is present and is treated, it is not unusual for a stage II displacement to progress to a stage I or to

a stage III displacement with no therapeutic procedures performed. When therapeutic procedures and a home exercise program are performed, they have been shown to be highly effective as a conservative, noninvasive treatment for a stage II displacement.[85–91] Signs and symptoms improved by these procedures are not the result of the disk's reducing to its normal position.[92] Rather, a return to functional movements of the mandible may be caused by elongation of the posterior attachment (PA) with further anterior displacement and advanced deformation of the disk, progressing from a stage II to a stage III displacement.[93] The condyle then is capable of functioning on the PA that has remolded to become fibrotic.[94] This change in the PA allows it to withstand loading from the condyle. However, in some patients, the PA does not remold, remolds inadequately, or remolds adequately for a time and then fails.[95] In such failed cases, an oral surgery consultation is indicated.

PHYSICAL THERAPY MANAGEMENT FOR TMD—A/M

The vast number of patients with TMD have both an arthrogenous and myogenous involvement. The interrelationship between arthrogenous and myogenous components is unclear.[96, 97] It is not unlikely that the arthrogenous and myogenous components are simply coexisting entities in a considerable number of patients.[96] As a general rule, if the patient's condition has both an arthrogenous and a myogenous component, the myogenous component should be treated first, except when *significant* inflammation or stage II displacement is present. These two conditions may require treatment at the same time the myogenous component is treated.

PHYSICAL THERAPY MANAGEMENT FOR TMD—M

The American Academy of Orofacial Pain lists six subset diagnoses for masticatory muscle disorders, such as myofascial pain, myositis, spasm, protective splinting, contracture, and neoplasia, which are applicable to TMD—M.[9] Fibromyalgia, also termed *myofascitis, myofibrositis,* or *fibrositis,* is often confused with myofascial pain.[98] Tests used to differentiate among the various masticatory muscle disorders and between myofascial pain and fibromyalgia have had poor reliability and validity. Attempts to differentiate the different muscle conditions are more academic and offer little clinical value. Even if reliability and validity were established for differentiating the various muscle conditions, the treatment(s) offered would be the same in most cases. This chapter condenses all masticatory muscle disorders in one classification, referred to as *masticatory muscle hyperactivity* (MMH). It is considered in the following discussion as a source of the patient's head and jaw symptoms.

Examination for Masticatory Muscle Hyperactivity

Symptoms associated with diurnal or nocturnal MMH range from pain or soreness to tightness and/or fatigue in the jaw and temple areas of the head. Some patients may have MMH symptoms only during the day and not at night. Other patients may not have symptoms during the day; symptoms may wake the patient at night or be present first thing in the morning.

Clinical examination for MMH involves digital palpation of the muscles of mastication. Numerous muscles are involved in the act of mastication. From a clinical point of view this chapter focuses on only the three muscles that are responsible for elevating the mandible—namely, the medial pterygoid, masseter, and temporalis muscles. The specificity of palpating the medial pterygoid is low because of the location of the medial pterygoid and the overlying of adjacent muscles to the medial pterygoid. Reliability and validity are better when palpating the temporalis and masseter muscles. This author relies on the masseter and temporalis as "scout muscles" to signify whether MMH is present. Palpation may reveal objective tightness of these muscles and/or the patient may subjectively state that he or she experiences tenderness or pain during the palpation examination. The amount of opening is not a reliable sign for diagnosis of MMH.

Treatment for Masticatory Muscle Hyperactivity

Oral Modification and Awareness

It is essential that patients are made aware of bad habits that require use of the muscles of mastication. Patients must be educated in how they can control and/or modify their bad habits.[99] Patient awareness of a problem over which he or she has some degree of control may be one of the essential and common components of a successful outcome.[100] Habits such as fingernail biting, or gum or ice chewing result in MMH if done repetitiously. The awareness and avoidance of such habits can therefore help in reducing MMH. Minimizing essential functional activities, such as talking, chewing food (nonchew diet), and drinking liquid (versus sucking fluid out of a straw), assists in reducing MMH.

Modalities

Modalities previously reviewed can also be used to decrease MMH. Superficial heat can be applied to the masseter and temporalis. Ultrasound and iontophoresis are limited to the masseter since hair may compromise the application of these modalities to the temporalis. When hyperactivity of intraoral muscles is suspected, intraoral electric stimulation rendered by a hand-held probe has been clinically helpful in achieving relaxation of intraoral muscles.[101]

Massage

Extraoral or intraoral massage or pressure point techniques may be offered to the muscles of mastication. The specific application of massage or pressure point techniques to the muscles is more an art than a science.

Therapeutic Exercises

Contracting one muscle or group of muscles causes reflex inhibition of the antagonist muscle(s). Contraction of the depressor muscles of the mandible causes a reciprocal inhibition of the elevator (antagonist) muscles. This can be done by having the patient place one fist under the chin to resist mouth opening. Questions of duration and the amount of resistance needed to initiate inhibition of the antagonist muscles in a dysfunctional state remain unanswered.[102, 103]

A maximum isometric contraction of a muscle can also induce relaxation of the contracting muscle. To inhibit the elevator muscles of the mandible effectively, the elevator muscles should be in a position of slight stretch. The patient positions the mouth slightly open and places the index and middle fingers of one hand over the lower central incisors. The patient attempts to close the mouth against an unyielding force: the fingers. For the elevator muscles to relax reflexly, a great amount of tension is required to stimulate the Golgi tendon organs (GTOs). Information on how long this relaxation/inhibition persists is limited.[104] I am concerned about performing a maximum isometric contraction of the elevator muscles. Depending on the degree of myofascial pain stemming from the elevator muscles and the degree of inflammation of the TMJ, such a maximum contraction often increases the patient's signs and symptoms. Good clinical decision making is mandated in this instance. I prefer minimal isometric contraction. Minimal contraction does not stimulate the GTOs. Minimal contraction gives the patient cortical awareness of the muscles contracting and then relaxing. Over time, this form of light isometric contraction may provide relaxation if done in conjunction with other forms of treatment.

Exercising the muscles of mastication for the purpose of increasing strength is the exception rather than the rule. I seldom find weak jaw muscles. The idea that a jaw muscle can be isolated so as to "test" it to see whether it is weak is difficult to accept. Even if the muscle can be isolated, a false-positive muscle testing result can be caused by (1) the patient's unwillingness to contract maximally, (2) pain that limits maximum contraction, and (3) pseudo-weakness secondary to reflex inhibition.[105, 106] Isometric exercise for the purpose of strengthening suspected jaw muscle weakness needs to be re-evaluated. However, muscle weakness can be suspected after strict immobilization, e.g., intermaxillary fixation, and may require instructing the patient on isometric, isotonic, and/or eccentric strengthening jaw exercises.

Neuromuscular Re-educational Exercises

If not a result of the oral habit(s) previously addressed, MMH is the result of bruxism. Bruxism and MMH are considered synonymous in this discussion. *Bruxism* has been defined as diurnal or nocturnal parafunctional activity, including clenching, bracing, gnashing, and/or grinding of the teeth.[19] At one time, stress was considered a leading cause of bruxism. Researchers have questioned the relationship between the stress-prone personality and bruxism, which may progress from normal behavior to abnormal behavior.[96, 107, 108] Though epidemiologic surveys indicate positive correlations between bruxism and TMD—A, any cause-and-effect relationship is still speculative.[96]

Since the cause of bruxism is unknown, the treatment becomes palliative. From the physical therapist's perspective, diurnal parafunction is controlled through a neuromuscular awareness exercise, known as *tongue up/teeth apart/breathe* (TTB). *Tongue up* is the normal rest position of the tongue.[26] Patients need to be educated about the normal rest position, which is up and forward with the tip of the tongue lightly touching the back side of the upper central incisors. The tongue in this position should help patients develop an awareness that their back teeth are slightly apart. Instructing and helping patients know how to breathe with the diaphragm will further encourage relaxation. Often, patients are observed breathing with their accessory muscles (e.g., scaleni and sternocleidomastoids), which only contributes to muscle hyperactivity. Motivating patients to perform TTB is largely fueled by the clinician's understanding of the physiologic mechanisms underlying TTB and the ability to demonstrate and communicate the application of this neuromuscular re-educational exercise in a meaningful way.[26]

Myofascial pain resulting from bruxism can be reduced through oral modification/awareness, modalities, massage, therapeutic, and neuromuscular re-educational exercises. In another approach to treating diurnal and nocturnal bruxism the physical therapist treats the cervical spine. Because the cervical spine's contribution to bruxism is theorized, the reader must draw his or her own conclusions. Managing bruxism by treating the cervical spine is discussed in the following section.

Cervical Spine Considerations

The cervical spine has been overlooked by the dental profession in both the clinical and research areas. Only recently has the dental profession considered the cervical spine in clinical practice. The Dental Practice Act Committee of the American Academy of Orofacial Pain convened in 1995 to study the scope of TMD/orofacial pain and dental practice. The term *TMD and orofacial pain* became useful to reflect the expanded scope of dental practice which now includes neurovascular and neuropathic pain management.[109] The committee concluded that the scope of dental practice for TMD and orofacial pain "is expanding beyond the teeth and oral cavity to include the diagnosis and treatment of disorders affecting the head and neck."[109] The term *orofacial pain* was judged to be too limiting because it implies anatomic limitations that are not consistent with the scope of dental practice.[109] To be consistent with contemporary practice, the term *head and neck pain management* is recommended to emphasize the expanding scope of dentistry.[109] Head and neck pain management encompasses TMD and orofacial pain.[109]

I believe viewing TMD as only a part of head and neck pain management is a step in the right direction. Physical therapists have been evaluating and treating patients' neuromuscular-skeletal involvement from this point of view for decades (e.g., treatment of medial knee pain may require supporting the arches of the foot, and relaxing back muscles may require stretching the hamstrings). However, my concern related to this expanding scope in dentistry is expressed in the following statement from the report of the Dental Practice Act Committee of the American Academy of Orofacial Pain:[109]

As a result of the comprehensive nature of dental education and the experience of clinical practice, only the dentist is able to assess whether intraoral pain, jaw pain, and facial pain originate from local causes or as a result of referred pain from cervical musculoskeletal structures, neurovascular pain, or neuropathic pain.

This position on the cervical spine is extremely narrow in thought and practice. The report goes on to state that dentists' main focus for evaluating and treating the cervical spine is trigger-point injections to the muscles.[109] Cervical musculoskeletal structures include not only muscles but soft tissue, facet joints, ligaments, disks, and neural tissues (i.e., nerve roots and peripheral nerves). *All of these cervical musculoskeletal tissues can be a source of cephalic symptoms, not just muscles.*[110–116] The cervical spine requires a comprehensive approach to evaluation and management. The medical doctor manages disease or pathosis stemming from the cervical spine as well as from the cranium, eyes, and ears. Fortunately for the patient, the vast majority of patients' symptoms originating in the cervical spine are of nondisease/nonpathologic origin.[117, 118] *It is the physical therapist who has the skills to perform a comprehensive evaluation of a nondiseased cervical spine condition.* Noninvasive treatment is thereby offered not only to the cervical muscles, but also to facet joints, central and peripheral nerves, and cervical disks. If the physical therapist is having difficulties managing the cervical spine, consultation with a medical professional is indicated.[119] The medical doctor can assist the physical therapist in the treatment of nonresponding muscle, facet joint, disk, and/or neural tissue involvement of the cervical spine.[119]

Head and neck pains are best evaluated by a team approach. For the nondiseased patient, the team must include the dental, medical, and physical therapy professions.

Prevalence of Cervical Spine Disorder Coexisting with TMD The coexistence of TMD and cervical spine disorder (CSD) is more prevalent than one might expect.[14, 15, 120–123] One study assessing the incidence of cervical pain/dysfunction in a TMD population found that cervical spine involvement is associated with TMD 70% of the time.[124] Another study indicates that bruxism is more common in patients with myofascial pain in both the muscles of mastication and the cervical spine.[125] A recent thesis by De Wijer concluded that patients with TMD report complaints in the neck area more frequently than controls, whereas patients with cervical spine disorder report more signs and symptoms of TMD than healthy controls.[15] When TMD is divided into TMD−M and TMD−A, neck and shoulder pain is more prevalent in TMD patients with a myogenous component than in TMD patients with an arthrogenous component.[126, 127] The coexistence of CSD and TMD−M complaints is real. The interrelationship as to cause and effect between CSD and TMD−M is still unknown. Clearly, research is needed to investigate whether such a cause-and-effect relationship exists between CSD and TMD.

There are two theories as to how a CSD may be a predisposing, precipitating, or perpetuating factor to bruxism. One theory is based on neurophysiologic influences of the tonic neck reflex on the muscles of mastication. The other theory suggests patients may brux in response to somatic pain originating from the cervical spine.

Bruxism Resulting from Tonic Neck Reflex Activity The role of the tonic neck reflex (TNR) in reflexly orienting the limbs in relationship to the head-body angle was described by Magnus in 1926.[128] Magnus,[129] in his classic work, analyzed the postural reaction of decerebrate quadrupeds when their heads were experimentally turned to an extreme right or left position. He found extension of the forelimb on the side toward which the head was turned and flexion of the opposite forelimb.

Localizing the origin of the TNR to a specific area and tissue began with Magnus and DeKleijn,[130] who had limited the receptive field for the TNR to the first three cervical segments of the spine. They showed that the decerebrate cat possessed TNR, which was not labyrinthine in origin but occurred secondary to activation of neck proprioceptors. The neck proprioceptors that are implicated consist of the facet joint receptors (the mechanoreceptors) and muscle spindle receptors.[131] In 1951 McCouch and colleagues[131] showed that the TNR of the decerebrate labyrinthectomized cat was not abolished when the muscle mass of the neck was sectioned. The TNR was abolished only after the facet joints in the upper cervical spine were denervated, demonstrating that *facet joint mechanoreceptors in the upper cervical spine* are the origin of the TNR. The effect of the TNR is to induce postural changes on trunk and upper/lower extrem-

ity musculature. Excellent reviews of the extensive body of literature on the mechanisms of TNR have been published.[132, 133] Pertinent to this discussion is the TNR influence on jaw muscle activity.

The TNR increases and decreases mandibular muscle tone through the trigemino-neck reflex, which consists of motor neurons located in the subnucleus caudalis and probably in the dorsal horn of the upper cervical spine.[134-136] This is verified when electric stimulation is applied to the central end of the ablated first cervical nerve and electromyographic activity is recorded from the masticatory muscles.[134] From these studies, *there appears to be a closely organized neurophysiologic reflex relationship between TNR activity and trigeminal motor neuron activity.*

A number of studies have confirmed that temporalis, masseter, suprahyoid, and infrahyoid muscle activity increases and decreases in response to extension and flexion of the head on the cervical spine.[134, 137-140] Changes in masticatory muscle activity in response to extension and flexion positions of the head on the neck can be explained by the neurophysiologic reflex relationship between TNR activity and trigeminal motor neuron activity. Changes in masticatory muscles may also occur in response to the gravitational pull on the mandible when the head assumes different positions on the neck. The effect of TNR on jaw muscle activity can be appreciated in a study that observed animals biting on hard objects, such as a bone or nut, between the molars.[134] When biting on the right molars, the animal rotated its head to the left and tilted right. Such head positioning facilitated the elevator muscles of the mandible through the TNR.[134]

In normal, real-life conditions TNR influences on muscle tone are expressed in complex postural responses that also reflect sensory information from other sources, such as vestibular, visual, somatic, and proprioceptive areas, all of which are likely to interact strongly with one another.[141] The existence of the trigemino-neck reflex is real, whereas the clinical significance of bruxism is theoretical. Can sustained, aberrant mechanoreceptor activity due to facet joint dysfunction in the upper cervical spine be sufficient to activate trigeminal motor neuron activity that would result in bruxism? Does treatment rendered to a dysfunctional cervical spine help to manage bruxism? Though the scientific response to both these questions is not known, the clinical answer to the latter is yes.

Bruxism Resulting from Somatic Pain
Although the stress-prone personality may no longer be considered the primary or only cause of bruxism, a patient's emotional state and response to environmental stress cannot be ignored as possible predisposing, precipitating, and perpetuating factors in bruxism. Another form of stress often overlooked is somatic stress, which can appear in the form of pain, experienced by the patient as the result of nociceptive afferent activity stemming from dysfunctional muscles, facet joints, and so on, of the cervical spine. The simplified concept that I am proposing is that patients may brux in response to a "pain in the neck."

This concept may be appreciated in the studies investigating cervical whiplash and temporomandibular joint injuries. It is clear that injuries to the TMJ can be attributed to direct impact of the mandible with hard structures, as well as direct impact with a deployed air bag. However, in cervical whiplash when there is no direct trauma to the mandible, injuries to the TMJ are still reported.[142, 143] The proposed cause-and-effect relationship is based on a series of forces acting on the mandible via the anterior neck muscles' tensing in response to posterior rotation of the cranium.[142] This movement is postulated to cause hypertranslation of the condyles. Condylar hypertranslation then results in damage to the TMJ structures and eventually causes disk displacement(s).[142] Several questions come to mind concerning the mechanism by which cervical whiplash has been theorized to cause injuries to the TMJ.

1. Were all the whiplash injuries the result of a rear-end impact, or were some the result of a side-impact injury? Does the postulated series of events previously described occur in a side-impact whiplash?
2. Whiplash can occur at an impact of 6 to 8 km/hr.[118] This impact subjects the cervical spine to a force of 4.5 G, which may result more in a compression-tension force than in a hyperextension-hyperflexion force.[118] The result is a

mild cervical spine injury. Can such a low impact initiate the postulated series of events previously described to injure the TMJ? Were the impact forces known in these studies?
3. Are the TMJ injuries recorded immediately post whiplash by magnetic resonance (MR) imaging? The majority of studies on whiplash and TMJ injuries do not record the interval between the date of the accident and time the MR imaging was done. In a recent article on this topic,[142] the time between the accident and the MR imaging ranged from a few days to more than 1 year. Only 15% of the 87 patients in this article received imaging within 1 to 30 days.[142]

The conclusion that "MR imaging clearly demonstrates the relationship between post MVA cervical whiplash and TMJ injuries"[142] is not warranted if these questions are not addressed. This is not to say that a higher incidence of disk displacements is seen in patients with postcervical whiplash. The mechanism postulated simply may be different.

It would be interesting to know how many whiplash patients brux. If bruxism (neuromuscular factors) is still one of several heterogeneous etiologic factors for disk displacements, could bruxism in these whiplash patients be a response to pain originating from the patient's neck? I will not go as far as to state that the cervical spine causes a disk displacement via bruxism. I am, however, suggesting that a symptomatic cervical spine can cause masticatory muscle hyperactivity that may be expressed as bruxism.

Summary Physical therapy diurnal management of masticatory muscle hyperactivity comprises oral modification/awareness exercises, modalities, massage, and mandibular and neuromuscular re-educational exercises. Physical therapy management of the symptomatic cervical spine is helpful in diurnal and nocturnal bruxism. Supporting the cervical spine with an appropriate cervical pillow either supine or side-lying also helps in the management of nocturnal bruxism. A number of patients have been observed to have a decrease in symptoms related to bruxism when no lifestyle or treatment changes occurred except that treatments were offered to the cervical spine.

The following section discusses the mechanism by which the cervical spine can be a source of two common cephalic symptoms: headache and dizziness.

Cervical Spine as a Source of Cephalic Symptoms

It is evident that serious disease or pathosis can cause cephalic symptoms that require a thorough neurologic and often otolaryngologic examination. It is just as evident that the cervical spine has not been recognized as it should as a source of non-diseased/pathologic cephalic symptoms. In order for the clinician to appreciate the cervical spine as a common source of cephalic symptoms, the neuroanatomic characteristics are now discussed.

The following is the neuroanatomic pathway explaining how nociceptive activity originating in the cervical spine tissues is perceived by the patient as symptoms in the head, face, and jaw areas.[110]

The spinal nucleus of the trigeminal nerve consists of three parts: pars oralis, par interpolaris, and pars caudalis. The pars caudalis extends caudally to merge with the grey matter of the spinal cord. The spinal tract of the trigeminal nerve descends to the level of at least C3 level and possibly as far as the C4 level. Fibers from the spinal tract terminate in the pars caudalis and in the upper three segments of the spinal cord. In the spinal cord, termination of the spinal tract of the trigeminal nerve overlaps that of the upper cervical nerves.

From the preceding description, Bogduk summarizes, "Terminals of the trigeminal nerve and the upper three cervical nerves ramify in a continuous column of grey matter formed by the pars caudalis of the spinal nucleus of the trigeminal nerve and the dorsal horns of the upper three cervical segments."[110] Bogduk states that this region of gray matter can legitimately be viewed as a single or combined nucleus, for which he prefers to use the term *trigeminocervical nucleus.*[110] Trigeminocervical nucleus incorporates the essential central nervous structures responsible for the transmission of pain. The trigeminocervical nucleus receives afferents from the trigeminal and upper cervical nerves. *This convergence of trigeminal and cervical afferents in the trigeminocervical nucleus is viewed by Bogduk as the nociceptive nucleus for the entire head and upper neck.*[110] Essentially, nociceptive information from the cervical spine tissues is transmitted to the trigeminocervical nucleus, which in turn gives the patient the perception of symptoms in the head, face, and jaw areas.[110, 116, 144–147] Numerous human studies have clearly demonstrated the existence of the trigeminocervical nucleus when experimental stimuli to the upper neck tissues produced referred pain in the head.[148, 149]

Common cervical spine tissues that can be a source of nociceptive information to the trigeminocervical nucleus would include those tissues innervated by cervical nerves C1, C2, C3, and C4. The more common tissues are the longus capitis and cervicis, the rectus capitis anterior and lateralis, and the posterior neck muscles: semispinalis capitis, longissimus capitis and splenius capitis, multifidus, sternocleidomastoid, and trapezius.[150] Facet joints innervated by C1, C2, C3, and C4 include the occipitoatlantal, C1–2, C2–3, and C3–4 facet joints.

In addition to the neuroanatomic connection explaining cephalic symptoms of cervical origin, there also is a peripheral nerve entrapment origin for cephalic symptoms. The greater occipital nerve (GON) is the main sensory nerve in the occipital area, deriving most of its fibers from the C2 nerve root.[150] Involvement of the C2 nerve root or greater occipital nerve has been collectively referred to as *occipital neuralgia.*[151] GON compression or irritation has been attributed to various causes, ranging from posttraumatic lesions and cervical degenerative arthrosis to muscle spasm in the upper cervical spine.[152–154]

Symptoms associated with GON entrapment would be located in the area innervated by cutaneous branches of the GON. Such complaints may be located in the occipital area, at the top of the skull, and/or around/in the ear or TMJ.[150]

HEADACHE

John Edmeads[155] points out that in order for the cervical spine to be a source of headaches, the following three conditions must be present:

1. There should be pain-sensitive structures within the neck.
2. There should be identifiable pathologic processes or physiologic dysfunction within the neck capable of serving as an adequate stimulus to the pain receptors in the cervical structures.
3. There should be identifiable neurologic pathways and mechanisms through which pain originating in the cervical structures may be referred to the head.

It appears from previous discussion that all of Edmeads' criteria are present for the cervical spine to be a source of headaches.

The term used to specify the cervical spine as the source of headaches is *cervicogenic*. It was first used by Sjaastad and associates in 1983.[156] *Cervicogenic* only indicates the region; it does not indicate the structure primarily affected.[156] Since 1983, numerous articles have appeared in the literature providing documentation of cervicogenic headache.[157–162] Only recently have relatively clear criteria for the diagnosis of cervicogenic headache been published.[162] The following are the primary criteria used to diagnose cervicogenic headache:[162–164]

1. Pain localized to neck and occipital region, which may project to the forehead, orbital region, temples, vertex, or ears
2. Pain precipitated or aggravated by special neck movements or sustained neck posture
3. At least one of the following:
   a. Resistance to or limitation of passive neck movements
   b. Changes in neck muscle contour, texture, tone, or response to active or passive stretching and contraction
   c. Abnormal tenderness of neck muscles

The examination by the dentist to diagnose nondiseased cervical spine involvement is covered later. Not included in the dental cervical spine examination are 3.a and 3.b, for practical reasons (patient positioning and manual skills of the clinician).

Cervical spine involvement needs to be considered even when other forms of headache have been implicated. Headaches that may be mistaken for cervicogenic headaches are the classic or common migraine, tension-type headache, and post-traumatic headache. Evidence suggests that cervicogenic headache is more common than migraine.[164] There is no doubt that diagnostic categories overlap because most headaches are diagnosed by location of symptoms.[165] The term *cervicogenic headache* is not suggested to supersede a more popular headache label (i.e., common migraine or tension-type headache). However, at the very least, cervical spine involvement should be considered as a primary feature or epiphenomenon.

DIZZINESS

Like headache, dizziness is a common complaint of patients that can originate in the cervical spine. Dizziness "is a general term, implying only the sense of a disturbed relationship to the space outside oneself."[166] *Vertigo* is the illusion of motion or position, either of the patient or of the patient's environment, and the term has been used more specifically to connote rotation.[167] Both *dizziness* and *vertigo* refer to a false sensation of motion of the body and in the discussion that follows are considered synonymous.[168] Dizziness often is described by the patient as unsteadiness, imbalance, floating, lightheadedness, and spinning.[166–168] Dizziness results from discrepancy or conflict in positional information from the cerebellum, vestibular nuclei, ears, eyes, proprioceptors, and other peripheral receptors.[110, 168] Troost[169, 170] identifies the cause of dizziness as either a peripheral (benign paroxysmal positional vertigo) or central disorder (ischemic or reflex vertigo). Pertinent to this discussion is reflex vertigo that contributes to dizziness.

Reflex cervical vertigo originates from neck proprioceptors whose input affects vestibular nucleus activity, resulting in dizziness.[110, 171] Bogduk states that "along with the eyes and labyrinths, the cervical vertebral column is an important source of proprioceptive information that influences the sense of balance, and it is well known, on clinical grounds, that cervical disease or injury can be accompanied by vertigo, but of a nature that does not imply vertebrobasilar insufficiency."[110] Neck proprioception originates from muscle spindles and mechanoreceptor activity in the cervical spine.[172]

Though orientation of the head in space is the special role of the vestibular apparatus, there is, as Cohen states,[173] "no conceivable way by which the semicircular canal or the otoliths can, by themselves, inform the brain of the angle formed by the head and the body." Orientation of the head to the body can be achieved only by neck proprioception. To have only the vestibular system indicating a position of the head in space, without information from the neck proprioceptors indicating the relationship of the head on the neck, would prove to be insufficient to function in the upright position.[173]

Vestibular catastrophes, such as vertigo and nystagmus, can be caused solely by abnormalities related to neck proprioceptors.[173] Various studies show that damage to deep cervical tissues, such as facet joints and neck muscles, produces a generalized ataxia, with symptoms of imbalance, disorientation, and motor incoordination.[174-176] Vertigo, ataxia, and nystagmus were induced in animals and humans by injecting local anesthetic into the neck.[177] The injections presumably interrupted the flow of afferent information from neck muscles and joint receptors. Hinoki,[178] through his experiments and clinical studies, suggests that vertigo after a whiplash injury may be due to overexcitation of the cervical soft tissues, such as muscles, ligaments, facet joints, and sensory nerves. Other seemingly unrelated symptoms, such as vomiting, tinnitus, and diminished hearing, could be related to cervical spine involvement.[171]

In conclusion, cephalic symptoms such as headaches and dizziness can have a variety of origins and may require input from a variety of health professionals. In all instances, however, the attentive clinician must address cervical spine involvement as one of the primary sources of neck and cephalic symptoms.

Dental Examination for Cervical Spine Disorder

Spinal research has largely focused on the lumbar spine. For this discussion, conclusions drawn about the lumbar spine are considered applicable to the cervical spine.

A clinician faces dilemmas in diagnosing and treating the lumbar and cervical spine. In many cases, it may be difficult or impossible to establish the correct diagnosis for a patient with spinal complaints.[179] An expert panel has estimated that a precise diagnosis probably cannot be determined for up to 80% to 90% of patients with spinal pain, depending in part on how we regard radiographic degenerative changes.[117] Clinical practice, despite the major advances in knowledge and technology, is largely an art.[179] What is known from clinical research is that the majority of patients seek help for *nonspecific* acute or chronic spinal complaints.[117] *Nonspecific* implies that no underlying disease can be established.[117]

Inspired in part by the Quebec Task Force publication, the medical and physical therapy professions have pursued research and clinical studies classifying patients having a nonspecific spinal involvement according to signs and symptoms (versus a radiologic diagnosis or physiopathologic hypothesis).[180-185] Classifying/diagnosing patients according to signs and symptoms should provide a direct treatment plan and a better understanding of treatment outcomes.[184-186] Physical therapists can also diagnose/classify patients according to signs and symptoms that identify the condition. A diagnosis based on symptoms and functional limitations can be the focus of the physical therapist's treatment and reassessment of the patient's condition.[21] Diagnosis by a physical therapist has been defined by Sahrmann:[20]

Diagnosis is the term that names the primary dysfunction toward which the physical therapist directs treatment. The dysfunction is identified by the physical therapist based on information obtained from the history, signs, symptoms, examination, and tests the therapist performs or requests.

Jette states, "The purpose of having a physical therapist establish a diagnosis is to name and communicate the primary impairment, disability, or handicap toward which the clinician directs his or her treatment within that professional's appropriate scope of practice."[21] A physical therapy diagnosis should not be used to reflect ownership of the condition.[21]

This author proposes the following classification and its subcategories for nonspecific complaints of the cervical spine. A similar list of categories has been published by the Quebec Task Force on Whiplash-Associated Disorders.[118]

Classification

   Movement Dysfunction of the Cervical Spine

Categories

1. Neck symptom(s) (central) without radiation
2. Neck symptom(s) with radiation into proximal upper extremity
   _____ L _____ R
   Radiation related to radiculopathy
   _____ Y _____ N
3. Neck symptom(s) with radiation into distal upper extremity
   _____ L _____ R
   Radiation related to radiculopathy
   _____ Y _____ N
   Neurologic signs _____ Y _____ N
4. Neck symptom(s) with cephalic radiation _____ L _____ R

Utilizing the categories should foster understanding and reduce confusion between the dental/medical professions and the physical therapy profession when discussing what the patient's problem is. Future examination methods that prove reliable and valid will specify the tissue(s) causing the patient's symptoms and functional limitations. Once the predictive value of tests is established, the preceding categories may have their own subcategories that name a specific tissue(s) that has undergone physiopathologic changes. An example is the following:

Classification

   Movement Dysfunction of the Cervical Spine

Category

   Neck symptom(s) with radiation cephalic to the left

Subcategories

C2–3 left facet joint dysfunction
Left occipital neuralgia
Muscle hyperactivity of the left suboccipital, levator scapulae, and trapezius muscles

---

Dentists can diagnose a nondiseased cervical spine condition on the basis of symptom locations. The following section indicates the minimum data a dentist should obtain through the history and physical examination for determining whether the patient has movement dysfunction of the cervical spine. The dentist may elect not to perform the examination and refer the patient to a physical therapist.

HISTORY

During the history interview the dentist should be alert to "red flags" suggesting a medical referral is indicated. Examples are a previous cancer history, trauma sufficient to cause a fracture, unexplained weight loss, intravenous drug abuse, and diplopia, dysarthria, dysphagia, and drop attacks with or without dizziness. The history interview also should include *mode of onset* (traumatic, insidious, iatrogenic), *progression of pain behavior* (pain better, worse, or unchanged), *past treatment and response to past treatment,* and *aggravating factors* (positions or movements of the cervical spine that increase or decrease the symptoms).

The following are symptoms that can result from cervical spine involvement. The list has been published by the Quebec Task Force on Whiplash-Associated Disorders.[118] These questions pertain to patients involved in a whiplash. However, I considered these same questions to be appropriate for those experiencing trauma from a nonwhiplash injury, as well as symptoms that have an insidious onset. I have placed the questions into three groups.

   Do you have any of the following symptoms?

Group One

Neck/shoulder pain
Reduced/painful neck movements

Headaches
Numbness, tingling, or pain in arm or hand
Dizziness/unsteadiness
Nausea/vomiting

Group Two

Difficulty in swallowing
Ringing in the ears
Memory problems
Problems in concentrating
Vision problems
Reduced/painful jaw movement

Group Three

Numbness, tingling, or pain in leg or foot
Lower back pain

Group one contains the key questions asked in order to diagnose "movement dysfunction of the cervical spine." These same questions allow the dentist to classify the patient into categories 1 to 4. Recording the patient's response to *group two* symptoms helps the clinician appreciate the role of the cervical spine as a source of symptoms normally thought to originate elsewhere. Medical exclusion of disease/pathosis as a source of *group two* symptoms makes the cervical spine a primary suspect. Patients experiencing *group two* symptoms should not be given false hope that the symptoms will diminish once the cervical spine condition is treated. Instead, a wait and see attitude should be applied. *Group three* symptoms are not as important for the dentist to ask about as they are for the physical therapist. They are listed here for completeness.

Patients can be asked to fill out a pain drawing (Fig. 10–1). The common pain drawing is used to describe presenting symptoms and can also be scored for research purposes according to the method of Margolis and associates.[187]

PHYSICAL EXAMINATION

The physical examination as illustrated in Figure 10–2 has been published by the Quebec Task Force on Whiplash-Associated Disorders.[118] I have modified several areas of the physical examination for use by the dentist. This examination is not intended to give the dentist a clear understanding of the absence or presence of radiculopathy, i.e., nerve root irritation/compression. Radiculopathy is included for completeness. The reader should refer to the reference for further understanding of radiculopathy.[119]

Completion of the history, pain drawing, and physical examination should provide the dentist with enough information to implicate the cervical spine as a source of the patient's head and neck symptoms, indicating a referral to a physical therapist. The following is a general overview of what the dentist should expect from the physical therapist in the management of movement dysfunction of the cervical spine.

Physical Therapy Management for Movement Dysfunction of the Cervical Spine

The following is a general overview of physical therapy management for movement dysfunction of the cervical spine. The reader is referred to the reference section for additional information on this topic.[188–195] As discussed in treatment of TMD, physical therapists seldom offer a single treatment option for a patient who has myriad tissue and functional involvements of the cervical spine. Treatment options considered by the physical therapist in the management of movement dysfunction of the cervical spine are the following:

- Patient education
- Sleeping postures
- Upright postures
- Exercise
- Cervical traction
- Cervical collar
- Manual therapy

The physical therapist's knowledge of anatomy, physiology, neurophysiology, and mechanics assists in the application of these treatment options. Cervical traction and cervical collar treatment are the only two options that are not offered to every patient. *Every* patient is educated about the condition along with precipitating and perpetuating factors that can aggravate it. *Every* patient is instructed on proper sleeping postures either supine or sidelying and if necessary the use of a cervical support. *Ev-*

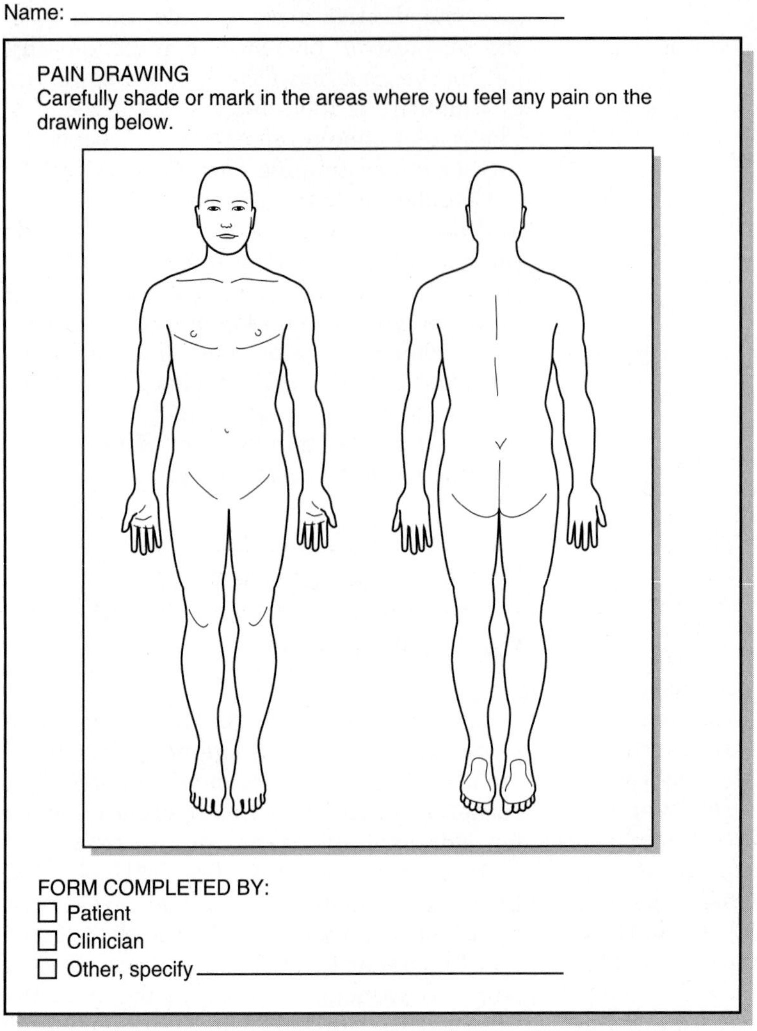

Name: ______________________

PAIN DRAWING
Carefully shade or mark in the areas where you feel any pain on the drawing below.

FORM COMPLETED BY:
☐ Patient
☐ Clinician
☐ Other, specify ______________________

FIGURE 10–1. Pain drawing.

ery patient is shown exercises to improve flexibility, strength, and endurance. *Every* patient receives manual therapy. Physical therapists have knowledge and skills in all treatment options listed. An area of special interest is the manual skills of the physical therapist.

Manual skills are incorporated into the examination and consist of palpation and passive mobility testing. Treatment via manual therapy may consist of hands-on, repetitive oscillations; steady stretch or high-velocity thrusts of joints; and application of various forms of soft tissue massage, muscle stretching, or shortening.[190] The potential therapeutic value of manual therapy revolves around its mechanical, neurologic, neurophysiologic, and psychological effects.[190–195] A comprehensive understanding of clinical viewpoints and scientific research on manual therapy can be obtained from the reference section.[190–199]

Chapter Summary

Guidelines for the management of TMD can be misleading, especially if the treatment under study is misunderstood. Research on the therapeutic value of physical therapy treatments must incorporate the role of the physical therapist in performing the treatments. This basic concept can help in future clinical and research studies that investigate the therapeutic value of physical therapy for TMDs.

Physical therapists play an important role in the conservative and noninvasive

Dental Examination of the Cervical Spine

Examination indicated but deferred to: ____PT and / or ____ MD

Date of Examination: Day _____ Month _____ Year _____

A. PAIN / LIMITATION

	No	Pain	Limitation
Flexion	____	____	____
Extension	____	____	____
Right rotation	____	____	____
Left rotation	____	____	____
Right lateral flexion	____	____	____
Left lateral flexion	____	____	____

B. PALPATORY TENDERNESS

_____ Yes
_____ No

If yes:	Left	Midline	Right
Cervical spine	____	____	____
Thoracic spine	____	____	____

Other, specify ______________________

C. NEUROLOGIC EXAMINATION

____ Normal or ...

	Sensory deficit Right	Sensory deficit Left	Motor weakness Right	Motor weakness Left	Decreased deep tendon reflexes Right	Decreased deep tendon reflexes Left
C5	____	____	____	____	____	____
C6	____	____	____	____	____	____
C7	____	____	____	____	____	____
C8	____	____	____	____	____	____
Other, specify	_____________		_____________		_____________	

D. DIAGNOSTIC TESTS

Plain radiographs
(Medical report available)
____ Yes ____ No

If yes:
____ Normal

____ Degenerative changes
Specify levels __________

Other specialized tests, specify:

____

____

F. MANAGEMENT PLAN

- Reassurance
  ____ Yes

- Activation
  ____ Return to usual activities ASAP

  ____ Delayed return to recreational activities

- Treatments
  ____ Medications, specify: ____________________________

  ____ Home care, specify: ____________________________

  ____ Referral to Physical Therapy: ______________________

  ____ Referral to a medical specialist: ___________________

E. DIAGNOSIS

CLASSIFICATION: Movement dysfunction of the cervical spine ____ Yes ____ No

If yes, patient categorized as:

__ 1. Neck symptom(s) (central) without radiation
__ 2. Neck symptom(s) with radiation into proximal upper extremity ___ L ___ R; Radiation related to radiculopathy ___Y___N
__ 3. Neck symptom(s) with radiation into distal upper extremity ___ L ___ R; Radiation related to radiculopathy ___Y___N
__ 4. Neck symptom(s) with radiation cephalic ___ L ___ R

REMARKS: ____

FIGURE 10–2. Form for dental examination of the cervical spine.

treatment of TMD: TMD—A, TMD—A/M, and TMD—M.

Subcategories of TMD—A that are diagnosed and treated by a physical therapist are inflammation, hypermobility, and hypomobility. Modalities for the treatment of inflammation have been covered, as well as the management of hypermobility. Hypomobility secondary to capsular tightness or a disk displacement without reduction can be managed by therapeutic procedures offered by a physical therapist. Physical therapy in the treatment of a disk displacement without reduction is gaining wider acceptance. Through the application of modalities, therapeutic procedures, and a home exercise program, a physical therapist can restore mobility of the mandible to a pain-free state with the disk remaining out of place. In conditions that do not respond to nonsurgical treatment for TMD, TMJ surgery and/or orthognathic surgery may be necessary. Postoperative physical therapy is important in pain control, promotion of healing, and restoration of functional mandibular movements.

Physical therapy management of TMD—M/bruxism focuses on oral modification, modalities, massage, and therapeutic and neuromuscular re-educational exercises. Decreasing symptoms and improving functional limitations associated with cervical spine involvement may also help reduce masticatory muscle hyperactivity. Theories that bruxism results from aberrant tonic neck reflex activity and cervical somatic pain have been discussed.

It is important to view TMD as only a component of head and neck pain management. Dentists cannot overlook the cervical spine as a major source of nondisease cephalic symptoms. Headaches, dizziness, as well as symptoms in the area of the eye, ear, and TMJ can originate in the cervical spine. Considering the number of muscles and facet joints of the cervical spine that can be a source of cephalic symptoms, the dentist alone cannot assess and treat referred pain from cervical musculoskeletal structures. A number of patients may unnecessarily continue to suffer from pain and functional limitations because the cervical spine was overlooked or treatments to the cervical spine were given by a clinician who did not have clinical skills or knowledge of a physical therapist.

The evaluation of the cervical spine that can be done by the dentist has been reviewed. The diagnosis of a nondiseased cervical spine is *movement dysfunction of the cervical spine*. Essentially, the diagnosis is made by the *exclusion* of disease/pathosis. The cervical spine evaluation primarily provides the clinician with functional information and a baseline to determine the effectiveness of treatment. A referral to a physical therapist is in order should the evaluation confirm the diagnosis of movement dysfunction of the cervical spine.

Physical therapists have various treatment options for managing the cervical spine. Manual therapy is a key treatment option. Should the physical therapist require assistance in managing nondiseased cervical spine–related complaints, he or she can consult a dentist and/or physician. Cervical pain secondary to inflammation of cervical dura, nerve roots, facet joints, or muscles may be relieved or reduced by localized injection by a medical doctor.

Patients experience multiple-tissue involvement that contributes to varying levels of symptoms and functional limitations of the head and neck. Whether or not the TMJ, muscles of mastication and occlusion, and cervical spine are interrelated or simply coexist remains to be seen. What is essential to head and neck pain management is a team approach consisting of a physical therapist, dentist, and physician. Physical therapists are key players in the conservative and noninvasive management of nondisease head and neck pains stemming from the TMJ, muscles of mastication, and cervical spine.

REFERENCES

1. Rothstein J, Delitto A, Scalzitti D: Understanding AHCPR Clinical Practice Guideline No. 14: Acute low back problems in adults. Prepared for the American Physical Therapy Association. J Am Phys Ther Assoc, Sept 1995, p 1.
2. Connolly J: AHCPR Guideline No. 14: Acute Low Back Problems in Adults: A commentary. Phys Ther Magazine 1995;3(9):89.
3. Bigos S, Bowyer O, Braen G, et al: Acute Low Back Problems in Adults. Clinical Practice Guideline No. 14. AHCPR publication 95 - 0642. Rockville, MD: Agency for Health Care Policy and Research, Public Health Service, US Department of Health and Human Services, 1994.
4. Tygiel PP: A critical analysis of the AHCPR acute low back pain guidelines. Orthop Pract 1995;7:3.
5. Ellis J: Concern still exists over guidelines for

treatment of acute low back pain. Phys Ther Bull July 21, 1995, p 10.

6. Woolf SH: Practice guidelines: A new reality in medicine. Part III. Impact on patient care. Arch Intern Med 1993;150:2464.

7. Judith Albino, Chairperson: National Institutes of Health Technology Assessment Conference on Management of Temporomandibular Disorders. April 29–May 1, 1996, Bethesda, MD.

8. Feine J, Widmer C, Lund J: Physical Therapy: A Critique. National Institutes of Health Technology Assessment Conference on Management of Temporomandibular Disorders. April 29–May 1, 1996, Bethesda, MD, p 75.

9. McNeil C (ed): Temporomandibular Disorders, Guidelines for Classification, Assessment and Management, ed 2. Lombard, IL, Quintessence, 1993.

10. Letter of communication from Marilyn M. Moffat, President of the APTA to William H. Hall, Director of Communications, National Institutes of Health. May 29, 1996. Letter on file with the American Physical Therapy Association.

11. A guide to physical therapist practice. Volume I: A description of patient management. Phys Ther 1995;75:707.

12. APTA House of Delegates Policies HOD #06-93-22-43, June 1996, APTA, Alexandria VA.

13. Okeson Jeffrey P: Current terminology and diagnostic classification schema. In: National Institutes of Health Technology Assessment Conference on Management of Temporomandibular Disorders. April 29–May 1, 1996, Bethesda, MD, p 21.

14. De Wijer A, Rob J, de Leeuw J, et al: Temporomandibular and cervical spine disorders: Self-reported signs and symptoms. Spine 1996;21:1638.

15. De Wijer A. Temporomandibular and cervical spine disorders. Dissertation, Utrecht University, The Netherlands, 1995. Pub Elinkwijk BV, Utrecht, The Netherlands.

16. McNamara JA Jr, Seligman DA, Okeson JP: The relationship of occlusal factors and orthodontic treatment to temporomandibular disorders. In Sessle BJ, Bryant PS, Dionne RA (eds): Temporomandibular Disorders and Related Pain Conditions. Seattle, IASP Press, 1995; pp 399–427.

17. Seligman DA, Pullinger AG: The role of intercuspal occlusal relationships in temporomandibular disorders: A review. J Craniomandibul Disord Facial Oral Pain 1991;5:96.

18. Seligman DA, Pullinger AG: The role of functional occlusal relationships in temporomandibular disorders: A review. J Craniomandibul Disord Facial Oral Pain 1991;5:265.

19. Okeson JP (ed): Orofacial Pain: Guidelines for Assessment, Diagnosis, and Management. Chicago: Quintessence, 1996.

20. Sahrmann S: Diagnosis by the physical therapist: A prerequisite for treatment. A special communication. Phys Ther 1988;68:703.

21. Jette A: Diagnosis and classification by physical therapists: A special communication. Phys Ther 1989;69:967.

22. Delitto A, Guccione A, Jette A, et al: Diagnosis in physical therapy. PT Magazine, June 1993, pp 58–65.

23. Dekker J, van Baar M, Curfs E, et al: Diagnosis and treatment in physical therapy: An investigation of their relationship. Phys Ther 1993;73:568.

24. Delitto A, Snyder-Mackler L: The diagnostic process: Examples in orthopedic physical therapy practice. Phys Ther 1995;75:203.

25. Fitsgerald G, McClure P, Beattle P: Issues in determining treatment effectiveness of manual therapy. Phys Ther 1994;74:227.

26. Kraus SL: Physical therapy management of TMD. In Kraus SL (ed): Clinics in Physical Therapy, Temporomandibular Disorders, ed 2. New York, Churchill Livingstone, 1994, p 161.

27. Brian R, Zarro V: Inflammation and repair and the use of thermal agents. In Michlovitz S (ed): Thermal Agents in Rehabilitation: Contemporary Perspectives in Rehabilitation, Philadelphia, FA Davis, 1990, p 1.

28. Benoit PW: History and physical examination for TMD. In Kraus SL (ed): Clinics in Physical Therapy, Temporomandibular Disorders, ed 2. New York, Churchill Livingstone, 1994, p 71.

29. Kraus SL: Evaluation and management of temporomandibular disorders. In Evaluation, Treatment and Prevention of Musculoskeletal Disorders. Minneapolis, The Saunders Group, 1993.

30. Michlovitz S (ed): Thermal Agents in Rehabilitation: Contemporary Perspectives in Rehabilitation, ed 2. Philadelphia, FA Davis, 1990.

31. Mannheimer JS: Physical therapy concepts in evaluation and treatment of the upper quarter: Therapeutic modalities. In Kraus SL (ed): TMJ Disorders: Management of the Craniomandibular Complex. New York, Churchill Livingstone, 1988, p 311.

32. Mannheimer J: Postoperative physical therapy protocols. In Kraus SL (ed): Clinics in Physical Therapy: Temporomandibular Disorders, ed 2. New York, Churchill Livingstone, 1994, p 277.

33. Ziskin MC, McDiarmid T, Michlovitz SL: Therapeutic ultrasound. In Michlovitz S (ed): Thermal Agents in Rehabilitation: Contemporary Perspectives in Rehabilitation, Philadelphia, FA Davis, 1990, p 134.

34. Stratton SA, Heckmann R, Francis RS: Therapeutic ultrasound: Its effect on the integrity of a nonpenetrating wound. J Orthop Sports Phys Ther 1984;5:278.

35. Munting E: Ultrasonic therapy for painful shoulders. Physiotherapy 1978;64:180.

36. Bierman W: Ultrasound in the treatment of scars. Arch Phys Med Rehabil 1954;35:209.

37. Michlovitz S: Cryotherapy: The use of cold as a therapeutic agent. In Michlovitz S (ed): Thermal Agents in Rehabilitation: Contemporary Perspectives in Rehabilitation. Philadelphia, FA Davis, 1990, p 63.

38. Travell J, Simons D: Myofascial Pain and Dysfunction: The Trigger Point Manual. New York, Williams & Wilkins, 1983.

39. Michlovitz S: Cryotherapy: Biophysical principles of heating and superficial heat agents. In Michlovitz S (ed): Thermal Agents in Rehabilitation: Contemporary Perspectives in Rehabilitation. Philadelphia, FA Davis, 1990, p 88.

40. Glass J, Stephen R, Jacobson C: The quality and distribution of radiolabeled dexamethasone delivered to tissue by iontophoresis. Int J Dermatol 1980;19:519.

41. Harris P: Iontophoresis: Clinical research in musculoskeletal inflammatory conditions. J Orthop Sports Phys Ther 1982;4:109.

42. Bertolucci L: Introduction of antiinflammatory drugs by iontophoresis: Double blind study. J Orthop Sports Phys Ther 1982;4:103.

43. Braun BL: Treatment of an acute anterior disk displacement in the temporomandibular joint. Phys Ther 1987;67:1234.

44. Lark M, Gangarosa C Sr: Iontophoresis: An effective modality for the treatment of inflammatory disorders of the temporomandibular joint and myofascial pain. J Craniomandibul Pract 1990;8:108.

45. Reid K, Dionne R, Sicard-Rosenbaum L, et al: Evaluation of iontophoresis applied dexamethasone for painful pathologic temporomandibular joints. Oral Surg Oral Med Oral Pathol 1994; 77:605.

46. Schiffman E, Braun B, Lindgren J, et al: Temporomandibular joint iontophoresis: A double-blind randomized clinical trial. J Orofac Pain 1996;10:157.

47. Mannheimer JS, Lampe GN: Clinical Transcutaneous Electrical Nerve Stimulation. Philadelphia, FA Davis, 1984.

48. Keith DA: Surgery of the Temporomandibular Joint. Boston, Blackwell Scientific Publications, 1988, pp 139–141.

49. Buckingham RB, Braun T, Harenstein DA, et al: Temporomandibular joint dysfunction syndrome: A close association with systemic joint laxity (the hypermobile joint syndrome). Oral Surg Oral Med Oral Pathol 1991;72:514.

50. Westling L, Mattiasson A: General joint hypermobility and temporomandibular joint derangement in adolescents. Ann Rheum Dis 1992;51:87.

51. Dijkstra PU, Lambert GM de Bont, Stegenga B, et al: Temporomandibular joint osteoarthrosis and generalized joint hypermobility. J Craniomandibul Pract 1992;10:221.

52. Akeson WH: An experimental study of joint stiffness. J Bone Joint Surg 1961;43A:1022.

53. Akeson WH, Amiel D, LaViolette D, et al: The connective tissue response to immobility: An accelerated ageing response. Exp Gerontol 1968;3:289.

54. Akeson WH, Amiel D, Woo S: Immobility effects of synovial joints: the pathomechanics of joint contracture. Biorheology 1980;17:95.

55. Salter RB, Simmonds DI, Malcolm BW, et al: The biological effect of continuous passive motion on the healing of full-thickness defects in articular cartilage. J Bone Joint Surg 1980;62A:1232.

56. Salter RB, Hamilton WH, Wedge JH, et al: Clinical applications of basic research on continuous passive motion for disorders and injuries of synovial joints, a preliminary report of a feasibility study. J Orthop Res 1983;3:325.

57. Toller P: Non-surgical treatment of the temporomandibular joint. Oral Sci Rev 1976;7:70.

58. Rasmussen OC: Description of population and progress of symptoms in a longitudinal study of temporomandibular arthropathy. Scand J Dent Res 1981;89:196.

59. Clark GT, Mulligan RA: A review of the prevalence of temporomandibular dysfunction. J Gerodontol 1986;3:231.

60. Greene CS, Turner C, Laskin DM: Long-term outcome of TMJ clicking in 100 MPD patients. J Dent Res 1982;61:218.

61. Turell J, Ruiz HG: Normal and abnormal findings in temporomandibular joints in autopsy specimens. J Craniomandibul Disord Facial Oral Pain 1987;1:257.

62. Hellsing G, Holmlund A: Development of anterior disk displacement in the temporomandibular joint: An autopsy study. J Prosthet Dent 1985;53:397.

63. Westesson PL, Eriksson L, Kurita K: Reliability of a negative clinical temporomandibular joint examination: Prevalence of disk displacement in asymptomatic temporomandibular joints. Oral Surg Oral Med Oral Pathol 1989;68:551.

64. Ribeio RF, Tallents RH, Katzberg RW, et al: The prevalence of disc displacement in symptomatic and asymptomatic volunteers aged 6 to 25 years. J Orofac Pain 1987;11:37.

65. Zamburlini I, Austin D: Long-term results of appliance therapies in anterior disk displacement with reduction: A review of the literature. J Craniomandibul Pract 1991;9:361.

66. Orenstein ES: Anterior repositioning appliances when used for anterior disk displacement with reduction—a critical review. J Craniomandibul Pract 1993;11:141.

67. Vichaichalermvong S, Nilner M, Panmekiate S, et al: Clinical follow-up of patients with different disc positions. J Orofac Pain 1993;7:61.

68. Moloney F, Howard JA: Internal derangements of the temporomandibular joint: Anterior repositioning splint therapy. Aust Dent J 1986;31:30.

69. de Leeuw R, Boering G, Stegenga B, et al: Clinical signs of TMJ osteoarthrosis and internal derangement 30 years after nonsurgical treatment. J Orofac Pain 1994;8:18.

70. Braun BL: The effect of physical therapy intervention on incisal opening after temporomandibular joint surgery. Oral Surg Oral Med Oral Pathol 1987;64:544.

71. Lehmann J, Masock A, Warren C, et al: Effect of therapeutic temperature on tendon extensibility. Arch Phys Med Rehabil 1970;51:481.

72. Warren C, Lehman J, Koblanski J: Heat and stretch procedures: An evaluation using rat tail tendon. Arch Phys Med Rehabil 1976;57:122.

73. Lentell G, Hetherington T, Eagan J, et al: The use of thermal agents to influence the effectiveness of a low-load prolonged stretch. J Orthop Sports Phys Ther 1992;16:200

74. Warren C, Lehmann J, Koblanski J: Elongation of rat tail tendon: Effect of load and temperature. Arch Phys Med Rehabil 1971;52:465.

75. McCarthy MR, Yates CK, Anderson MA, et al: The effects of immediate continuous passive motion on pain during the inflammatory phase of soft tissue healing following anterior cruciate reconstruction. J Orthop Sports Phys Ther 1993;17(2):96–101

76. Salter RB: The biological concept of continuous passive motion of synovial joints: The first 18 years of basic research and its clinical application. Clin Orthop 1989;242:12.

77. Gossman MR, Sharmann SA, Rose SJ: Review of length-associated changes in muscle. Phys Ther 1979;62:1799.

78. McCarthy MR, O'Donoghue PC, Yates CK, et al: The clinical use of continuous passive motion in physical therapy. J Orthop Sports Phys Ther 1992;15:132.

79. McCarty WL, Darnell MW: Rehabilitation of the temporomandibular joint through the application of motion. J Craniomandibul Pract 1993;11:289.

80. Osborn JW: The disc of the human temporomandibular joint: Design, function and failure. J Oral Rehabil 1985;12:279.

81. Wright V, Dowson D, Longfield M: Joint stiffness - its characterization and significance. Biomed Eng 1969;4:8.

82. Randall T, Portney L, Harris BA: Effects of joint

mobilization on joint stiffness and active motion of the metacarpal-phalangeal joint. J Orthop Sports Phys Ther 1992;16:30.

83. Stromberg D, Wiederhielm CA: Viscoelastic description of a collagenous tissue in simple elongation. J Appl Physiol 1969;26:857.

84. LaBan MM: Collagen tissue: Implications of its response to stress in vitro. Arch Phys Med Rehabil 1962;43:461.

85. Chung S-C, Kim H-S: The effects of the stabilization splint on the TMJ closed locked. J Craniomandibul Pract 1993;11:95.

86. Farrar WB: Characteristics of the condylar path in internal derangements of the TMJ. J Prosthet Dent 1978;39:319.

87. Murakami K-I, Segami N, Moriya Y, et al: Correlation between pain and dysfunction and intraarticular adhesions in patients with internal derangement of the temporomandibular joint. J Oral Maxillofac Surg 1992;50:705.

88. Dolwick MF, Katzberg RW, Helms CA: Internal derangements of the temporomandibular joint: Fact or fiction? J Prosthet Dent 1983;49:415.

89. Martini G, Martini M, Carano A: MRI study of a physiotherapeutic protocol in anterior disk displacement without reduction. J Craniomandibul Pract 1996;14:216.

90. de Leeuw R, Boering G, Stegenga B, et al: Radiographic signs of temporomandibular joint osteoarthrosis and internal derangement 30 years after nonsurgical treatment. Oral Surg Oral Med Oral Pathol 1995;79:382.

91. Mongini F, Ibertis F, Manfredi A: Long-term results in patients with disc displacement without reduction treated conservatively. J Craniomandibul Pract 1996;14:301.

92. Scapino RP: The posterior attachments: Its structure, function, and appearance in TMJ imaging studies, Part 1. J Craniomandibul Disord Facial Oral Pain 1991;5:83.

93. Scapino RP: Histopathology of the disc and posterior attachment. In Disc Displacement, Internal Derangements of the TMJ. In Palacios E (ed): Magnetic Resonance Imaging of the Temporomandibular Joint. Stuttgart, Georg Thieme Verlag, 1990.

94. Van Dyke AR, Goldman SM: Manual reduction of displaced disk. J Craniomandibul Pract 1990;8:350.

95. Minagi S, Nozaki S, Sato T, et al: Manipulation techniques for treatment of anterior disk displacement without reduction. J Prosthet Dent 1991;65:686.

96. Labbezoo F, Lavigne G: Do bruxism and temporomandibular disorders have a cause-and-effect relationship? J Orofac Pain 1997;11:15.

97. Mao J, Stein R, Osborn J: Fatigue in human jaw muscles: A review. J Orofac Pain 1993;7:135.

98. Russell JI (ed): Clinical overview and pathogenesis of the fibromyalgia syndrome, myofascial pain syndrome, and other pain syndromes. J Musculoskeletal Pain 1996;4.

99. Lawerence ES, Razook SJ: Nonsurgical Management of Mandibular Disorders. In Kraus S (ed): Clinics in Physical Therapy, Temporomandibular Disorders, ed 2. New York, Churchill Livingstone, 1994, p 125.

100. Schnurr RF, Rollman GB, Brooke RI: Are there psychologic predictors of treatment in temporomandibular joint pain and dysfunction? Oral Surg Oral Med Oral Pathol 1991;72:550.

101. Bertolucci LE: Physical therapy post-arthroscopic TMJ management (update). J Craniomandibul Pract 1992;10:130.

102. Smith AM: The coactivation of antagonist muscles. Can J Physiol Pharmacol 1981;59:733.

103. Burke D: Critical examination of the case for or against fusimotor involvement in disorders of muscle tone. In Desmedt JE (ed): Motor Control Mechanisms in Health and Disease. New York, Raven Press, 1983, p 133.

104. Tanigawa MC: Comparison of the hold-relax procedure and passive mobilization on increasing muscle length. Phys Ther 1972;52:725.

105. DeAndrade J, Grant C, Dixon A: Joint distention and reflex muscle inhibition in the knee. J Bone Joint Surg 1965;47(A):313.

106. Larsson L, Thilander B: Mandibular positioning, the effect of pressure on joint capsule. Acta Neurol Scand 1964;40:131.

107. Hathaway KM: Behavioral and psychosocial management. In Pertes RA, Gross SG (eds): Clinical Management of Temporomandibular Disorders and Orofacial Pain. Chicago, Quintessence, 1995.

108. Slater M, Brooke RI, Merskey GF, et al: Is the temporomandibular pain and dysfunction syndrome a disorder of the mind? Pain 1983;17:151.

109. Robert Rosenbaum, Committee Chairman: The scope of TMD / orofacial pain (head and neck pain management) in contemporary dental practice. J Orofac Pain 1997;11:78.

110. Bogduk N: Cervical causes of headache and dizziness. In Grieve G (ed): Modern Manual Therapy. New York, Churchill Livingstone, 1986, p 289.

111. Everett N: Functional Neuroanatomy, ed 6. Philadelphia, Lea & Febiger, 1972.

112. Kerr F: Mechanism, diagnosis and management of some cranial and facial pain syndromes. Surg Clin North Am 1963;43:951.

113. Kerr F, Olafson R: Trigeminal and cervical volleys. Arch Neurol 1961;5:171.

114. Kerr F: A mechanism to account for frontal headache in cases of posterior fossa tumors. J Neurosurg 1961;18:605.

115. Kerr F: Structural relation of the trigeminal spinal tract to upper cervical roots and the solitary nucleus in the cat. Exp Neurol 1961;4:134.

116. Allen ME (ed): Musculoskeletal pain emanating from the head and neck. J Musculoskeletal Pain 1996;4.

117. Spitzer WO (ed): Scientific approach to the assessment and management of activity-related spinal disorders. A monograph for Clinicians Report of the Quebec Task Force on Spinal Disorders. Spine 1987;12(7).

118. J. David Cassidy, Editorial Coordinator: Scientific monograph of the Quebec Task Force on Whiplash-Associated Disorders: Redefining "whiplash" and its management. Spine 1995;20(85).

119. Lester JP, Windsor RE, Dreyer, SJ: Medical management of the cervical spine. In Kraus SL (ed): Clinics in Physical Therapy: Temporomandibular Disorders, ed 2. New York, Churchill Livingstone, 1994, p 413.

120. Braun BL, DiGiovanna A, Schiffman E, et al: A cross-sectional study of temporomandibular joint dysfunction in post-cervical trauma patients. J Craniomandibul Disord Facial Oral Pain 1992;6:24.

121. Clark GT: Examining temporomandibular disorder patients for craniocervical dysfunction. J Craniomandibul Pract 1983;2:55.

122. De Laat A, Meuleman H, Stevens A: Relation between functional limitations of the cervical spine and temporomandibular disorders (abstract). J Orofac Pain 1993;1:109.

123. Kirveskari P, Alanen P, Karskela V, et al: Association of functional state of stomatognathic system with mobility of cervical spine and neck muscle tenderness. Acta Odontol Scand 1988;46:281.

124. Padamsee M, Mehtan N, Forgione A, et al: Incidence of cervical disorders in a TMD population. (IADR; Abstract No. 680). J Dent Res 1994;73.

125. Isaccsson G, Linde C, Isberg A: Subjective symptoms in patients with temporomandibular joint disc displacement versus patients with myogenic craniomandibular disorders. J Prosthet Dent 1989;61:70.

126. Lobbezoo-Scholte AM: Diagnostic subgroups of craniomandibular disorders. PhD dissertation, Utrecht University, The Netherlands, 1993.

127. DeLeeuw JRJ: Psychosocial aspects and symptom characteristics of craniomandibular dysfunction. PhD dissertation, Utrecht University, The Netherlands, 1993.

128. Magnus R: Some results of studies in the physiology of posture. Lancet 1926;2:531.

129. Magnus R: Korperstellung, pp xiii, 740, Berlin, 1924, Julius Springer, Animal Posture, Croonian Lecture. Proc R Soc B 98(690):339–353.

130. Magnus R, DeKleijn A: Die Abhangigkeit des Tonus der Extremitatenmuskeln von der Kopfstellung. Pflugers Arch 1912;145:455.

131. McCouch G, Deering I, Ling T: Location of recepters for tonic neck reflexes. J Neurophysiol 1951;14:191.

132. Wilson VJ: The tonic neck reflex: Spinal circuitry. In Peterson B, Richmond F (eds): Control of Head Movement. New York, Oxford University Press, 1988.

133. Pompeiano O: The tonic neck reflex: Supraspinal control. In Peterson B, Richmond F (eds): Control of Head Movement. New York, Oxford University Press, 1988.

134. Funakoshi M, Amano N: Effects of the tonic neck reflex on the jaw muscles of the rat. J Dent Res 1973;52:668.

135. Sumino R, Nozaki S, Katoh M: Trigemino-neck reflex. In Kawamura Y, Dubner R (eds): Oral-Facial Sensory and Motor Functions. Tokyo, Quintessence Books, 1981, p 81.

136. Wyke BD: Neurology of the cervical spinal joints. Physiotherapy 1979;65:72.

137. Funakoshi M, Fujita N, Takehana S: Relations between occlusal interference and jaw muscle activities in response to changes in head position. J Dent Res 1976;55:684.

138. Bratzlavsky M, Vander Eecken H: Postural reflexes in cranial muscles in man. Acta Neurol Belg 1977;77:5.

139. Mohl N: Head posture and its role in occlusion. NY State Dent J 1976;42:17.

140. Forsberg CM, Hellsing E, Linder-Aronson S, et al: EMG activity in neck and masticatory muscles in relation to extension and flexion of the head. Eur J Orthod 1985;7:177.

141. Aiello I, Rosati G, Sau GF, et al: Tonic neck reflexes on upper limb flexor tone in man. Exp Neurol 1988;101:41.

142. Garcia R, Arrington JA: The relationship between cervical whiplash and temporomandibular joint injuries: An MRI study. J Craniomandibul Pract 1996;14:233.

143. Kronn E: The incidence of TMJ dysfunction in patients who have suffered a cervical whiplash injury following a traffic accident. J Orofac Pain 1993;7:209.

144. Everett N: Functional Neuroanatomy, ed 6. Philadelphia, Lea & Febiger, 1972.

145. Kerr F: Mechanism, diagnosis and management of some cranial and facial pain syndromes. Surg Clin North Am 1963;43:951.

146. Kerr F, Olafson R: Trigeminal and cervical volleys. Arch Neurol 1961;5:171.

147. Kerr F: Structural relation of the trigeminal spinal tract to upper cervical roots and the solitary nucleus in the cat. Exp Neurol 1961;4:134.

148. Feistein B, Langton J, Jameson R, et al: Experiments on referred pain from deep somatic tissues. J Bone Joint Surg 1954;36A:981.

149. Bogduk N, Marsland A: C3 headaches. Paper presented at the International Meeting on Pain and Regional Anaesthesia. Australian Pain Society, Perth, February, 1983.

150. Bogduk N: The clinical anatomy of the cervical dorsal rami. Spine 1982;7:319.

151. Cox C, Cocks G: Occipital neuralgia. J Med Assoc State Ala 1979;48:23.

152. Saadah H, Taylor F: Sustained headache syndrome associated with tender occipital nerve zones. Headache 1987;27:201.

153. Jansen J, Markakis E, Rama B, et al: Hemicranial attacks or permanent hemicrania—a sequel of upper cervical root compression. Cephalalgia 1989;9:123.

154. Magnusson T, Ragnarsson T, Bjornsson A: Occipital nerve release in patients with whiplash trauma and occipital neuralgia. Headache 1996;36:32.

155. Edmeads J: The cervical spine and headache. Neurology 1988;38:1874.

156. Sjaastad O, Saunte C, Hovdahl H, et al: "Cervicogenic" headache: An hypothesis. Cephalalgia 1983;3:249.

157. Sjaastad O, Fredriksen T, Stolt-Nielsen A: Cervicogenic headache, C2 rhizopathy, and occipital neuralgia: A connection? Cephalalgia 1986;6:189.

158. Pfaffenrath V, Dandekar R, Pollmann W: Cervicogenic headache - the clinical picture, radiological findings and hypotheses on its pathophysiology. Headache 1987;27:495.

159. Fredriksen T, Hovdal H: "Cervicogenic headache": Clinical manifestation. Cephalalgia 1987;7:147.

160. Fredriksen T, Fougner R, Tangerud A, et al: Cervicogenic headache: Radiological investigations concerning head/neck. Cephalalgia 1989;9:139.

161. Jaeger B: Are "cervicogenic" headaches due to myofascial pain and cervical spine dysfunction? Cephalalgia 1989;9:157.

162. Classification and diagnostic criteria for headache disorders, cranial neuralgias and facial pain, ed 1. International Headache Society. Cephalalgia 1988;8(suppl 7):61.

163. Olesen J (ed): Classification and Diagnostic Criteria for Headache Disorders, Cranial Neuralgias and Facial Pain. Copenhagen: The International Headache Society, 1990.

164. Nilsson N: The prevalence of cervicogenic headache in a random population sample of 20–59 year olds. Spine 1995;20:1884.

165. Rose F: Headache: Definition and classification. In Vinken PJ, et al (eds): Handbook of Clinical Neurology, Vol 48, No 4: Headache. New York, Elsevier, 1986, p 1.

166. Smith D: Dizziness, a clinical perspective. Neurol Clin 1990;8:199.
167. Adams R, Victor M: Principles of Neurology, ed 3. New York, McGraw-Hill, 1985.
168. Brown J: A systemic approach to the dizzy patient. Neurol Clin 1990;8:209.
169. Troost B: Dizziness and vertigo in vertebrobasilar disease, Part I. Stroke 1980;11(3):301–303.
170. Troost B: Dizziness and vertigo in vertebrobasilar disease, Part II. Stroke 1980;11(4):413–415.
171. De Jong J, Bles W: Cervical dizziness and ataxia. In Bles W, Brandt T (eds): Disorders of Posture and Gait. Amsterdam, The Netherlands, Elsevier, 1986, p 1856.
172. Abrahams V: The physiology of neck muscles: Their role in head movement and maintenance of posture. Can J Physiol Pharmacol 1977;55:332.
173. Cohen L: Role of eye and neck proprioceptive mechanisms in body orientation and motor coordination. J Neurophysiol 1961;24:1.
174. Manzoni D, Pompeiano O, Stampacchia G: Tonic cervical influences on posture and reflex movements. Arch Ital Biol 1979;117(2):81.
175. Cope S, Ryan GMS: Cervical and otolith vertigo. J Laryngol 1959;73:113.
176. Gray LP: Extralabyrinthine vertigo due to cervical muscle lesions. J Laryngol 1956;70:352.
177. De Jong PTVM, De Jong JMBV, Cohen B, Jong-kees LBW: Ataxia and nystagmus induced by injection of local anesthetics in the neck. Ann Neurol 1977;1:240.
178. Hinoki M: Vertigo due to whiplash injury: A neurological approach. Acta Otolaryngol Suppl (Stockh) 1985;419:9.
179. Liang M, Andersson G, Bombardier C, et al: Strategies for outcome research in spinal disorders. Spine 1994;19(S):2037S.
180. Coste J, Paolaggi J, Spira A: Classification of nonspecific low back pain. II. Clinical diversity of organic forms. Spine 1992;17:1038.
181. Guccione A: Physical therapy diagnosis and the relationship between impairments and function. Phys Ther 1991;71:499.
182. DeRosa C, Porterfield J: A physical therapy model for the treatment of low back pain. Phys Ther 1992;72:261.
183. Delitto A, Cibulka M, Erhard R, et al: Evidence for use of an extension-mobilization category in acute low back syndrome: A prescriptive validation pilot study. Phys Ther 1993;73:216.
184. Dekker J, van Baar M, Curfs E, et al: Diagnosis and treatment in physical therapy: An investigation of their relationship. Phys Ther 1993;73:568.
185. Riddle D, Rothstein J: Intertester reliability of McKenzie's classification of the syndrome types present in patients with low back pain. Spine 1993;18:1333.
186. McKenzie R: The Lumbar Spine: Mechanical Diagnosis and Therapy. Waikanae, New Zealand, Spinal Publications, 1981.
187. Margolis RB, Tail RC, Krause SJ: A rating system for use with patient pain drawings. Pain 1986;25:57.
188. Kraus SL: Cervical spine influences on the management of TMD. In Kraus SL (ed): Clinics in Physical Therapy: Temporomandibular Disorders, ed 2. New York, Churchill Livingstone, 1994, p 325.
189. Grieve's Modern Manual Therapy. Boyling & Palastangat. 1994; New York, Churchill Livingstone.
190. Zusman M: Spinal manipulative therapy: Review of some proposed mechanisms, and a new hypothesis. Aust J Physiother 1986;32.
191. Korr (ed): The Neurobiologic Mechanisms in Manipulative Therapy. New York, Plenum Press, 1978.
192. Idczak R (ed): Aspects of manipulative therapy. Proceedings of a Multidisciplinary International Conference on Manipulative Therapy, Lincoln Institute of Health Sciences, Melbourne, Aug 1979.
193. Rothstein J (ed): Manual therapy: Special issue. Phys Ther 1992;72.
194. Goldstein M (ed): The Research Status of Spinal Manipulative Therapy. U.S. Department of Health, Education, and Welfare. DHEW Publication No. (NIH) 76-998. NINCDS Monograph No. 15, 1975.
195. Manipulative Physiotherapists Association of Australia, 7th Biennial Conference. Nov 27–30, 1991, Blue Mountains, New South Wales. Published by Manipulative Physiotherapists Association, Australia, North Fitzroy Victoria, Australia. Scientific Programme Convenor, Jenny McConnell.
196. Bogduk N: A scientific approach to cervical diagnosis. Proceedings from the Fourth Biennial Conference of Manipulative Therapist Association of Australia, Brisbane, May 22–25, 1985, pp 151–158.
197. Grieve G (ed): Modern Manual Therapy of the Vertebral Column. New York, Churchill Livingstone, 1986, pp 270–282.
198. Jull G, Bogduk N, Marsland A: The accuracy of manual diagnosis for cervical zygoapophyseal joint pain syndrome. Med J Aust 1988;148:223.
199. Shepard K, Jensen G, Schmoll B, et al: Alternative approaches to research in physical therapy: Positivism and phenomenology. Phys Ther 1993;73:88.

CHAPTER

11

The Role of Occlusion in Temporomandibular Disorders

Ross H. Tallents • Scott I. Stein • Mark E. Moss

A patient suffering from facial pain is often evaluated through the "eyes" of the clinician's specialty. Examination of a patient with temporomandibular joint (TMJ) pain by an orthodontist, an oral and maxillofacial surgeon, a prosthodontist, or a general dentist may result in treatment strategies that differ significantly. It is critical that the best possible result be attained with the least cost and discomfort to the patient, as well as the best prognosis for recovery. It is also critical that when patients with facial pain are evaluated the clinician think "differential diagnosis" and not label the patient as a temporomandibular dysfunction (TMD) patient. This will reduce the possibility of unnecessary or inappropriate dental treatments.

The guidelines for the assessment, diagnosis, and management of TMD from the American Academy of Orofacial Pain categorize the factors associated with the development of pain and dysfunction.[1] They are divided into factors that increase the risk (predisposing), cause the onset (initiating), and enhance the progression (perpetuating) of developing a TMJ disorder. This chapter evaluates the occlusal factors (dental and skeletal) that relate to the development of pain and dysfunction associated with TMD. The need for orthognathic surgery is also evaluated from a TMJ pain and dysfunction viewpoint.

Dentistry has been of the opinion that occlusion (dental and skeletal) is the most important predisposing factor in the development of TMJ disorders. The etiology, diagnosis, and treatment of TMJ pain and dysfunction are controversial. A multifactorial etiology has been suggested, which usually implies that the profession is unsure about the specific etiology. Clinical examination often reveals features (e.g., deep bite, skeletal abnormalities, dental occlusal factors, plain film x-ray findings) thought to be the "cause" of the patient's pain. One must be cautious when making associations between clinical observations and etiological factors (predisposing, initiating, or perpetuating) in the development of TMJ pain and dysfunction. The major problem in many clinical studies is that a control sample is not available for clinical and statistical comparison.

There are varying opinions as to the contribution of occlusion (malocclusion) in the development of mandibular dysfunction. Presently there are no studies that suggest that orthodontics, restorative dentistry, or oral and maxillofacial surgery prevents an individual from developing symptoms or promotes the development of symptoms. In this chapter we explore the various occlusal features and attempt to draw some conclusions as to why they may or may not contribute to TMD. The observations here are confined to skeletal and dental relationships, how they may be altered by treatment, and whether this is related to a decrease in symptoms. Various risk factors are summarized, as well as differential diagnoses when indicated.

Pertinent literature is reviewed and the

results compared with dental and skeletal variables obtained in our study of 82 asymptomatic volunteers and 263 symptomatic patients with intraarticular TMJ disorders. Asymptomatic volunteers responded to a solicitation for inclusion in the study. All volunteers were accepted into the study following completion of a TMJ subjective questionnaire documenting the absence of jaw pain, joint noise, and locking and a positive history for TMD and a clinical TMJ and dental examination for the absence of signs and symptoms commonly associated with TMD or internal derangement. All symptomatic subjects had localized jaw joint pain and/or pain on movement or when eating. Vertical opening and right and left mandibular movements were measured and recorded.

All study participants had bilateral high-resolution magnetic resonance imaging (MRI) scans in the sagittal (closed and opened) and coronal (closed) planes to evaluate the TMJs for the presence or absence of disk displacement. Each study participant was classified as normal MRI (no disk displacement) or having disk displacement (DD). The study participants were divided into the following four groups:

1. Asymptomatic, normal MRI (Fig. 11–1)
2. Asymptomatic, with disk displacement on MRI (Figs. 11–2 and 11–3)
3. Symptomatic, with normal MRI (see Fig. 11–1)
4. Symptomatic, with disk displacement on MRI (see Figs. 11–2 and 11–3)

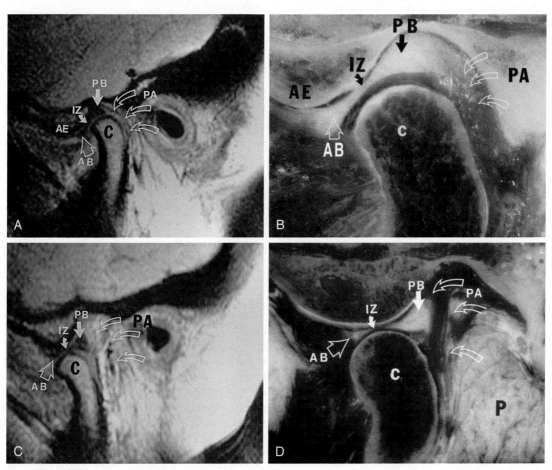

FIGURE 11–1. Closed and open sagittal magnetic resonance scan and cadaver sections of a temporomandibular joint with normal disk position. A representative cadaver section is presented for familiarization of the anatomy. *A,* Closed sagittal scan of a joint with normal disk position. *B,* Closed sagittal cadaver section of a joint with normal disk position. Note the homologies with *A. C,* Sagittal scan of the joint in *A* in the open jaw position. The disk is located between the condyle and the articular eminence and has a bow-tie configuration. *D,* Open sagittal cadaver section of a joint with normal disk position. Note the homologies with *C.* AB, anterior band *(large open arrow);* AE, articular eminence; c, condyle; IZ, intermediate zone *(small curved arrow);* P, parotid gland; PA, posterior attachment *(large curved open arrows);* PB, posterior band *(solid large arrow).*

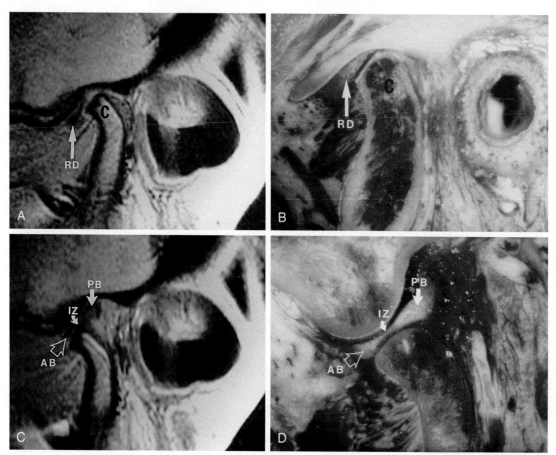

FIGURE 11–2. Closed and open sagittal magnetic resonance scan and cadaver sections of a temporomandibular joint with a displaced disk. *A*, Closed sagittal scan of a joint with disk displacement. There is a remodeled disk *(solid arrow)* anterior to the condyle. The bow-tie configuration seen in Figure 11–1*A* and *B* is not present. *B*, Closed sagittal cadaver section of a joint similar to the one in *A*. There is a remodeled disk *(solid arrow)* anterior to the condyle. The posterior attachment is thin at the superior aspect of the condyle. *C*, Sagittal scan of the joint in *A* in the open-jaw position. Note that the disk is interposed between the condyle and the articular eminence, similar to the scan in Figure 11–1*B*. This represents disk displacement with reduction. *D*, Open sagittal cadaver section of a joint similar to the one in *C*. Note the anatomic similarities between them. AB, anterior band *(large open arrow)*; IZ, intermediate zone *(small curved arrow)*; PB, posterior band *(solid large arrow)*; RD, remodeled disk.

Subjects were collapsed into groups based on the presence or absence of disk displacement because it has been demonstrated that the type and severity of disk displacement are not correlated with pain.[2]

Critical questions relating to the contribution of each variable or group of variables are posed at the beginning of each section, and conclusions are drawn.

Anterior Controls

There are three critical questions with respect to the overlap of the anterior teeth: (1) Does an increase (deep bite) or decrease (open bite) in vertical overlap of the incisors predispose a patient to intraarticular TMJ disorders? (2) Does an increase (retrognathic) or decrease (prognathic) in the horizontal overlap of the incisors predispose a patient to intraarticular TMJ disorders? and (3) If there is a predisposition, does correction decrease the risk of developing intraarticular TMJ disorders or decrease symptoms? The risk and correction are dealt with in the orthodontic and orthognathic section.

It has been suggested that excessive horizontal and/or vertical overlap of the anterior teeth "predisposes" an individual to the development of mandibular dysfunction.[3, 4] The problem in attempting to verify this suggestion is the lack of suitable longitudinal studies. Whether the overlap observations are a result of sampling bias, a cause of dysfunction, or secondary to degenerative changes in the skeletal and dental relationships due to disk displacement is unknown. Inferences can be drawn only indirectly without longitudinal studies. Earlier reports[5–10] present conflicting opinions. They suggest that increased overlap (horizontal or vertical) of the anterior teeth is responsible for the development of mandibular dysfunction. However, these studies *do not have adequate controls*.

Mohlin and Kopp[11] demonstrated no such relationship. Likewise, Pullinger and colleagues[12] demonstrated no relationship between deep bite and position of the condyle in the glenoid fossa. It has also been suggested that increased vertical overlap of the anterior teeth is associated with joint sounds[13] and masticatory muscle tenderness.[14, 15] The majority of studies do not support these associations.[16–24]

A decrease in vertical overlap—in particular, skeletal anterior open bite—has been associated with condylar changes such as osteoarthritis (OA) and degenerative joint disease (DJD),[25–27] and with rheumatoid arthritis.[26, 28] The possible etiology of skeletal open bite is considered in the discussion in this section. The implications of surgical correction of anterior open bite are discussed in the orthognathic surgery section.

Increased horizontal overlap of anterior teeth has been associated with TMD symptoms[18, 22] and osteoarthritic changes.[25, 29] Other studies failed to provide evidence of horizontal overlap associations with TMD.[13, 19–21, 23, 24, 29–33] There are several reasons why this might occur. An epidemiologic study that examines the general population for symptoms is unlikely to have a large number of open bites or class II division I malocclusions. Patients presenting for orthognathic surgery are more likely to have these occlusal and skeletal features. The study of Link and Nickerson[34] demonstrated this skew in distribution. Dibbets and associates[35] followed a group of children with changing craniofacial morphology. They suggested that when there are objective signs of dysfunction and skeletal changes similar to those found by Link and Nickerson,[34] asymmetry and retrognathia are observed. These two studies reinforce the need to understand the source of the sample.

An example of sampling bias was demonstrated by Williamson,[36] who evaluated 304 children from ages 6 to 16 years and found that there was a high prevalence of class II subjects in his pain group. There was an

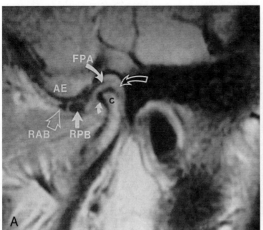
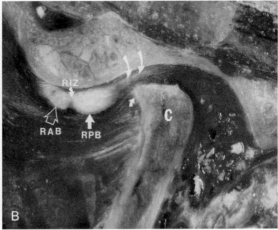

FIGURE 11–3. Closed sagittal magnetic resonance scan and cadaver section of a temporomandibular joint with a displaced disk. *A,* Closed sagittal scan of a joint with chronic disk displacement. There is a remodeled deformed disk anterior to the condyle. The intermediate zone (IZ) is not clearly visualized. There is a fibrotic posterior attachment (FPA) superior to the condylar head *(large curved solid arrow).* The posterior attachment (PA) posterior to the condyle has a bright signal *(large curved arrow).* There is a small osteophyte on the anterior aspect of the condyle *(small arrow). B,* Closed sagittal cadaver section of a joint with chronic disk displacement similar to the joint in *A.* There is a remodeled deformed disk anterior to the condyle. The IZ *(curved small arrow)* is clearly visualized. There is an FPA superior to the condylar head *(large curved solid arrow).* The PA posterior to the condyle is not fibrotic *(large curved arrow).* There is a small osteophyte on the anterior aspect of the condyle *(small arrow).* RAB, remodeled anterior band *(open large arrow);* RPB, remodeled posterior band *(solid large arrow).*

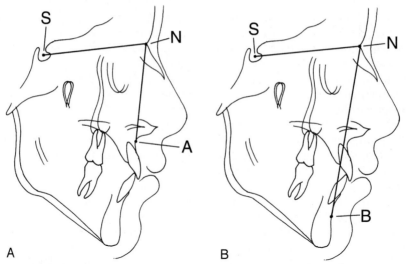

FIGURE 11–4. *A,* The angle SNA represents the anterior-posterior position of the maxilla to the cranial base. *B,* The angle SNB represents the anterior-posterior position of the mandibular denture base to the cranial base. S, sella; N, nasion; A, A-point; B, B-point.

equal number of class II subjects among his controls. The age of the subject is also important when evaluating incisal relationships. There is a higher probability of a younger subject (before growth spurts) presenting with a deeper bite.[37, 38]

Seligman and Pullinger[14] showed that horizontal overlap greater than 5 mm is very uncommon in a healthy nonpatient population. In this adult symptomatic sample, there was a significant number of patients with overlap greater than 5 mm. This may suggest either that they always had this trait or that it occurred as a result of some progressive skeletal changes. Again, this reinforces the need to know the demographics of a sample and compare the experimental group with controls.

Ronquillo and coworkers[39] found no strong relationship between the overlap of the incisors, condyle position, and arthrographic findings of the TMJ. Analysis of variance demonstrated a relationship between distal condyle position, disk displacement without reduction, and decreased vertical overlap of the incisors, indicating some tendency toward open bite. This study did not have a control sample.

Stein and colleagues[40] demonstrated an increase in horizontal overlap when asymptomatic controls with normal disk positions were compared with symptomatic patients with bilateral DJD. The mean horizontal overlap for asymptomatic controls with normal joints was 3.1 mm (SD ± 1.2 mm); for the bilateral DJD group, it was 5.3 mm (SD ± 2.8 mm). They also demonstrated a shorter posterior face height, a higher mandibular plane angle, and a more retrusive SNA and SNB (Fig. 11–4) in symptomatic TMD patients. These measurements suggest a retruded mandible in the presence of a retruded maxilla. This would produce a more convex facial profile. These findings

TABLE 11–1.	**Mean Age and Degree of Overlap for Asymptomatic Volunteers and Symptomatic Patients**		
	N	**Mean Age in Years (X ± SD)**	**Horizontal Overlap (mm) (X ± SD)**	**Vertical Overlap (mm) (X ± SD)**
Volunteer normal joint	55	27.8 (7.60)	2.65 (1.09)	3.22 (1.47)
Volunteer disk displacement	27	26.6 (9.47)	3.26 (1.85)	3.19 (1.83)
Symptomatic normal joint	42	29.2 (11.22)	3.03 (1.64)	3.37 (1.55)
Symptomatic disk displacement	221	30.19 (13.07)	3.41 (2.00)	3.35 (1.74)

TABLE 11–2.	**Horizontal Overlap of Asymptomatic Volunteers and Symptomatic Patients and Prevalence of Overlap**				
	N	**% < 4 mm**	**% ≥ 4 mm**	**Odds Ratio**	**P Value**
Volunteer normal joint	55	96.4	3.6	—	—
Volunteer disk displacement	27	74.1	25.9	9.3	.049
Bilateral symptomatic normal joints	42	83.3	16.7	5.3	.037
Symptomatic disk displacement	221	77.4	22.6	7.7	.001

Chi-square = 9.208, df = 1, P = .049 for volunteers with normal joints versus volunteers with disk displacement.
Chi-square = 4.804, df = 1, P = .037 for volunteers with normal joints versus symptomatic normal joints.
Chi-square = 10.384, df = 1, P = .001 for volunteers with normal joints versus symptomatic patients with disk displacement.

are similar to those of Link and Nickerson[34] but not as profound as in a sample of patients presenting for orthognathic surgery.

The characteristics of 82 asymptomatic volunteers with no TMD complaints and 263 symptomatic patients are summarized in Table 11–1. All study participants had bilateral high-resolution MRI in the sagittal (closed and opened) and coronal (closed) planes to evaluate the TMJs for the presence or absence of internal derangement.[41] On the basis of these findings, each study participant was then classified as normal MRI (no internal derangement) or having disk displacement: disk displacement with reduction (DDR), disk displacement with no reduction (DDN), or DDN and DJD. In the succeeding sections, these data are used for comparison to selected papers in the literature with acceptable controls.

Horizontal overlap of 4 mm or greater was compared in symptomatic patients and controls (Table 11–2). In the asymptomatic subjects with DD, 26% (odds ratio = 9.3, P = .049) had horizontal overlap equal to or greater than 4 mm. In symptomatic subjects with normal joints, 17% had that degree of horizontal overlap (odds ratio = 5.3, P =

.037), and in subjects with DDR or DDN with or without DJD, 23% did (odds ratio = 7.7, P = .001). The same trends were found in subjects with horizontal overlap of 3 mm or greater.

The occurrence of vertical overlap of 4 mm or greater is demonstrated in Table 11–3. There were no significant differences among the groups. The same trends were found in vertical overlap of 3 mm or greater.

DISCUSSION

Cachiotti and associates[21] found no differences between symptomatic patients and symptom-free controls in terms of horizontal and vertical overlap of the incisors. Pullinger and coworkers[42] suggested that DDN/DJD, OA, and myalgia groups were positively associated with increased horizontal overlap. Increase in vertical overlap was associated only with DDR.

In a study by Stein and colleagues,[40] increase in vertical overlap (2.8 mm for asymptomatic volunteers versus 3.6 mm for patients with bilateral DDR) was positively associated with bilateral DDR. The axial

TABLE 11–3.	**Vertical Overlap of Asymptomatic Volunteers and Symptomatic Patients and the Prevalence of Overlap**				
	N	**% < 4 mm**	**% ≥ 4 mm**	**Odds Ratio**	**P Value**
Volunteer normal joint	55	80.0	20.0	—	—
Volunteer disk displacement	27	74.1	25.9	1.4	.578
Bilateral symptomatic normal joints	42	80.9	19.1	0.94	1
Symptomatic disk displacement	221	77.8	22.1	1.14	.73

Chi-square = 0.37, df = 1, P = .578 for volunteers with normal joints versus volunteers with disk displacement.
Chi-square = 0.014, df = 1, P = 1 for volunteers with normal joints versus symptomatic normal joints.
Chi-square = 0.122, df = 1, P = .856 for volunteers with normal joints versus symptomatic patients with DD.

inclination of the incisors on a cephalometric film was also more upright (128 degrees for asymptomatic volunteers versus 137 degrees for patients with bilateral DDR) when compared with asymptomatic volunteers and symptomatic patients with intraarticular TMJ disorders (Fig. 11–5).

Several authors have suggested a relationship between deep bite and distal shift of the mandible.[43, 44] They suggested that in 30% to 40% of their patients, the mandible shifted anteriorly after orthodontic treatment. Thuer and associates[45] evaluated class II division 2 patients under orthodontic treatment and found no anterior mandibular positioning with proclination of the incisors and bite opening. Gianelly and coworkers[46] reported no difference in the position of the condyles between class II malocclusion patients with steep incisors and a deep bite and class II patients without these characteristics. These studies suggest no correlation between the steepness of the bite and/or deep bite inducing the condyles to move distally.

Pullinger and colleagues[42] demonstrated a higher prevalence of open bite in DDR, DDN/DJD, primary OA, and myalgia patients. Our study had only three open bites, so comparisons could not be made. In a separate study of 614 consecutive symptomatic patients with intraarticular TMJ disorders examined in the department of orthodontics and TMJ disorders from 1987 to 1993, 32 subjects had anterior open bites.[47] Twenty-seven of 32 (84%) had disk displacement confirmed by MRI. Fourteen of 27 (52%) had degenerative changes on both tomographic and MRI examinations.

Riolo and associates[18] suggested that open bite was positively associated with TMD and muscle tenderness. They also suggested that excessive or negative horizontal overlap was more likely to be associated with joint tenderness. Angle class II molar relationship was positively associated with joint noise. These data suggest that there is a degree of retrognathia or open bite in a TMD sample.

The data in Tables 11–2 and 11–3 and the findings of Pullinger and colleagues[42] suggest that a small but significant portion of a TMD sample has increased horizontal overlap as compared with a control sample. These data also suggest a tendency toward open bite. There are two possible explanations for these findings: The horizontal overlap of these individuals may have always been larger, or these findings represent degenerative changes in the condyle (arthritic changes), possibly related to DD. Pullinger and colleagues[42] suggest that some patients have primary OA that is probably not related to disk displacement. This premise is based on the fact that some patients had no history of clicking, locking, or TMD problems before examination. Recent studies of asymptomatic adults[48] and adolescents and young adults[49–51] suggest that disk displacement is a common finding, even in the absence of symptoms. This might suggest that OA is progressing in volunteers without pain, clicking, or locking. Schellhas and coworkers[52] suggested that major skeletal remodeling occurs in the presence of disk displacement. The skeletal asymmetry or retrognathia did not occur over a short period. There were probably long-standing de-

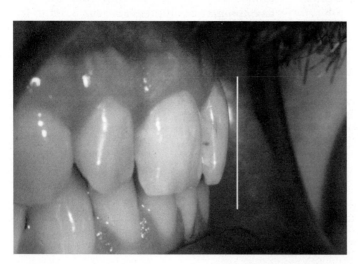

FIGURE 11–5. The position of the maxillary incisors in patients with bilateral disk displacement with reduction is more upright, as depicted by the white line.

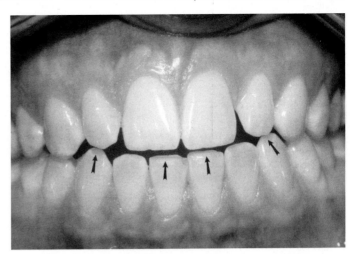

FIGURE 11–6. Twenty-three-year-old woman with anterior open bite at the time of clinical examination. Note the wear facets on the mandibular anterior teeth *(arrows)*. Bilateral magnetic resonance imaging scans demonstrated bilateral disk displacement without reduction and degenerative joint disease.

rangements, which would account for the severe degenerative changes seen in their patients. Kuwahara and Maruyama[53, 54] suggest that condylar atrophy is associated with younger individuals and internal derangements or OA of the TMJ. They also suggest that one or both lower missing first molars are associated with condylar atrophy. Two case studies demonstrate the need to suspect intracapsular derangements when patients present with anterior open bite.

CASE 1

This patient was examined for bilateral TMJ pain (Fig. 11–6). There was no audible joint noise and no history of jaw locking. Dental examination revealed a small anterior open bite. There are many causes of open bite, such as mouth breathing and enlarged tonsils and adenoids. Careful examination of the anterior teeth revealed wear facets on the canines. There were also facets and erosion on the mandibular incisors, suggesting that these teeth had been in contact previously. The patient was not aware of any acute changes in the occlusion of the anterior teeth. This suggests that changes in the occlusion had been occurring over a long period. There was probably a vertical and a horizontal component to these changes. An MRI demonstrated disk displacement without reduction associated with bilateral degenerative joint disease. This supports the contention that DJD may produce changes in the anteroposterior relationship of the maxillary and mandibular dental arches. The presence of wear on the lower anterior teeth

should alert the clinician to the possibility of degenerative changes in the TMJs in some open-bite cases. This also suggests that the open bite may be a result of the DJD, not the cause, even if the subject does not have pain. These relationships are discussed in the orthognathic section.

CASE 2

This patient presented with bilateral TMJ pain (Fig. 11–7). Some faceting was seen on the right mandibular canine and the maxillary lateral incisors. There was not much wear on the mandibular central and lateral incisors, and there was a suggestion of mamelons on the four incisors. This wear pattern suggests that the patient previously had minimal overlap of the incisors. The patient's open bite was now approximately 2 mm. The MRI demonstrated bilateral disk displacement without reduction associated with degenerative joint disease.

These two cases emphasize the need to be suspicious when patients present with open bites. In the absence of another explanation (e.g., adenoids, tonsils, tongue thrust), joint derangements should be suspected. The patients here had pain, but one should also be suspicious in asymptomatic subjects with no pain. Kerstens and associates[55] demonstrated that patients undergoing orthognathic surgery, with no previous symptoms, may exhibit TMD after surgical treatment. The open bite or large horizontal overlap of the incisors should be viewed as a risk factor before the initiation of ortho-

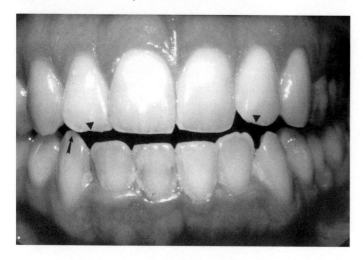

FIGURE 11–7. Thirty-five-year-old woman with bilateral temporomandibular joint pain. Contrast this patient to the one in Figure 11–6. There is minimal suggestion of wear facets and some suggestion of mamelons on the anterior teeth. This patient also had bilateral disk displacement without reduction and degenerative joint disease.

dontic, prosthodontic, routine oral surgery (e.g., third molar extraction), or orthognathic surgery. The etiology of the open bite can be explored by performing tomograms, looking for degenerative changes. Roberts and colleagues[56] demonstrated that 47% of symptomatic patients with DDN have degenerative changes ($P < .05$). This suggests that tomograms would pick up less than half of patients with DDN. Another tool that has been suggested to be highly correlated with disk displacement is the position of the condyle in the fossa with tomography. Brand and coworkers[57] found disk position prediction based on condyle position to be accurate in 63% of 243 subjects. They concluded that anterior disk position failed to alter condyle position more frequently than condylar retropositioning occurred in the absence of anterior disk displacement. Kamelchuk and associates[58] suggested that tomography as a diagnostic test of abnormal disk position had a sensitivity of 0.43, a specificity of 0.80, and a positive predictive value of 0.64. They stated that tomography is inappropriate as a diagnostic test for prediction of the type of internal derangement. Only when there is DJD can the clinician feel comfortable with the diagnosis of disk displacement in the absence of other signs and symptoms. Clinicians should not be apprehensive about treatment but should inform patients that there is a risk for the development of TMJ pain.

CONCLUSIONS

This literature review suggests that there may be a relationship between increased horizontal overlap of the incisors and disk displacement. This relationship is probably related to disk displacement and arthritic changes in the TMJs. It is important to note that this represents only 16% to 25% of symptomatic TMD patients and volunteers with disk displacement. The strength of this relationship will be determined only with longitudinal studies.

Coupling of the Anterior Teeth

The question of the superiority of one type of anterior contact (canine versus group function) over another has been debated in the literature. There is no scientific evidence regarding the impact of these occlusal schemes on either the success or failure of restorative dentistry treatment outcomes or on the prevention of TMJ disorders. These findings *should not detract* from sound restorative dentistry provided by the supporters of any occlusal concept; they merely suggest that one cannot claim success or failure based on a given philosophy.

Schuyler[59] is credited with the introduction of bilaterally balanced occlusion. Later, Schuyler and others[60–62] suggested that the concept of balanced occlusion be replaced with unilateral balanced occlusion or group function. A review of these developments from 1905 to 1990 is presented by Thornton.[63] To date, there has been no scientific evidence to support the use of one occlusal scheme over another.

Our study, which evaluates the prevalence of disk displacement in symptomatic and asymptomatic subjects, supports the contention that group function may be more prevalent in asymptomatic volunteers. Table 11–4 compares asymptomatic volunteers with symptomatic patients with intraarticular TMJ disorders. In the volunteers with normal joints, there is a higher prevalence of group function (65%) on the right side. In all other groups, there is a more or less equal distribution.

DISCUSSION

There is only one published study that attempted to evaluate the effect of the different occlusal schemes without changing the vertical dimension of occlusion.[64] In this study, the effect of group function versus canine guidance on electromyographic activity in jaw elevator muscles and related mandibular movement was investigated in 12 asymptomatic subjects. Simultaneous recordings during unilateral chewing and parafunctional tasks were analyzed quantitatively. When a naturally acquired group function was temporarily and artificially changed into a dominant canine guidance, a significant general reduction of elevator muscle activity was observed when subjects exerted full isometric tooth-clenching efforts in a *lateral* mandibular position. Unilateral chewing produced no significant alterations in the activity or coordination of the muscles when an artificial canine guidance was introduced. The results suggest that canine-protected occlusions do not significantly alter muscle activity during mastication but significantly reduce muscle activity during lateral movement. These data suggest that canine-protected occlusion might eliminate bruxism. A paper by Holmgren and coworkers[65] suggested that although pain scores were lowered, bruxing habits remained when symptomatic patients wore splints. In 61% of patients, the active wear facets on the splints were observed at every visit (2-week intervals), and in 31% they occurred from time to time. Similar findings were reported by Gentz[66] and Kydd and Daily,[67] who found that an occlusal splint did not stop nocturnal bruxism.

These studies imply that alteration of the occlusal scheme decreases muscle activity and pain in an experimental situation, but placement of a splint (a change in the occlusal scheme) does not eliminate bruxing habits.[64] Therefore, caution should be observed when restoring occlusions under the assumption that parafunctional movements will be eliminated.

CONCLUSIONS

Our study found that there is no increase in the prevalence of canine guidance in asymptomatic volunteers (see Table 11–4), which suggests that the occlusal scheme does not exert a preventive effect. In fact, on the right side, there seems to be a shift toward group function. These results suggest that altering the occlusal scheme prob-

TABLE 11–4.	Distribution of Subjects with Canine versus Group Function in Symptomatic and Asymptomatic Patients				
	Canine Guidance Left	**Canine Guidance Right**	**Group Function Left**	**Group Function Right**	**Total**
Volunteer normal joint	18 (33%)	19 (35%)	37 (67%)	36 (65%)	55
Volunteer disk displacement	9 (33%)	12 (44%)	18 (67%)	15 (56%)	27
Symptomatic normal joint	20 (48%)	17 (40.5%)	22 (52%)	25 (59.5%)	42
Symptomatic disk displacement	98 (44%)	115 (52%)	123 (56%)	106 (48%)	221

Right side canine:
Chi-square = 0.755, df = 1, P = .385 for volunteers with normal joints versus volunteers with disk displacement.
Chi-square = 0.549, df = 1, P = .359 for volunteers with normal joints versus symptomatic normal joints.
Chi-square = 5.394, df = 1, P = .020 for volunteers with normal joints versus symptomatic patients with disk displacement, with the asymptomatic volunteers having more group function.
Left side canine:
Chi-square = 0.003, df = 1, P = 1 for volunteers with normal joints versus volunteers with disk displacement.
Chi-square = 2.216, df = 1, P = .148 for volunteers with normal joints versus symptomatic normal joints.
Chi-square = 2.439, df = 1, P = .129 for volunteers with normal joints versus symptomatic patients with disk displacement.

ably has little effect on oral habits or the development of intraarticular TMJ disorders and therefore should be recommended with caution for the prevention of parafunctional activity.

Missing Posterior Teeth

There are three critical questions with respect to missing teeth: (1) Is there an increased risk of OA and intraarticular TMJ disorders? (2) Does replacement of missing teeth decrease the risk of or cure intraarticular TMJ disorders? and (3) Are there biochemical and/or neurochemical factors that may induce pain related to the teeth (extraction, cracked teeth, endodontics) or unrelated to extraction and/or endodontics.[7]

Loss of molar support has been correlated with osteoarthritic changes.[68-73] One must keep in mind that the prevalence of osteoarthritic changes and tooth loss increases with age. Subsequent studies have demonstrated that these associations *decrease* when the data are controlled for age.[75, 77] Studies of nonpatient populations do not provide sufficient evidence of an association between TMD and loss of molar support.[77-82]

Witter and colleagues,[87] in a 6-year follow-up of patients with an absence of molar support, suggested that loss of posterior teeth does not increase the risk of TMD. They also suggested that removable partial dentures do not prevent TMD and do not improve oral function. Lederman and Clayton[89] found dysfunction in 68% of 50 patients with fixed partial dentures in all posterior quadrants. These observations pose two problems: restorative dentistry is not justified as a solution for TMD, and even if a symptomatic patient is restored, he or she may continue to have pain. There are other possible etiologies for facial pain in a patient with missing posterior teeth. The presence of disk displacement or neuropathy from extractions, root canals, or fractured teeth may represent multiple risk factors. The following studies support the possible contribution of nerve damage and/or neuropathy.[90-99] There are several animal studies that suggest that manipulation of the teeth (extraction, extirpation, and high occlusal contacts) induces changes in the TMJ.[93-96] Kubo[100] evaluated the uptake of

horseradish peroxidase in the monkey TMJ synovium after occlusal alterations. He found an increase in horseradish peroxidase in the type A synovial cells and also some degeneration of the cells. This suggests that a high occlusal contact is capable of producing cellular changes in response to occlusal insult. Correlation in the human condition is lacking, but there is some indirect evidence that is discussed in the retruded contact position–intercuspal position (RCP-ICP) section.

There have been several other studies evaluating neural disruptions after extractions or experimental dental nerve lesions. Fried and associates[92] studied anterograde horseradish peroxidase tracing and immunohistochemistry of trigeminal ganglion tooth pulp neurons after dental nerve lesions in the rat. They demonstrated that with extraction, fracture, and partial removal of the roots of the mandibular left molar, there were long-term cytochemical changes that affected trigeminal ganglion neurons. They also demonstrated that calcitonin gene-related peptide–positive neurons were much reduced in the trigeminal ganglion, suggesting partial or complete neuronal death. This represents changes capable of affecting trigeminal ganglion neuron conduction.

Another possible cause of pain in an extraction site is neuralgia-inducing cavitational osteonecrosis (NICO).[97, 98] These lesions were first described by Black[101] as soft bone or hollow bone cavities. They are often referred to as Ratner cysts.[102] A more elaborate discussion of the etiology occurs later.

Gobel and Binck[93] demonstrated that degenerative changes occurred in the subnucleus caudalis after tooth pulp extirpations in the cat. They demonstrated that primary nerve endings in laminae 2 and 3 of the spinal trigeminal nucleus degenerate over a more protracted period, gradually losing their synaptic vesicles and synaptic connections.

In a subsequent study, Gobel[94] extirpated the tooth pulp in mandibular teeth unilaterally in the cat. He demonstrated that injury to the distal branches of the primary trigeminal neurons resulted in trans-synaptic degenerative changes in the dendritic arbors of second-order neurons, which destroyed fine-caliber high-order dendrites in laminae 1 and 2.

Ueno[95] evaluated the uptake of horseradish peroxidase in the TMJ synovium of rats following unilateral extraction of molars. He demonstrated that the uptake of horseradish peroxidase in type A synovial cells decreased as the experimental time increased. The decrease suggests that degenerative changes may have occurred in these cells.

Clements and colleagues[96] evaluated the pulpal projections to the trigeminal subnucleus caudalis in the rat. Using cholera toxin conjugated to horseradish peroxidase, they demonstrated that immunoreactive fibers extended into laminae 1 to 3 caudally and were present in the border zone between laminae 4 and 5. The results demonstrate that these fibers coexist with the fibers of the TMJ. This suggests that if there is convergence (teeth, TMJ), there is the possibility that tooth pain might mask itself as TMJ pain.

Another possible reason for chronic sensory input is periodontal disease. This should be considered in the differential diagnosis, because the area of the brain stem is the subnucleus intermedius and caudalis, the domain of the TMJ and the teeth. Hamba and coworkers[104] injected interleukin-1B into the gingiva and tooth pulp of the rat. There was an upregulation of c-fos proto-oncogene in the subnucleus intermedius and caudalis in the nuclei responsible for pain relay and pain inhibition of nociception. The pattern for the gingiva was almost matched to the pattern of tooth pulp stimulation. This suggests that periodontal disease is capable of producing sensory input similar to teeth and the TMJ and may have

to be addressed before considering treatment directed at jaw joint pain.

Although these studies may seem unrelated to TMD, they should make us aware of the multiple possible etiologies of facial pain. When we evaluate patients with missing teeth and make the association between missing teeth and TMJ problems, it may not be loss of posterior support that contributes to the development of jaw joint and/or muscle pain. Here, care must be taken in the selection of words. If the term TMD is used, the assumption will be that TMJ dysfunction is always related to posterior tooth loss. Neuronal degeneration (deafferentation, neuropathy) may be contributing to the individual's pain. This is one reason why a patient may continue to have pain in spite of appropriate treatment.

We often see patients with a history of mandibular molar removal, followed by removal of premolar(s) and subsequently the second molar. Quite often we cannot explain why this individual's pain continues. A possible explanation is that there has been neuronal degeneration (apoptosis), producing altered neuronal transmission that makes the individual perceive pain (possibly phantom pain) even though the primary insult (abscess, caries, fracture) is gone. The presence of missing, endodontically treated, and/or cracked teeth in conjunction with disk displacement may represent multiple risk factors that must be carefully evaluated before the initiation of treatment. This is most important in patients with multiple failed attempts at conservative treatment.

Tables 11–5 and 11–6, comparing volun-

TABLE 11–5.	Prevalence of Missing Lower Posterior Teeth on the Left Side			
	None	**One Missing Lower Left Tooth**	**None**	**Two Missing Lower Left Teeth**
Volunteer normal joint	46 (83.6%)	9 (16.4%)	53 (96.3%)	2 (3.7%)†
Volunteer disk displacement	20 (74.1%)	7 (25.9%)	27 (100%)	0 (0.0%)
Symptomatic normal joint	29 (69.0%)	13 (31.0%)	38 (90.5%)	4 (9.5%)
Symptomatic disk displacement	144 (65.2%)	77 (34.8%)*	191 (86.4%)	30 (13.6%)‡

One missing tooth:
Chi-square = 1.054, df = 1, P = .337 for volunteers with normal joints versus volunteers with disk displacement.
Chi-square = 2.890, df = 1, P = .141 for volunteers with normal joints versus symptomatic normal joints.
*Chi-square = 7.010, df = 1, P = .008 for volunteers with normal joints versus symptomatic patients with disk displacement.
Two missing teeth:
Chi-square = 1.006, df = 1, P = 1 for volunteers with normal joints versus volunteers with disk displacement.
Chi-square = 1.422, df = 1, P = .398 for volunteers with normal joints versus symptomatic normal joints.
†Chi-square = 4.244, df = 1, P = .039 for volunteers with normal joints versus symptomatic patients with disk displacement.
‡P <.05.

TABLE 11–6.	Prevalence of Missing Lower Posterior Teeth on the Right Side				
	None	**One Missing Lower Right Tooth**	**None**	**Two Missing Lower Right Teeth**
Volunteer normal joint	46 (83.6%)	9 (16.4%)*	52 (98.2%)	1 (1.8%)
Volunteer disk displacement	20 (74.1%)	7 (25.9%)	26 (96.3%)	0 (3.7%)
Symptomatic normal joint	28 (66.7%)	14 (33.3%)*	37 (88.1%)	5 (11.9%)*
Symptomatic disk displacement	156 (70.6%)	65 (29.4%)*	194 (87.8%)	27 (12.2%)*

One missing tooth:
Chi-square = 1.054, df = 1, P = .337 for volunteers with normal joints versus volunteers with disk displacement.
Chi-square = 3.791, df = 1, P = .059 for volunteers with normal joints versus symptomatic normal joints.
Chi-square = 3.821, df = 1, P = .061 for volunteers with normal joints versus symptomatic patients with disk displacement.
Two missing teeth:
Chi-square = 0.271, df = 1, P = 1 for volunteers with normal joints versus volunteers with disk displacement.
Chi-square = 4.175, df = 1, P = .082 for volunteers with normal joints versus symptomatic normal joints.
Chi-square = 5.224, df = 1, P = .022 for volunteers with normal joints versus symptomatic patients with disk displacement.
*P <.05.

teers with normal joints and symptomatic patients with disk displacement, demonstrate an increase in the prevalence of missing teeth in symptomatic patients with intraarticular TMJ disorders. The significance increases with two missing teeth. This suggests that disk displacement and missing teeth might represent multiple risk factors, and the associated pain may come from one or both conditions.

A series of papers has renewed the interest in "bone cavities." There is increasing evidence that impairment of blood supply to the marrow spaces produces ischemia and multiple small intramedullary infarcts over time.[91, 92, 97–99] Multiple quadrants of the jaw are often involved at different times or simultaneously. There are often systemic risk factors, including pregnancy, use of oral contraceptives or estrogen supplements, protein C and S deficiency, and plasminogen deficiency. The clinician should be aware of these entities when patients are refractory to conservative treatment. It may be necessary to perform additional radiographic studies (computed tomography, radiopaque dye into the sinuses, periapical films, [99]technetium-MDP) for differential diagnosis of the persistent pain.[99]

DISCUSSION

Pullinger and colleagues[42] demonstrated a higher prevalence of missing posterior teeth in DDR, OA with a history of DD, and primary OA patients. They also suggested

that when there are five missing posterior teeth, the odds ratios were greater than 2:1.

When patients are seen for the evaluation of TMJ disorders, at a minimum Panorex and bite-wing radiographs should be taken to aid in the elimination of odontologic etiology. We prefer a full series of periapical films and bite wings. This does not completely eliminate the possibility of an odontologic cause but aids in the elimination of inappropriate treatment directed at TMJ pain.

We present three cases that demonstrate the importance of a differential diagnosis for the elimination of an odontologic etiology and discuss the reason for the problems with clinical presentation of the patients.

CASE 3

A 34-year-old woman made an emergency visit with painful right-sided clicking (Fig. 11–8). At that time, she had a maxillary full-coverage occlusal splint that had not given pain relief. She complained of right-sided pain while chewing in the area of the TMJ. A complete examination was not done at this time. She was instructed to take nonsteroidal anti-inflammatory drugs (NSAIDs) and use warm, moist soaks in the area of the TMJ. She was scheduled for a full mouth series of periapical films because there were no films available from the previous clinician. When the films were taken, a periapical radiolucency was seen on the mesial buccal root of the mandibular right first molar. This tooth was not mobile or tender to percussion, nor was a fistula present. The patient did not want to have root canal

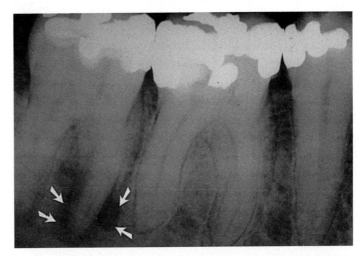

FIGURE 11–8. Mandibular right periapical radiograph of a patient with painful clicking of the temporomandibular joint. The periapical radiolucency can be seen around the mesial root *(arrows)*. Subsequent extraction relieved all pain, even though the clicking persisted.

therapy, and the decision was made to extract the tooth. She was given an appointment 2 weeks later for an examination of her chief complaint: right-sided jaw joint pain. At that visit, she stated that she had no jaw joint pain. She was scheduled for follow-up 3 months later, and there was no pain. This enforces the need for evaluation of the oral structures as a potential source of pain.

CASE 4

An 18-year-old woman presented with right-sided jaw joint pain and audible joint noise, suggestive of DDR. At the initial examination, she stated that there was right-sided headache and photophobia to such an extent that she had to go into a dark room when the headaches began. She had a previous Panorex that was negative, and no other films were taken at that time. Dental examination revealed an anterior open bite and mandibular asymmetry to the right side. She had been receiving splint and pharmacologic management (NSAIDs) by her dentist and a neurologist that had not changed her pain symptoms. It was decided to perform an MRI on the TMJs because of the failure of conservative treatment. The scan demonstrated DDN on the right side. She returned for the follow-up visit after the scan and stated that she had a "bump" over the maxillary right second molar. A periapical radiograph was taken that was not definitive for a periapical abscess, even though there was some thickening of the periodontal ligament space (Fig. 11–9). The patient declined root canal therapy and had the tooth removed. All pain was relieved, and she has been pain free for 3 years.

CASE 5

A 35-year-old man had a long history of right-sided jaw pain. Root canals were performed on several teeth on the right side, the teeth were subsequently extracted, and the pain was still present. The clinical appearance of the patient's left side can be seen in Figure 11–10A at the initial examination. At this time, he stated that his face hurt on the right side from the angle of the mandible to the TMJ. The teeth were not tender to palpation. The patient was not seen for 6 months, and on his return visit, the remaining teeth were removed. He still had pain on the right side. The outlines of the extraction sites could be seen on the Panorex film (Fig. 11–10B), which might suggest neurogenically induced cavitational osteonecrosis. An examination was done

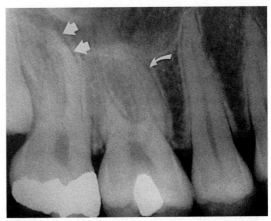

FIGURE 11–9. Maxillary right periapical radiograph of a patient with pain in the right temporomandibular joint. This patient had pain on function and pointed to the right joint as the source of most of the pain. Extraction of the second molar relieved all pain.

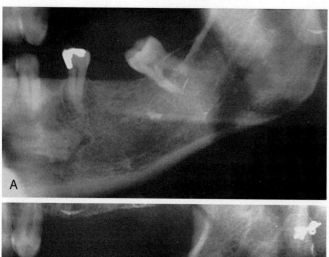

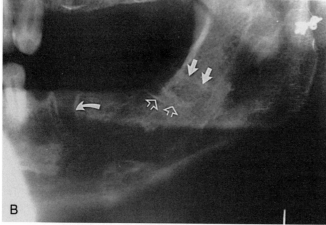

FIGURE 11–10. *A*, Panorex of the right mandible of a subject with long-standing right-sided temporomandibular joint pain. *B*, Panorex 6 months later shows lucent areas at the extraction sites.

at this time, including a mandibular block. The pain did not change. An MRI was performed on the right side, which demonstrated DDN. Local anesthesia was introduced into the TMJ area, and most of the pain was gone. There has been no subsequent follow-up on this patient.

These cases demonstrate the importance of differential diagnosis to rule out odontologic and neurologic problems, even in the presence of jaw joint pain.

TMJ pain seems to be associated with posterior tooth loss. Ishimaru and associates[105] reported on the effect of unilateral posterior malocclusion on TMJ intraarticular pathology in sheep. Two other studies suggested that there is an increase in degenerative changes in young patients with missing posterior molars and DD.[53, 54] They found that the extraction of the maxillary left posterior teeth in the presence of OA accelerated the osteoarthritic changes. When OA was induced by scraping the condylar head and the teeth were *not* extracted, the osteoarthritic process was not as severe.

This suggests that loss of posterior teeth may represent a risk factor in the presence of internal derangement of the TMJ and may explain the higher prevalence of OA with missing posterior teeth, as suggested by Kopp.[70] This does not explain the presence or absence of pain in this group. This may also be one explanation of why there is often no reduction of pain after the replacement of missing posterior teeth and why there is no decrease in the risk of developing TMJ pain, as suggested by some authors.[75–89]

One aspect of missing posterior teeth is decrease in function. Pirttiniemi and colleagues[109] and Shaw and Molyneux[110] evaluated altered function in the rat and rabbit, respectively. Rats were fed a soft diet after weaning, and the incisors were shortened regularly to keep them out of occlusion. The controls were fed a hard diet. Immunohistochemical techniques and image analysis were employed to investigate deposition of pro–type I collagen and type II collagen and the thickness of articular cartilage layers in the mandibular condyle. The total number of chondroblasts was reduced by 35% at the age of 50 days in the soft-diet compared with the hard-diet animals. The results show that deposition of type I and II collagens, thickness of the cartilage cell layers, and number of chondrocytes are sensitive to alterations in loading.

Shaw and Molyneux[110] evaluated the effect of reduced functional dentition (no incisal contacts) on the development of the mandibular disk in young rabbits by measuring cell proliferation within the disk following tooth extraction. Maxillary and mandibular incisor teeth were extracted from 18 animals at 5 weeks of age. Eighteen age- and sex-matched control rabbits with intact dentitions were treated in parallel. In the absence of incisor teeth, reflex gnawing and incising failed to develop, resulting in altered jaw movements and muscle force requirements. The mitotic rate in the anterior band was reduced significantly ($P = .0117$). The rates for the intermediate and posterior bands were not significantly affected. There was an associated reduction in alveolar bone mass and deformation of the developing craniomandibular complex. These observations suggest that altered function affects bone and disk development in the rabbit.

Therefore, it may not be the missing tooth or teeth as much as the long-term effect of the missing units or altered jaw function that may be associated with TMD or facial pain in the presence of multiple risk factors (e.g., DD, missing posterior teeth).

CONCLUSION

The literature does not support the notion that replacement of posterior teeth decreases the risk of TMJ pain. The risk of OA, when data are controlled for age, does not correlate with the development of TMJ pain. The recent studies of Ishimaru and coworkers[105] and others[53, 54] suggest that OA will be more severe in the absence of posterior teeth, but how this may equate to the development of joint pain is unknown. The studies of Shaw and Molyneux[110] and Pirttiniemi and colleagues[109] suggest that there are morphologic changes in developing animals with hypofunction. These data suggest that alteration of function, missing teeth, diet consistency, or lack of incisal contacts may influence development within the TMJ.

Molar Classification

The critical question when evaluating the anteroposterior position of the maxillary and mandibular molars is whether symptomatic patients with intraarticular TMJ disorders demonstrate a major shift toward class II or class III molar relationships. The skeletal and dental relationship of the dental arches is a function of (1) the position of the maxilla (A point, see Fig. 11–4A); nasion–A-point (NA) to Frankfort horizontal (FH) [Lande's angle], Fig. 11–11; (2) the position of angulation of the anterior teeth; (3) the position of the mandible (B point, see Fig. 11–4B; pogonion, nasion pogonion (NP) to FH [facial angle], Fig. 11–12; and (4) the first molar relationship. Each of these measurements gives a different impression of the anteroposterior relationship of the dental arches. Rosenblum[111] provided insight into the problems of using skeletal landmarks. From a dental viewpoint, we use the horizontal and vertical overlap of the anterior teeth and the molar position as a guide for taxonomy.

There have not been many studies classifying the anteroposterior relationship of the mandibular and maxillary first molars. Blake,[112] in an unpublished thesis from the

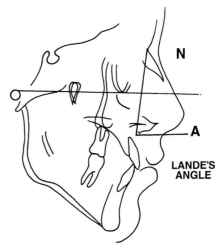

FIGURE 11–11. Lande's angle represents the position of the maxillary denture base in relation to the Frankfort horizontal plane.

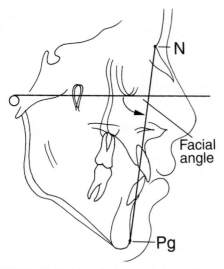

N

Facial
angle

Pg

FIGURE 11–12. Facial angle represents the position of the chin to the Frankfort horizontal plane.

University of Washington, and studies by Pullinger and colleagues[113] and de Latt and van Steenberghe[115] suggest that 22% to 26% of nonpatients have class II molar relationships and 4% to 9% have class III molar relationships. In studies by Pullinger[113] and Solberg[116] and their associates, it is suggested that 68% of a nonpatient population have class I molar relationships, 15% have class II division 1, 4% have class II division 2, and 13% have class III. In Blake's study,[112] 22% of controls had class II molar relationships (17% class II division 2 and 5% class II division 1). Among symptomatic patients, 42% had class II molar relationship (30% class II division 1 and 12% class II division 2).

Our study demonstrates no major differences in the molar classification (Tables 11–7 and 11–8). There were 46 not classified (1.8% in the asymptomatic volunteers ver-

sus 16.4% in the symptomatic patients with DD) because of right missing molars. In Table 11–7, it can be seen that there is no major shift to class II division 1 (14.8% versus 21.2%) or division 2 (3.7% versus 7.1%). This suggests that the differences in horizontal (anteroposterior) relationships are subtle enough that there is no major effect on right molar position. The left molar relationship is demonstrated in Table 11–8. There is an increase in the prevalence of class II division 1 subjects (15.4% versus 24.6%; $P = .048$).

DISCUSSION

Although there are no major differences in molar relationships between volunteers and symptomatic patients, the low prevalence should not suggest a lack of correlation. Careful examination of previous studies[112–116] suggests that nonpatients present with class II division 1 15% to 17% of the time. Twenty-two to thirty percent of symptomatic patients[112, 113, 115] are class II division 1. Our study found 21% class II division 1 on the right side and 25% on the left side (see Tables 11–7 and 11–8). This suggests that the differences in horizontal (anteroposterior) relationships are subtle enough that there is no major effect on right molar position. Table 11–2 demonstrates an increase in the horizontal overlap equal to or greater than 4 mm in the TMD patients compared with the asymptomatic volunteers (16.7% to 22.6% versus 3.6%). The mean horizontal overlap was 2.65 ± 1.09 mm for asymptomatic volunteers and 3.41 ± 2.00 mm for symptomatic patients with disk displacement. Although there is a sta-

| TABLE 11–7. | Prevalence of Right First Molar Classification |

	Class I	Class II/1	Class II/2	Class III	Total	No. Classification	Total
Volunteer normal joint	39 (72.2%)	8 (14.8%)	2 (3.7%)	5 (9.3%)	54	1	55
Volunteer disk displacement	17 (68.0%)	3 (12.0%)	2 (8.0%)	3 (12.0%)	25	2	27
Symptomatic normal joint	22 (61.1%)	8 (22.2%)	1 (2.8%)	5 (13.9%)	36	6	42
Symptomatic disk displacement	121 (65.8%)	39 (21.2%)	13 (7.1%)	11 (6.0%)	184	46	221

Chi-square = 0.89, df = 3, P = .827 for volunteers with normal joints versus volunteers with disk displacement.
Chi-square = 1.53, df = 3, P = .674 for volunteers with normal joints versus symptomatic normal joints.
Chi-square = 2.54, df = 3, P = .468 for volunteers with normal joints versus symptomatic patients with disk displacement.
P <.05.

TABLE 11–8.	Prevalence of Left First Molar Classification

	Class I	Class II/1	Class II/2	Class III	Total	No. Class	Total
Volunteer normal joint	37 (71.2%)	8 (15.4%)	1 (1.9%)	6 (11.5%)	52	3	55
Volunteer disk displacement	16 (61.5%)	4 (15.4%)	2 (7.7%)	4 (15.3%)	26	1	27
Symptomatic normal joint	21 (58.3%)	7 (19.4%)	1 (2.8%)	7 (19.4%)	36	6	42
Symptomatic disk displacement	115 (64.3%)	44 (24.6%)	13 (7.3%)	7 (3.9%)	179	42	221

Chi-square = 1.94, df = 3, P = .585 for volunteers with normal joints versus volunteers with disk displacement.
Chi-square = 1.70, df = 3, P = .048 for volunteers with normal joints versus symptomatic normal joints.
Chi-square = 7.87, df = 3, P = .048 for volunteers with normal joints versus symptomatic patients with disk displacement.

tistical difference between the groups, it represents only 16% to 25% of the sample (see Table 11–2). In Table 11–8, there are differences between volunteers and symptomatic patients with disk displacement. There are fewer class I subjects and an increase in the prevalence of class II divisions 1 and 2. Although significant, this represents only a small increase in class II.

CONCLUSIONS

The changes seen in symptomatic patients with intraarticular TMJ disorders demonstrate an increase in class II molar relationships on the left side. There seems to be a slight retrusion (16% to 25%) in the incisal relationships, but not sufficient enough to produce a major change in molar relationships or retrusion of the mandible to produce class II division 1 incisal relationships.

Discrepancy between RCP and ICP

There are three critical questions with reference to the retruded contact position and the intercuspal position contacts: (1) Is the prevalence of an RCP-ICP discrepancy greater in symptomatic patients with intraarticular TMJ disorders as opposed to asymptomatic volunteers? (2) Does an uneven initial contact (in the vertical plane) produce pain and lead to the development of TMJ pain? and (3) Does removal of this RCP-ICP discrepancy decrease or eliminate TMJ symptoms?

Solberg and coworkers[116] and Helkimo[117] both described RCP-ICP discrepancies. They suggested that these occur in 67% to 98% of subjects in epidemiologic studies. Pullinger and colleagues[113] demonstrated a prevalence of 71% in a nonpatient population. It has also been suggested that an asymmetric slide occurs more frequently in TMD patients. Several studies reported this frequency to be between 15% and 33%.[116–118] Pullinger and colleagues[113] reported that 26% of subjects in a nonpatient population had asymmetric slides. Solberg and coworkers[116] and de Latt and van Steenberghe[115] reported slides of greater than 1 mm in 9% to 10% of patients with mandibular dysfunction. Pullinger and colleagues[113] found that 10% of their nonpatient population had a slide of 1 mm or greater. Cacchiotti and associates[21] demonstrated similar findings in subjects with and without TMJ disorders. The current literature *does not strongly support* the role of dental occlusion as an etiologic factor of TMD from the standpoint of RCP-ICP slides.[119] The literature *does suggest* that provocation-type studies (acute interference) consistently cause muscle and TMJ pain in humans. These provocation-type studies can be divided into two categories: studies that introduce a lateral occlusal interference, and those that introduce a vertical occlusal interference. Rugh and colleagues[120] described the placement of a lateral occlusal interference in 10 subjects that caused a lateral and forward deflection of the dental occlusion. This study suggested that this deflective occlusal contact did not induce the bruxing out but did cause TMJ pain in 4 of 10 subjects.

Riise and Sheikholeslam[121] suggested that vertical occlusal interference is capable of producing changes in muscle activity as early as 1 hour after insertion in humans. After 48 hours, there was a significant increase in activity in the anterior temporal muscle. This increase persisted until the interference was removed 1 week later and had almost completely disappeared 1 week after removal.

Randow and coworkers[122] suggested that a vertical occlusal interference causes TMJ and/or muscle pain. They placed a vertical occlusal interference in eight volunteers in both the RCP and the ICP. Signs and symptoms of TMD developed over a period of 2 weeks and persisted in one subject for 9 months after the interference was removed. Subjects developed clenching, changes in chewing patterns, periodontal tenderness, headache, muscle tension, clicking, and tenderness of the TMJ. They also experienced difficulty in jaw opening. All the previously stated symptoms did not occur in each patient. Two subjects did not develop any pain or dysfunction.

These studies suggest that there is inconsistent agreement between the introduction of various occlusal contacts and the development of mandibular dysfunction. They do suggest that a vertically high contact *does* induce pain that often disappears with removal.

There is no doubt, from clinical experience, that a high occlusal contact frequently produces pain. Pain usually ceases when this contact is removed. In some patients who have had high restorations (high fillings, crowns) placed, the pain persisted even when the high contact was removed. Whether a chronic occlusal discrepancy will alter the sensation (sensory input) and produce plastic changes in the central nervous system is unknown. Theoretically, if experimental hyperocclusal contacts cause pain

and dysfunction in humans, we should be able to measure this by the change in production of neurotransmitters in the trigeminal main sensory nucleus and spinal trigeminal tract (substance P, calcitonin gene-related peptide) and dynorphin gene expression (c-fos) in experimental animals. It has been shown that these substances increase in models of experimental arthritis or when capsaicin is injected into a joint.[123] One could postulate that a high occlusal contact represents a chronic noxious stimulus that increases sensory input, which may be reflected by an increase in neurotransmitter production in the trigeminal main sensory nucleus and spinal trigeminal tract. This increase in neurotransmitters has the potential to lead to alterations in the afferent processing in the trigeminal complex, neuronal toxicity, and alteration of the modulation of sensory input, resulting in hyperalgesia and pain. These experiments have not been systematically performed in an animal model.

In our study, the distribution of RCP-ICP slides can be seen in Table 11–9. There are no significant differences among the four studied groups. This brings up some interesting questions. If the discrepancy between RCP and ICP in asymptomatic individuals is no different from that in symptomatic individuals, we must question the validity of this observation as an etiologic or a contributing factor in the development of intraarticular TMJ disorders.

The distribution of the direction of the slides is listed in Table 11–10. It can be noted that there are no differences among the groups. This suggests that neither anterior nor lateral slides are more prevalent in producing intraarticular TMJ disorders. Uneven right or left contact in RCP (Table 11–11) is not more prevalent in symptomatic

TABLE 11–9.	**Prevalence of a Slide from the Retruded Contact Position to the Intercuspal Position**		
	None	**<1 mm**	**>1 mm**
Volunteer normal joint	30 (54.6%)	12 (21.8%)	13 (23.6%)
Volunteer disk displacement	17 (63.0%)	4 (14.8%)	6 (22.2%)
Symptomatic normal joint	27 (64.3%)	11 (26.2%)	4 (9.5%)
Symptomatic disk displacement	115 (52.0%)	49 (22.2%)	57 (25.8%)

Chi-square = 0.695, df = 2, P = .707 for volunteers with normal joints versus volunteers with disk displacement.
Chi-square = 3.28, df = 2, P = .194 for volunteers with normal joints versus symptomatic normal joints.
Chi-square = 0.136, df = 2, P = .934 for volunteers with normal joints versus symptomatic patients with disk displacement.
$P <.05$.

TABLE 11–10.	Prevalence of Symmetry/Asymmetry of the Slide from the Retruded Contact Position to the Intercuspal Position			
	None	**Straight**	**Right**	**Left**
Volunteer normal joint	30 (54.6%)	15 (27.3%)	4 (7.2%)	6 (10.9%)
Volunteer disk displacement	17 (63.0%)	7 (25.9%)	1 (3.7%)	2 (7.4%)
Symptomatic normal joint	27 (64.3%)	8 (19.1%)	4 (9.5%)	3 (7.1%)
Symptomatic disk displacement	114 (51.6%)	60 (27.2%)	32 (14.5%)	15 (6.8%)

Chi-square = 0.842, df = 3, P = .839 for volunteers with normal joints versus volunteers with disk displacement.
Chi-square = 1.57, df = 3, P = .665 for volunteers with normal joints versus symptomatic normal joints.
Chi-square = 2.81, df = 3, P = .422 for volunteers with normal joints versus symptomatic patients with disk displacement.
$P < .05$.

patients with DD. There was a tendency for the symptomatic but normal patients to exhibit more bilateral-even initial contacts in RCP.

DISCUSSION

In studies that contained a control group, there was no statistically significant difference in occlusal observations. Cacchiotti and associates[21] found no differences in the RCP-ICP discrepancy when comparing a nonpatient sample with a patient sample. They also found no differences in the direction of the slide, whether it was in an anterior or a lateral direction. The same is true of the study by Pullinger and colleagues,[42] with the exception of subjects with DDR, primary OA, and myalgia. They also recorded slides that were greater than 1 mm but broke them down into 2-, 3-, 4-, 5-, and 6-mm slides and demonstrated that patients with DDR, primary OA, and myalgia had greater RCP-ICP discrepancies. This may be an expression of condylar changes (OA) producing arthrosis (remodeling), which has been suggested by Stein,[40] Dibbetts,[35] Shellhas,[206] and Link and Nickerson.[207]

Occlusal adjustment to remove RCP-ICP and/or vertical interferences has long been recommended for the treatment of TMD. Studies have suggested that the use of occlusal adjustment to alter nocturnal electromyographic activity is not reliable. Therefore, occlusal adjustment has not been recommended for the treatment of bruxism.[124, 125] Occlusal adjustment has been demonstrated to have an effect on the signs and symptoms of TMD.[126–129] Another study recommended more conservative treatment with a stabilization splint and home exercises.[130] Occlusal adjustment may be appropriate when an occlusal interference has been introduced from a recent restoration. Adjustment may be considered when it is obvious that it will improve mandibular stability, when there are obvious occlusal discrepancies noted by the patient, or when symptoms have decreased after stabilization splint treatment. There are no known preventive measures for TMJ dysfunction.[2] There are no long-term studies that suggest that prophylactic occlusal adjustment will prevent the development of TMD, although this has been suggested by a longitudinal study in children.[131]

There are some interesting studies that suggest that alterations in occlusion might induce changes in the TMJ.

TABLE 11–11.	Initial Contact in the Retruded Contact Position		
	None	**Right**	**Left**
Volunteer normal joint	16 (29.0%)	15 (27.3%)	24 (43.7%)
Volunteer disk displacement	7 (25.9%)	10 (37.0%)	10 (37.0%)
Symptomatic normal joint	25 (59.5%)	11 (26.2%)	6 (14.3%)
Symptomatic disk displacement	92 (41.6%)	49 (22.2%)	80 (36.2%)

Chi-square = 0.821, df = 2, P = .663 for volunteers with normal joints versus volunteers with disk displacement.
Chi-square = 11.862, df = 2, P = .003 for volunteers with normal joints versus symptomatic normal joints.
Chi-square = 2.91, df = 21, P = .223 for volunteers with normal joints versus symptomatic patients with disk displacement.
$P < .05$.

To date, no animal model is acceptable for the study of TMJ pain and the effects of dental occlusion (malocclusion) and alterations of the dental occlusion. The only study to evaluate manipulation within the TMJ was performed by Broton and Sessle.[132] They placed normal saline, hypertonic saline, potassium chloride, and histamine into the TMJs of cats. They found increases in electromyographic activity in the temporal, digastric, and genioglossus muscles with histamine, potassium chloride, and hypertonic solutions. This suggests that the products of tissue injury (inflammation) are capable of producing TMJ pain. Kubo[100] did a study evaluating the effect of a high occlusal contact in monkeys.[100] He found an increase in immunoreactive type A synovial cells containing horseradish peroxidase. This suggests that a high occlusal contact may be capable of producing changes in the synovial cells in response to the occlusal insult. Correlation to the human condition is lacking.

CONCLUSIONS

It seems that there are very minor differences in the prevalence of RCP-ICP discrepancies in asymptomatic volunteers and symptomatic subjects. The second question related to uneven initial contacts suggests that patients with symptomatic but normal joints are less likely to have uneven initial contacts in RCP. This observation is difficult to interpret and requires further study.

The literature suggests that in animal models, a high occlusal contact produces synovial changes[100] and extraction of posterior teeth in the presence of OA produces a more severe arthritis.[105] There is also an increase in the prevalence of OA in patients with DD and missing posterior teeth.[53, 54] The reversibility of these effects is unknown; therefore, occlusal adjustment should be approached with caution when the exact etiology of a patient's pain has not been established. In clinical practice, one should consider minor occlusal adjustment only after splint therapy has been performed *and there has been relief or significant relief of symptoms.* Splint therapy, which provides bilateral, even occlusal contacts in centric relation–centric occlusion and anterior guidance, should be viewed as differential diagnosis. If symptoms are reduced over a 3- to 6-month period, this provides some justification for minor occlusal adjustment. There is some justification for occlusal adjustment, supported by provocation studies.[120, 122]

Non–Working Side Contacts

There has been much debate about the contribution of non–working side contacts (balancing side contacts) and TMJ pain. The critical questions are: (1) Is there a greater prevalence of non–working side contacts in symptomatic patients than in asymptomatic volunteers? and (2) Does the removal of non–working side contacts as a dental treatment in symptomatic patients decrease symptoms? These questions can be answered only if the prevalence in asymptomatic subjects is compared with that in symptomatic patients and provocation studies are evaluated.

In a study of young adults with non–working side interferences and no signs or symptoms of TMD, it has been suggested that the masticatory system has an adaptive capacity.[133] Magnusson and Enbom[134] found that the insertion of a non–working side contact bilaterally resulted in various subjective symptoms and clinical signs of dysfunction in many but not all subjects during a 2-week period. In a control group, the application of the interference was only simulated. Some subjects developed both subjective symptoms and clinical signs of dysfunction, even though no interference was placed. The introduction of a non–working side contact by Ingerval and Carlsson[135] produced a decrease in postural masseter and temporal muscle activity.

In our study, the symptomatic patients with normal joints and symptomatic patients with DD had fewer non–working side interferences compared with the volunteers with normal joints (Tables 11–12 and 11–13).

DISCUSSION

These results are confusing when considering non–working side contacts as an etiology of TMJ pain, and it can be concluded that there is no simple relationship between signs and symptoms of TMD and non–working side contacts. These results agree with the observations of Agerberg and Sand-

TABLE 11–12.	Non–Working Side Interferences for Asymptomatic Volunteers and Symptomatic Patients (Right Side)			
Group‡	0	1	>1	Total
1	11 (20%)*	23 (41.82%)	21 (38.18%)	55
2	7 (25.93%)	12 (44.44%)	8 (29.63%)	27
3	28 (66.67%)*	11 (26.19%)	3 (7.14%)	42
4	110 (49.77%)†	72 (32.58%)	39 (17.65%)	221

Chi-square = 0.694, df = 2, P = .707 for volunteers with normal joints versus volunteers with disk displacement.
*Chi-square = 23.831, df = 2, P = .001 for volunteers with normal joints versus symptomatic normal joints.
†Chi-square = 18.540, df = 2, P = .001 for volunteers with normal joints versus symptomatic patients with disk displacement.
‡Group 1, asymptomatic volunteer with normal joint; group 2, asymptomatic volunteer with disk displacement; group 3, symptomatic volunteer with normal joint; group 4, symptomatic volunteer with disk displacement.

strom.[136] They found the prevalence of non–working side interferences to be 88% to 89% in a nonpatient population consisting of 60 teenagers and 80 young adults (compare to Group 1, Tables 11–12 and 11–13 in our study). These subjects had at least one unilateral non–working side contact. It was concluded that such interferences could not be established as an etiology for TMD. Hochman and associates[137] found non–working side contacts in 94% of 96 symptomatic patients, which suggests that these contacts are common. Kirveskari and co-workers[138] also offered support by suggesting that most studies are unable to find interference-free subjects among asymptomatic subjects. Magnusson and colleagues[139] in a longitudinal 10-year follow-up study of 84 subjects, found a 32% increase in non–working side interferences. Egermark and Ronnerman[140] concluded that although there was a high prevalence of occlusal interferences during orthodontic treatment, this was of little importance in the development of TMD. Minagi and coworkers[141] found a significant correlation between the *absence* of non–working side contacts and

an increasing prevalence of joint sounds with age. They suggested that certain types of non–working side contacts may be protective of the TMJ.

CONCLUSIONS

In our study, the symptomatic patients had fewer non–working side interferences than the volunteers with normal joints (see Tables 11–12 and 11–13). It can be concluded that there is a high prevalence of non–working side contacts in symptomatic and asymptomatic subjects and that addition or removal of these contacts in volunteers gives no clear indication that they are completely responsible for the development of TMJ pain.

Orthodontic Treatment

The critical question is whether orthodontic treatment decreases or increases the risk of developing intraarticular TMJ disor-

TABLE 11–13.	Non–Working Side Interferences for Asymptomatic Volunteers and Symptomatic Patients (Left Side)			
Group‡	0	1	>1	Total
1	12 (21.82%)*	23 (41.82%)	20 (36.36%)	55
2	5 (18.52%)	14 (51.85%)	8 (29.63%)	27
3	25 (59.52%)*	10 (23.81%)	7 (16.67%)	42
4	113 (51.13%)†	64 (28.96%)	44 (19.91%)	221

Chi-square = 0.740, df = 2, P = .691 for volunteers with normal joints versus volunteers with disk displacement.
*Chi-square = 14.466, df = 2, P = .001 for volunteers with normal joints versus symptomatic normal joints.
†Chi-square = 15.807, df = 2, P = .001 for volunteers with normal joints versus symptomatic patients with disk displacement.
‡Group 1, asymptomatic volunteer with normal joint; group 2, asymptomatic volunteer with disk displacement; group 3, symptomatic volunteer with normal joint; group 4, symptomatic volunteer with disk displacement.

ders. Several controlled long-term studies have been completed evaluating the effect of orthodontic treatment and the prevalence of TMJ disturbances. Sadowsky and Polson[142] compared 96 post-treatment adolescent patients from Illinois and 111 post-treatment patients from Rochester with 103 and 111 untreated subjects, respectively. Patients were examined for a minimum of 10 years after the completion of orthodontic procedures. There were no differences between subjects and controls with respect to TMJ pain, tenderness, discomfort, or joint sounds. They concluded that comprehensive fixed appliance therapy in adolescent subjects did not increase or decrease the risk of developing TMD in this 10-year period.

Larsson and Ronnermen[143] studied 23 patients who had undergone extensive orthodontic treatment 10 years earlier. The prevalence of mandibular dysfunction in the treated group was lower than a reference value in the general population. There was no association between extensive tooth movement and occurrence of symptoms. The authors stated, "In view of the severe malocclusions which all patients in this study had previously exhibited, the low prevalence of functional disturbances suggests that orthodontic treatment prevents rather than causes such disturbances." It may be more appropriate to state that orthodontics neither increases nor decreases the risk of developing TMD.

Janson and Hasund[144] evaluated 60 orthodontically treated subjects 5 years after retention. These subjects included four premolar extraction as well as nonextraction cases. Orthodontically treated subjects had fewer functional problems than those with untreated malocclusions. The authors stated, "There does not appear to be a functional risk in orthodontic treatment of Angle Class II division 1 malocclusion."

Dibbets and van der Weele,[145] in a 10-year longitudinal study, reported that symptoms during orthodontic treatment were most likely age-related and not due to treatment. Symptoms were the same after 10 years for patients treated with the activator and Begg appliances. These findings support the concept that orthodontic treatment does not induce TMJ dysfunction.

Helm and colleagues[146] compared 758 nonorthodontically treated subjects with 83 orthodontically treated subjects. The pres-

TABLE 11–14.	Prevalence of Orthodontic Treatment	
	Orthodontics	**No Orthodontics**
Volunteer normal joint	18 (37%)	37 (63%)
Volunteer disk displacement	6 (22%)	21 (78%)
Symptomatic normal joint	10 (24%)	32 (76%)
Symptomatic disk displacement	57 (25%)	164 (75%)

There are no significant differences between having and not having orthodontic treatment ($P > .05$).

ence of pain, tenderness, clenching, headaches, clicking, and tooth loss was evaluated. They found no significant differences, with the exception of tooth loss. It was also concluded that morphologic untreated malocclusions did not predispose to tooth loss or functional disorders of the masticatory system up to age 30.

Siebert[147] examined two groups of children; 98 individuals not yet treated orthodontically, and 114 who had previously undergone orthodontic treatment. Eighty percent of the untreated children and 60% of the orthodontically treated children had TMJ and muscle tenderness.

Dahl and associates[148] reported no differences in the presence of TMJ symptoms in 19-year-olds who were treated orthodontically compared with a nontreated group. In a cephalometric analysis of an orthodontically treated and untreated sample, Apt and coworkers[149] found no significant differences when comparing angular and linear measurements, skeletal type, horizontal and vertical overlap, and the presence of TMJ symptoms. Peltola and colleagues[150] suggested that there were no significant differences between orthodontically treated patients and nonorthodontically treated subjects in terms of reported TMD symptoms. They reported that there were more degenerative findings on Zonographic radiographs in the orthodontically treated subjects.

In our study (Table 11–14), the prevalence of having orthodontic treatment is approximately equal across the four diagnostic groups. From an epidemiologic standpoint, it seems that having orthodontic treatment neither protects against nor causes the development of TMJ pain.

DISCUSSION

Several studies have been performed to investigate the implication of orthodontic treatment and the initiation of symptoms of mandibular dysfunction.[142–149, 151, 152] Given the number of individuals receiving orthodontic treatment today, greater numbers of individuals presenting for treatment of TMD will have had such treatment. When comparing the subjective, objective, and cephalometric parameters, there are no drastic differences between patients with TMJ pain and control samples.

CONCLUSIONS

One must conclude that having orthodontic treatment neither hinders nor accelerates the development of mandibular dysfunction. Peltola and colleagues[150] reported more degenerative findings on Zonographic radiographs in orthodontically treated subjects. This study deserves further clarification to determine whether these patients with degenerative changes were at risk before orthodontic treatment (e.g., mandibular asymmetry, retrognathia). The presence of skeletal deviations at the initiation of orthodontic treatment should alert the clinician, because they are often associated with degenerative changes in the TMJ. Kuwahara and Maruyama[53] suggested that condylar atrophy was closely related to craniomandibular disorders, especially to DD or OA of the TMJ. These findings in an asymptomatic patient may represent a relative risk of developing jaw joint pain.

Condyle Position

The two critical questions are: (1) Is there an association between the position of the condyle in the articular fossa and intraarticular TMJ disorders? and (2) Does altering the position of the condyle result in positive treatment outcomes compared with not changing the position of the condyle? Observations concerning condyle position have been addressed in several studies. The distribution of anterior, concentric, and posterior condylar position in normal asymptomatic volunteers[153–155] and symptomatic patients[154–161] has been evaluated. Blaschke and Chase[155] reported wide variation in the position of the condyle within the mandibular fossa in asymptomatic volunteers. Madsen[156] made similar observations in asymptomatic volunteers. Pullinger[154, 160] studied condylar position in 74 asymptomatic joints representing a "normal" population using tomography. Condyles were found to be concentric in 43%, posterior in 27%, and anterior in 30% (Table 11–15). In TMD patients, Pullinger and colleagues[161] found that the position of the condyles was skewed toward the posterior; 29% of the condyles were concentric, 54% were posterior, and 17% were anterior.

Bean and Thomas[159] found little or no difference in joint space narrowing between asymptomatic (N = 100) and symptomatic (N = 200) patients using the transcranial projection. Twenty-seven percent of the symptomatic patients had anterior and posterior joint space narrowings. In the asymptomatic group, 30% had anterior and posterior joint space narrowings.

Ronquillo and associates[157] evaluated 170 joints (using tomography), with arthrographic confirmation of disk position. There

TABLE 11–15.	Distribution of Condyle Position in Selected Studies		
	Anterior (%)	Concentric (%)	Posterior (%)
Pullinger[160] asymptomatic	30	43	27
Blaschke[155] asymptomatic	14	58	28
Pullinger[161] symptomatic	17	29	54
Ronquillo[157] symptomatic	15	39	46
Pullinger[154] clicking	9	20	71
Ronquillo[157] clicking	15	24	61

Summarized from references 154, 155, 157, 160, 161.

was a statistically significant number of patients with distally positioned condyles (61%) in the DDR group (clicking) as compared with the other diagnoses (symptomatic normals and DDN).

Table 11–15 compares previous studies of asymptomatic and symptomatic subjects. In the symptomatic population, there are more distal condyle positions. Ronquillo demonstrated that in a symptomatic population, the major shift of condyle position comes from the DDR subgroup. Comparing Ronquillo's[157] "clicking" and Pullinger's[154] "clicking" groups suggests that a skew toward the distal is influenced by individuals with the diagnosis of a reducing disk displacement. This contention is supported further by Ronquillo's[157] observations in the symptomatic normal and DDN groups, which demonstrate similar distributions of posterior, concentric, and anterior condyle positions.

Our study (Table 11–16) demonstrates that there is a higher prevalence of symptomatic DDR and DDN patients with distal condyle positions. It must be noted, however, that when compared with volunteers with normal joints, this represents a shift of 18% to 24% of the respective sample. There is still 51% to 58% of the respective sample with concentric or anterior condyle positions. This emphasizes the need to review all objective and subjective data before making a definitive diagnosis. There is no longitudinal study that evaluates treatment outcomes when a condyle position is changed from posterior to concentric or anterior to concentric in symptomatic subjects with DDN or normal joints. There are several studies in symptomatic patients with DDR that suggest that moving the condyle anterior to establish more normal anatomic relationships does reduce pain.[162–164] This does not mean that moving a distal condyle

to a more concentric position for any patient with a distal condyle position (e.g., a symptomatic patient with DDN or a normal but symptomatic joint) will produce a therapeutic effect. Maloney and Howard[165] suggested that if anterior repositioning splints are discontinued, the success rate will be only 35% at 3 years. This suggests that when the condyle position is changed in a symptomatic patient with DDR, this position must be maintained, or pain will return. This does not suggest that the same is true for a symptomatic patient with DDN or a normal but symptomatic joint. There are presently no controlled studies evaluating this treatment concept.

DISCUSSION

It can be concluded that a symptomatic population has more distal condyle positions. The fallacy here is that condyle position has shifted distally in response to joint abnormality. Ronquillo and associates[157] showed that in nonreducing patients and symptomatic normals, concentric and anterior condyles dominated. Whether the position of the condyle is a dependable predictor of joint abnormality should be questioned. Brand and colleagues[57] found that disk position prediction, based on condyle position, was accurate in 63% of 243 subjects. They concluded that anterior disk position failed to alter condyle position more frequently than condylar retropositioning occurred in the absence of anterior disk displacement. Kamelchuk and coworkers[58] suggested that tomography as a diagnostic test of abnormal disk position had a sensitivity of 0.43, a specificity of 0.80, and a positive predictive value of 0.64. They stated that tomography

TABLE 11–16.	Distribution of Condyle Position in the Study Groups			
	Anterior	**Concentric**	**Posterior**	**Total**
Volunteer normal joint	38 (36.5%)	42 (40.4%)	24 (23.1%)*	104
Symptomatic normal joint	29 (33.3%)	36 (41.4%)	22 (25.3%)	87
Symptomatic DDR	24 (23.1%)	37 (35.6%)	43 (41.3%)*	104
Symptomatic DDN	13 (20.3%)	20 (31.3%)	31 (48.4%)†	64

*Chi-square = 8.87, df = 2, P = .0119 for volunteers with normal joints versus symptomatic patients with disk displacement with reduction (DDR).

†Chi-square = 12.12, df = 2, P = .0023 for volunteers with normal joints versus symptomatic patients with disk displacement without reduction (DDN).

TABLE 11–17.	All Joints with DDR Compared with Asymptomatic Volunteers	
	Distal Condyle Position	**Not Distal Condyle Position**
Disk displacement with reduction	43	61
No disk displacement (asymptomatic volunteers)	24	80

Cells in Table 11–16 have been collapsed to create this table.
Sensitivity (TP/TP + FP) = 43/43 + 24 = .64.
Specificity (TN/TN + FN) = 80/80 + 61 = .56.
FN, false negative; FP, false positive; TN, true negative; TP, true positive.

TABLE 11–19.	All Joints with a Symptomatic but Normal Joint Compared with Asymptomatic Volunteers	
	Distal Condyle Position	**Not Distal Condyle Position**
Symptomatic normal	22	65
No disk displacement (asymptomatic volunteers)	24	80

Cells in Table 11–16 have been collapsed to create this table.
Sensitivity (TP/TP + FP) = 22/22 + 24 = .33.
Specificity (TN/TN + FN) = 80/80 + 65 = .54.
FN, false negative; FP, false positive; TN, true negative; TP, true positive.

is inappropriate as a diagnostic test for predicting the type of internal derangement.

Two-by-two tables were constructed from Table 11–16 to evaluate the power of the observations that were significant in subjects with and without disk displacement (Tables 11–17 to 11–19). In subjects with DDR the sensitivity was 0.64, in those with DDN it was 0.56, and in symptomatic normals it was 0.33. This suggests the ability of a distal condyle to predict disk displacement to be low. In subjects with DDR the specificity was 0.56, in those with DDN it was 0.65, and in symptomatic normals it was 0.55. This suggests a high prevalence of distal condyle position in subjects without disk displacement.

An observation concerning the position of the condyle at any point in time is simply an observation, and the staging of a pathologic process cannot be assumed. No study, with the exception of that by Gianelly and colleagues,[166] has documented condyle position before and after orthodontic treatment and demonstrated no changes in condyle position during the treatment period.

CONCLUSIONS

It may be concluded that observations of the position of the condyle in symptomatic patients may be a matter of chance rather than a dependable predictor of the staging of the joint derangement or the result of treatment procedures. There is an increase in distal condyles in symptomatic patients, which is approximately 18% to 24% in patients with disk displacement. It is not a great enough shift of the data to be a good predictor. This has been demonstrated by Kamelchuk and coworkers[58] and in Tables 11–17 to 11–19. The effect of treatment procedures can be confirmed only if pretreatment plain films are taken before the initiation of treatment procedures (orthodontics, prosthodontics, and/or oral surgery).

Orthognathic Surgery and TMJ Ramifications

TMD and orthognathic surgery (OS) are two of the most involved and complicated treatment problems in dentistry. Patients in need of treatment for TMJ signs and symptoms or requiring OS present the treating

TABLE 11–18.	All Joints with DDN Compared with Asymptomatic Volunteers	
	Distal Condyle Position	**Not Distal Condyle Position**
Disk displacement with reduction	31	33
No disk displacement (asymptomatic volunteers)	24	80

Cells in Table 11–16 have been collapsed to create this table.
Sensitivity (TP/TP + FP) = 31/31 + 24 = .564.
Specificity (TN/TN + FN) = 80/80 + 33 = .650.
FN, false negative; FP, false positive; TN, true negative; TP, true positive.

clinician with unique situations. A chief complaint of TMJ pain in a patient who also has a dentofacial deformity for which OS is indicated is one of the most difficult case types in which to achieve an acceptable result. Patients presenting with a dentofacial deformity for which OS is planned who have some TMJ signs or symptoms pose an equally complicated problem.

The critical questions that arise when treating a patient with or without TMJ signs and symptoms who also has a dentofacial deformity that requires OS are:

1. What impact does OS have on the TMJ pain complaints of a patient presenting with a chief complaint of pain in the TMJ who also has a dentofacial deformity requiring OS?
2. What impact does OS have on the TMJ pain complaints of a patient presenting with a dentofacial deformity as a chief complaint who also has some clinical TMJ signs and symptoms?
3. What impact does OS have on the TMJ pain complaints of a patient with dentofacial deformities and no TMJ signs and symptoms?
4. What effect, if any, does disk displacement have on mandibular asymmetry, OS relapse, and TMJ signs or symptoms pre- and postoperatively?

The discussion of these four questions includes issues such as the effect of the type of surgical procedure, the type of fixation used, and the presence or absence of TMJ internal derangement. Although the literature is sparse and in most cases retrospective in nature, it is worth reviewing in context of these issues.

Few studies have dealt with the outcomes of OS patients whose primary complaint was pain and discomfort from TMJ signs and symptoms. None have been prospective in scope. One reason for this may be that most TMJ treatment schemes stress noninvasive, reversible procedures prior to the more involved nonreversible procedures such as disk repair, meniscotomy, or OS.[167] The success of self-management or reversible treatment modalities during acute periods of TMJ pain probably limits the patient population requiring nonreversible types of treatment.[168] Furthermore, the lack of evidence showing the benefit of certain occlusal schemes or the unequivocal, repeated prevalence of specific skeletal and or dental malrelationships in TMD patients may have limited the use of OS (and other nonreversible procedures) as a treatment modality for TMJ pain.[168–176]

This is not to say that there have not been treatment outcome reports of patients whose primary complaints were of TMJ signs and symptoms who also were in need of and underwent OS. Tucker and Thomas[167] and Piecuch and colleagues[177] presented individual cases of TMD patients presenting with short-face syndrome (vertical maxillary hypoplasia) who were eventually treated with maxillary disimpaction surgery who had remarkable cessation of TMJ symptoms postoperatively.

Unfortunately, most studies do not separate patients with TMJ signs and symptoms as a chief complaint as clearly as do the two previously cited case reports. Karabouta and Martis[178] examined 280 OS patients with mandibular deformities and found 40.8% of the patients (114) to have one or more TMJ symptoms. They found that some patients had such severe TMJ symptoms that they presented for treatment of their TMJ problem and not their dentofacial deformity. Unfortunately, they were not followed as a single group in the report of results in this study.

Magnusson and others[179] studied 20 patients with dentofacial deformities requiring OS. TMJ pain-dysfunction was a common reason for requesting treatment. All patients were examined preoperatively with both subjective and objective testing, including both self-report of TMJ symptoms and the use of the Helkimo index. Follow-up observations were performed 1 week after intermaxillary fixation removal and 6 months, 1 year, and 2.5 years after surgery. There was a statistically significant reduction in the clinical dysfunction index; however, there was no report, on an individual basis, of which patients felt better or worse after treatment. Furthermore, there were no controls.

The lack of studies examining TMJ signs and symptoms in patients treated with concomitant OS suggests that we have to use studies that examine OS patients who also have TMJ signs or symptoms to draw inferences on the effect of OS on TMJ pain. This is where a clinician's ability to draw solid conclusions becomes confusing. There are several variables to consider: surgical technique, type of fixation, type of surgery, presence or absence of internal derangement, and length of follow-up. Not surprisingly, results vary tremendously. For example, Kerstens and associates[180] studied 480 OS patients pre- and postoperatively and found that 16.2% had one or more TMJ symptoms preoperatively. They found that 66% of these patients reported a reduction or resolution of these symptoms. However, they also found that 11.5% of the preoperatively asymptomatic patients developed TMJ symptoms postoperatively.

Laskin and others[171] surveyed 116 oral and maxillofacial surgery training programs to determine the prevalence of TMJ signs and symptoms prior to OS. They also wanted to find out how many of the preoperatively asymptomatic patients developed TMJ signs and symptoms after surgery. The responses were so varied that the authors concluded that until further data are collected it is unclear whether any association exists between skeletal disharmonies and mandibular dysfunction, and therefore it is "impossible to conclude whether orthognathic correction procedures are specific and therapeutic for patients who have concurrent TM disorders."

White and Dolwick[181] studied the prevalence and variance of TMD in 75 OS patients retrospectively. They found that 37 (49.3%) of the patients had had some signs or symptoms prior to surgery. After surgery, 33 (89.1%) of the symptomatic patients had improved function and reduction or resolution of their symptoms, 1 (2.7%) showed no change, and 3 (8.1%) got worse. In the asymptomatic presurgical group, 3 (7.9%) developed TMJ signs and symptoms postoperatively. This means that 7 (9.3%) had TMJ symptoms postsurgically. Although the authors were pleased with the overall improvement of symptoms, they concluded that "on an individual basis, currently it is impossible to predict whether orthognathic surgery will alleviate symptoms of TMD."

Upton and colleagues[182] retrospectively studied 102 OS patients. Fifty-five (53%) reported presurgical TMJ signs and symptoms. Postsurgical follow-up demonstrated that 43 (78%) reported that symptoms improved after completion of treatment for their dentofacial deformity, 9 (16%) reported

no change, and 3 (5%) reported that their symptoms were worse postoperatively. Four (8.5%) of the 47 patients who had had no pretreatment TMJ signs and symptoms developed some after OS treatment. Overall, 16 (15.6%) had postsurgical TMJ symptoms. In the authors' discussion, they stated that "surgical repositioning of the maxillomandibular skeleton may lead to resolution or improvement of TMJ pain-dysfunction symptoms in an *unpredictable* number of patients."

TYPES OF SURGERY

Maxillary

When specific types of orthognathic surgical procedures are analyzed for their effect on TMJ signs and symptoms, similar conflicting reports emerge (Table 11–20). Kahnberg[183] studied superior maxillary repositioning for the correction of open bite and vertical maxillary excess. Eleven patients were screened clinically and anamnestically and were found to be free of TMJ symptoms. In over 60%, TMJ symptoms developed postoperatively during a 6- to 12-month follow-up.

Herbosa and others[184] studied 29 patients undergoing maxillary impaction surgery for the correction of vertical maxillary hyperplasia. They found that 11 of 29 (37.9%) patients showed TMJ signs and symptoms presurgically. The 12-month postoperative findings showed that only 6 of 29 (20.7%) of the patients were symptomatic, a 55% decrease. This reduction was not statistically significant even though it was a marked reduction. The authors did not state whether the six patients reporting symptoms postoperatively were symptomatic or asymptomatic preoperatively.

Egermark-Eriksson and associates[185] studied patients (N = 22) undergoing anteroinferior repositioning of the maxilla and found a slight improvement of TMJ-related symptoms postoperatively, which was not statistically significant.

Mandibular

Setback

Astrand and colleagues[186] published one of the first comprehensive retrospective re-

| TABLE 11–20. | Summary of Orthognathic Studies |

Study	No. of Subjects	Presurgical Symptoms (%)	Postsurgical No Symptoms (%)	Postsurgical Improved (%)	Postsurgical Not Improved or Worse (%)	Presurgical No Symptoms/ Postsurgical Symptoms (%)	Total No. of Subjects with Symptoms Postsurgically (%)	Type of Surgery
Kerstens and others (1989)[180]	480	78 (16.3)	403 (84.0)	53 (66.6)	26 (33.3)	47 (11.7)	73 (15.2)	Various
Upton and others (1984)[182]	102	55 (53)	47 (47)	43 (78)	12 (21)	4 (8.5)	16 (15.7)	Various
Karabouta and Martis (1985)[178]	280	114 (40.8)	166 (52.9)	102 (90)	12 (11.1)	6 (3.7)	18 (6.4)	Various, BSSO
White and Dolwick (1992)[181]	75	37 (49.3)	38 (50.7)	33 (89)	3 (7.9)	3 (7.9)	7 (9.3)	Various
Kahnberg (1988)[183]	13	(0)	13 (100)	*	7 (60)	7 (60)	7 (60)	Maxillary impaction
Herbosa and others (1990)[184]	29	11 (37.9)	18 (62)	5 (45)	*	*	60 (20.7)	Maxillary impaction
Egermark-Eriksson and others (1988)[185]	18	7 (38.8)	11 (61.1)	3 (42.9)	*	*	4 (22.2)	Maxillary inferior repositioning
Pepersack and Chausse (1978)[188]	67	*	*	*	*	*	20 (29.9)	Mandibular setback
Freihofer and Petresevic (1975)[189]	43	*	*	*	*	*	16 (37.2)	Mandibular advancement

*Data not presented in study.
BSSO, bilateral sagittal split osteotomy.

views of mandibular OS. They studied 55 patients with mandibular prognathism treated with oblique sliding osteotomy of the mandibular rami to allow for mandibular setback. Six-month follow-up showed seven patients to have TMJ symptoms; five patients eventually resolved. Two of the seven patients complaining of TMJ symptoms 6 months after surgery reported that they had had symptoms prior to surgery. No statistical analysis was performed on this group of patients regarding TMJ signs or symptoms.

Wisth[187] retrospectively examined two groups of patients with mandibular prognathism. One group had been operated on with oblique vertical ramus osteotomy for mandibular setback surgery 10 years previously. The other group did not undergo surgery and acted as controls. The authors reported that 71% of the untreated controls reported subjective TMJ symptoms. Twenty-six percent of the treated group reported functional disturbances and symptoms.

Pepersack and Chausse[188] studied prognathic patients treated with mandibular setback surgery at 5-year follow-up. Results showed that 20 of 67 patients had TMJ signs or symptoms. No report of presurgical patient evaluation was given.

Advancement

Freihofer and Petresevic[189] retrospectively studied 43 patients treated with mandibular sagittal split osteotomy for advancement of the mandible. The 5-year follow-up found 16 patients complaining of TMJ clicking, and only 1 of these complained of pain. No presurgical reports on TMJ signs or symptoms were reported.

Hackney and others[190] studied 18 consecutive patients treated with bilateral sagittal split osteotomy (BSSO) for the advancement of the mandible. TMJ dysfunction was studied by physical examination and by history immediately after surgery (T1) and 6 to 12 months postoperatively (T2). Results showed that three patients had TMJ pain at T1; one of these resolved at T2. Four patients had a click at T1, and three had resolved at T2. Two subjects that were asymptomatic preoperatively developed clicks postoperatively. The authors concluded that there were no significant differences between T1 and T2 in number of patients experiencing pain or clicks.

Rodrigues-Garcia and associates[191] examined 124 patients requiring BSSO mandibular advancement surgery for the correction of class II malocclusion. These patients were not seeking treatment for TMD, but many either reported some TMJ signs or symptoms presurgically or were found to have TMJ signs or symptoms during the presurgical examination. Three indices were used for TMJ evaluation: craniomandibular index (CMI), dysfunction index (DI), and muscle index (MI). Patients were evaluated 2 weeks presurgically, 1 week postsurgically, and 6 weeks, 6 months, 1 year, and 2 years postoperatively. The authors found a statistically significant decrease in both CMI and MI values as well as a statistically significant reduction in self-reports of subjective facial pain and pain on opening.

Ochs and others[192] may have summarized the effect of OS on TMJ pain best when they stated that "it is uncertain what impact orthognathic surgery has on a patient's TMJ signs or symptoms. The general trend in the literature suggests that a significant number of patients with dentofacial deformity and TMJ disorders will experience an improvement in their symptoms after surgery." However, "during preoperative consultation, it is important to remember that on an individual basis, it is impossible to determine whether orthognathic surgery will lead to a resolution of the TMJ disorder."

FIXATION TYPE AND CONDYLE POSITION

With the development of rigid internal fixation (RIF) for stabilization of BSSO of the mandible, questions arose regarding the effect of this technique versus wire (non-RIF) on TMJ signs and symptoms. Several authors have demonstrated the difficulty in maintaining the presurgical position of the mandibular condyles when mandibular setbacks or advancements are performed in conjunction with RIF.[193-195] This is also a problem when wire fixation is used; however, the ability for self-correction is dramatically reduced when RIF is used.[196]

Two problems have been addressed in the literature regarding RIF: the maintenance of intercondylar width and angle and the

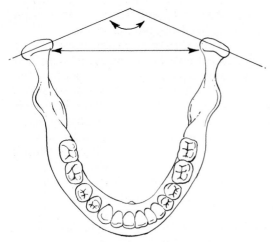

FIGURE 11–13. Maintenance of intercondylar width, angle, and presurgical condylar position is a major concern during mandibular procedures.

control and maintenance of the presurgical position of the condyle (Fig. 11–13). Consequently, techniques have been developed to control the proximal mandibular segment in relation to the contralateral segment as well as to the glenoid fossa so that the condyle finishes in a position closely approximating its presurgical starting point (Fig. 11–14).[194, 196, 197] Clinicians treating OS patients are interested in any type of procedure that may alter the condyle-fossa relationship.

Several studies have examined the effect of RIF on TMJ signs and symptoms, and several have compared RIF with non-RIF methods.

One of the benefits of RIF has been the reduced time in intermaxillary fixation that patients have to spend postoperatively as compared to those who have non-RIF. There is good evidence to suggest that patients treated with RIF do better in terms of maintenance of the position of the condyle and healing and have less relapse than those treated with the combination of non-RIF and several weeks of intermaxillary fixation.[198–202] These studies have been countered by authors claiming an increase in prevalence of TMJ signs and symptoms with the use of RIF.[29]

Most investigators comparing the effect of RIF with non-RIF procedures on TMJ signs and symptoms have found either no change or a reduction of symptoms.[198, 201] Some have actually shown an improvement in TMJ signs and symptoms with the use of RIF as compared to non-RIF.[202] However, some studies suggest that condylar position may be altered by RIF and subsequently play a part in the development or exacerbation of TMJ signs and symptoms. Most studies show that with careful planning and surgical technique, changes in condyle position are readily adapted to.

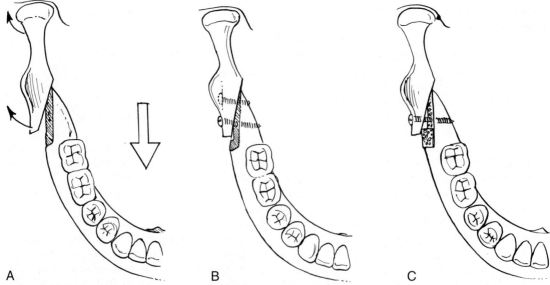

A B C

FIGURE 11–14. *(A)* Bilateral sagittal split osteotomy in combination with anterior or posterior positioning of the tooth-bearing segment can cause changes in the presurgical position of the condyle. Positional screws *(B)* and bone shims *(C)* have both been used to prevent lateral displacement of the condylar segment. (Adapted from Proffit WR, Fields HW: Contemporary Orthodontics, ed 2. St. Louis, Mosby, 1993.)

Perhaps the definitive study on the effect of RIF versus non-RIF on TMD has come from a multicenter prospective study by Nemeth and associates.[203] These investigators examined 127 patients in need of class II correction by means of BSSO. They were divided randomly to receive RIF or non-RIF. TMJ signs and symptoms were analyzed using the CMI. Patients were followed and examined 2 years after BSSO. Their findings clearly showed no difference in the effect of RIF and non-RIF on TMJ signs and symptoms and that RIF did not increase the risk of TMJ signs and symptoms.

Although it is important to determine how TMJ signs and symptoms will be affected by type of surgical movement as well as type of surgical fixation, an equally important factor to examine is the type of skeletal deformity that the patient has. More important to our discussion is whether there is a specific dentofacial deformity that is more likely to present with TMJ signs and symptoms preoperatively or postoperatively.

CRANIOFACIAL MORPHOLOGY, INTERNAL DERANGEMENT, AND TMJ SIGNS AND SYMPTOMS

Several authors have examined OS patients both pre- and postoperatively and have found that patients presenting with high mandibular plane angles, class II malocclusion featuring retrognathia, open bite with vertical maxillary excess, and retrognathia are more likely to have TMJ signs and symptoms preoperatively and are more likely to develop or maintain them postoperatively.[181, 204–207] Kahnberg[183] studied 13 patients who had maxillary impaction for correction of open bite with vertical maxillary excess. None had clinical or anamnestic TMJ signs or symptoms preoperatively. Over 60% of the patients developed TMJ symptoms during the 6- to 30-month follow-up period.

Kerstens and others[180] studied 480 OS patients both pre- and postoperatively and found that retrognathic patients with low- and normal-angle mandibles were more likely to have preoperative TMJ signs and symptoms and were more likely to show improvement of these symptoms postoperatively. However, the group of patients who

had BSSO and LeFort I maxillary impaction as treatment for high-angle mandibular retrognathism had the highest postsurgical incidence of TMJ signs and symptoms.

Kerstens and colleagues[205] studied 206 patients who underwent OS in combination with orthodontic treatment. They found that 12 patients suffered condylar atrophy during postsurgical follow-up and that all 12 had the same skeletal pattern—high mandibular plane angle and class II retrognathia with open bite—and that all were treated with BSSO and LeFort I osteotomy. Nine (75%) of these patients had TMJ signs or symptoms presurgically. Four (33%) of the original 12 complained that their pain was worse after surgery, 6 (50%) found no improvement, and 2 (16%) reported that their pain was better.

When Bouwman and associates[208] studied 158 OS patients prone to condylar resorption (as determined by the fact that all had absolute mandibular deficiency and a high mandibular plane angle), 24 (26.4%) of the 91 treated with intermaxillary fixation showed signs of condylar resorption, whereas only 8 (11.9%) of the 67 treated without intermaxillary fixation showed signs of condylar resorption postoperatively. Their results suggest that avoiding intermaxillary fixation in OS patients with retrognathia and a high mandibular plane angle may help minimize postoperative TMJ signs and symptoms as well as relapse due to condylar resorption.

White and Dolwick[181] examined the prevalence and variance of TMJ dysfunction in OS patients. They studied 75 patients retrospectively and found that 49.3% had preoperative TMJ signs and symptoms. TMJ dysfunction was found to be significantly more prevalent in patients with class II skeletal dentofacial deformities.

The obvious trend in these previously reviewed studies suggests that the craniofacial morphology of certain patients may be a clue to the treating clinician that there is a potential for pre- and postoperative risk of TMJ signs and symptoms. The etiology of this facial type has been suggested by many authors and may be closely related to internal derangement of the TMJ; however, no prospective longitudinal studies have been conducted that unequivocally show this link.[205, 207–213]

Boering[214] and Dibbets and others[209] have

shown the effect of TMJ remodeling on craniofacial development and morphology in adolescent and adult patients. Patients showing x-ray deformities of the TMJs had distinct morphologies featuring shorter corpus, smaller posterior facial heights, and a profile that appeared to be more class II division 1. When these mandibles were studied to assess their growth pattern, it was shown that they were backward rotating and formed antegonial notches.

Bjork and Skieller[215] conducted a 25-year longitudinal study on normal and abnormal growth of the mandible. Mandibles that had normal growth showed a forward rotation. Nearly every mandible showing a backward rotation featured some form of condylar problem. It is interesting to note that Bjork and Skeiller[215] alluded to the fact that these mandibles may have an effect on the morphology of other parts of the developing face when they stated that "it is not known to what extent maxillary growth is primarily affected. It is obvious, however, from the maxillary implants and from the inclination of the anterior surface of the zygomatic process that there was increasing backward rotation of the maxillary corpus, probably secondary to the rotation of the mandibular corpus."

Stringert and Worms[204] compared cephalometric data from a group of 62 subjects with documented internal derangements with a sample of 102 subjects from a normative sample. It is important to note that this normative sample did not undergo hard or soft tissue imaging to document the presence or absence of internal derangement. The results documented an increased proportion of "high plane" or hyperdivergent subjects in the experimental group. There was a decrease in the proportion of "low plane" or hypodivergent subjects in the experimental group. When the experimental subjects were segregated for the presence or absence of trauma, there was no difference in the proportion of subjects in any vertical or anteroposterior skeletal pattern subgroup. There was a tendency, based solely on descriptive statistics, for the nontrauma group to exhibit an increased proportion of subjects with "division 2"-type incisal relationships (n = 5). It must be noted that these were not necessarily skeletal class II, division 2 individuals but only that their incisal relationships (axial inclination) were below

the mean with reference to the sella-nasion cranial base. Also, the frequency (n = 5) was insufficient for statistical comparisons.

Schellhas and Keck[210] presented a case report on 10 patients who had originally presented for a consultation for abnormal occlusion or cosmetic facial deformity, or both. There was 1 male and 9 females. All patients were studied by clinical examination, TMJ radiography, and either arthrography or MRI. An attempt was made to correlate occlusal deficits—such as asymmetric anterior open bite, bilateral open bite, and developing retrognathia—with radiologic observations of condyle destruction, articular surface collapse, and loss of condylar vertical dimension (posterior face height). It should be noted that the MRI findings were not longitudinal in nature and therefore did not correlate with changes over time.

Link and Nickerson[207] examined 39 patients referred for OS. Patients had either class I open bite, class I on one side and class II contralaterally, or class II bilaterally with or without open bite. Patients who were evaluated by arthrography (n = 35) or who had clearly deformed condyles as seen on transpharyngeal radiographs (n = 4) were included in the study. The mean patient age was 29 years. Condylar morphology was defined by transpharyngeal radiography and classified as being normal, small, or deformed. The 24 deformed joints evaluated by arthrography had disk displacement without reduction. Condyles with small morphology and 80% of condyles with normal morphology also had an internal derangement. The six patients with mandibular deviation had either small or deformed condyles with internal derangement on the side to which the mandible deviated. The six contralateral joints had normal bony morphology. In the patients with deviation, those who had normal morphology and a normal disk were class I on the ipsilateral side and class II on the contralateral joint with internal derangement. The other three patients with deviation all had bilateral internal derangement, but the more advanced derangement was on the side that demonstrated the greater degree of class II molar relationship and the small or deformed condyle. Of the 30 symmetric class II (with or without open bite) patients, 43% had bilateral deformed condyles or a combination of deformed and small condyles. All open-bite patients and 88% of the patients with class II malocclusion had bilateral derangements. The patients with facial deviation offered the greatest support for the hypothesis that internal derangement has a significant influence on craniofacial morphology. The three patients with unilateral disk displacement had mandibular deviation to the side with disk displacement. The patients with bilateral disk displacement had mandibular deviation toward the side with the more advanced displacement.

Schellhas and associates[206] retrospectively evaluated 100 patients presenting for OS with retrognathic facial skeletal morphology with or without lateral chin displacement and open bite. There were 85 females and 15 males age 11 to 65. The authors stressed that it was the skeletal deformities that were of primary concern. All subjects had MRI of the TMJs owing to the suspected role of internal derangement in cases of unstable occlusion and facial asymmetry. Patients were divided into stable and unstable groups based on the presence or absence of changes in their facial contour or occlusion, or both, in the 24 months prior to the investigation. However, it should be noted that the groups were based on patients' responses to a questionnaire and not on clinical observations over the previous 24-month period. Sixty-one patients denied pain, and 45 denied any mechanical TMJ symptoms such as clicking, locking, and masticatory dysfunction in a routine questionnaire. Results of this study showed that all of the 58 patients with unstable facial deformity or occlusal disturbances, or both, had internal derangement of at least one joint. The degree of joint degeneration and remodeling directly paralleled the deviation of facial deformity in most cases. Thirty of 42 patients with stable deformities were found to have internal derangements of at least one TMJ. When lateral deviation of the chin was evident clinically, it was noted to be uniformly toward the smaller condyle or the more degenerated TMJ. Two patients showed an enlarged condyle. In these patients, diagnosed with condylar hyperplasia, the chin was deviated away from the enlarged condyle toward the smaller condyle, which had internal derangement. The authors warn that skeletal abnormalities such as retrognathia and fa-cial asymmetry with or without malocclusion may represent underlying TMJ internal derangement in OS candidates. They cite Nickerson and Moystad,[216] who stated that pain-free, nonclicking TMJs may have internal derangements that may be the cause of skeletal remodeling. This has also been suggested by Roberts and colleagues.[217]

Schellhas and others[211] studied 128 consecutive children suspected of having TMJ disease because of inflammatory (pain), mechanical, or structural symptoms such as retrognathia and mandibular asymmetry. They were retrospectively examined with radiographic studies (submentovertex, anteroposterior, jaw-protruded facial, and lateral closed-mouth radiographs, as well as closed- and open-mouth lateral TMJ tomograms) and MRI. Results showed that lateral deviation of the chin was always toward the smaller and more degenerated TMJ. MRI findings showed that 112 of 128 children exhibited at least one joint with internal derangement. Eighty-five had bilateral derangements. Fifty-six of 60 retrognathic patients were found to have joints with internal derangement. Advanced stages of TMJ derangement were almost invariably noted in cases of severe retrognathia or lateral asymmetry.

Hatala and others[218] evaluated the effect of unilateral disk displacement on growth changes in the New Zealand white rabbit. Fifteen female rabbits (age 10 weeks) were included in the study. Five experimental rabbits had surgically created anterior disk displacement, five had no surgery, and five controls had sham surgery. The five rabbits that had sham surgery showed no condylar deformity. The linear measurements were not done for these animals because only histology was evaluated for this group. The rabbits were sacrificed at 22 weeks of age, and the mandibles were hemisected and radiographed. Cephalograms were digitized and analyzed by conventional methods. The gross appearance showed shortening and flattening of the articulating surface in the experimental group (Fig. 11–15). No significant shortening and flattening was found in the control groups (Fig. 11–16). These observations suggest that surgically created internal derangement can produce altered growth in the mandible.

A paper addressing the subject of inter-

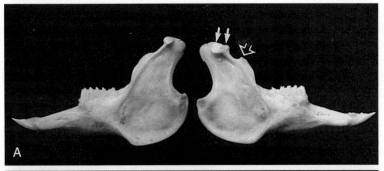

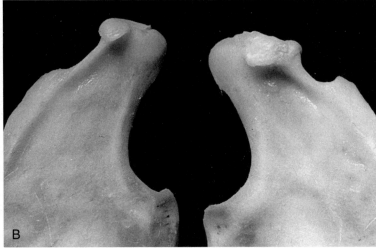

FIGURE 11–15. *A,* Sagittal view of an experimental side and contralateral side of one animal. *Solid arrows* show the flattening and irregular surface of the anterior condylar surface of the side that had surgically created anterior disk displacement. The *open arrow* demonstrates the altered morphology of the coronoid process. *B,* Close-up of the ramus, condylar head, and coronoid process. Note the irregular surface of the condylar head on the experimental side as compared to the contralateral side.

nal derangement and craniofacial form was published by Brand and colleagues.[212] This group compared 23 female volunteers with bilateral normal TMJs, diagnosed with MRI, with 24 female TMD patients with various internal derangements, also diagnosed with MRI. All patients were adults, no attempt was made to group patients with internal derangements by specific diagnosis, and no patients with degenerative joint disease (DJD) were included in the study. Each female in the study had lateral cephalometric radiographs. Twenty-four landmarks were used to generate 23 angular and 26 linear measurements. Results showed that the patients with internal derangement had significantly smaller maxillas and mandibles.

Stein[213] studied 198 consecutive patients from the Temporomandibular Disorders Clinic at the Eastman Dental Center and 80 asymptomatic volunteers. Each subject had had a standard lateral cephalometric radiograph and had been studied with bilateral TMJ MRIs. Right and left full-profile TMJ laminographic radiographs were obtained for 128 of the patients and each of the volunteers. The asymptomatic volun-

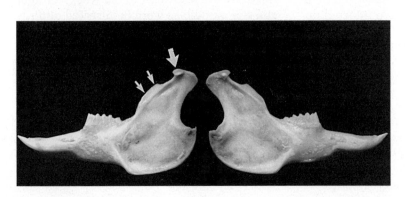

FIGURE 11–16. Sagittal view of a control animal. Note the smooth surface of both condylar heads *(solid large arrow)* and the symmetric shape of the coronoid process *(small arrows).*

teers were examined and determined to have no subjective or objective symptoms of TMD. Groups were divided according to MRI diagnosis of their TMJs (normal, internal derangement, DJD). Groups were also divided by sex owing to significant gender differences that became apparent during statistical analysis. Table 11–21 shows that the female patients with bilateral DJD had a shorter sella-nasion (69.5 mm versus 73.4 mm) and a shorter basion-nasion (Ba-N) (106 mm versus 110.4 mm); a more retrusive maxillary sella-nasion-A point (SNA) (78.9 degrees versus 83.1 degrees) and mandibular denture base sella-nasion-B point (SNB) (75.2 degrees versus 79.6 degrees); a steeper mandibular plane (30.5 degrees versus 24.5 degrees); a larger Y-axis (63.1 degrees versus 58.1 degrees); and a greater overjet (5.2 mm versus 3.1 mm). There was a more divergent relationship of palatal plane to the occlusal plane (11.3 degrees versus 6.3 degrees), Frankfort horizontal plane to occlusal plane (10.8 degrees versus 5.5 degrees), and palatal plane to mandibular plane (31 degrees versus 25.2 degrees). There was also a shorter posterior face height (45.6 mm versus 47.1 mm), giving a retrognathic appearance. The male patients with bilateral DJD and unilateral internal derangement showed similar mandibular characteristics in terms of reduced facial angle and mandibular denture base, as well as increased mandibular plane angle and Y-axis. The male patients with internal derangement showed divergence of palatal plane, occlusal plane, and mandibular plane, similar to that seen in the female patients.

The laminographic data showed that there was more mandibular asymmetry in the female patients with *unilateral* internal derangement and DJD than in the female volunteers with bilateral normal joints. Furthermore, the data generated from the group with unilateral DJD show that the side with joint degeneration was asymmetric (shorter ramal height) as compared to the side without DJD and that the differences can be traced to the mandibular ramus, body, effective length, and gonial angle. Much of the significant deviation in skeletal form was limited to the mandible and its relation to other craniofacial structures. There was also some suggestion that patients affected by more severe forms of unilateral internal derangement showed greater side-to-side differences (4.6 mm versus 1.5 mm for ramus height and 5.2 mm versus 2.1 mm for effective length) for mandibular measurements than did other groups of subjects (Table 11–22 and Fig. 11–17).

The studies previously presented suggest a link between craniofacial development and internal derangement of the TMJ. Furthermore, they suggest that internal derangement may lead to specific types of craniofacial morphology, which include high mandibular plane angles, mandibular retrognathia with or without open bite, and facial asymmetry in both the growing and the nongrowing patient and that these types of patients frequently present for OS. It should be clearly pointed out that each of these studies represents a simple static snapshot in time; they do not show actual dynamic change with time. Once again, it must be

TABLE 11–21.	Cephalometric Analysis: Values for Selected Measurements for Female Bilateral Normal Volunteers and Bilateral DDN/DJD Patients

Cephalometric Analysis	Bilateral Normal	Bilateral DDN/DJD
Cranial base		
S-N (mm)	73.4*	69.5*
Ba-N (mm)	110.4*	106.0*
Skeletal pattern		
Maxillary		
SNA	83.1*	78.9*
Mandibular		
SNB	79.6*	75.2*
Mandibular Plane	24.5*	30.5*
Y-axis	58.1*	63.1*
Intermaxillary		
FH-OP (Occlusal cant)	5.5*	10.8*
PP-OP	6.3*	11.3*
PP-MP	25.2*	31*
Denture pattern		
Intermaxillary		
Horizontal overlap	3.1*	5.2*
Vertical relations		
Ar-Go (lower posterior face height)	47.1*	45.6*

*$P < .05$.
DDN, disk displacement without reduction; DJD, degenerative joint disease; S-N sella-nasion; Ba-N, basion-nasion; SNA, sella-nasion-A point; SNB, sella-nasion-B point; FH, Frankfort horizontal plane; OP, occlusal plane; PP, palatal plane; MP, mandibular plane; Ar-Go, articular-gonion.

TABLE 11–22.	Laminographic Measurements for Mean Side-to-Side Differences for Female Bilateral Normal Volunteers and Unilateral DDN/DJD Patients

Laminographic Measurements	Bilateral Normal	Unilateral DDN/DJD
Ramus	1.5*	4.6*
Effective length	2.1*	5.2*

*$P < .05$.
DDN, disk displacement without reduction; DJD, degenerative joint disease.

reiterated that the ability to determine whether a connection truly exists between disk displacement and craniofacial form will come only from longitudinal, prospective studies.

The points raised in this chapter suggest that further prospective research is needed to help elucidate the full effect of OS (type of osteotomy and fixation) on TMJ signs and symptoms. Furthermore, patients in need of OS may represent a risk factor either for having TMJ signs and symptoms prior to surgery or for developing them postsurgically.

Summary

This chapter has evaluated dental and skeletal variables of patients presenting with and without TMJ pain. The profession has always looked at dental occlusion (uneven contacts in centric relation, discrepancies between centric relation and centric occlusion, deep bite, open bite, tooth contacts in lateral jaw movement) as specific etiologies of TMJ pain and dysfunction. The present review suggests the following.

Anterior Controls There is an increase in horizontal overlap of the anterior teeth in symptomatic TMD patients. This increase is more profound when the subjects have bilateral DJD. This suggests that some of the horizontal changes in symptomatic patients (and probably nonpatients) are directly related to internal derangements of the TMJs.

Coupling of the Anterior Teeth There does not seem to be a strong relationship between the type of anterior guidance (canine versus group function) and the presence or absence of TMJ pain and dysfunction. The literature also suggests that bruxing habits may not be eliminated by changing the occlusal scheme.

Missing Posterior Teeth The literature does not support the notion that replacement of missing teeth will decrease the risk of or cure TMJ disorders. Missing teeth do seem to be associated with pain in or around the TMJ and mandible. These observations require further investigation.

Molar Class There does not seem to be a major shift to class II division 1 or 2 in symptomatic patients. Although there are isolated instances when it seems obvious that class II division 1 has a high prevalence among symptomatic patients, this may be because of how the sample is obtained (i.e., OS studies).

Discrepancy between Centric Relation and Centric Occlusion There do not seem to be major differences in the prevalence of RCP-ICP contacts in symptomatic patients. This suggests that adjustment of the occlusion to eliminate RCP-ICP contacts should be done only when splint therapy has decreased pain or the source of the interfering contact is obvious to the clinician or the patient.

Non–Working Side Contacts Symptomatic patients had fewer non–working side contacts than did asymptomatic volunteers. Therefore, it is difficult to consider removal of these contacts as part of therapy unless they are noted to be a nuisance.

Orthodontic Treatment There does

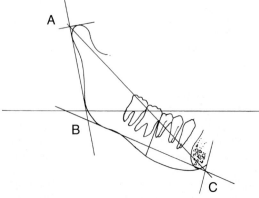

FIGURE 11–17. Mandibular ramus length *(A–B)*, body length *(B–C)*, and effective length *(A–C)*.

not seem to be a correlation between the presence or absence of TMJ symptoms and having or not having orthodontic treatment. Therefore, a clinician cannot suggest to a patient that orthodontic therapy will alleviate TMJ symptoms or prevent symptoms from developing at a later date.

Condyle Position There seems to be a slight shift to a more distal condyle position in symptomatic patients with disk displacement. This shift represents about 18% to 24% of the symptomatic patients with disk displacement. The data presented here suggest that symptomatic patients with disk displacement tend to have an increase in the prevalence of condyles located distally. The construction of two-by-two tables for calculations of sensitivity and specificity in our data and by Kamelchuk and colleagues[58] suggest that the position of the condyle is not a good predictor of the presence or absence of joint derangement.

The alteration of condyle position, as a treatment procedure, has been tested in patients with DDR and demonstrates that pain can be altered with this procedure. There are no studies demonstrating alteration of condyle position in symptomatic patients with DDN or symptomatic normal joints. Therefore, there are no treatment outcome data to support the hypothesis that alteration of the position of the condyle (i.e., moving it from distal to concentric) for the purposes of altering joint loading is acceptable. There is some evidence to support changes in condyle position in patients with documented evidence of DDR.

REFERENCES

1. Okeson JP: Orofacial Pain: Guidelines for Assessment, Diagnosis and Management. Chicago: Quintessence, 1996, p 119.
2. Schiffman EL, Fricton JR, Haley DP, Shapiro BL: The relationship between the level of mandibular pain and dysfunction and stage of temporomandibular joint internal derangement. J Dent Res 1992;71:1812–1815.
3. Stack BC, Funt LA: Temporomandibular dysfunction in children. J Pedod 1977;1:240.
4. Owen AH: Orthodontic/orthopedic treatment of craniomandibular pain dysfunction. Part 2. Posterior condylar displacement. J Craniomandib Pract 1985;3:344–349.
5. Franks AS: The dental arch of patients presenting with temporomandibular joint dysfunction. Br J Oral Surg 1967;5:157–166.
6. Roth RH: Temporomandibular pain-dysfunction and occlusal relationships. Angle Orthod 1973;43:136–153.
7. Berry DC, Watkinson AC: Mandibular dysfunction and incisor relationship. Br Dent J 1978; 44:74–77.
8. Ricketts RM: Clinical implications of the temporomandibular joint. Am J Orthod 1966;52:416–439.
9. Bell WE: Clinical Managements of Temporomandibular Joint Disorders. Chicago, Year Book Medical Publishers, 1982, pp 71–74.
10. Liebman M, Gazit C, Lilos P: Mandibular dysfunction in 10–18 year olds as related to morphologic occlusion. J Oral Rehabil 1985;12:209–214.
11. Mohlin B, Kopp S: A clinical study on the relationship between malocclusion, occlusal interferences and mandibular pain and dysfunction. Swed Dent J 1978;12:105–112.
12. Pullinger AG, Solberg WK, Hollander L, Peterson A: Relationships of mandibular condylar position to dental occlusion factors in an asymptomatic population. Am J Orthod 1987;91:200–206.
13. Runge ME, Sadowsky C, Sakols EL, DeGole EA: The relationship between temporomandibular joint sounds and malocclusion. Am J Orthod Dentofacial Orthop 1989;96:36–42.
14. Seligman DA, Pullinger AG: The role of the intercuspal relationships in temporomandibular disorders: A review. J Craniomandib Disord Facial Oral Pain 1991;5:96–106.
15. Seligman DA, Pullinger AG, Solberg WK: Temporomandibular disorders. Part III: Occlusal and articular factors associated with muscle tenderness. J Prosthet Dent 1988;59:483–489.
16. Solberg WK, Flint RT, Brantner JP: Temporomandibular joint pain and dysfunction: A clinical study of emotional and occlusal components. J Prosthet Dent 1972;28:412–422.
17. Roberts CA, Tallents RH, Katzberg RW, et al: Comparison of internal derangements of the TMJ with occlusal findings. Oral Surg Oral Med Oral Pathol 1987;63:645–650.
18. Riolo ML, Brandt D, Ten Have TR: Associations between occlusal characteristics and signs and symptoms of TMJ dysfunction in children and young adults. Am J Orthod Dentofacial Orthop 1987;92:467–477.
19. Shiau YY: Incidence of temporomandibular disorders in teenagers of Taiwan. J Dent Res 1989; 68:740.
20. Gunn SM, Woolfold BW, Faja BW: Malocclusion and TMJ symptoms in migrant children. J Dent Res 1987;66:253.
21. Cacchiotti D, Plesh O, Bianchi P, et al: Signs and symptoms in samples with and without temporomandibular disorders. J Craniomandib Disord Facial Oral Pain 1991;5:167–172.
22. Heloe B, Heiberg AN, Krogstad BS: A multiprofessional study of patients with myofascial pain dysfunction syndrome I. Acta Odontol Scand 1980;38:109–117.
23. Heloe B, Heloe LA: Characteristics of a group of patients with temporomandibular joint disorders. Community Dent Oral Epidemiol 1975;3:72–79.
24. Pedersen A, Hansen H-J: Internal derangement of the temporomandibular joint in 211 patients: Symptoms and treatment. Community Dent Oral Epidemiol 1987;15:339–343.
25. Pullinger AG, Seligman DA: The degree to which attrition characterizes differentiated patient groups of temporomandibular joint disorders. J Orofacial Pain 1993;7:196–208.
26. Tegelberg A, Kopp S: Clinical findings in the sto-

matognathic system for individuals with rheumatoid arthritis and osteoarthritis. Acta Odontol Scand 1987;45:65–75.

27. Williamson EH, Hall JT, Zwemer JD: Swallowing patterns in human subjects with and without temporomandibular dysfunction. Am J Orthod Dentofacial Orthop 1990;98:507–511.

28. Akerman S, Kopp S, Nilner M, et al: Relationship between clinical and radiologic findings of the temporomandibular joint in rheumatoid arthritis. Oral Surg Oral Med Oral Pathol 1988;66:639–643.

29. Tsolka P, Fenlon MR, McCullock AJ, et al: A controlled clinical electromyographic and kinesiographic assessment of craniomandibular disorders in women. J Orofacial Pain 1994;8:80–89.

30. Schiffman EL, Fricton JR, Heley D: The relationship of occlusion, parafunctional habits and recent life events to mandibular dysfunction in a non-patient population. J Oral Rehabil 1992; 19:201–223.

31. Lieberman NU, Gazit E, Fuchs C, et al: Mandibular dysfunction in 10–18 year old school children as related to morphologic malocclusion. Oral Rehabil 1985;12:209–214.

32. Castaneda R, McNeill C, Noble W: Biomechanical factors in TMJ osteoarthritis. J Dent Res 1988;67:124.

33. Castaneda R, McNeill C, Guerrero A: Biomechanics in TMJ osteoarthritis. J Dent Res 1989; 68:259.

34. Link JL, Nickerson JW: Temporomandibular joint internal derangements in an orthognathic surgery population. Int J Adult Orthod Orthognath Surg 1992;7:161–169.

35. Dibbets JMH, Van der Weele LT, Uildriks AKJ: Symptoms of TMJ dysfunction: Indicators of growth patterns? J Pedod 1985;9:265–284.

36. Williamson EH: Temporomandibular dysfunction in pretreatment adolescent patients. Am J Orthod 1977;72:429–433.

37. Humerfelt A, Slagsvold O: Changes in occlusion and craniofacial pattern between 11 and 25 years of age. Trans R Soc Ortho 1972;2:113–122.

38. Björk A, Palling M: Adolescent changes in sagittal jaw relation, alveolar prognathy and incisal inclination. Acta Odontol Scand 1955;12:201–232.

39. Ronquillo HI, Guay J, Tallents RH, et al: Comparison of internal derangements with condyle position: Horizontal and vertical overlap and angle class. J Craniomandib Disord 1988;3:137–140.

40. Stein S, Tallents RH, Hatala MA, et al: The effect of TMJ internal derangement on craniofacial morphology. Paper presented at the annual winter meeting of the Rochester Section of the AADR, 1996.

41. Katzberg WR, Westesson PL, Tallents RH, et al: Temporomandibular joint: Magnetic resonance assessment of rotational and sideways disc displacements. Radiology 1988;169:741–748.

42. Pullinger AG, Seligman DA, Gornbein JA: A multiple logistic regression analysis of the risk and relative odds of temporomandibular disorders as a function of common occlusal features. J Dent Res 1993;72:968–979.

43. Erickson LP, Hunter WS: Class II, division 2 treatment and mandibular growth. Angle Orthod 1985;55:215–224.

44. Swann GC: The diagnosis and interception of class II, division 2 malocclusion. Am J Orthod 1954;40:325–340.

45. Thuer U, Ingerval B, Burgin W, Demisch A: No posterior mandibular displacement in Angle class II, division 2 malocclusion as revealed with electromyography and sirognathography. Eur J Orthod 1992;14:162–171.

46. Gianelly AA, Hunter JC, Boffa J: Condylar position and class II deep bite, no-overjet malocclusion. J Orthod Dentofacial Orthop 1989;96:428–432.

47. Hatala MA, Ribeiro R, Tallents RH, et al: The prevalence of open bite in symptomatic temporomandibular joint dysfunction patients. In preparation.

48. Tallents RH, Katzberg RW, Murphy WC, Proskin H: Magnetic resonance imaging findings in asymptomatic volunteers and symptomatic TMD patients. J Prosthet Dent 1996;75:529–533.

49. Ribeiro R, Tallents RH, Katzberg RW: The prevalence of disc displacement in symptomatic and asymptomatic volunteers from 6 to 25 years. J Orofacial Pain 1997;11:37–47.

50. Hans MG, Liederman J, Goldberg J, et al: A comparison of clinical examination, history and magnetic resonance imaging for identifying orthodontic patients with temporomandibular joint disorders. Am J Orthod Dentofacial Orthop 1992;101:54–59.

51. Davant TS, Green CS, Perry HT, Lautenschlager EP: A quantitative computer assisted analysis of disc displacement in patients with internal derangement using sagittal view magnetic resonance imaging. J Oral Maxillofac Surg 1993;51:974–979.

52. Shellhas KP, Piper MA, Omlie MR: Facial skeleton remodeling due to temporomandibular joint degeneration: An imaging study of 100 patients. AJNR Am J Neuroradiol 1990;11:541–551.

53. Kuwahara T, Maruyama T: Relationship between condylar atrophy and tooth loss in craniomandibular disorders. J Osaka Univ Dent Sch 1992;32:91–96.

54. Kuwahara T, Maruyama T: Condylar atrophy in craniomandibular disorders. J Osaka Univ Dent Sch 1992;32:84–90.

55. Kerstens HTC, Tuinzing DB, van der Kwast WAM: Temporomandibular joint symptoms in orthognathic surgery. J Craniomaxillofac Surg 1989;17:215–218.

56. Roberts CA, Tallents RH, Katzberg WR, et al: Correlation of clinical parameters to the arthrographic depiction of TMJ internal derangements. Oral Surg Oral Med Oral Pathol 1988;66:32–36.

57. Brand JW, Whinery JG, Anderson QN, Keenan KM: Condyle position as a predictor of temporomandibular joint internal derangement. Oral Surg Oral Med Oral Pathol 1989;67:469–476.

58. Kamelchuk L, Nebbe B, Baker C, Major P: Adolescent TMJ tomography and magnetic resonance imaging: A comparative study. J Orofacial Pain 1997;11:321–327.

59. Schuyler CH: Factors of occlusion applicable to restorative dentistry. J Prosthet Dent 1953;3:772–782.

60. Muhleman HR, Savdir S, Rateitschak KH: Tooth mobility—its causes and significance. J Periodontol 1965;36:148–153.

61. Glickman I: Inflammation and trauma from occlusion, co-destructive factors in chronic periodontal disease. J Periodontol 1963;34:5–10.

62. Hillam DG: Stress in the periodontal ligament. J Periodontal Res 1973;8:51–56.

63. Thornton LJ: Anterior guidance: Group function/canine guidance: A literature review. J Prosthet Dent 1990;64:479–482.

64. Belser UC, Hannam AG: The influence of altered working-side occlusal guidance on masticatory muscles and related jaw movement. J Prosthet Dent 1985;53:406–413.

65. Holmgren K, Sheikholeslam A, Riise C: Effect of a full arch maxillary occlusal splint on parafunctional activity during sleep in patients with nocturnal bruxism and signs and symptoms of craniomandibular disorders. J Prosthet Dent 1993;69:293–297.

66. Gentz R: Apparatus for recording bruxism during sleep. Swed Dent J 1972;65:327–342.

67. Kydd WL, Daly C: Duration of nocturnal tooth contacts during bruxism. J Prosthet Dent 1985;53:717–721.

68. Akerman S, Kopp S, Nilner M, et al: Relationship between clinical and radiologic findings of the temporomandibular joint in rheumatoid arthritis. Oral Surg Oral Med Oral Pathol 1988;66:639–643.

69. Tegelberg A, Kopp S: Clinical findings in the stomatognathic system for individuals with rheumatoid arthritis and osteoarthritis. Acta Odontol Scand 1987;45:65–75.

70. Kopp S: Clinical findings in temporomandibular joint osteoarthrosis. Scand J Dent Res 1977;5:434–443.

71. Martinez M, Aguilar N, Barghi N, et al: Prevalence of TMJ clicking in subjects with missing posterior teeth. J Dent Res 1984;63:345.

72. Barghi N, Aguilar CD, Martinez C, et al: Prevalence of types of temporomandibular joint clicking in subjects with missing posterior teeth. J Prosthet Dent 1987;57:617–620.

73. Holmlund A, Helsing G, Axelsson S: The temporomandibular joint: A comparison of clinical and arthroscopic findings. J Prosthet Dent 1989;62:61–65.

74. Holmlund A, Axelsson S: Temporomandibular joint osteoarthrosis: Correlation of clinical and arthroscopic findings with degree of molar support. Acta Odontol Scand 1994;52:214–218.

75. Whittaker DK, Jones JW, Edwards PW, et al: Studies on the temporomandibular joint of an eighteenth-century London population (Spitalfields). J Oral Rehabil 1990;17:89–97.

76. Widmalm SE, Westesson P-L, Kim I-K, et al: Temporomandibular joint pathology related to sex, age and dentition in autopsy material. Oral Surg Oral Med Oral Pathol 1994;78:416–425.

77. Pekkarinen V, Yli-Urpo A: Helkimo's indices before and after prosthetic treatment in selected cases. J Oral Rehabil 1987;14:35–42.

78. Helkimo M: Studies on function and dysfunction of the masticatory system. III: Analysis of anamnestic and clinical recordings of dysfunction with the aid of indices. Swed Dent J 1974;67:165–182.

79. Swanljung O, Rantanen T: Functional disorders of the masticatory system in southwest Finland. Community Dent Oral Epidemiol 1979;7:177–182.

80. Kirveskari P, Alanen P: Association between tooth loss and TMJ dysfunction. J Oral Rehabil 1985;12:189–194.

81. Wilding RJC, Owen CP: The prevalence of temporomandibular joint dysfunction. in edentulous non–denture wearing individuals. J Oral Rehabil 1987;14:175–182.

82. Pullinger AG, Baldioceda F, Bibb CA: Relationship of TMJ articular soft tissue to underlying bone in young adult condyles. J Dent Res 1990;69:1512–1518.

83. Muir CB, Goss AN: The radiologic morphology of asymptomatic temporomandibular joints. Oral Surg Oral Med Oral Pathol 1990;70:349–354.

84. Lundeen TF, Scruggs RR, McKinney MW, et al: TMJ symptomatology among denture patients. J Craniomandib Disord Facial Oral Pain 1990;4:40–46.

85. Leake JL, Hawkins R, Locker D: Social and functional impact of reduced posterior dental units in older adults. J Oral Rehabil 1994;21:1–10.

86. DeBoever JA, Adriaens PA: Occlusal relationship in patients with pain-dysfunction symptoms in the temporomandibular joint. J Oral Rehabil 1983;10:1–7.

87. Witter DJ, De Haan AFJ, Kayser AF, VanRossum GM: A 6 year follow-up study of oral function in shortened dental arches. Part I: Craniomandibular dysfunction and oral comfort. J Oral Rehabil 1994;21:113–125.

88. Witter DJ, De Haan AFJ, Kayser AF, VanRossum GM: A 6 year follow-up study of oral function in shortened dental arches. Part II: Craniomandibular dysfunction and oral comfort. J Oral Rehabil 1994;21:353–366.

89. Lederman KH, Clayton JA: Restored occlusions. Part II: The relationship of clinical and subjective symptoms to varying degrees of TMJ dysfunction. J Prosthet Dent 1982;47:303–309.

90. Bouquot JE, Roberts AM, Person P, Christian J: Neuralgia inducing cavitational osteonecrosis (NICO): Osteomyelitis in 224 jawbone samples from patients with facial neuralgia. Oral Surg Oral Med Oral Pathol 1992;73:307–319.

91. Bouquot JE, Christian J: Long term effects of jawbone curettage on pain of facial neuralgia. J Oral Maxillfac Surg 1995;53:387–397.

92. Fried K, Arvidsson J, Robertson B, Pfaller K: Anterograde horseradish peroxidase tracing and immunohistochemistry of the trigeminal ganglion tooth pulp neurons after dental nerve lesions in the rat. Neuroscience 1991;43:269–278.

93. Gobel S, Binck JM: Degenerative changes in primary trigeminal axons in the neurones of the nucleus caudalis following tooth pulled extirpations in the cat. Brain Res 1977;132:347–354.

94. Gobel S: An electron microscopic analysis of the trans-synaptic effects of peripheral nerve injury subsequent to tooth pulp extirpations of neurons in laminae I and II of the medullary dorsal horn. J Neurosci 1984;4:2281–2290.

95. Ueno S: The uptake of horseradish peroxidase in the temporomandibular joint synovium of the rat following unilateral extraction of molars. J Dent Res 1982;61:516–520.

96. Clements JR, Magnusson KR, Hautman J, Beitz AJ: Rat tooth pulp projections to spinal trigeminal subnucleus caudalis are glutamate-like immunoreactive. J Comp Neurol 1991;309;281–288.

97. Glueck CJ, McMahon RE, Bouquot JE, et al: Thrombophilia, hyperfibrinolysis and osteonecrosis of the jaws. Oral Surg Oral Med Oral Pathol 1996;81:557–566.

98. Bouquot JE: Ischemia and infarction of the jaws—the "phantom" pain of NICO. J Craniomandib Pract 1994;12:138–139.

99. Roberts AM, Person P, Chandran NB, Hori JM: Further observations on dental parameters of trigeminal and atypical facial neuralgias. Oral Surg Oral Med Oral Pathol 1984;58:121–129.

100. Kubo Y: The uptake of horseradish peroxidase in monkey temporomandibular joint synovium after occlusal alteration. J Dent Res 1987;66:1049–1054.

101. Black GV: A Work on Special Dental Pathology, ed 2. Chicago, Medico-Dental, 1920.

102. Ratner EJ, Person P, Kleinman DJ, et al: Jawbone cavities and trigeminal and atypical facial neuralgias. Oral Surg Oral Med Oral Pathol 1979;48:3–20.

103. Roberts AM, Person P: Etiology and treatment of idiopathic trigeminal and atypical facial neuralgias. Oral Surg Oral Med Oral Pathol 1979;48:298–308.

104. Hamba M, Muro M, Hiraide T, Ozawa H: Expression of c-fos-like protein in the rat brain after injection of interleukin-1-beta into the gingiva. Brain Res Bull 1994;34:61–68.

105. Ishimaru J, Handa Y, Kurita K, Goss AN: The effect of occlusal loss on normal and pathological temporomandibular joints: An animal study. J Craniomaxillofac Surg 1994;22:95–102.

106. Ishimaru J, Goss AN: A model for osteoarthritis of the temporomandibular joint. J Oral Maxillofac Surg 1992;50:1191–1195.

107. Bosanquet A, Ishimaru J, Goss AN: Effect of experimental disc perforation in sheep temporomandibular joints. Int J Oral Maxillofac Surg 1991;20:177–181.

108. Ishimaru J, Handa Y, Kurita K, Goss AN: Effect of marrow perforation on the sheep temporomandibular joint. Int J Oral Maxillofac Surg 1992;21:239–242.

109. Pirttiniemi P, Kantomaa T, Salo L, Tuominen M: Effect of reduced articular function on deposition of type I and type II collagens in the mandibular condyle cartilage of the rat. Arch Oral Biol 1996;41:127–131.

110. Shaw RM, Molyneux GS: The effects of mandibular hypofunction on the development of the mandibular disc in the rabbit. Arch Oral Biol 1994;39:747–752.

111. Rosenblum R: Class II malocclusion: Mandibular retrusion or maxillary protrusion? Angle Orthod 1995;65:49–62.

112. Blake SR: Study of the incidence of malocclusion and facial characteristics in high school students in Seattle, age 15–20. Thesis, Department of Orthodontics, School of Dentistry, University of Washington, Seattle, 1954.

113. Pullinger AG, Seligman DA, Solberg WK: Temporomandibular disorders. Part I: Functional status, dentomorphologic features, and sex differences in a non-patient population. J Prosthet Dent 1988;59:228–235.

114. Melnick AK: A cephalometric study of mandibular asymmetry in a longitudinally followed sample of growing children. Am J Orthod Dentofacial Orthop 1992;101:355–366.

115. de Latt A, van Steenberghe D: Occlusal relationships and temporomandibular joint dysfunction. Part I: Epidemiologic findings. J Prosthet Dent 1985;54:835–842.

116. Solberg WK, Woo MW, Houston JB: Prevalence of mandibular dysfunction in young adults. J Am Dent Assoc 1979;98:25–34.

117. Helkimo M: Studies on function and dysfunction of the masticatory system. Swed Dent J 1974;67:1–18.

118. Hansson T, Nelner M: A study of the occurrence of symptoms of disease of the temporomandibular joint masticatory musculature, and related structures. J Oral Rehabil 1975;2:313–324.

119. Seligman DA, Pullinger AG: Association of occlusal variables among refined TM patient diagnostic groups. J Craniomandib Disord Facial Oral Pain 1989;3:227–236.

120. Rugh JD, Barghi N, Drago CJ: Experimental occlusal discrepancies and nocturnal bruxism. J Prosthet Dent 1984;51:548–553.

121. Riise C, Sheikholeslam A: The influence of experimental interfering occlusal contacts on the postural activity of the anterior temporal and masseter muscles in young adults. J Oral Rehabil 1982;9:419–425.

122. Randow K, Carlsson K, Edlund I, Oberg T: The effect of an occlusal interference on the masticatory system: An experimental investigation. Odont Revy 1976;27:245–256.

123. Kyrkanides S, Tallents RH, Macher DJ, et al: Expression of sP and CGRP in the trigeminal nuclear complex in an animal TMJ pain model. Paper presented at the Allen Brewer Upstate Prosthodontic Conference, Eastman Dental Center, Rochester, NY, June 12, 1997.

124. Kardachi BJR, Bailey JO, Ash MM: A comparison of biofeedback and occlusal adjustment on bruxism. J Periodontol 1978;49:367–372.

125. Bailey JO, Rugh JD: Effect of occlusal adjustment on bruxism as monitored by nocturnal EMG recordings. J Dent Res 1980;59:317.

126. Clark GT, Adler RC: A critical evaluation of occlusal therapy: Occlusal adjustment procedures. J Am Dent Assoc 1985;110:743–750.

127. Magnusson T, Carlsson GE: Occlusal adjustment in patients with residual or recurrent signs of mandibular dysfunction. J Prosthet Dent 1983;49:706–710.

128. Vallon D, Ekberg EC, Nilner M, Kopp S: Short term effect of occlusal adjustment on craniomandibular disorders including headaches. Acta Odontol Scand 1991;49:89–96.

129. Vallon D, Ekberg EC, Nilner M, Kopp S: Occlusal adjustments in patients with craniomandibular disorders including headaches. A 3 and 6 month follow-up. Acta Odontol Scand 1995;53:55–59.

130. Wenneberg B, Nystrom T, Carlsson GE: Occlusal equilibration and other stomatognathic treatment in patients with mandibular dysfunction and headache. J Prosthet Dent 1988;59:478–483.

131. Kirveskari P, Alanen P, Jämsä J: Association between craniomandibular disorders and occlusal interferences in children. J Prosthet Dent 1992;67:692–696.

132. Broton JG, Sessle BJ: Reflex excitation of masticatory muscles induced by algesic chemicals applied to the temporomandibular joint of the cat. Arch Oral Biol 1988;33:741–747.

133. Ingervall B, Carlsson GE: Masticatory muscle activity before and after elimination of balancing side occlusal interference. J Oral Rehabil 1982;9:183–192.

134. Magnusson T, Enbom L: Signs and symptoms of mandibular dysfunction after introduction of experimental balancing-side interferences. Acta Odontol Scand 1984;42:129–135.

135. Ingerval B, Carlsson GE: Masticatory muscle activity before and after elimination of balancing side occlusal interference. J Oral Rehabil 1982;9:183–192.

136. Agerberg G, Sandstrom R: Frequency of occlusal interferences: A clinical study in teenagers and young adults. J Prosthet Dent 1988;59:212–217.

137. Hochman N, Ehrlich J, Yaffe A: Tooth contact during dynamic lateral excursions in young adults. J Oral Rehabil 1995;22:221–224.

138. Kirveskari P, Alanen P, Jamsa T: Association between craniomandibular disorders and occlusal interferences. J Prosthet Dent 1989;62:66–69.

139. Magnusson T, Carlsson GE, Egermark I: Changes in clinical signs of craniomandibular disorders from the age of 15 to 25 years. J Orofacial Pain 1994;8:207–215.

140. Egermark I, Ronnerman A: Temporomandibular disorders in the active phase of orthodontic treatment. J Oral Rehabil 1995;22:613–618.

141. Minagi S, Watanabe H, Sato T, Tsuru H: The relationship between balacing-side occlusal contact patterns and temporomandibular joint sounds in humans: Proposition of the concept of balancing-side protection. J Craniomandib Disord Facial Oral Pain 1990;4:251–256.

142. Sadowsky C, Polson AM: Temporomandibular disorders and functional occlusion after orthodontic treatment: Results of two long-term studies. Am J Orthod 1984;86:386–390.

143. Larsson E, Ronnerman A: Mandibular dysfunction symptoms in orthodontically treated patients ten years after completion of treatment. Eur J Orthod 1981;3:89–94.

144. Janson M, Hasund A: Functional problems in orthodontic patients out of retention. Eur J Orthod 1981;3:173–179.

145. Dibbets J, van der Weele L: Orthodontic treatment in relation to symptoms attributed to dysfunction of the temporomandibular joint. Am J Orthod 1987;91:193–199.

146. Helm S, Kreiborg S, Solow B: Malocclusion at adolescence related to self-reported tooth loss and functional disorders in adulthood. Am J Orthod 1984;85:393–400.

147. Siebert G: Zur Frage okklusaler Interferenzer bei Jugendlischen. Dtsch Zahnartzl 1975;30:539–543.

148. Dahl BL, Krogstad BS, Ogaard B, Eckersberg T: Signs and symptoms of craniomandibular disorders in two groups of 19-year-old individuals, one treated orthodontically and the other not. Acta Odontol Scand 1988;46:89–93.

149. Apt K, Goldin B, Sommers E, Tallents R: Orthodontics as possible etiology of TMJ dysfunction. Abstract presented at the Farrar-Norgaard Society meeting, Rochester, NY, August 1989.

150. Peltola JS, Kononen M, Nystrom M: A follow-up study of radiographic findings in the mandibular condyles of orthodontically treated patients and associations with TMD. J Dent Res 1995;74:1571–1576.

151. Geering-Gaerny J, Rakosi T: Initwl symptome von Kiefergelenk-storungen bei Kindern im alter von 8-14 Jahren. Schweiz Monatsschr Zahnkeilkd 1971;81:691–712.

152. Sadowsky C, BeGole E: Long term status of temporomandibular joint function and functional occlusion after orthodontic treatment. Am J Orthod 1980;78:201–212.

153. Blaschke D, Blaschke T: Normal TMJ bone relationships in centric occlusion. J Dent Res 1981;60:98–104.

154. Pullinger A: The significance of condyle position in normal and abnormal temporomandibular joint function. In Clark G, Solberg W (eds): Perspectives in Temporomandibular Disorders. Chicago, Quintessence, 1987, pp 89–103.

155. Blaschke D, Chase DC: Differences in TMJ condyle-temporal relationships in normal men and women. J Dent Res 1984;63:266.

156. Madsen B: Normal variation in anatomy, condylar movements and arthrosis of the TMJ. Acta Radiol Diagn 1966;4:273–288.

157. Ronquillo HI, Guay J, Tallents RH, et al: Tomographic analyses of mandibular condyle position as compared to arthrographic findings of the temporomandibular joint. J Craniomandib Disord 1988;2:59–64.

158. Katzberg R, Keith DA, Guralnick WC, TenEick WR: Internal derangements of the temporomandibular joint: An assessment of condylar position in centric occlusion. J Prosthet Dent 1983;49:250–254.

159. Bean L, Thomas C: Significance of condylar positions in patients with temporomandibular disorders. J Am Dent Assoc 1987;114:76–77.

160. Pullinger AG, Solberg WK, Hollander L, Peterson A: Relationships of mandibular condyle position to dental occlusion factors in an asymptomatic population. Am J Orthod Dentofacial Orthop 1987;91:200–206.

161. Pullinger AG, Solberg WK, Hollender L, Guichet D: Tomographic analysis of mandibular condyle position in diagnostic subgroups of temporomandibular disorders. J Prosthet Dent 1986;55:723–729.

162. Tallents RH, Katzberg WR, Roberts CA, et al: Use of protrusive splint therapy in anterior disk displacement of the temporomandibular joint: A 1 to 3 year follow-up. J Prosthet Dent 1990;63:336–341.

163. Lundh H, Westesson PL, Kopp S, Tillstrom BA: Anterior repositioning splint in the treatment of temporomandibular joint with reciprocal clicking: Comparison with a flat occlusal splint and untreated control group. Oral Surg Oral Med Oral Pathol 1985;60:131–136.

164. Summer JD, Westesson PL: Mandibular repositioning can be effective in treatment of reducing TMJ disc displacement: A long-term clinical and MR follow-up. J Craniomandib Pract 1997;15:107–120.

165. Maloney F, Howard JA: Internal derangements of the temporomandibular joint. III. Anterior repositioning splint therapy. Aust Dent J 1986;31:30–39.

166. Gianelly AA, Hughes HM, Wohigemuth P, Gildea G: Condylar position and extraction. Am J Orthod Dentofacial Orthop 1988;93:201–205.

167. Tucker MR, Thomas PM: Temporomandibular pain and dysfunction in the orthodontic surgical patient: Rationale for evaluation and treatment sequencing. Int J Adult Orthod Orthognath Surg 1986;1:11–22.

168. Greene CS, Marbach JJ: Epidemiologic studies of mandibular dysfunction: A critical review. J Prosthet Dent 1982;48:184–190.

169. Mohlin B, Koop S: A clinical study on the relationship between malocclusions, occlusal interferences and mandibular pain and dysfunction. Swed Dent J 1978;2:105–112.

170. Roberts CA, Tallents RH, Katzberg RW, et al: Comparison of internal derangements of the TMJ with occlusal findings. Oral Surg Oral Med Oral Pathol 1987;63:645–650.

171. Laskin DM, Ryan WA, Greene CS: Incidence of temporomandibular symptoms in patients with major skeletal malocclusions: A survey of oral and maxillofacial surgery training programs. Oral Surg Oral Med Oral Pathol 1986;61:537–541.

172. Dahlberg G, Petersson A, Westesson PL, Eriksson L: Disk displacement and temporomandibular joint symptoms in orthognathic surgery patients. Oral Surg Oral Med Oral Pathol Oral Radiol Endod 1995;79:273–277.

173. Solberg WK, Flint RT, Brantner JP: Temporomandibular joint pain and dysfunction: A clinical study of emotional and occlusal components. J Prosthet Dent 1972;28:412–422.

174. Clarke G: Occlusion and myofacial pain dysfunction: Is there a relationship? J Am Dent Assoc 1982;104:443–446.

175. Seligman DA, Pullinger AG, Solberg WK: Prevalence of dental attrition and its association with factors of age, gender, occlusion and TMJ symptomatology. J Dent Res 1988;67:1323–1333.

176. Droukas B, Lindee C, Carlsson GE: Occlusion and mandibular dysfunction: A clinical study of patients referred for functional disturbances of the masticatory system. J Prosthet Dent 1985;53:402–406.

177. Piecuch J, Tideman H, Dekoomen H: Short-face syndrome: Treatment of myofascial pain dysfunction by maxillary disimpaction. Oral Surg 1980;49:112–116.

178. Karabouta I, Martis C: The TMJ dysfunction syndrome before and after sagittal split osteotomy of the rami. J Oral Maxillofac Surg 1985;13:185–188.

179. Magnusson T, Ahlborg G, Finne K, et al: Changes in temporomandibular joint pain-dysfunction after surgical correction of dentofacial anomalies. Int J Maxillofac Surg 1986;15:707–714.

180. Kerstens HC, Tuinzing DB, van der Kwast WA: Temporomandibular joint symptoms in orthognathic surgery. J Craniomaxillofac Surg 1989;17:215–218.

181. White CS, Dolwick MF: Prevalence and variance of temporomandibular dysfunction in orthognathic surgery patients. Int J Adult Orthod Orthognath Surg 1992;7:1–14.

182. Upton LG, Scott RF, Hayward JR: Major maxillomandibular malrelations and temporomandibular joint pain-dysfunction. J Prosthet Dent 1984;51:686–690.

183. Kahnberg KE: TMJ complications associated with superior repositioning of the maxilla. J Craniomandib Pract 1988;6:312–315.

184. Herbosa EG, Rotskoff KS, Ramos BF, Ambrookian HS: Condylar position in superior maxillary repositioning, and its effect on the temporomandibular joint. J Oral Maxillofac Surg 1990;48:690–696.

185. Egermark-Eriksson I, Kahnberg KE, Ridell A: Longitudinal study of function and dysfunction in the stomatognathic system after maxillary osteotomy with anterior inferior repositioning of the maxilla. J Craniomandib Pract 1988;6:239–244.

186. Astrand P, Bergljung L, Nord PG: Oblique sliding osteotomy of the mandibular rami in 55 patients with mandibular prognathism. Int J Oral Surg 1973;2:89–101.

187. Wisth PJ: Mandibular function and dysfunction in patients with mandibular prognathism. Am J Orthod 1984;85:193–198.

188. Pepersack WJ, Chausse JM: Long term follow up of the sagittal splitting technique for correction of mandibular prognathism. J Oral Maxillofac Surg 1978;6:117–140.

189. Freihofer HP, Petresevic D: Late results after advancing the mandible by sagittal splitting of the rami. J Oral Maxillofac Surg 1975;3:250–257.

190. Hackney FL, Van Sickels JE, Nummikoski PV: Condylar displacement and temporomandibular joint dysfunction following bilateral sagittal split osteotomy and rigid fixation. J Oral Maxillofac Surg 1989;47:223–227.

191. Rodgrigues-Garcia R, Sakai S, Rugh JD, et al: Effects of major Class II occlusal corrections on temporomandibular signs and symptoms. J Orofacial Pain 1998;12:185–192.

192. Ochs MW, LaBlanc JP, Dolwick MF: The diagnosis and management of concomitant dentofacial deformity and temporomandibular disorder. Oral Maxillofac Surg Clin North Am 1990;2:669–690.

193. Kundert M, Hadjfanghelou O: Condylar displacement after sagittal splitting of the mandibular rami. J Oral Maxillofac Surg 1980;8:223–227.

194. Luhr GH: The significance of condylar position using rigid fixation in orthognathic surgery. Clin Plast Surg 1989;16:147–156.

195. Will LA, Joondeph DR, Hohl TH, West RA: Condylar position following mandibular advancement: Its relationship to relapse. J Oral Maxillofac Surg 1984;42:578–588.

196. Epker BN, Wylie GA: Control of the condylar-proximal mandibular segments after sagittal split osteotomies to advance the mandible. Oral Surg Oral Med Oral Pathol 1986;62:613–617.

197. Schwestka R, Engelke D, Kubein-Meesenburg D: Condylar position control during maxillary surgery: The condylar positioning appliance and three-dimensional double splint method. Int J Adult Orthod Orthognath Surg 1990;5:161–165.

198. Paulus GW, Steinhauser EW: A comparative study of wire osteosynthesis versus bone screws in the treatment of mandibular prognathism. J Oral Surg 1982;54:2–6.

199. Moenning JE, Bussard DA, Lapp TH, Garrison BT: A comparison of relapse in bilateral sagittal split osteotomies for mandibular advancement: Rigid internal fixation (screws) versus inferior border wiring with anterior skeletal fixation. Int J Adult Orthod Orthognath Surg 1990;5:175–182.

200. Buckley MJ, Tulloch JF, White RP Jr, Tucker MR: Complications of orthognathic surgery: A comparison between wire fixation and rigid internal fixation. Int J Adult Orthod Orthognath Surg 1989;4:69–74.

201. Souyris F: Sagittal splitting and bicortical screw fixation of the ascending ramus. J Oral Maxillofac Surg 1978;6:198–203.

202. Timmis DP, Aragon SB, Van Sickels JE: Masticatory dysfunction with rigid and nonrigid osteosynthesis of sagittal split osteotomies. J Oral Surg 1986;62:119–123.

203. Nemeth DZ, Rodrigues-Garcia RCM, Rugh JD, et al: Effects of rigid vs wire fixation with BSSO on signs and symptoms of temporomandibular disorders. 1997; submitted for publication.

204. Stringert HG, Worms FW: Variations in skeletal and dental patterns in patients with structural and functional alterations of the temporomandibular joint: A preliminary report. Am J Orthod 1986;89:285–297.

205. Kerstens HC, Tuinzing DB, Golding RP, van der Kwast WA: Condylar atrophy and osteoarthrosis after bimaxillary surgery. Oral Surg Oral Med Oral Pathol 1990;69:274–280.

206. Schellhas KP, Piper MA, Bessette RW, Wilkes CH: Mandibular retrusion, temporomandibular joint derangement and orthognathic surgery planning. Plast Reconstr Surg 1992;90:218–232.

207. Link JL, Nickerson JW Jr: Temporomandibular joint internal derangements in an orthognathic surgery population. Int J Adult Orthod Orthognath Surg 1992;7:161–169.

208. Bouwman JPB, Kerstens HCJ, Tuinzing DB: Condylar resorption in orthognathic surgery. The role of intermaxillary fixation. Oral Surg Oral Med Oral Pathol 1984;78:138–141.

209. Dibbets JM, Van Der Weele LT, Uildriks AKJ: Symptoms of TMJ dysfunction: Indicators of growth patterns? J Pedodontics 1985;9:265–284.

210. Schellhas KP, Keck RJ: Disorders of skeletal occlusion and temporomandibular joint disease. Northwest Dentistry 1989;68:35–39.

211. Schellhas KP, Pollei SR, Wilkes CH: Pediatric internal derangements of the temporomandibular joint: Effect on facial development. Am J Orthod Dentofacial Orthop 1993;104:51–59.

212. Brand JW, Nielson KJ, Tallents RH, et al: Lateral cephalometric analysis of skeletal patterns in patients with and without internal derangement of the temporomandibular joint. Am J Orthod Dentofacial Orthop 1995;107:121–128.

213. Stein SI: A comparison of craniofacial morphology of TMD patients and asymptomatic volunteers [senior research thesis]. Rochester, NY, Eastman Dental Center, Department of Orthodontics, 1995.

214. Boering G: Arthrosis deformans van het kaakgewricht. Leiden, Stafleu en Tholen, 1966.

215. Bjork A, Skieller V: Normal and abnormal growth of the mandible. A synthesis of longitudinal cephalometric implant studies over a period of 25 years. Eur J Orthod 1983;5:1–46.

216. Nickerson JW Jr, Moystad A: Observations on individuals with radiographic bilateral condylar remodeling. J Craniomandib Pract 1983;1:20–37.

217. Roberts CA, Tallents RH, Katzberg RW, et al: Comparison of internal derangements of the TMJ with occlusal findings. Oral Surg Oral Med Oral Pathol 1987;63:645–650.

218. Hatala MP, Macher DJ, Tallents RH, et al: Effect of a surgically created disc displacement on mandibular symmetry in growing rabbits. Oral Surg Oral Med Oral Pathol 1996;82:625–633.

CHAPTER

12

Orthognathics and the Temporomandibular Joint

Ronald H. Roth

The temporomandibular joints (TMJs) are the foundation of occlusion. It is impossible to obtain a stable and healthy result in orthodontics or orthognathics with unstable joints that are recontouring and changing. When we change the occlusion, we affect the position of the condyles and the stability of the joints. We must be aware of the relationship between these factors so that we know how best to treat both the joints and the occlusion, as well as when not to treat.

Although there is an abundance of literature on occlusion and the TMJs, much of it is seriously flawed. Many of the studies used inadequate sample sizes, incorrect techniques, unskilled operators, and inappropriate measuring devices. In addition, many of the wrong factors were studied to determine the relationship between occlusion and the TMJs. One can go into the literature and find articles to support whatever one cares to believe. In addition, a number of prominent people in dentistry have taken the position that because no one has proved to their satisfaction that there is an association between occlusion and temporomandibular disorders (TMDs), an association does not exist. There is no justification for this stance, for lack of proof is not proof of a lack of association. In fact, TMDs are multifactorial problems. Unfortunately, TMD has become the catch-all term for all head, neck, and jaw pain.

Review of the Literature

Most studies that failed to show a relationship between occlusion and TMDs did not use instrumentation and did not study factors that would be expected to correlate with joint- or occlusion-related problems. For example, the studies of Pullinger and Seligman[1-4] found no definite relationship between TMDs and occlusion. They surveyed 222 dental and oral hygiene students in a three-part study with questionnaires, clinical examinations, and dental casts. They evaluated factors such as the centric slide at the occlusal level, which can be very misleading as to what is actually going on at the condylar level. They also examined condylar position on oriented tomograms of the joints relative to symptoms and found no significant correlation statistically. However, condylar position on radiographs is only a gross measurement of position. In addition, the subjects' teeth were not in occlusion when the tomograms were taken. It is necessary to have the teeth in occlusion to note the effects of occlusion on condylar position.

In their review of the literature, McNamara and colleagues[5] found a relatively low association between occlusal factors and the signs and symptoms of TMDs. However, because of the factors studied and the manner in which they were studied (hand-held dental casts, retruded contact position–intercuspal contact position [RCP-ICP] slides intraorally, tomograms), one would be unlikely to find a correlation even if it did exist. No attempt was made to override the effects of the neuromusculature when manipulating the mandible.

Based on some of the classic literature, it

is evident that an ideally positioned condyle is one positioned upward and forward against the posterior slope of the eminence, with the disk interposed. Moffett,[6] Sicher,[7] and others[8–10] described how the histologic structures of the joint are designed to withstand heavy loads with the condyles in this position. The resultant vector of the elevator muscles is directed anterosuperiorly.[9] Williamson and coworkers,[11, 12] Girardot,[13] and Wood and associates[14] showed this in their studies; Lundeen and Gibbs,[15] using the gnathic replicator, showed that the action of healthy musculature positions the condyles in this upward and forward position. Use of the gnathic replicator demonstrated how the condyles move to and from this position during the chewing cycle in a good occlusion.

Electromyographic studies found that masticatory muscle function is disrupted by occlusal interferences that prevent the seating of the condyles in centric relation.[16–18] As explained later in this chapter, attaining this position through treatment is essential to achieving healthy joints and stable results. Kirveskari and colleagues[19] showed in a large, prospective, double-blind study that occlusal equilibration consistently relieved TMJ symptoms over the long term. Equilibration was performed to eliminate centric interferences in children, and long-term follow-up was done. This well-done study provided conclusive evidence of the relationship between occlusion and the TMJ, yet it is never quoted by the naysayers. Crawford, in comparing subjects with ideal occlusions with a random sample of subjects matched by age and sex, showed an exceptionally high correlation between TMD symptoms and displacement of the condyles in maximum intercuspation of the teeth.[20]

Arnett and coworkers[21, 22] described the biochemical and biomechanical relationships between occlusion and the TMJ, as well as a number of other factors. Hatcher and associates[23, 24] explored the response of joint tissue to stress and strain through the use of imaging techniques and mechanical computer modeling. In all these studies, occlusion was determined to be one of the factors involved in joint remodeling and degenerative joint disease. I rely heavily on these scholarly, yet clinically oriented resources, along with personal clinical experience, for much of what is presented in this chapter.

Presentation of the Clinical Problem

It seems obvious that the basis for the occlusion between the mandible and the maxilla is the condyles and the TMJs. Most orthognathic surgeons realize that failure to place the condyles properly results in some form of failure shortly after (within months of) surgery. The mandible is supported in its position by the TMJs, and joint failure results in change in the occlusal relationship and a failed result.

There is not much doubt that condylar resorption is a major problem, even for well-trained orthognathic surgeons and orthodontists. It is the leading cause of surgical failure. Therefore, it behooves us to understand the nature and causes of joint resorption and the conditions that surround it.

We may be presented with several different scenarios:

1. A patient with head, neck, and/or jaw pain.
2. A patient who has responded well to repositioning splint therapy, whose joints are comfortable and stable, but who requires surgical correction of the jaw relationship to establish a decent functional occlusion.
3. A patient who is relatively asymptomatic and is looking for aesthetic improvement of the face and teeth.
4. A patient who has suffered a traumatic injury.

The questions are: Can we reasonably predict condylar resorption? Can we prevent condylar resorption? Can we wisely select candidates for treatment, and if so, how do we go about doing this? Can we solve TMJ problems by fixing the occlusion? Can we eliminate or reduce the incidence of disappointing experiences for our patients?

In order to do this, we need to understand the mechanisms at work and the interrelationships between a number of factors. We must ascertain the status of the TMJs, make a good differential diagnosis, and determine whether orthognathic treatment is appropriate for the patient and what the risk factors are. We do this by taking a thorough history, performing a complete clinical examination, and obtaining appropriate imaging studies. This information must then be integrated with a conceptual model of how the patient's joints will tend to respond to the various factors present in the individual case.

Initial Evaluation

The first step is to determine whether the patient's problem is in fact related to the TMJs and/or the occlusion. The rule of thumb is to rule out everything else first. There are many conditions that mimic temporomandibular dysfunction and may cause head and neck pain or what appears to be joint or muscle pain—nasopharyngeal tumors, parotid tumors, neurologic tumors, sialolithiasis, temporal arteritis, vascular headaches or migraines, referred pain, dental pathology, and psychological disturbances, to name a few. The dangerous and life-threatening conditions need to be ruled out first. We must also look at other physical problems that may have a bearing on the muscles of mastication and mandibular posture. Back problems, leg length problems, and neck problems may result in poor head and body posture, causing constant muscle contraction and pain in the muscles of the head and neck and the muscles of mastication. Numerous systemic conditions also mimic TMDs, and it is important to recognize them.

I generally divide patients into two broad categories: those who have a clear-cut relationship between the muscles of mastication, the TMJs, and the occlusion, and those who do not. This may sound like an oversimplification, but those patients without a clear-cut relationship between their symptoms and the dental structures are usually not good candidates for orthognathic or orthodontic procedures to solve their pain or dysfunction problems. In other words, after getting a thorough history and doing the clinical examination, some relationship between symptoms and the dental structures should be apparent before contemplating treatment of the occlusion, the joints, or both. Patients who are good candidates for treatment usually have symptoms in the

joints (clicking, crepitation, or pain in the joints themselves, and a history to match the symptoms) and in the muscles of mastication and problems with occlusion. The history and the clinical examination usually tell you most of what you need to know. Imaging either confirms or denies the condition in most instances.

It is a good idea to read the history first to get a good idea of the chain of events leading up to the patient's visit and to have this information in the correct chronologic order. This tends to direct the examination toward either proving or disproving any tentative diagnosis that may have been assumed.

If the patient does not have clear-cut signs and symptoms related to the TMJs, the muscles of mastication, and the occlusion, there is usually a "pain from other causes" component. It is at this point that one needs to do a differential diagnosis as to the cause of the pain, rather than leaping to the conclusion that the pain is related to the occlusion and/or the TMJs. If, however, there is a relationship between the signs and symptoms and the TMJs, the muscles of mastication, and the occlusion, one needs to determine the status of the TMJs. The presence or absence of muscle pain or tenderness, tenderness of the joints, noises in the joints, limitation of opening, deviation of opening or closing, limitation of movement, character of movement, and relationship to pain or sounds during movement may all give clues to the status of the joints.

Based on the clinical impression, appropriate imaging should be obtained. Various plain films of the joints are useful, but most desirable are oriented tomograms using a submental vertex view to measure the angle of the condylar poles to ensure that the central beam is aligned with the condylar axis. Three cuts should be made, and tomograms of the coronal view of the joints should also be obtained. If there is doubt about the position of the articular disk, magnetic resonance imaging (MRI) should be performed to determine the status of the disks.

To quote Hatcher and colleagues[23]: "To maximize the diagnostic yield from imaging, there must be knowledge of both the biologic process and the temporal relationship of the condition under study compared to its resultant image pattern. Unfortunately, there have been more advances in the development of imaging modalities than in determining the clinical significance of the image findings or image evaluation." They go on to say, "Optimal loading of the articular tissues is required to sustain their health; either excessive or deficient loads on these tissues may result in tissue injury." The imaging either confirms or denies the clinical suspicions gained from the history and the examination.

The initial evaluation of the occlusion should be done from articulator-mounted models in centric relation position. The interocclusal registrations should be obtained after deprogramming with a device such as a bite plane for several days beforehand if the patient is in pain or it is difficult to manipulate the mandible. Longer-term, full-time repositioning splints (centric relation position) should be instituted to determine the full extent of the discrepancy.

Patients can be prone to condylar degeneration, and we must learn to look for the attributes of such a predilection. Arnett and coworkers[21, 22] described 12 factors that lead to condylar resorption and thus tend to increase the likelihood of what they call "dysfunctional remodeling": biochemical factors—sex and age (females aged 12 to 26 most vulnerable), autoimmune factors (the arthritides), hyperparathyroidism, estrogen factor (mediates bone metabolism), prolactin (pregnancy occurrence), corticosteroids (previous use); and biomechanical factors—condylar compression (can be caused by orthodontics and orthognathics), internal derangement, parafunction (resulting in ischemic reperfusion), macrotrauma, and unstable occlusion (condyles not properly seated against disk and eminence within the fossae). Hatcher and colleagues'[23] imaging interpretation and work on stress and strain as related to TMJ remodeling and joint degeneration complement nearly everything described by Arnett and coworkers.[21, 22, 25]

Clinical Approach

Basically, once major systemic problems have been ruled out and a clear-cut relationship between the symptoms and the muscles of mastication, the TMJs, and the occlusion established, we need to evaluate and

diagnose the status of the joints. We can divide these problems into three main categories: neuromuscular problems and myofascial pain, progressive condylar resorption, and degenerative joint disease. However, in many instances, these categories represent progression along a continuum of joint degeneration. That is why a complete and accurate chronologic history is essential.

Tomographic evaluation using properly oriented tomograms reveals the following: gross condylar position, condyle size, condyle shape, condylar cortex, and eminence shape. MRI illustrates disk position and disk shape and reveals any soft tissue masses that are present.

A complete list of symptoms (e.g., sounds, pain, headache, limitation of motion) is needed. In addition, any relevant habits; airway status; previous treatment such as orthodontics, orthognathics, or extensive restorations; and any trauma or recent occlusal change must be noted. What does the patient do when the symptoms occur, and is it effective? Who, if anyone, has the patient seen for treatment? What was the treatment? How many times has the patient been treated?

The occlusion should be studied from centrically related mounted casts on an anatomic articulator. If the patient has been in pain, the musculature is sensitive or painful, or the mandible is difficult to manipulate, a repositioning splint should be worn full time for 10 to 14 days before taking interocclusal registrations to mount the models. The mounted models will give a much more accurate picture of the occlusion and the actual condition present.

From these records, as well as the clinical examination, a thorough chronologic history, and imaging, one can usually determine the status of the joints, locate the point in the continuum where the patient is at present, and assess whether the patient is prone to condylar resorption.

Hatcher and colleagues[24] state that remodeling of the joints is a response to heavy destructive joint loads and is an attempt to establish, through the remodeling process, more optimal joint loading. This may be why a joint that has been stabilized with splint therapy may undergo degenerative changes during orthodontic or orthognathic treatment. The stresses may have been optimized with splint use, but the treatment modalities create excessive forces and lead to tissue breakdown. Orthodontic treatment is microloading of the joints over an extended period, whereas orthognathic treatment is macroloading over a short period. The two together in a receptive host will surely result in dysfunctional remodeling during and after treatment.

The question becomes whether a particular patient is a good candidate for orthodontic or orthognathic treatment. For instance, a female patient aged 22 years presents with internal derangement of both TMJs and a displaced disk without reduction; some remodeling of the condyles, showing signs of "bird beaking"; a severe class II open-bite malocclusion with procumbent lower anteriors; a steep mandibular plane angle; protrusive upper incisors; a maxillary excess and anteroposterior midface deficiency; an obtuse nasolabial angle; and a history of clicking, followed by limited opening and disappearance of the clicking. The clicking appeared during orthodontic treatment, and sometime after treatment the closed lock occurred. This patient is a poor candidate for treatment. She has one biochemical factor for dysfunctional condylar resorption (female between 12 and 26 years of age) and one biomechanical factor for condylar resorption (internal derangement). Degenerative changes in the bony architecture have already occurred. In addition, the facial appearance suggests the probability of a multiple-piece LeFort I procedure with mandibular advancement and genioplasty. It would probably also require four-bicuspid extraction, with orthodontic treatment over 21 to 24 months to close the extraction sites. So there is the possibility of prolonged condylar compression with the orthodontics and with the mandibular surgery (advancement, hardware, condylar displacement). Although most would contemplate treatment of this patient, she would be an extremely poor risk and a likely candidate for progressive condylar resorption, which would appear to be a latent relapse.

We must assess the status of the TMJs in all patients and formulate a picture of the biochemical and biomechanical factors that are or will be at work. We must make a value judgment as to the feasible treatment options and present them to the patient and significant others and let them make the final decision in light of the risks involved.

Treating the Patient with Temporomandibular Disorder

As stated before, we cannot assume that because the patient presents for treatment and has a malocclusion, correction of the malocclusion will solve the problem. It may be necessary to test the response to a change in occlusion and condylar position with a centric splint that is worn full time and adjusted initially every few days, then once a week, then once every several weeks to deprogram the neuromuscular system and see if consistent relief of symptoms is attained. Before splint wear, appropriate tomograms of the joints should be obtained to monitor any change in joint recontouring.

We usually attempt to stabilize the condylar position in centric relation if possible, as this provides a stable base if occlusal treatment, orthodontics, or orthognathic surgery is indicated. If the joints are deranged and seating of the condyles is painful, or if the joints start resorbing on a centric splint, we discontinue it. At that point, however, a forward position splint or a condylar distraction splint may be used, but only for relief of symptoms. This is usually accompanied by a course of physical therapy, biofeedback training, and/or pain management. I am very hesitant to attempt to treat the occlusion in the presence of internally deranged joints that exhibit resorption with the use of a centric splint.

In certain cases, joint repair may be attempted by doing disk plication surgery or diskectomy. This will not necessarily yield a normal functioning joint or stop degenerative joint disease, but in a fair number of cases, the patient gets along better and the joints become stable enough to contemplate orthognathic correction of the occlusion. However, it is advisable to test this response with centric splint therapy for 6 to 12 months, using tomographic comparisons at different times to judge the stability of the occlusion on the splint (minimal or no need for adjustment) and the stability of the joints. A radionuclide scan may be obtained to see whether there is bone exchange activity in the joints. When all clinical parameters indicate that the joints are stable and the patient is reasonably comfortable, then treatment can be considered.

Whenever possible, elimination of mandibular surgery is desirable, even if it leads to a minor degree of facial compromise. If this is not possible, orthodontic preparation should be as rapid and atraumatic as possible. About 3 months before surgery, centric splint therapy should be used to stabilize the joints and test their stability.

The surgical procedure should include a fixation technique that maintains the osteotomy gaps so as not to torque the condyles and cause condylar compression. Bivector seating of the condyles into a superior-anterior relation in the fossa is desirable, and excess loading from hardware should be avoided. Large advancements (>8 mm) should also be avoided whenever possible. Semirigid fixation with flexible plates is probably the best way to maintain condylar positioning without compression. Rigid or semirigid fixation without intermaxillary fixation is preferable. The immobilization and potential clenching during intermaxillary fixation can cause the start of degenerative changes on a receptive host.

At the conclusion of orthodontics and orthognathics, the orthodontist should stabilize the tooth positions as soon as possible with retention devices and then revert to splint therapy to restabilize the joints. A centric splint should be worn 24 hours a day and adjusted at first every day or two, then once a week, and then every several weeks or when the patient is either uncomfortable or feels that the splint is out of adjustment.

Repositioning and recontouring should be monitored with mandibular position indicator (MPI) (SAM instrument system) or condylar position indicator (CPI) (Panadent instrument system) readings and tomograms. Once the joints are stabilized, hinge axis recordings and mandibular movement recordings should be done, and the mounted models evaluated for equilibration and/or restorative dentistry. It has been my experience that symptoms recur in patients with TMDs unless the occlusion is corrected to the most minute detail. Orthodontics per se does not do this well enough. Other modalities such as equilibration or restorative dentistry must be used to refine the occlusion in most cases.

Summary

The term *TMD* is nondescriptive. It is applied to all patients with head and neck pain, TMJ problems, or both and implies that all these patients have the same condition. Generalized statements regarding TMD patients are usually erroneous and confusing. Each patient should be evaluated to determine the most likely cause of the problem. If the chief complaint is pain or joint problems, it is necessary to test the response of the occlusion and the stability of the joints with full-time, long-term (6 months to a year or more) splint use before entering a course of orthodontics and orthognathic surgery.

TMJ problems are multifactorial, and occlusion is one of those factors. There is no justification to assume that occlusion is not part of the problem. Some TMJ myofascial problems can be successfully treated by proper correction of the occlusion. Other TMJ problems must be corrected surgically, and some TMJ problems cannot be corrected.

There are certain identifiable factors that make an individual prone to condylar resorption.[21-23] It is possible through the use of an accurate history, clinical examination, and appropriate imaging to determine whether an individual is a candidate for treatment. The joint status of all patients should be determined before treatment, as many relatively asymptomatic patients may be prone to degenerative joint disease if unfavorable joint loading occurs. We need to identify these high-risk patients before proceeding with treatment and discuss the risks and potential problems with them. The joints should be stabilized with full-time centric splint wear and monitored appropriately before making the decision to proceed with treatment. Attention to minimizing condylar compression (especially in patients prone to resorption) and accurate seating of condyles at surgery is advisable.

REFERENCES

1. Pullinger AG, Seligman DA, Solberg WK: Temporomandibular disorders. Part II. Occlusal factors associated with temporomandibular joint tenderness and dysfunction. J Prosthet Dent 1988; 59:363–367.
2. Pullinger AG, Solberg WK, Hollender L, Guichet

D: Tomographic analysis of mandibular condyle position in diagnostic subgroups of temporomandibular disorders. J Prosthet Dent 1986;55:723–729.

3. Pullinger AG, Solberg WK, Hollender L, Petersson A: Relationship of mandibular condylar position to dental occlusion factors in an asymptomatic population. Am J Orthod Dentofacial Orthop 1987;91:200–206.

4. Seligman DA, Pullinger AG, Solberg WK: Temporomandibular disorders. Part III. Occlusal and articular factors associated with muscle tenderness. J Prosthet Dent 1988;59:483–489.

5. McNamara JA Jr, Seligman DA, Okeson JP: Occlusion, orthodontic treatment, and temporomandibular disorders: A review. J Orofac Pain 1995;9:73–90.

6. Moffett BC Jr, Johnson LC, McCabe JB, et al: Il rimodellamento articolare dell'articolazione temporomandibolare nell'uomo adulto. Minerva Stomat 1969;18:611–630.

7. Sicher H: Sicher's Oral Anatomy, ed 7. St. Louis, CV Mosby, 1980, p 178.

8. Gilboe DB: Centric relation as the treatment position. J Prosthet Dent 1983;50:685–689.

9. Okeson JP: Management of Temporomandibular Disorders and Occlusion, ed 3. St. Louis, CV Mosby, 1993.

10. Rees L: The structure and function of the mandibular joint. Br Dent J 1954;96:125–133.

11. Williamson EH, Evans DL, Barton WA, Williams BH: The effect of bite plane use on terminal hinge axis location. Angle Orthod 1977;47:25–33.

12. Williamson EH, Steinke RM, Morse PK, Swift TR: Centric relation: A comparison of muscle-determined position and operator guidance. Am J Orthod 1980;77:133–145.

13. Girardot RA: Condylar displacement in patients with TMJ dysfunction. CDS Review 1989;89(8):49–55.

14. Wood DP, Floreani KJ, Galil KA, Teteruck WR: The effect of incisal bite force on condylar seating. Angle Orthod 1994;64:53–62.

15. Lundeen HC, Gibbs CH: Advances in Occlusion. Boston, MA, John Wright PSG Inc., 1982, pp 2–32.

16. Naeije M, Hansson TL: Short-term effect of the stabilization appliance on masticatory muscle activity in myogenous craniomandibular disorder patients. J Cranio Disord 1991;5:245–250.

17. Ramfjord SP: Bruxism, a clinical and electromyographic study. J Am Dent Assoc 1961;62:21–44.

18. Ramfjord SP: Dysfunctional temporomandibular joint and muscle pain. J Prosthet Dent 1961;11:353–374.

19. Kirveskari P, Alanen P, Jamsa T: Association between craniomandibular disorders and occlusal interferences in children. J Prosthet Dent 1992;67:692–696.

20. Crawford SD: Condylar axis position, as determined by the occlusion and measured by the CPI instrument, and signs and symptoms of temporomandibular dysfunction. Angle Orthodont 1999;69:103–116.

21. Arnett GW, Milam SB, Gottesman L: Progressive mandibular retrusion—idiopathic condylar resorption. Part I. Am J Orthod Dentofacial Orthop 1996;110:8–15.

22. Arnett GW, Milam SB, Gottesman L: Progressive mandibular retrusion—idiopathic condylar resorption. Part II. Am J Orthod Dentofacial Orthop 1996;110:117–127.

23. Hatcher DC, McEvoy SP, Mah RT, Faulkner MG: Distribution of local and general stresses in the stomatognathic system. In McNeill C (ed): Science and Practice of Occlusion. Carol Stream, IL, Quintessence, 1997, pp 259–270.

24. Hatcher DC, Blom RJ, Baker CG: Temporomandibular joint spatial relationships: Osseous and soft tissues. J Prosthet Dent 1986;56:344–353.

25. Arnett GW, Tamborello JA: Progressive class II development—female idiopathic condylar resorption. Oral Maxillofac Surg Clin 1990;2:699–716.

Morphologic Changes of the Temporomandibular Joint Associated with Orthognathic Surgery

G. William Arnett • Stephen B. Milam
Lawrence Gottesman • C. MacDonald Worley, Jr.

Orthognathic surgery may be associated with morphologic changes of the temporomandibular joint (TMJ). Three possible responses are morphostasis, morphoadaptation, and morphodegeneration. Morphostasis is characterized by a lack of change in joint hard and soft tissues. Morphoadaptation is manifested by focal remodeling, maintenance of ramus height, normal mandibular growth (if growth occurs postsurgically), and postsurgical B point stability. Morphodegeneration is distinguished by total condylar remodeling, loss of ramus height, decreased mandibular growth (if growth occurs postsurgically), and postsurgical bite relapse of B point. The key question is, what causes the change in the TMJ morphology following orthognathic surgery?

TMJ morphologic changes may be evidenced by clinical and/or radiographic methods. Radiographically, changes in condylar shape, density, or size may be apparent. Soft tissues of the joint also change simultaneously, although we generally describe these changes in terms of condyles for lack of a simple, inexpensive way of quantifying them. Clinically, late changes in the occlusion may be associated with postsurgical condylar morphologic change. A review of all forms of B point relapse is necessary to explain morphologic condylar relapse. Posterior B point relapse and attendant occlusal relapse can occur at only two anatomic locations after bilateral sagittal osteotomy advancement: the osteotomy site or the TMJ. B point relapse occurs at the osteotomy site via slippage, the TMJ via condylar sag,[1-6] and the TMJ via morphologic change.[7-13]

Osteotomy Slippage

Osteotomy slippage occurs before osteotomy union in response to paramandibular connective tissue (PMCT) stretch, which produces force and pulls the tooth-bearing fragment posteriorly after advancement. The PMCT consists of skin,[1] subcutaneous tissue,[1] muscle,[1, 14-20] and periosteum.[1] When stretched, these tissues are under tension, forming a vector that pulls the tooth-bearing fragment posteriorly toward the presurgical position. Counteracting the PMCT vector are osteosynthesis hardware (bicortical screws, superior border wires, inferior border wires, circummandibular wires or plates with unicortical screws), skeletal suspension,[21, 22] and the condyle, if it is seated in the glenoid fossa. The hardware, skeletal suspension, and condyle support system function to hold the tooth-bearing fragment in the advanced position, countering the pull of the PMCT. When osteotomy union occurs, the osteotomy then supports B point in the new anterior position.

Wire osteosynthesis is associated with early relapse, as reported in stability studies.[2–4, 8, 23, 24] This may indicate an increase in osteotomy slippage when found with a seated condyle. Bicortical screws are associated with less osteotomy slippage, as evidenced by early B point stability recorded in multiple studies.[8, 24–26]

Condylar Sag

The term *condylar sag,* as used in the literature, refers to a condyle that is positioned inferior or anterior-inferior to the glenoid fossa seated position and, because of this position, has no ability to support B point in the advanced position.[1–5, 23, 27, 28] This definition is inadequate because a condyle contacting posteriorly, medially, or laterally is also positioned inferiorly and, by the preceding definition, is in condylar sag.[8] These condyles are positioned inferiorly but contact the rim of the glenoid fossa medially, laterally, or posteriorly and therefore support B point. The form of condylar sag that is nonsupportive of B point should be renamed *noncontact condylar sag.* With *contact condylar sag,* the condyle is inferior but contacts the fossa medially, laterally, or posteriorly and thus supports B point in the advanced position.

Morphologic Change and Late Relapse

Arnett and colleagues recently published a series of papers regarding morphologic changes of the condyles following orthognathic surgery.[8, 9, 29–31] Their proposed classification system comprises two main categories that attempt to explain both morphoadaptation and morphodegeneration following orthognathic surgery: host adaptive capacity factors and mechanical compression.[29, 30]

HOST ADAPTIVE CAPACITY FACTORS

Several host adaptive capacity factors have been identified.[29, 30]

HOST ADAPTIVE CAPACITY FACTORS

Age
Systemic illnesses
Hormones: estrogen, prolactin, corticosteroids

Age

Severe morphodegeneration typically occurs in the second and third decades. What factor or factors are responsible are still unidentified. The mean age of morphodegeneration as reported in the literature is 20.5 years old.

Systemic Illnesses

These illnesses may include autoimmune disorders, endocrine disorders, nutritional disorders (e.g., anorexia nervosa), metabolic diseases, infectious diseases, cardiovascular diseases, blood dyscrasias, and excessive psychological stress.

Hormones

Hormonal factors may have a marked influence on remodeling of the mandibular condyle.

Estrogen

Arnett and Tamborello reported on 10 female patients with idiopathic condylar resorption.[9] Forty other patients (all female) with severe condylar resorption (condylysis) have been reported in the literature.[9, 32–39] These clinical experiences indicate that some women may be predisposed to morphodegeneration of the TMJ.

Abubaker and coworkers studied human

TMJs for estrogen and progesterone receptors using an immunohistochemical method.[40] They found that 72% of symptomatic women and only 14% of asymptomatic women had immunodetectable estrogen receptors in tissue specimens obtained from their TMJs. They concluded: "It is feasible to speculate that the concurrent presence of these receptors and specific circulating hormone levels will lead to connective tissue alterations in the TMJ disk, causing some structural changes in this tissue."

The exact role of estrogen in the pathogenesis of TMJ disease (i.e., dysfunctional remodeling) is unclear. Estrogen inhibits cartilage synthesis in animal models of osteoarthritis.[41] Estrogen also increases the production of specific cytokines that have been implicated in inflammatory joint diseases.[42–44]

Prolactin

Prolactin, a hormone responsible for initiating postpartum milk letdown, can exacerbate cartilage and bone degradation in animal models of inflammatory arthritides.[45] It is likely that prolactin contributes to the accelerated condylysis that has been observed in some pregnant women.

In summary, it appears that the female predisposition to dysfunctional remodeling of the TMJ may be attributed, in part, to the modulation of the biologic responses of articular tissues to functional loading by sex hormones.

Corticosteroids

Corticosteroids have been reported to cause joint resorption.[46–50] It is conceivable that changes in corticosteroid levels may, in some individuals, initiate mandibular condylar resorption and attendant progressive class II malocclusion.

MECHANICAL COMPRESSION

Several sources of TMJ compression have been identified as causing or contributing to morphoadaptation and morphodegeneration.[29, 30]

COMPRESSIVE FACTORS

Occlusal therapy
Internal derangement
Parafunction
Macrotrauma
Unstable occlusion

Soft tissue and osseous changes are seen with all sources of compressive loading. Soft tissues of the TMJ typically undergo a rapid physical transformation when subjected to chronic or excessive mechanical forces. In separate studies, Isberg and Isacsson[51] and Furstman[52] depicted the soft tissue alterations associated with compressive events. Isberg and Isacsson observed a flattening of the posterior band of the articular disk, with changes in its collagen fiber orientation, when the mandibular condyle was displaced posteriorly for 5 weeks.[51] Furstman created unstable occlusion in rats by adding vertical occlusal interferences unilaterally.[52] This manipulation led to an increased deposition of fibrous connective tissue and osteoid matrix on the articular surface of the glenoid fossa. In addition, an increased thickness and disorientation of collagen fibers of the articular disk were observed.

Ultimately, joint soft tissue changes may contribute to osseous remodeling. Multiple studies have assessed the osseous changes associated with condylar compression.[8, 9, 53–60] These studies have shown consistent osseous resorption of the postglenoid spine and posterior condylar surface when the condyle is posteriorized and compressed in the glenoid fossa. Similarly, Arnett and colleagues[8] demonstrated morphologic changes of the mandibular condyle associated with posteriorization and medial or lateral condylar torquing during orthognathic surgery.

The morphology of the TMJ appears to be very sensitive to functional loading. Mongini tomographically demonstrated condylar changes following occlusal equilibration.[61] Peltola found a greater variation in condylar shape among orthodontically treated patients compared with controls.[62] These morphologic changes presumably represent normal functional remodeling stimulated by changes in mechanical stresses imposed on the TMJ following occlusal equilibration or orthodontic therapy.

Mechanical factors may occur in isolation or may be interrelated, interdependent, and coexistent. When two or more biomechanical factors coexist, morphologic change is more likely to occur. Additionally, when the host adaptive capacity is limited, morphologic changes are accentuated when mechanical factors are active.

Occlusal Correction Compression

Occlusal treatment is associated with both late condylar changes and B point regression. Biomechanical and intraoperative condyle position changes have been identified as causative. Coexisting remodeling stimuli (internal derangement, parafunction, macrotrauma, unstable occlusion, hormones, systemic diseases, or neurogenic conditions) may accentuate condylar remodeling, producing dysfunction.

Because of the nature of orthognathic surgery, gross positional changes of the mandibular condyle can occur, producing gross condylar morphologic changes. Orthodontic and prosthetic care may also produce condyle position changes, but generally not to the same extent as orthognathic surgery. Orthodontic mechanics used to correct skeletal malocclusions (e.g., class III and II elastics, cross-arch elastics) may be capable of greater condyle position changes and associated compression with resorption.

Ellis and Hinton[60] studied rigid and wire-fixated sagittal osteotomies of the mandible in monkeys and observed resorption of the postglenoid spine and posterior aspect of the condyle associated with posteriorization of the condyle when rigid fixation was used. They believed that with rigid fixation of the osteotomy sites, the condyles were displaced in a posterior direction from soft tissue (muscle, skin) resistance to the advanced mandible. Because the mandibular condyles provide posterior support for the mandible, these reactive forces were presumably transferred to articulating structures within the joint, leading to the observed remodeling. They concluded that condylar resorption after orthognathic surgery is probably related to biomechanical compression.

Arnett and colleagues[8] tomographically studied 61 orthognathic surgery patients to determine the effects of surgically induced condyle position change on the morphology of the mandibular condyle. They found that intraoperative position changes led to morphodegeneration and late mandibular relapse. They identified either the surgeon (direction and force) or the hardware as producing the intraoperative condyle position changes and compression.

Arnett and colleagues[8] also identified two types of intraoperative condylar change: posterior condylar change (PCC) and medial-lateral condylar change (MLCC). In both instances, the condyles and disk tissues are compressed against the fossa wall. In response to compression, remodeling of the joint structures (which causes B point relapse[8, 9]) may begin from 9 to 18 months after surgery. Many relapse studies do not follow patients this long and therefore do not note this relapse. As remodeling occurs, the condyle seats superiorly, resulting in B point and dental relapse over the long term.

In the group that underwent PCC, all the condyles were seated in an identical fashion.[8] The condylar seating technique for the sagittal osteotomies was heavy posterosuperior pressure on the vertical portion of the proximal fragment. The net vector of this force was posterosuperior on the condyle, and the high-low wires were active in pushing and holding the condyle in a posterosuperior position in the glenoid fossa.

A study by Jankelson and Abib[63] demonstrated how orthognathic surgery may place the condyle posteriorly with this seating technique. Male human subjects were subjected to changes in the terminal hinge position of the condyle based on forces applied posteriorly to the chin. The individuals in the study group were awake and semi-upright. When 5 pounds of pressure was applied to the chin with a "gnathoretrusive" device, the condyles were retruded 0.71 mm in the glenoid fossa. With 15 pounds of pressure, the condyle retruded 1.16 mm. These findings refute the inviolate nature of the posterior border position of the mandible and indicate that the posterior border position (centric relation) is actually related to the amount of force applied to the chin, which overrides the resistance of the tendons, ligaments, muscles, and capsule. With orthognathic surgery (under general anesthesia in the supine position), the effects of posteriorly directed, excessive force on the condyles may change condyle position, as in the Jankelson group.

The Arnett study seems to verify this assumption: 19 of 26 condyles moved posteriorly when seated with the posterior vector.[8] This group of patients had early B point stability and late B point relapse secondary to condylar resorption. Resorption was verified tomographically. Animal studies have been published that demonstrate this remodeling phenomenon in response to condylar posteriorization.[54, 55, 60, 64]

In the Arnett group that underwent MLCC, all the condyles were seated in an identical fashion, and bivector seating of the condyles was achieved.[8] Following seating, the condylar and tooth-bearing fragments were modified to produce a large contact area. At that point, a clamp was placed across the two fragments to stabilize the condyle in the bivector position. Three transcutaneous screws were then placed to secure the fragments together. With this technique, medial or lateral torque and compression were produced. The torquing was produced during clamping and/or when the screws closed the gap between the segments, torquing the condyles. As the gap was closed, rotation occurred at the first contact point and the condyle torqued to the medial or lateral aspect of the fossa, creating compression. Compression produces good early stability but can cause late relapse similar to posterior compression as condylar remodeling occurs. Condylar torque is frequently associated with bicortical screws in the literature.[65–70] By avoiding osteotomy gap closure, potential condylar torquing can be minimized.

Articular Disk–Condyle Malrelationships

When internal derangement and morphologic alteration occur concurrently, the internal derangement may produce condylar morphologic change by compression. Condylar translation is markedly decreased with anterior disk displacement without reduction. Under this condition, impaired translation of the mandibular condyle may be attributed to a physical obstruction of condylar movement by the displaced articular disk. The obstruction produces compressive forces that are imparted to contacting structures of the joint. Therefore, internal derangement may produce condylar remodeling by contributing to compressive loading of articular tissues. This notion is supported by multiple studies that have shown that condylar remodeling is more likely to be associated with anterior disk displacement without reduction than with reduction.[33, 71–74]

Parafunction

Parafunction may produce compression that is capable of initiating condylar resorption[75–79] or enhancing resorption caused by other factors that initiate this process. Intracapsular pressures have been recorded from symptomatic TMJs that have approached 200 mm Hg with clenching.[80] These intracapsular pressures exceed the estimated capillary perfusion pressure and can therefore impair blood flow to intracapsular tissues, leading to loss of temporomandibular tissue volume, which causes mandibular retrusion.

Macrotrauma

Macrotrauma may also promote condylar resorption.[8, 9, 37, 53] Macrotrauma consists of one episode (compression or stretch) of large-magnitude force that is transmitted to articular structures of the TMJ. The force is generally of a sufficient magnitude that it is acutely injurious to affected articular tissues. The occlusion is not altered at the time of the macrotrauma. TMJ alterations occur over time following the macrotrauma, leading to progressive mandibular retrusion. Resorption of this nature has been associated with removal of third molars,[9] blows to the lower jaw without fracture,[9, 37] orthognathic surgery,[9, 53, 81] joint surgery,[81] whiplash,[81] and protrusive splint therapy.[81]

Unstable Occlusion

Unstable occlusion may contribute to condylar resorption. Two forms of occlusion exist independent of Angle classification: stable and unstable. A stable occlusion does not deflect the condyle position during interdigitation of the dentition regardless of

Angle classification. An unstable occlusion produces compressive deflection of the condyle during interdigitation of the teeth regardless of Angle classification. Furstman described disorientation of collagen fibers in the articular disk and severe osteosclerotic changes of the mandibular condyle that are associated with the loss of occlusal stability.[52] Gazit and Ehrlich and their colleagues also observed structural changes of the TMJ that were associated with unstable occlusion, including bone resorption and fibrocartilage calcification.[82, 83] Posteriorization of the mandibular condyle secondary to occlusal changes (i.e., unstable occlusion) may lead to postglenoid spine and posterior condylar resorption.[8, 9, 51, 53-56] Additionally, Rasmussen found that TMJ arthropathy, when followed over time, generally ended with resolution of symptoms and signs. A small group of patients in the Rasmussen study—those who were missing posterior teeth and/or posterior stops—did not have resolution of symptoms and signs.[84] It may be that these patients are representative of the effects of unstable occlusion.

Treatment of Morphodegeneration (Condylar Resorption)

Treatment for condylar resorption is threefold: control or eradication of the cause, stabilization of the unstable occlusion and TMJ (healing), and correction of the resultant occlusal deformity. Identification and treatment of the etiology may be difficult when host adaptive capacity is a factor.

Mechanical stresses are probably the most common source of condylar resorption. Occlusal therapy and possible attendant compression of the TMJ should be recognized as causing condylar resorption, especially in combination with decreased host adaptive capacity. Retreatment of the occlusion is generally successful unless recompression of the TMJ occurs.

Arnett and colleagues[9, 29, 30, 53] proposed a treatment protocol for patients who have undergone resorption with resulting unstable occlusion. This protocol consists of orthodontic preparation for surgery followed by anti-inflammatory medications, stabilizing splints, and precise orthognathic sur-

gery that does not reload the joints. Without this protocol before orthognathic surgery, further condylar resorption routinely occurs.[9]

REFERENCES

1. Epker BN, Wessberg GA: Mechanisms of early skeletal relapse following surgical advancement of the mandible. Br J Oral Surg 1982;20:175–182.
2. Ive J, McNeill RW, West RA: Mandibular advancement: Skeletal and dental changes during fixation. J Oral Surg 1977;35:881–886.
3. Kohn MW: Analysis of relapse after mandibular advancement surgery. J Oral Surg 1978;36:676–684.
4. Lake SL, McNeill RW, Little RM, West RA: Surgical mandibular advancement: A cephalometric analysis of treatment response. Am J Orthod 1981;80:376–394.
5. Sandor GKB, Stoelinga PJW, Tideman H, Leenen RJ: The role of intraosseous osteosynthesis wire in sagittal split osteotomies for mandibular advancement. J Oral Maxillofac Surg 1984;42:231–237.
6. Will LA, West RA: Factors influencing the stability of the sagittal split osteotomy for mandibular advancement. J Oral Maxillofac Surg 1989;47:813.
7. Worms FW, Speidel TM, Bevis RR, Waite DE: Posttreatment stability and esthetics of orthognathic surgery. Angle Orthod 1980;50:251–273.
8. Arnett GW, Tamborello JA, Rathbone JA: Temporomandibular joint ramifications of orthognathic surgery. In Bell WH (ed): Modern Practice in Orthognathic and Reconstructive Surgery. Philadelphia, WB Saunders, 1992, pp 522–593.
9. Arnett GW, Tamborello JA: Progressive class II development—female idiopathic condylar resorption. Oral Maxillofac Surg Clin North Am 1990;2:699–716.
10. Doyle MG: Stability and complications in 50 consecutively treated surgical-orthodontic patients: A retrospective longitudinal analysis from private practice. Int J Adult Orthod Orthognath Surg 1986;1:23–36.
11. LaBlanc JP, Turvey T, Epker BN: Results following simultaneous mobilization of the maxilla and mandible for the correction of dentofacial deformities: Analysis of 100 consecutive patients. Oral Surg Oral Med Oral Pathol 1982;54:607–612.
12. Phillips RM, Bell WH: Atrophy of mandibular condyles after sagittal ramus split osteotomy: Report of case. J Oral Surg 1978;36:45–49.
13. Weinberg S, Craft J: Unilateral atrophy of the mandibular condyle after closed subcondylar osteotomy for correction of mandibular prognathism. J Oral Surg 1980;38:366–368.
14. Poulton DR, Ware WH: Surgical-orthodontic treatment of severe mandibular retrusion. Am J Orthod 1971;59:244.
15. Poulton DR, Ware WH: Surgical-orthodontic treatment of severe mandibular retrusion II. Am J Orthod 1973;63:237.
16. Finn RA, Throckmorton GS, Bell WH, Legan HL: Biomechanical considerations in the surgical correction of mandibular deficiency. J Oral Surg 1980;38:257.
17. Guernsey LH: Stability of treatment results in class II malocclusion corrected by full mandibular advancement surgery. Oral Surg 1974;37:668.

18. Guernsey LH, DeChamplain RW: Sequelae and complications of the intra-oral sagittal osteotomy in the mandibular rami. Oral Surg 1971;32:176.

19. McNeill RW, Hooley JR, Sundberg RI: Skeletal relapse during intermaxillary fixation. J Oral Surg 1973;31:212.

20. Steinhauser EW: Advancement of the mandible by sagittal ramus split and suprahyoid myotomy. J Oral Surg 1973;31:516.

21. Ellis E III, Gallo WJ: Relapse following mandibular advancement with dental plus skeletal maxillomandibular fixation. J Oral Maxillofac Surg 1986;44:509.

22. Mayo KH, Ellis E III: Stability of the mandible after advancement and use of dental plus skeletal maxillomandibular fixation: An experimental investigation in *Macaca mulatta*. J Oral Maxillofac Surg 1987;45:243.

23. Schendel SA, Epker BN: Results after mandibular advancement surgery: An analysis of 87 cases. J Oral Surg 1980;38:265–282.

24. Watzke IM, Turvey TA, Phillips C, Proffit WR: Stability of mandibular advancement after sagittal osteotomy with screw or wire fixation: A comparative study. J Oral Maxillofac Surg 1990;48:108–121.

25. Van Sickels JE, Flanary CM: Stability associated with mandibular advancement treated by rigid osseous fixation. J Oral Maxillofac Surg 1985;43:338.

26. Van Sickels JE, Larsen AJ, Thrash WJ: Relapse after rigid fixation of mandibular advancement. J Oral Maxillofac Surg 1986;44:698–702.

27. Epker BN: Modifications in the sagittal osteotomy of the mandible. J Oral Surg 1977;35:157–159.

28. Epker BN, Wolford LM: Modified sagittal ramus osteotomy. In Dentofacial Deformities, Surgical-Orthodontic Correction. St. Louis, CV Mosby, 1980, pp 78–79.

29. Arnett GW, Milam SB, Gottesman L: Progressive mandibular retrusion—idiopathic condylar resorption. Part I. Am J Orthod Dentofacial Orthop 1996;110:8–15.

30. Arnett GW, Milam SB, Gottesman L: Progressive mandibular retrusion—idiopathic condylar resorption. Part II. Am J Orthod Dentofacial Orthop 1996;110:117–127.

31. Arnett GW, Tamborello JA: Condylar movement during intermaxillary fixation sagittal osteotomy. In Clinical Congress on Orthognathic Challenges: Predictability, Stability and Complications. AAO/AAOMS Clinical Congress Scientific Abstract Session, Anaheim, CA, 1986.

32. Kent JN, Carlton DM, Zide MF: Rheumatoid disease and related arthropathies. Oral Surg Oral Med Oral Pathol 1986;61:423–439.

33. Link JJ, Nickerson JW: Temporomandibular joint internal derangements in an orthognathic surgery population. Int J Adult Orthod Orthognath Surg 1992;7:161–169.

34. Goodwill CJ, Steggles BG: Destruction of the temporomandibular joints in rheumatoid arthritis. Ann Rheum Dis 1966;25:133–136.

35. Caplan HI, Benny RA: Total osteolysis of the mandibular condyle in progressive sclerosis (scleroderma). Oral Surg Oral Med Oral Pathol 1978;46:362–366.

36. Lanigan DT, Myall RWT, West RA, McNeill RW: Condylysis in a patient with mixed vascular disease. Oral Surg Oral Med Oral Pathol 1979;48:198–204.

37. Ogden GR: Complete resorption of the mandibular condyles in rheumatoid arthritis. Br Dent J 1986;160:90.

38. Ramon Y, Samra H, Oberman M: Mandibular condylosis and apertognathia as presenting symptoms in progressive systemic sclerosis (scleroderma). Oral Surg Oral Med Oral Pathol 1987;63:269–274.

39. Dick R, Jones DN: Temporomandibular joint condyle changes in patients undergoing chronic haemodialysis. Clin Radiol 1973;24:72–76.

40. Abubaker AO, Arslan W, Sotereanos GC: Estrogen and progesterone receptors in the temporomandibular joint disk of symptomatic and asymptomatic patients. J Oral Maxillofac Surg 1993;5:1096–1100.

41. Rosner IA, Goldberg VM, Getzy L, Moskowitz RW: Effects of estrogen on cartilage and experimentally induced osteoarthritis. Arthritis Rheum 1979;22:52–58.

42. Ralston SH, Russell RG, Gowen M: Estrogen inhibits release of tumor necrosis factor from peripheral blood mononuclear cells in postmenopausal women. J Bone Miner Res 1990;5:983–988.

43. De M, Sanford TR, Wood GW: Interleukin-1, interleukin-6, and tumor necrosis factor alpha are produced in the mouse uterus during the estrous cycle and are induced by estrogen and progesterone. Dev Biol 1992;151:297–305.

44. Cutolo MA, Sulli A, Barone A, et al: Macrophages, synovial tissue and rheumatoid arthritis [review]. Clin Exp Rheumatol 1993;11:331–339.

45. Whyte A, Williams RO: Bromocriptine suppresses postpartum exacerbation of collagen-induced arthritis. Arthritis Rheum 1988;31:927–928.

46. Susami T, Kuroda T, Yano Y, Nakamura T: Growth changes and orthodontic treatment in a patient with condylolysis. Am J Orthod Dentofacial Orthop 1992;102:295–301.

47. Rabey GP: Bilateral mandibular condylysis—a morphanalytic diagnosis. Br J Oral Surg 1977–78;15:121–134.

48. Silbermann M, Livne E: Age-related degenerative changes in the mouse mandibular joint. J Anat 1979;129:507–520.

49. Furstman L, Bernick S, Zipkin I: The effect of hydrocortisone and fluoride upon the rat's mandibular joint. J Oral Therap Pharm 1965;1:515–525.

50. Pellicci PN, Zolla-Pazners S, Rabhan WM, Wilson PD: Osteonecrosis of the femoral head associated with pregnancy: A report of three cases. Clin Orthop Rel Res 1984;185:59–63.

51. Isberg AM, Isacsson G: Tissue reactions of the temporomandibular joint following retrusive guidance of the mandible. J Craniomandib Pract 1986;4:143–148.

52. Furstman L: The effect of loss of occlusion upon the temporomandibular joint. Am J Orthod 1965;51:245–261.

53. Arnett GW: A redefinition of bilateral sagittal osteotomy (BSO) advancement relapse. Am J Orthod Dentofacial Orthop 1993;104:506–515.

54. Janzen EK, Bluher JA: The cephalometric, anatomic and histological changes in *Macaca mulatta* after application of a continuous acting retraction force in the mandible. Am J Orthod 1965;51:823–855.

55. Ramfjord SP, Hiniker JJ: Distal placement of the mandible in adult rhesus monkeys. J Prosthet Dent 1966;16:491–502.

56. Adams CD, Merkle MC, Norwick KW, et al: Dentofacial remodeling produced by intermaxillary forces in *Macaca mulatta*. Arch Oral Biol 1972;17:1519–1535.

57. Joho J-P: The effects of extraoral low-pull traction of the mandibular dentition of *Macaca mulatta*. Am J Orthod 1973;64:555.

58. Shimozuma K: Effects of vertical forces on the dentofacial complex of *Macaca irus*. Nippon Kyosei Shika Gakkai Zasshi 1982;41:413–449.

59. Asano T: The effects of mandibular retrusive force on the growing rat mandible. Am J Orthod 1986;90:464.

60. Ellis E III, Hinton RJ: Histologic examination of the temporomandibular joint after mandibular advancement with and without rigid fixation: An experimental investigation in adult *Macaca mulatta*. J Oral Maxillofac Surg 1991;49:1316–1327.

61. Mongini F: Condylar remodeling after occlusal therapy. J Prosthet Dent 1980;43:568–577.

62. Peltola JS: Radiologic variations in mandibular condyles of Finnish students, one group orthodontically treated and the other not. Eur J Orthod 1993;15:223–227.

63. Jankelson B, Abib F: Effect of variation in manipulative force on the repetitiveness of centric relation registration: A computer-based study. J Am Dent Assoc 1986;113:59–62.

64. Adams CD, Meikle MC, Norwick KW, Turpin DL: Dentofacial remodeling produced by intermaxillary forces in *Macaca mulatta*. Arch Oral Biol 1972;17:1519–1535.

65. Hackney FL, Van Sickels JE, Nummikoski PV: Condylar displacement and temporomandibular joint dysfunction following bilateral sagittal split osteotomy and rigid fixation. J Oral Maxillofac Surg 1989;47:223.

66. Kundert M, Hadjianghelou O: Condylar displacement after sagittal splitting of the mandibular rami. J Maxillofac Surg 1980;8:278–287.

67. Lund E, Sindet-Pedersen S: Postoperative changes after bilateral mandibular osteotomies: A computed tomography study. Oral Surg Oral Med Oral Pathol 1989;67:588.

68. Spitzer W, Rettinger G, Sitzmann F: Computerized tomography examination for the detection of positional changes in the temporomandibular joint after ramus osteotomies with screw fixation. J Maxillofac Surg 1984;12:139–142.

69. Timmis DP, Aragon SB, Van Sickels JE: Masticatory dysfunction with rigid and nonrigid osteosynthesis of sagittal split osteotomies. Oral Surg Oral Med Oral Pathol 1986;62:119–123.

70. Tuinizing DB, Swart IGN: Lagerveranderunben des caput mandibulae bei verwendung von zugschrauben nach sagittaler osteotomie des unterkiefers. Dtsch Z Mund Kiefer Gesichtschir 1978;2:94–96.

71. Nickerson JW Jr, Boering G: Natural course of osteoarthritis as it relates to internal derangement of the TMJ. Oral Maxillofac Clin North Am 1989;1:27–45.

72. Westesson P-L, Eriksson L, Kurita K: Reliability of negative clinical temporomandibular joint examination: Prevalence of disk displacement in asymptomatic joint. Oral Surg Oral Med Oral Pathol 1989;68:551–554.

73. Westesson P-L: Structural hard-tissue changes in temporomandibular joints with internal derangement. Oral Surg Oral Med Oral Pathol 1985;59:220–224.

74. Eriksson L, Westesson P-L: Clinical and radiological study of patients with anterior disc displacement of the temporomandibular joint. Swed Dent J 1983;7:55–64.

75. Bell WE: Temporomandibular Disorders: Classification, Diagnosis, Management, ed 3. Chicago, Year Book Medical Publishers, 1990, pp 339–341.

76. Gibbs CH, Mahan PE, Manderlia A, et al: Limits of human bite strength. J Prosthet Dent 1986;56:226–229.

77. Bates RE Jr, Gremillion HA, Stewart CM: Degenerative joint disease. Part I. Management and diagnosis considerations. Cranio 1993;11:284–290.

78. Mahan PE, Alling CC: Occlusion and occlusal pathofunction. In Mahay PE, Alling CC: Facial Pain, ed 3. Philadelphia and London, Lea & Febiger, 1991, pp 187–193.

79. Gray RJH: Pain dysfunction syndrome and osteoarthritis related to unilateral and bilateral temporomandibular joint symptoms. J Dent 1986; 14:156–159.

80. Nitzan DW: Intra-articular pressure in the functioning human temporomandibular joint and its alteration by uniform elevation of the occlusal plane. J Oral Maxillofac Surg 1994;52:671–679.

81. Schellhas KP, Wilks CH, Fritts HM, et al: MR of osteochondritis dissecans and avascular necrosis of the mandibular condyle. AJNR Am J Neuroradiol 1989;190:3–12.

82. Gazit D, Ehrlich J, Kohen Y, Bab I: Effect of occlusal (mechanical) stimulus on bone remodeling in rat mandibular condyle. J Oral Pathol 1987; 16:395–398.

83. Ehrlich J, Jaffe A, Shanfeld JL, et al: Immunohistochemical localization and distribution of cyclic nucleotides in the rat mandibular condyle in response to an induced occlusal condyle change. Arch Oral Biol 1980;25:545–549.

84. Rasmussen OC: Description of population and progress of symptoms in a longitudinal study of temporomandibular arthropathy. Scand J Dent Res 1981;89:196–203.

Intrajoint Therapy

CHAPTER

Arthroscopy

Anders B. Holmlund

Development of Temporomandibular Joint Arthroscopy

The first arthroscopic examination was performed by Takagi in 1918.[1] Using a pediatric cystoscope, he performed arthroscopy of the knee joint on a cadaver. In 1921, Bircher described the first arthroscopic examinations in Europe.[2] However, these reports were poorly accepted and did not encourage further studies. The main objection concerned illumination problems. In these first prototypes, illumination was provided by a small lamp at the end of the arthroscope. The risk of damaging the bulb and spreading the glass fragments inside the joint was considerable. Moreover, the lamp was in the way and impaired viewing. It was therefore a long time before the next step forward was taken by Watanabe,[3] a protégé of Takagi's. In 1957, he introduced the first specially designed arthroscope. However, the illumination problems had not been solved, and the real breakthrough came with the commercial introduction of the flexible fiber-light cable in the early 1970s. Another invention, the Hopkins rod-lens telescope, was also introduced commercially in the 1970s and constituted a significant improvement in optics.

The first report on temporomandibular joint (TMJ) arthroscopy was published by Ohnishi in 1975, following the strong Japanese tradition in the field of arthroscopy.[4] He used the recently developed No. 24 Watanabe 1.7-mm telescope with improved fo-

cusing ability. Previously, the rigid telescopes could not focus at a distance less than 3 mm from the end of the arthroscope. In 1980, Ohnishi's experiences with TMJ arthroscopy were published in English,[5] and this was the beginning of TMJ arthroscopy. Other reports followed, such as those of Murakami in Japan, Holmlund in Sweden, and McCain, Kaminishi, and Sanders in the United States. TMJ arthroscopy is now an important aid in the diagnosis and treatment of temporomandibular disorders (TMD).

The term *arthroscopy* comes from the two Greek words *arthros* (joint) and *scopein* (to view) and simply means to look directly into the joint. Arthroscopy has two basic indications: diagnosis and treatment. The indications have gradually evolved for each joint, but the same basic arthroscopic principles and instruments are used, regardless of which joint is to be examined. However, the special anatomy and function of the TMJ must be considered.

Anatomic Considerations

TEMPOROMANDIBULAR JOINT ANATOMY

The functional anatomy of the TMJ is described elsewhere in this book (Volume 4, Chapter 1). However, there are some special considerations with regard to the arthroscopic procedure that should be mentioned. The joint is divided by the disk into an upper and a lower compartment. The volume of the upper compartment is about twice as large as that of the lower compartment. The kinetics of the TMJ is a combination of rotation and sliding movements whereby the disk-condyle complex slides down the eminence. In most TMD, this sliding movement is impaired. If translation is completely impaired, the joint space is almost totally closed, making a safe puncture of the joint impossible. Fortunately, in patients with chronic locking or even rheumatoid arthritis, this is not the case, and the space is large enough to permit safe puncture of the joint. If no translation is demonstrated on radiographs or at clinical examination, arthroscopy should not be attempted because it will damage the joint structures. In the lateral and medial areas, the capsule and disk attachment fuse and become attached to the lateral and medial poles of the condyle. Puncture of the upper compartment involves only penetration of the lateral capsule, whereas puncture of the lower compartment involves penetration of both the capsule and the disk ligament. Puncture of the lower compartment thus always involves the slight risk of damaging the lateral disk attachment and consequently displacing the disk medially. The TMJ capsule is almost membrane thin in the anterior and anteromedial parts. This must be considered while distending the joint. Irrigation, if performed with too much pressure, may cause rupture of the anterior and medial capsules, with subsequent extravasation of fluid into the surrounding tissues. The better-developed lateral capsule is usually resistant to the trocar during puncture. The insertion in the glenoid fossa of the posterior disk attachment varies considerably. In some cases, the attachment also has an anterior insertion in the deepest part of the glenoid fossa. It is important not to perform a lateral puncture of the joint too far posteriorly because of increased risk of damage to and bleeding in the posterior disk attachment. Occasionally, the roof of the glenoid fossa is paper thin. According to the author's experience with TMJ arthroscopy over 15 years, accidental penetration into the middle cranial fossa should be almost impossible if the proper technique and instruments are used. However, patients with advanced rheumatic disease associated with major erosions of the articular cartilage and bone may be at risk; in such cases, a radiographic examination with tomograms is necessary.

The TMJ is surrounded by important anatomic structures—the temporal vessels and tympanic membrane posteriorly, and the facial nerve inferiorly and anteriorly on the lateral side. The chorda tympani is close to the medial capsule, and the maxillary artery is located somewhat inferior to the joint on the medial side. Puncture of the TMJ must be planned with great care to avoid damaging these structures. However, it is relatively safe to insert the instruments from the lateral side between the temporal vessels posteriorly and the temporal branch of the facial nerve anteriorly.

ARTHROSCOPIC ANATOMY

It is important to learn the normal arthroscopic anatomy. Even in joints with pronounced pathologic changes, there are areas of normal anatomy that are the main landmarks and references.

When performing arthroscopy, the natural color of the intraarticular tissues may be distorted, for several reasons. The arthroscopic examination is performed with the joint distended by gas or fluid. Gas distention gives a brighter image, but because heat is increased, the vascularity may be affected. Moreover, fibrillation of the cartilage and disk may escape detection because, with gas distention, the tissues adhere. Distention is therefore usually performed with fluid, such as saline solution. This reduces the heat, but it may also affect the vascularity, depending on the temperature of the irrigation fluid. If fluid at room temperature (which is most common) is used, this will reduce the vascularity of the synovial lining. The color of the tissue will also be slightly opaque when fluid is used. However, fibrillation of fibrocartilage and disk will be accurately displayed.

The tissue color may also be distorted by the light cables and light sources used. Fiber light cables give a slight yellow discoloration to the tissue, owing to a higher absorption in the blue part of the spectrum. Fluid light cables provide a more accurate image, but these are rather impractical for clinical use. Optimally, the light source should provide a color temperature of 5000 to 6000 K in order not to distort the tissue color.

Because all these factors must be considered, there is a real need for proper training in diagnostic arthroscopy.

Upper Compartment

The synovial lining is well developed in the posterior part of the glenoid fossa. The posterior disk attachment has a smooth, sometimes slightly folded appearance (Fig. 14–1*A*). The vascularity is discrete, especially if irrigation fluid at room temperature is used. The posterior band of the disk frequently seems to protrude and, in contrast to the posterior disk attachment, is not vascular (Fig. 14–1*B*). However, the boundary between the disk and its attachments is not clear-cut. The anteroposterior orientation of the collagen bundles can sometimes be visualized. The normal disk and fibrocartilage appear white to slightly yellow in color, with a smooth surface (Fig. 14–1*C*). The boundary between the anterior band of the disk and the anterior disk attachment is usually well defined. The vascularity of the latter is even more discrete than that of the posterior disk attachment. The anterior capsule is thin, almost membrane-like (Fig. 14–1*D*). The anterior half of the medial capsule is also extremely thin and almost translucent (Fig. 14–1*E*). Posteriorly, the medial capsule, reinforced with fibrous tissue, serves as another important anatomic landmark during TMJ arthroscopy (Fig. 14–1*F*).

Laterally, the recess between the disk and the lateral capsule may be rather deep and narrow and, in many cases, is difficult to inspect.

Lower Compartment

In general, vascularity is less apparent in the lower compartment. The posterior recess is deep, and the capsule is attached to the condylar neck (Fig. 14–1*G*). Laterally and medially, there are narrow recesses between the condylar head and the disk, and in some cases the disk attachments can be seen. The central area contains the posterosuperior part of the condylar head and the central part of the disk (Fig. 14–1*H*). Because the joint space is extremely narrow in this part, one cannot move the arthroscope

into the anterior recess without damaging the fibrocartilage and disk. The anterior part of the lower compartment contains the functional (and therefore more interesting) part of the condyle. The anterior capsule is extremely thin and directly overlies the upper belly of the lateral pterygoid muscle (Fig. 14–1*I*). The anterior recess is small and difficult to puncture without a great risk of damaging internal joint structures or muscle insertions near the joint.

Indications for Diagnostic Arthroscopy

Many TMDs are difficult to diagnose. The reasons for this are numerous. The TMJ has an anatomic position under the skull base, which complicates clinical and radiographic examinations, and the close relationship between jaw muscles and joint structures complicates the interpretation of clinical signs and symptoms caused by muscle hyperactivity alone or by organic joint disease. Moreover, projection of pain from other areas, such as the cervical part of the spine, may be mistaken for TMJ pain.

A careful case history and clinical examination are of great importance in TMJ diagnosis. Neither arthroscopy nor any other supplementary technique (radiography, magnetic resonance imaging [MRI]) can substitute for a thorough clinical examination. Moreover, these supplementary techniques are invasive or costly. Such methods should therefore be regarded as important adjuncts to the clinical examination and can confirm or (perhaps more important in the field of TMD) refute a tentative diagnosis. Whether arthroscopy should be performed is often determined by what the other techniques, such as computed tomography (CT) and MRI, cannot achieve. One definite advantage of arthroscopy is that diagnosis and therapy can be performed simultaneously. It is also possible to perform biopsies.

The indications for diagnostic arthroscopy are as follows:

1. Internal derangement
2. Osteoarthritis
3. Arthritides
4. Pseudotumors
5. Post-traumatic complaints

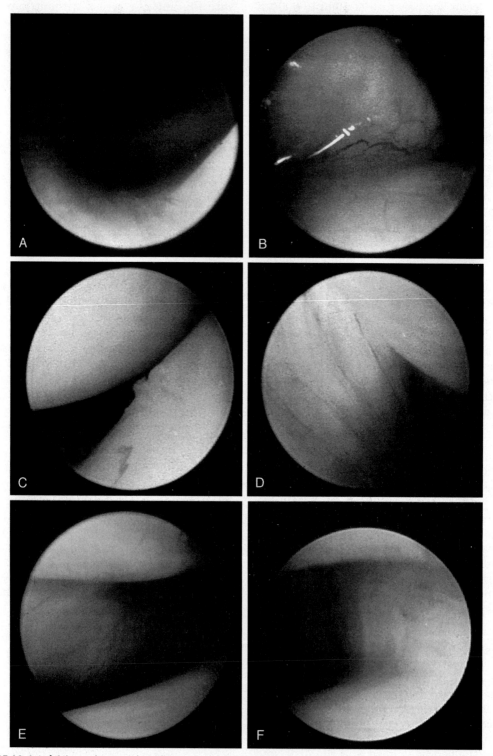

FIGURE 14–1. Left joint under normal conditions. *A,* Upper compartment; posterior disk attachment. *B,* Upper compartment; posterior band of the disk. *C,* Upper compartment; central part of the disk and posterior slope of the eminence. *D,* Upper compartment; anterior capsule and anterior part of the eminence. *E,* Upper compartment; anterior part of the medial capsule, inferior part of the eminence, and anterior part of the disk. *F,* Upper compartment; posterior part of the medial capsule. The glenoid fossa is above, the disk below.

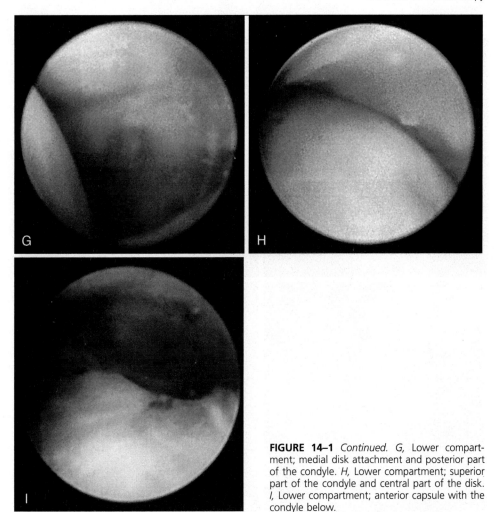

FIGURE 14–1 *Continued. G,* Lower compartment; medial disk attachment and posterior part of the condyle. *H,* Lower compartment; superior part of the condyle and central part of the disk. *I,* Lower compartment; anterior capsule with the condyle below.

Internal derangement (disk derangement, disk displacement) is the most common reason for surgical intervention. This condition has been studied extensively in recent decades, and definite clinical signs and symptoms have been reported, although the etiopathogenesis has not been clarified. Two variants have been described. The first is associated primarily with painful clicking or catching of the TMJ. The clinical signs and symptoms are well defined and correlate closely with findings during open surgery.[6] Although the arthroscopic examination can sometimes confirm the clicking, this is usually not the case, because irrigation reduces friction. Almost no intraarticular findings are present, and the anatomy is generally normal. Occasionally, the surface of the disk may show remodeling. Little, if any, inflammation is present. Degenerative changes are uncommon and minor in the

fibrocartilage and disk. More definite arthroscopic signs are found in the second variant—so-called chronic locking. In these cases, a degenerative process typically develops in the posterior part of the disk and the posterior disk attachment. Arthroscopically, there is a loss of the well-defined boundary between the disk and the posterior disk attachment, with softening and hyperemia of the disk (Fig. 14–2A). Usually one sees only mild inflammation, although in about 20% of cases the inflammation is more severe, with synovial hyperplasia.[7] Arthrotic changes are infrequent in the fibrocartilage; if present, they are usually slight.

The late stage of osteoarthritis correlates well with clinical signs (crepitation)[8] and radiographic features (sclerosis, flattening, erosions).[9] However, arthroscopy more accurately reveals the severity of cartilage and

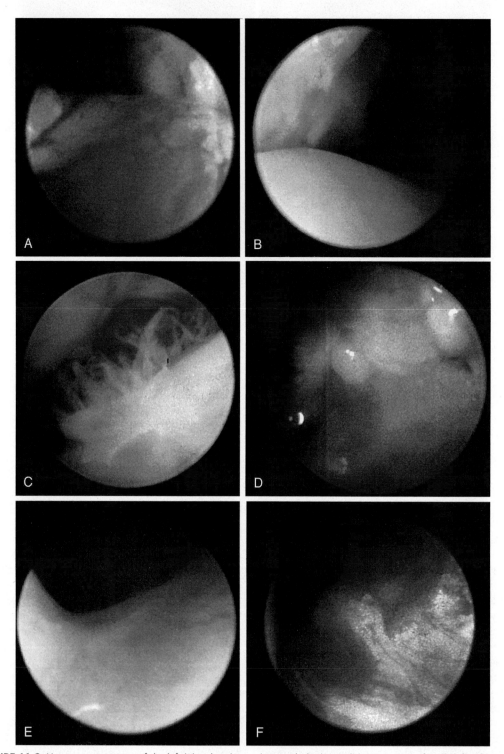

FIGURE 14–2. Upper compartment of the left joint showing various pathologic conditions. *A,* Loss of well-defined boundary between the posterior band of the disk and the posterior disk attachment. The area shows capillary hyperemia. *B,* Slight fibrillation of the fibrocartilage on the posterior slope of the eminence. The disk, below, is unaffected. *C,* Pronounced fibrillation of the central part of the disk. *D,* Close view of the fibrocartilage in the glenoid fossa showing arthrotic lesions and remodeling. *E,* Capillary hyperemia in the posterior disk attachment. *F,* Synovial hyperplasia in the posterior disk attachment.

disk involvement and of associated inflammation[9] (Fig. 14–2*B–D*). This information is important for choosing intraarticular pharmacotherapy—steroids or hyaluronan. It may also provide additional information as to whether open surgery should be performed.

The TMJ may also be involved in arthritides—in particular, rheumatoid arthritis, psoriatic arthritis, and pelvospondylitis. An early diagnosis of TMJ involvement is important. However, clinical signs and symptoms are nonspecific, and proposed radiographic features (erosions) are also found in joints with osteoarthritis and are demonstrated rather late in the disease process. Arthroscopy provides reliable information on the degree of inflammation and cartilage involvement[10, 11] (Fig. 14–2*E* and *F*). In the chronic stage, fibrosis seems to be an important diagnostic marker.[10] A synovial biopsy, readily obtained during arthroscopy, has been found to aid the diagnosis further, particularly in patients with generalized joint disease.[11] Because lysis and lavage can be done simultaneously and have proved highly effective, arthroscopy should definitely be considered in patients with arthritides. In rarer conditions, such as crystal-induced arthritis (gout and pseudogout), arthroscopy may be the only way to make a correct diagnosis.

Pseudotumors, such as synovial chondromatosis and pigmented villonodular synovitis, are best diagnosed with arthroscopy, because clinical signs and symptoms frequently resemble those of internal derangement, osteoarthritis, or arthritis. In patients with synovial chondromatosis, numerous loose cartilage bodies can be visualized almost blocking the joint space. These loose bodies are not always detectable with CT and MRI.[12] In patients with pigmented villonodular synovitis, typical synovial projections with pigmentation are found.

Arthroscopy is indicated in some patients with post-traumatic complaints, particularly insurance cases.

Contraindications

Absolute contraindications are bony ankylosis, advanced resorption of the glenoid fossa, infection in the joint area, and malignant tumors. Relative contraindications are patients at increased risk for hemorrhage, patients at increased risk for infection, and fibrous ankylosis.

In TMJs in which the tomograms indicate advanced resorption of the glenoid fossa, diagnostic arthroscopy should be avoided because of the risk of accidental perforation into the middle cranial fossa. In patients having an infection in the soft tissues surrounding the joint, there is a considerable risk of spreading an extraarticular infection into the joint. However, in cases of infectious arthritis, it may be desirable to perform an arthroscopic puncture of the joint to establish drainage and irrigate the joint. In cases of suspected malignant tumors, diagnostic arthroscopy should be avoided because of the risk of spreading malignant cells with the irrigation fluid.

Patients at increased risk of bleeding should be carefully evaluated and prepared before arthroscopy to prevent this complication, which may lead to hemarthrosis. Patients at increased risk of infection (e.g., immunodeficient patients) must also be carefully assessed, especially with regard to the need for prophylactic antibiotic therapy. Diagnostic arthroscopy should be avoided in joints with pronounced fibrotic ankylosis.

Preoperative Care

First, the physical condition of the patient should be reevaluated and decisions about prophylactic treatment implemented.

Diagnostic TMJ arthroscopy can be performed under local anesthesia. The patient should be told that the anesthetic almost invariably affects the upper branches of the facial nerve. The author has found after performing about 500 TMJ arthroscopies under local anesthesia that this transient, mild side effect is well tolerated by patients. Although diagnostic TMJ arthroscopy can be performed without sedation, most patients prefer to be given intravenous sedation. Midazolam, a relatively short-acting benzodiazepine, has good pharmacologic properties and also relaxes the jaw muscles. Patients should be asked to remove earrings and contact lenses before arthroscopy.

Plain radiographs or orthopantographs do not provide sufficiently detailed anatomic information about the TMJ. Plain radiographs should therefore be supplemented with tomograms. In routine cases, sagittal tomography is adequate, but CT is necessary for more advanced cases. Tomography is better than MRI for evaluating the anatomy of the bones. MRI may provide valuable information on disk position and disk deformation, but there is still a lack of studies regarding the diagnostic accuracy of MRI. In cases of suspected tumors, however, MRI may be the only choice.

Preoperative radiographic examination may consist of one or more of the following:

- Axial or frontal projection
- TMJ orthopantograph
- Corrected sagittal tomogram (or equivalent)

The axial (submentovertical) projection—always performed with sagittal tomography—shows information on the inclination of the condyle in the frontal plane. A frontal (anteroposterior) projection may be used instead. The TMJ orthopantograph provides an image of the translation in both TMJs at the same time. The corrected sagittal tomogram accurately shows the bony anatomy of the condyle, the eminence, and the glenoid fossa. Recently, orthopantographs with programs for tomography as well have been developed and are valuable in outpatient clinics.

Diagnostic Arthroscopy Equipment

Several publications have described the basic equipment for diagnostic TMJ arthroscopy.[13, 14] Figure 14–3 shows a suitable set of instruments. Most telescopes have a diameter of about 2 mm, but ultrathin telescopes have recently been developed with a diameter of about 0.7 mm. However, such a reduction in diameter also results in a loss of optical quality. In contrast, too large a telescope is difficult to move inside the joint. More important than the diameter is the quality of the optical system. A rod-lens telescope (Karl Storz GmbH & Co, Tuttlingen, Germany) has proved superior to other models. For diagnostic purposes, the telescope should have a direction of view of 30 degrees. The field of

vision is thereby much increased simply by rotating the instrument.

The arthroscopic sheath should fit properly on the telescope so that it just overlaps the telescope at the tip, thereby protecting the lens. The sharp and blunt trocar should fit the sheath and extend slightly over it at the tip. A 1.2-mm disposable standard needle is suitable for outflow.

Routine examinations can be performed with light from a halogen lamp. However, a xenon cold-light fountain, which provides light with more accurate color purity, is better when photographs and videotapes are needed for publication and teaching purposes.

The light cable connects the telescope to the light source. Although a so-called fluid cable provides the best color, it is fairly rigid and therefore impractical for routine clinical use. A fiber-light cable, which is more flexible, is therefore used. Some color distortion (too much yellow) must be expected because of higher absorption in the blue part of the spectrum.

Photographic slides are better than those obtained in video recordings (see Figs. 14–1 and 14–2). However, video has improved greatly during the last decade; it is excellent for teaching purposes, facilitates case review, and facilitates file documentation. Moreover, sterility can be better maintained with videoscopy.

Arthroscopic Procedure

ANESTHESIA

Routine diagnostic arthroscopy and minor arthroscopic surgery can be performed under local anesthesia. Arthroscopy under local anesthesia is more cost-effective than that under general anesthesia. No assistant is required to manipulate the jaw, and the patient can move the mandible normally.

Excellent anesthesia of the joint area is achieved by blocking the auriculotemporal nerve posterior to the condyle and infiltrating the subcutaneous tissue lateral to the joint (3 to 4 mL of lidocaine/epinephrine, 10 mg/mL). Local anesthesia can be combined with intravenous sedation, using a short-acting benzodiazepine such as midazolam. In patients with markedly impaired TMJ

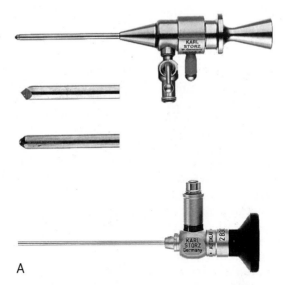

A

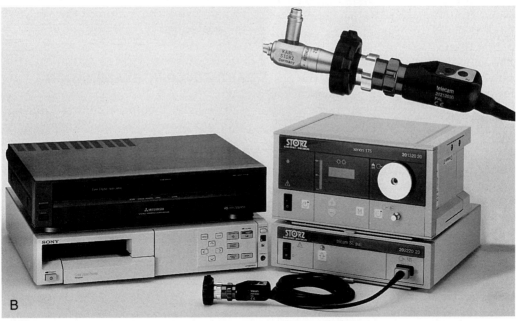

B

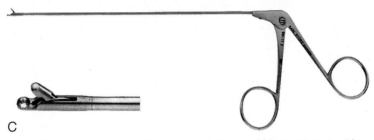

C

FIGURE 14–3. *A,* Rod-lens 30-degree telescope with sheath and sharp and blunt trocars. *B,* Video camera, light source, video recorder, and video printer. *C,* Biopsy forceps. Notice the cup form of the jaws, which avoids compression of the material.

mobility and in patients for whom more advanced arthroscopic surgery is planned, general anesthesia is preferred.

PUNCTURE

The arthroscopic examination should be performed with the patient in a supine position to reduce the risk of inducing a vasovagal reaction. The technique for puncture has been described in several publications.[13, 14]

First, the upper compartment is distended with 2 mL of lidocaine, which is injected slowly until resistance is felt. Additional injections of the anesthetic block any sensory input from branches of the posterior deep temporal and masseteric nerves supplying the anterior part of the TMJ. If no resistance is encountered after the injection of 3 mL, the distention should be stopped, because this suggests the occurrence of leakage through the capsule into the surrounding tissue.

The so-called inferolateral approach is usually used to gain good access to the posterior part of the upper compartment of the TMJ (Fig. 14–4). With this approach, access to the anterior recess is somewhat limited. However, from a diagnostic point of view, it is particularly important to examine the posterior part of the joint. This is also the best approach for puncturing the lower compartment. Alternative approaches to the upper compartment include the endaural and anterolateral approaches (see Fig. 14–4). The former may give a better view of the lateral part of the upper compartment; the latter provides better access to the anterior recess of the upper compartment.

It is questionable whether the lower compartment should be punctured at all. Even if the puncture is successful, only the posterior nonfunctional parts of the disk and condyle are visualized, and there is always at least some risk of damaging the lateral disk attachment. Routine puncture of the lower compartment should therefore be avoided.

The telescope should always be used to ensure that the arthroscopic sheath has been correctly placed. An outflow portal is then created (inferolateral approach) about 5 mm anterior to and slightly below the arthroscopic sheath. Continuous irrigation is performed using isotonic saline solution. For more prolonged arthroscopic surgery, Ringer's solution may be a better alternative because it has been found to protect the chondrocytes and maintain the synthesis of proteoglycans.

ARTHROSCOPIC EXAMINATION

The light should be adjusted during the arthroscopic examination. When examining the fibrocartilage, more light is reflected, which blinds the optical unit (so-called white-out). The light must therefore be reduced. In contrast, when examining the disk attachments and the capsule, where the vascularity may be marked, much light is absorbed and more light is needed. Video-controlled light sources are now available that permit automatic adjustment of light.

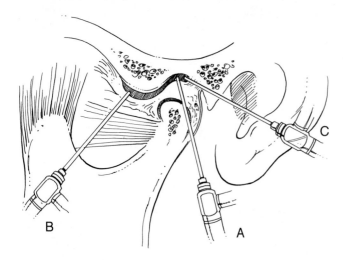

FIGURE 14–4. Puncture directions for the upper compartment of the temporomandibular joint. *A*, Inferolateral approach. *B*, Anterolateral approach. *C*, Endaural approach.

The arthroscopic examination begins with identification of the arthroscopic landmarks—the boundary between the disk and the posterior disk attachment (see Fig. 14–1*B*), the medial capsule (see Fig. 14–1*E* and *F*), the inferior part of the eminence (see Fig. 14–1*C*), and the anterior capsule if possible (see Fig. 14–1*D*). The arthroscope should always be moved slowly and gently between the various landmarks. Rotation of the arthroscope increases the field of vision considerably. The outflow should be monitored continually; if the needle becomes obstructed, considerable extravasation may occur in a short time. The irrigation pressure should be kept constant and low. In a small joint such as the TMJ, this is best performed with a syringe by the assisting nurse. A total irrigation volume of 30 mL is usually sufficient for diagnostic arthroscopy.

Magnification of the structures by the telescope may be a problem. The amount of magnification depends on the distance between the object viewed and the arthroscope. A ratio of 1:1 is obtained at a distance of 20 to 25 mm, which means that magnification is always present in a small joint such as the TMJ. Use of a graded probe inserted through a second portal is very valuable.

In the upper compartment, the examiner should first identify the posterior disk attachment and the posterior part of the disk (see Fig. 14–1*A* and *B*). The posterior disk attachment is the predominant location for inflammation and should be thoroughly examined for signs of inflammation such as increased vascularity, capillary hyperemia, villi, or synovial hyperplasia (see Fig. 14–2*A*, *E*, and *F*). Loss of the well-defined boundary between the posterior part of the disk and the posterior disk attachment indicates degenerative changes usually found in joints with chronic locking and osteoarthritis. During alternate opening and closing movements, any elongation of the posterior disk attachment is revealed. The arthroscope should then be moved more medially to visualize the medial capsule (see Fig. 14–1*E* and *F*). After withdrawing the arthroscope slightly, it is directed anteromedially; when the mouth is closed slightly, it will slip under the eminence into the anterior recess (see Fig. 14–1*D*). However, in about one third of cases, it may be difficult to reach the anterior recess. Force should

never be used in these cases, because it will damage the fibrocartilage. From a diagnostic point of view, the anterior recess is of minor importance; pathologic changes are almost never found there.

During withdrawal of the arthroscope, the temporal cartilage and disk surface should be evaluated (see Fig. 14–1*C*). Signs of osteoarthritis, such as fibrillation, lesions in the fibrocartilage, and denuded subchondral bone, may be located mainly on the posterior slope of the eminence (see Fig. 14–2*B*). Disk perforations are usually detected in the lateral, central, and posterior parts (see Fig. 14–2*C*). The lateral capsule is difficult to examine. This problem may be overcome to some extent by using an endaural approach. A retrograde optic (120 degrees) can also be used.

In some cases, the lower compartment can be examined through a large disk perforation from the upper compartment.

The arthroscopic examination is completed by thorough irrigation to remove any blood clots. Excess fluid is then removed by suctioning through the arthroscopic sheath. The small skin incision is closed with surgical tape.

SYNOVIAL BIOPSY

Although arthroscopy is very accurate for diagnosing synovitis, recent studies indicate that a synovial biopsy may also be of value. Current indications for synovial biopsy include suspected arthritides or benign tumors.

In the knee, biopsy under direct arthroscopic control is best because of the wide variation within the joint. It is therefore necessary to use a second portal for the biopsy forceps. In small joints such as the TMJ, a so-called semiblind technique is sufficient.[15] First the area for obtaining the biopsy must be selected; then the arthroscopic sheath is fixed in that position, and the telescope is removed. Then the biopsy forceps is inserted, the sheath slightly withdrawn, the forceps opened, and the biopsy performed. The correct location should be confirmed through the telescope. Recent studies in the TMJ have shown that the semiblind technique has the same high accuracy as biopsy under direct visual control.[16]

The type of biopsy forceps used is important. The forceps must be cup-shaped with sharp edges, in order to cut the tissue precisely without compressing the specimen. A suitable biopsy forceps is shown in Figure 14–3C.

Postoperative Care

Diagnostic arthroscopy under local anesthesia has many advantages compared with that performed under general anesthesia, and the patient is ready to go home after only an hour's rest in the clinic. Any anesthetic effects on branches of the facial nerve have usually disappeared by then.

If arthroscopic surgery has been performed simultaneously, the patient is given a training program. A physiotherapist is contacted if needed. Control of any parafunctional habits is maintained postoperatively.

Information about hygiene and food is given to the patient. In case of postoperative pain, a mild analgesic is prescribed.

Prophylactic antibiotics may be given to patients at high risk for infection (e.g., those with immunodeficiency, heart valve prosthesis). Normally, however, there is no need for prophylactic antibiotics.

Complications

Intraoperative and postoperative complications are seldom associated with diagnostic arthroscopy. This accords with data in the orthopedic literature regarding knee joint arthroscopy.[17] However, it should be emphasized that a complication in the TMJ area can be disastrous for the patient. A few such complications have been reported concerning damage to the middle ear and the facial nerve.[18, 19] In arthroscopic surgery, particularly the more complicated procedures, the risk of complications is obviously greater. Adequate knowledge of the external and internal anatomy of the TMJ is a prerequisite for clinical use of the arthroscope. Preoperative radiographic examination should include tomograms. Training on cadavers is recommended. Experience with open TMJ surgery facilitates the management of complications.

VASCULAR INJURY

The TMJ is surrounded by a dense vascular network, and collateral circulation in the area is extensive. It is therefore not as vulnerable as the hip with regard to avascularity, and surgical interruption of the vessels usually does not damage the joint structures. Carter and Testa noted hemorrhagic complications in 1.8% of cases in a survey of 2225 TMJ arthroscopies.[20] In about 80%, the temporal vessels were involved.

Vascular malformations, such as arteriovenous fistulae, resulting from TMJ arthroscopy are unlikely, but they have been reported.[21, 22]

If well-designed trocars are used, these rarely cause bleeding during puncture of the TMJ. More often it is the outflow needle that causes bleeding, especially if the needle is difficult to position. The bleeding is usually venous in origin and easily controlled using a tamponade. In persistent cases, the cutaneous incision can be extended slightly and the source of bleeding ligated or controlled with cautery. Intraarticular bleeding may occur in more advanced arthroscopic surgery. The protocol suggested by McCain is appropriate.[23] All instruments are removed, and the condyle is moved to the compartment where bleeding has occurred and kept there for about 5 minutes. The instruments are then reinserted to irrigate and débride clots that may have formed. If this procedure does not work, the joint must be opened and the bleeding controlled.

Intraarticular hemorrhage is common in trauma to the mandible.[24] However, the accumulated blood is resorbed within a few weeks.[24] Thus, the risk of developing arthrofibrosis because of intraarticular hemorrhage is low.

EXTRAVASATION

Excessive extravasation of irrigation fluid into the surrounding tissue sometimes occurs. In prolonged arthroscopic surgery the risk is greater, and cases of extensive edema in the upper airway with subsequent postobstructive pulmonary edema have been reported.[25] Neurapraxia of both motor and sensory nerves may also develop. If the surgeon continually checks the outflow, this is unlikely.

SCUFFING

The cartilage may be scuffed by the trocar during puncture. The scuffed fibrocartilage should not be mistaken for arthrotic changes. This lesion can be avoided if the trocar is directed toward the crest of the glenoid fossa until it touches the bone. The sharp trocar is then exchanged for a blunt one, which is directed slightly inferiorly to slip into the upper compartment.

BROKEN INSTRUMENTS

Instruments that break during arthroscopic manipulation are an unpleasant complication. Such complications have been reported by McCain and de la Rua[26] and Tarro.[27] This reinforces the need for the surgeon to be trained in open TMJ surgery, because this may be the only way to retrieve a broken instrument. For many reasons, a broken instrument should not be left in place. It may be potentially dangerous, and it may be blamed for a poor result. This complication can be avoided by using correct technique and impeccable instruments.

A protocol for arthroscopic retrieval of broken instruments has been recommended by McCain and de la Rua:[26]

1. Stop the procedure and maintain the position of the arthroscope and working cannulas.
2. Keep the broken object in view.
3. Check the inflow bags to maintain sufficient irrigation and to prevent collapse of the joint from lack of fluid.
4. Record and measure the depth of the instrument with a scored cannula.
5. Have adequate instruments available for removal.
6. Adjust inflow to ensure optimal visibility.
7. Radiograph the joint if the object cannot be located.
8. Consider fluoroscopic assistance to localize the object if it cannot be found arthroscopically.
9. Remove the object.

OTOLOGIC COMPLICATIONS

A few otologic complications have been noted in association with TMJ arthroscopy. Van Sickels and colleagues reported a case of perforation of the tympanic membrane and partial dislocation of the malleus.[18] Applebaum and coworkers described three patients who largely lost their hearing.[19] Such serious complications can be avoided only by proper training in TMJ anatomy and practice on cadavers before the clinical use of TMJ arthroscopy.

The influence of TMJ arthroscopy on normal hearing has been evaluated by audiometric measurements pre- and postoperatively.[28, 29] Both studies indicate that the risk of adverse effects on hearing is extremely low.

INTRACRANIAL DAMAGE

Damage to intracranial structures during TMJ arthroscopy has been reported.[30, 31] The roof of the glenoid fossa can be extremely thin, but the author's autopsy studies indicate that it takes considerable force to penetrate the roof of the glenoid fossa, even with a sharp trocar. In patients whose cartilage and bone show marked destruction (e.g., advanced rheumatoid arthritis), great caution must be exercised, and routine radiographic examination should be supplemented with CT.

INFECTION

In an extensive review of 3146 patients (4831 joints) by McCain and colleagues in 1992,[32] the frequency of infection was low (15 cases; 0.3%). This brings into question the common use of prophylactic antibiotics. The author has performed more than 500 TMJ arthroscopies without using any antibiotics, and no patient has developed an infection. Considering recent reports on the increase in bacterial resistance to antibiotics, routine use of antibiotic prophylaxis is not advisable.

Arthroscopy is not indicated if an infection exists in the area of intended puncture. However, in suppurative arthritis, arthroscopic drainage and lavage can be helpful, and specimens can be taken for culture.

NERVE INJURY

Injuries to nerves are almost never associated with TMJ arthroscopy. In more than 4800 TMJ arthroscopies, McCain and colleagues reported only three cases (0.06%) with permanent nerve damage.[32] Thus the frequency is about the same as that reported for knee joint arthroscopy. The auriculotemporal and facial nerves are most often involved. Excessive extravasation of irrigation fluid may rarely have a transient effect on the infraorbital, inferior alveolar, and lingual nerves.

Accuracy of Diagnostic Arthroscopy

One limitation of diagnostic TMJ arthroscopy is that, for reasons previously mentioned, only the upper compartment can be examined. Therefore, an important question is whether pathology of the lower compartment is also reflected in the upper compartment. Regarding the main pathologic changes—inflammation and degeneration—changes in the upper and lower compartments seem to correlate well. However, lesions of the condyle cannot be detected, except when a large disk perforation gives access to the lower compartment through the perforation.

The diagnostic accuracy of TMJ arthroscopy has been evaluated in autopsy studies and in patients. In 1985, Holmlund and Hellsing evaluated the accuracy of reported morphologic changes in autopsy specimens.[33] The results indicated a high accuracy. In 1989, Holmlund investigated the sensitivity and specificity of the arthroscopic diagnosis of osteoarthrosis and synovitis.[34] The arthroscopic findings correlated with those of subsequent open surgery. In 1987, Goss and associates reported a close agreement between the arthroscopic and macroscopic findings regarding disk displacement during subsequent open surgery.[35] Several studies correlating arthroscopic findings with histologic and immunohistochemical findings in synovial biopsies show close agreement regarding inflammation.[7, 11, 15, 16, 36] The arthroscopic diagnosis of synovitis should be based on the presence of capillary hyperemia and synovial hyperplasia.[15]

Arthroscopic Surgery

In the field of orthopedic surgery, arthroscopic procedures have increasingly replaced open joint surgery. The duration of the postoperative period and the frequency of complications have thereby been reduced.

However, arthroscopic surgery of the TMJ is more difficult. The anatomic position limits its use, and the small size and the anatomy of the joint often provide limited access for instruments. The introduction of new instruments with small dimensions, and particularly the surgical laser, has increased the possibility of doing arthroscopic surgery on the TMJ. However, one should keep in mind that the increased access to the joint provided by small instruments does not necessarily mean that the procedure is effective. Many new instruments are ineffective as far as working capacity. An increased risk of broken instruments must also be considered. The complexity of the procedure can make it rather time-consuming, and some advanced arthroscopic procedures may take even longer than open surgery.

EQUIPMENT

In addition to the instruments described for diagnostic arthroscopy, the following instruments can be used:

- Forceps, knives, and scissors
- Mini-shavers
- Surgical lasers

For diagnostic arthroscopy, the optimal direction of view of the telescope is 30 degrees. However, for arthroscopic surgery, the direction of view of the telescope should be less than 10 degrees to facilitate instrumentation (Fig. 14–5).

Mini-shavers have been used to smooth the surfaces of the disk and fibrocartilage. The shaver blades must not be too small, because the fibrocartilage and disk are rather tough tissues. Bipolar cautery has been used to coagulate tissue in case of synovial bleeding or to cut the tissue. How-

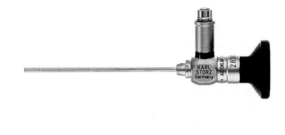

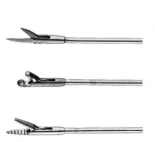

FIGURE 14–5. A 0-degree telescope suitable for arthroscopic surgery. Small-diameter scissors and forceps must be of high quality.

ever, both the mini-shavers and cautery have now been replaced by the surgical laser.

In laser surgery, the wavelength of the transmitted light is most important. The energy of lasers with a wavelength in the far infrared spectrum, such as the carbon dioxide laser, is largely absorbed by water. The tissues in the joint have a high water content, which would make this laser ideal, because most of the laser energy is absorbed by the superficial layers of tissue. The thermal damage zone is minimal, less than 70 μm. However, because of its long wavelength (10.6 μm), it cannot be transmitted through a fiber light cable without distortion. It is therefore not practical for arthroscopic surgery. The neodymium:yttrium-aluminum-garnet (Nd:YAG) laser operates at a wavelength of 1.06 μm. Owing to its short wavelength, the laser beam transmits easily through a flexible light cable; as a free beam, it also passes through water without being absorbed. The tissue penetration exceeds the tissue effect seen during surgery by 3 to 5 mm. The Nd:YAG laser is excellent for coagulation. However, because the thermal damage zone is too large, it is not ideal for the TMJ. The holmium:YAG laser is a better alternative; it operates at a wavelength of 2.1 μm. The thermal damage zone is about 0.5 mm, making this laser ideal for the TMJ. The working capacity is too low in

the knee, but in a small joint such as the TMJ, this is not a problem.

TECHNIQUE

As mentioned previously, minor surgical procedures, such as lysis and lavage or partial synovectomy, may be performed under local anesthesia with or without sedation. However, if more advanced and prolonged procedures, such as disk repositioning and suturing, are planned, these are best performed under general anesthesia.

The draping technique is the same as for open TMJ surgery. The assistant can mobilize the mandible intraorally with the thumb through the sterile drapes. A less effective but common technique is to place a towel clamp at the angle of the mandible.

Arthroscopic surgery is best performed under direct visual control through the telescope. Two methods are used: a double-cannula technique and the so-called triangulation technique. A double cannula needs only one portal, but the diameter of the instrument is about 4 mm, and access to the various joint compartments is therefore fairly limited. However, with the introduction of arthroscopic lasers, this problem may soon be overcome. Recently, an optic of about 2 mm with an inbuilt channel for the laser fiber was designed.[37]

Triangulation requires an extra entry for instrumentation, but it gives better access. This technique has been described by McCain and colleagues.[30, 38] Various portals can be used in combination (see Fig. 14–4). The inferolateral approach gives the best access to the posterior part of the joint, the anterolateral approach the best access to the anterior part, and the endaural approach the best access to the lateral part of the joint. Triangulation is more invasive, and the risk of complications is therefore slightly greater. The instruments may also be more difficult to keep in the correct position, and this technique requires a well-trained assistant. In general, more advanced arthroscopic procedures call for great skill and training on cadavers before their clinical use can be recommended. Experience in open TMJ surgery is a prerequisite for correct handling of complications.

PROCEDURES

Lavage

In patients with osteoarthritis of the knee, irrigation of the joint with isotonic saline solution or Ringer's solution has been found to be effective for providing pain relief and improving function.[39–45] In osteoarthritis and synovial joint disease, one finds an accumulation of microcartilaginous debris and inflammatory products. A thorough lavage removes these irritating products, thus relieving symptoms and resulting in more favorable conditions for repair.

The procedure is relatively easy to perform and requires few instruments. In its simplest form, a 1.2-mm needle is used for outflow. It should be positioned in the anterior recess of the upper compartment. The irrigation is performed with a syringe and a 0.6-mm needle placed in the posterior recess of the upper compartment. While slowly injecting a total of 100 mL of isotonic saline solution, one must constantly check the outflow. The patient may move the jaw during the irrigation.

Lavage is particularly effective in patients with severe inflammation (e.g., rheumatoid arthritis), as indicated in a recent study.[45] However, a good treatment outcome has also been reported in patients with internal derangement of the TMJ.[39–44] Nitzan and associates proposed an interesting explanation for this.[39] In patients with TMJ locking, a vacuum effect and increased synovial fluid viscosity cause the disk to adhere to the eminence. The lavage procedure therefore decompresses the upper compartment.

Lavage is also frequently performed in combination with diagnostic arthroscopy. The arthroscopic examination is highly accurate regarding inflammation and provides a sound base for the determination of which procedure should be performed. The lavage procedure is performed using the outflow needle for irrigation and the arthroscopic sheath for outflow. The greater outflow (compared with simple lavage) makes the lavage procedure more efficient.

TMJ lavage is a quick and noninvasive method with hardly any complications. It can be performed in an outpatient clinic and costs very little. It should be considered as the first treatment alternative in patients with internal derangement, osteoarthritis, and arthritis of the TMJ.

Lysis

Fibrotic bands are infrequent in patients with TMJ internal derangement.[10] In patients with osteoarthritis and arthritides, fibrosis resulting from repeated inflammatory episodes may be more severe and require lysis or removal to improve function. The lysis can be performed blindly, using a blunt trocar with sweeping movements from anterior to posterior (Fig. 14–6). However, it is better to use the holmium:YAG laser under direct arthroscopic control, as described by Koslin.[46]

Lysis of fibrotic bands can be effective in some patients with marked fibrosis. However, the procedure is always combined with lavage (which has a 70% to 80% success

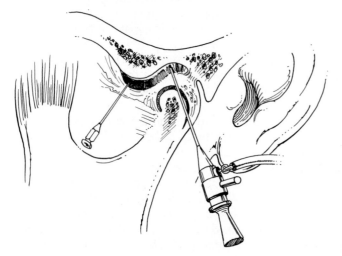

FIGURE 14–6. Lysis of fibrotic bands using the blunt trocar in sweeping movements from anterior to posterior.

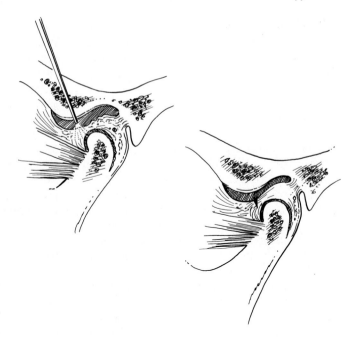

FIGURE 14–7. Anterior release and repositioning of the disk using laser technique.

rate alone) and sometimes with a steroid injection as well. It has therefore been difficult to assess the efficacy of lysis alone. Reported success rates for lysis and lavage range between 50% and 90%,[47, 48] which also suggests considerable variation in the design of these studies.

Lateral Capsule Release

During open TMJ surgery, it has been observed that translation of the disk-condyle complex improves when the lateral capsule is incised. The improvement may be due to decompression of the upper compartment (the disk is thickened and interferes with the capsule, the capsule has been thickened and interferes with the disk, or both the capsule and the disk have been thickened). Arthroscopically, the release procedure is accomplished by using the blunt trocar with sweeping movements from anterior to posterior (see Fig. 14–6). The procedure can also be performed using a miniblade or a laser, but it then requires direct arthroscopic control via an endaural approach.[49] Good short-term results have been reported.[50] However, because the procedure was combined with both lysis and lavage in the studies available, its clinical relevance should be further evaluated in clinical trials.

Disk Repositioning

Disk repositioning focuses on the imaging findings of a displaced disk in patients with chronic locking of the TMJ. It is also an attractive principle for restoring the disk and repositioning it instead of performing diskectomy. The latter procedure has therefore been used extensively in open TMJ surgery. A wedge is cut out in the elongated posterior attachment of the disk, and the disk is then sutured back into its normal (superior) position on the condyle. Most studies report success rates between 80% and 95%.[51] However, postoperative MRI has failed to show long-term improvement after the procedure, and the disk may become displaced again.[52, 53]

A few studies have reported on arthroscopic disk repositioning.[54, 55] First an anterior release is performed with a laser; the disk is then pushed posteriorly and held in position while a suture is passed through the posterior part of the disk and tied to either the anterior wall of the meatus or the subcutaneous tissue posterior to the joint. This technique requires considerable skill and is time-consuming. The technique of passing the suture through the avascular portion of the disk is questionable. A better alternative may be to create scar tissue with the laser in the posterior disk attachment and thereby stabilize the disk in a correct position (Fig. 14–7).[46]

Good short-term results have been reported with disk suturing,[54] but there is a need for long-term outcome studies using MRI.

Synovectomy

It is an attractive principle to intervene early in the disease process in patients with arthritides and to remove areas of focal granulation in the synovial lining to prevent spread to the fibrocartilage. Controversy exists regarding the long-term effect of arthroscopic synovectomy in the knee. However, it has been shown to reduce pain and improve function for up to 5 years.[56]

Synovectomy should be performed under direct arthroscopic control using a holmium:YAG laser that vaporizes the tissue, which is then removed by irrigation. At present, there are few outcome studies regarding the TMJ.

Débridement and Abrasion

Joints with osteoarthritis and arthritides frequently display irregularities of the fibrocartilage and disk. These irregularities may interfere with the smooth functioning of the joint, in which case they must be removed. They can be removed with a minishaver. However, the use of a shaver in a small joint such as the TMJ requires considerable surgical skill, and removal should always be done under direct arthroscopic control to avoid complications such as damage to vessels and nerves close to the joint capsule. The holmium:YAG laser is a better alternative for débridement because of improved access to the more distant parts of the joint.

Abrasion arthroplasty has been discussed in the orthopedic literature, but much controversy exists regarding its efficacy. The procedure for the TMJ was described by Quinn in a preliminary study.[57] It must be further evaluated.

Restriction

TMJ hypermobility or recurrent luxation can also be treated arthroscopically. This method focuses on producing scar tissue in the posterior disk attachment, thereby limiting forward translation of the disk-condyle complex (see Fig. 14–7). One way of creating this scar tissue is to inject a sclerosing solution subsynovially in the posterior disk attachment.[58] Another possibility is to use cautery or lasers.[59] A third method is to pass a suture through the posterior part of the disk and then tie it to the anterior wall of the meatus.[60] Short-term outcome studies have shown good results with all three methods.[59, 60] However, no long-term evaluation has been published.

Intraarticular Pharmacotherapy

Intraarticular injections with corticosteroids and hyaluronan have been used in combination with TMJ arthroscopy. Both these drugs alleviated pain and improved mandibular function in patients with chronic arthritis.[61] Moreover, hyaluronan seems to have a good effect on clicking joints.[62]

At the end of arthroscopic procedures, corticosteroids are usually injected. However, in the TMJ, this always entails some extravasation of the steroid through the portals created, which may cause atrophy of the subcutaneous tissue. It is therefore better to inject easily dissolvable steroids into small joints such as the TMJ or to wait 1 week before doing this.

Hyaluronan should also be injected strictly intra-articularly, because an extra-articular injection causes severe pain.

POSTOPERATIVE CARE

In addition to what has been mentioned previously about diagnostic arthroscopy, the patient must be instructed individually regarding postoperative training, depending on the type of procedure performed. In patients with chronic locking who have undergone lysis and lavage, more intensive training should be recommended; in those who have had disk repositioning and restriction procedures, training should be introduced gradually.

As regards outcome evaluation, various recommendations have been published that should be followed.[63] In clinical practice, the American Association of Oral and Maxillofacial Surgeons 1984 criteria for success are sufficient. The length of the follow-up period should be at least 1 year.

Summary

As in the field of orthopedic surgery, arthroscopy has become an important method for the diagnosis and treatment of TMD. Its accuracy in diagnosing TMD is high. Simultaneous biopsy can be performed to improve diagnostic accuracy. Complications are minor and infrequent. The various new surgical methods show good short-term results. The application of surgical lasers to the TMJ has extended the possibilities for arthroscopic surgery. Some arthroscopic procedures, such as lysis and lavage, can be done under local anesthesia in an outpatient clinic. Arthroscopy is cheaper than open TMJ surgery because it means shorter hospitalization and little if any sick leave for the patient. Finally, arthroscopy provides unique possibilities for research to elucidate the complicated etiopathogenesis of TMDs.

REFERENCES

1. Takagi K: Practical experiences using Takagi's arthroscope. J Jpn Orthop Assoc 1939;14:359.
2. Bircher E: Die Arthroendoskopie. Zentralbl Chir 1921;48:1460.
3. Watanabe M, Takeda S, Ikeuchi H: Atlas of Arthroscopy. Tokyo, Igaku Shoin, 1969.
4. Ohnishi M: Arthroscopy of the temporomandibular joint [in Japanese]. J Jpn Stomatol 1975;42:207.
5. Ohnishi M: Clinical application of arthroscopy in the temporomandibular joint diseases. Bull Tokyo Med Dent Univ 1980;27:41.
6. Holmlund A, Gynther G, Axelsson S: Diskectomy in treatment of internal derangement of the temporomandibular joint. Oral Surg Oral Med Oral Pathol 1993;76:266.
7. Holmlund A, Gynther G, Reinholt FP: Disk derangement and inflammatory changes in the posterior disk attachment of the temporomandibular joint: A histologic study. Oral Surg Oral Med Oral Pathol 1992;73:9.
8. Holmlund AB, Axelsson S: Temporomandibular arthropathy: Correlation between signs and symptoms and arthroscopic findings. Int J Oral Maxillofac Surg 1996;25:178.
9. Holmlund A, Hellsing G: Arthroscopy of the temporomandibular joint: A comparative study of arthroscopic and tomographic findings. Int J Oral Maxillofac Surg 1988;17:128.
10. Holmlund AB, Gynther G, Reinholt FP: Rheumatoid arthritis and disk derangement of the temporomandibular joint: A comparative arthroscopic

study. Oral Surg Oral Med Oral Pathol 1992;73:273.
11. Gynther GW, Holmlund AB, Reinholt FP, Lindblad S: Temporomandibular joint involvement in generalized osteoarthritis and rheumatoid arthritis: A clinical, histologic and immunohistochemical study. Int J Oral Maxillofac Surg 1997;26:10.
12. Holmlund A, Reinholt F, Bergstedt H: Synovial chondromatosis of the temporomandibular joint. Oral Surg Oral Med Oral Pathol 1992;73:266.
13. Holmlund A: Temporomandibular joint arthroscopy. In Parisien JS (ed): Current Techniques in Arthroscopy. Philadelphia, Current Medicine, 1994, p 33.
14. Bonell L, Buoncristiani RD, Koslin M, et al: Instrument development. In McCain JP (ed): Principles and Practice of Temporomandibular Joint Arthroscopy. St. Louis, Mosby, 1996, p 11.
15. Gynther GW, Holmlund AB, Reinholt FP: Synovitis in internal derangement of the temporomandibular joint. J Oral Maxillofac Surg 1994;52:913.
16. Carls FR, von Hochstetter A, Makek M, Engelke W: Diagnostic accuracy of TMJ arthroscopy in correlation to histological findings. J Craniomaxillofac Surg 1995;23:75.
17. Small NC: Complications in arthroscopic surgery performed by experienced arthroscopists. J Arthroscopic Rel Surg 1988;4:215.
18. Van Sickels JE, Nishioka GJ, Hegewald MD: Middle ear injury resulting from TMJ arthroscopy. J Oral Maxillofac Surg 1987;45:962.
19. Applebaum EL, Berg LF, Kumar A, Mafee MF: Otologic complications following temporomandibular joint arthroscopy. Ann Otol Rhinol Laryngol 1988;97:675.
20. Carter JB, Testa L: Complications of TMJ arthroscopy: A review of 2,225 cases: Review of the 1988 annual scientific sessions abstracts. J Oral Maxillofac Surg 1988;46:M14–M15.
21. Moses JJ, Topper D: Arteriovenous fistula: An unusual complication associated with arthroscopic TMJ surgery. J Oral Maxillofac Surg 1990;48:1220.
22. Carls FR, Engelke W, Locher MC, Sailer HF: Complications following arthroscopy of the temporomandibular joint: Analysis covering a 10-year period (451 arthroscopies). J Craniomaxillofac Surg 1996;24:12.
23. McCain JP: Arthroscopy of the human TMJ. J Oral Maxillofac Surg 1988;46:648.
24. Goss AN, Bosanquet AG: The arthroscopic appearance of acute temporomandibular joint trauma. J Oral Maxillofac Surg 1990;48:780.
25. Hendler BH, Levin LM: Postobstructive pulmonary edema as a sequela of temporomandibular joint arthroscopy: A case report. J Oral Maxillofac Surg 1993;51:315.
26. McCain JP, de la Rua H: Foreign body retrieval: A complication of TMJ arthroscopy. J Oral Maxillofac Surg 1989;47:1221.
27. Tarro A: Instrument breakage associated with arthroscopy of the temporomandibular joint: Report of a case. J Oral Maxillofac Surg 1989; 47:1226.
28. Jones JL, Horn KL: The effect of temporomandibular joint arthroscopy on ear function. J Oral Maxillofac Surg 1989;47:1022.
29. McCain JP, Goldberg HM, de la Rua H: Preoperative and postoperative audiologic measurements in patients undergoing arthroscopy of the TMJ. J Oral Maxillofac Surg 1989;47:1026.
30. McCain JP, de la Rua H, le Blanc N: Puncture

technique and portals of entry for diagnostic and operative arthroscopy of the TMJ. J Arthroscopy Rel Surg 1991;7:221.

31. Murphy MA, Silvester KC, Chan TYK: Extradural haematoma after temporomandibular joint arthroscopy: A case report. Int J Oral Maxillofac Surg 1993;22:332.

32. McCain JP, Sanders B, Koslin MG, et al: Temporomandibular joint arthroscopy: A 6-year multicenter retrospective study of 4,831 joints. J Oral Maxillofac Surg 1992;50:926.

33. Holmlund A, Hellsing G: Arthroscopy of the temporomandibular joint: An autopsy study. Int J Oral Maxillofac Surg 1985;14:169.

34. Holmlund A: Diagnostic accuracy of temporomandibular joint arthroscopy: A comparison of findings during arthroscopy and arthrotomy. Oral Maxillofac Surg Clin North Am 1989;1:79.

35. Goss AN, Bosanquet A, Tideman H: The accuracy of temporomandibular joint arthroscopy. J Craniomaxillofac Surg 1987;15:99.

36. Merrill RG, Yih WY, Langan MJ: A histologic evaluation of the accuracy of TMJ diagnostic arthroscopy. Oral Surg Oral Med Oral Pathol 1990;70:393.

37. Ogi N, Kurita K, Toyama M, Maki I: Thin fiber TMJ arthroscope with inner channel for laser lysis of fibrous adhesion [abstract]. International Symposium on TMJ Arthroscopy and Arthroscopic Surgery, San Diego, 1995.

38. McCain JP, de la Rua H: A modification of the double puncture technique in temporomandibular joint arthroscopy. J Oral Maxillofac Surg 1990;48:760.

39. Nitzan DW, Dolwick MF, Martinez GA: Temporomandibular joint arthrocentesis: A simplified treatment for severe, limited mouth opening. J Oral Maxillofac Surg 1991;49:1163.

40. Dimitroulis G, Dolwick MF, Martinez A: Temporomandibular joint arthrocentesis and lavage for treatment of closed lock: A follow-up study. Br J Oral Maxillofac Surg 1995;33:23.

41. Murakami K, Hosaka H, Moriya Y, et al: Short-term treatment outcome study for the management of temporomandibular joint closed lock: A comparison of arthrocentesis to nonsurgical and arthroscopic lysis and lavage. Oral Surg Oral Med Oral Pathol 1995;80:253.

42. Fridrich KL, Wise JM, Zeitler DL: Prospective comparison of arthroscopy and arthrocentesis for temporomandibular joint disorders. J Oral Maxillofac Surg 1996;54:816.

43. Hosaka H, Murakami K, Goto K, Iizuka T: Outcome of arthrocentesis for temporomandibular joint closed lock at 3 years follow-up. Oral Surg Oral Med Oral Pathol Oral Radiol Endod 1996;82:501.

44. Nitzan DW, Samson B, Better H: Long-term outcome of arthrocentesis for sudden-onset, persistent, severe closed lock of the temporomandibular joint. J Oral Maxillofac Surg 1997;55:151.

45. Gynther GW, Holmlund A: Efficacy of arthroscopic lysis and lavage in patients with temporomandibular joint symptoms and generalized osteoarthritis or rheumatoid arthritis. J Oral Maxillofac Surg (submitted for publication).

46. Koslin M: Part 3—electrosurgery and laser technology. In McCain JP (ed): Principles and Practice of Temporomandibular Joint Arthroscopy. St. Louis, Mosby, 1996, p 24.

47. Perrott DH, Alborzi A, Kaban LB, Helms CA: A prospective evaluation of the effectiveness of temporomandibular joint arthroscopy. J Oral Maxillofac Surg 1990;48:1029.

48. Holmlund A, Gynther G, Axelsson S: Efficacy of arthroscopic lysis and lavage in patients with chronic locking of the temporomandibular joint. Int J Oral Maxillofac Surg 1994;23:262.

49. Moses JJ, Poker ID: Temporomandibular joint arthroscopy: The endaural approach. J Oral Maxillofac Surg 1989;18:347.

50. Moses JJ, Poker ID: TMJ arthroscopic surgery: An analysis of 237 patients. J Oral Maxillofac Surg 1989;47:790.

51. Merrill RG: Historical perspectives and comparisons of TMJ surgery for internal disc derangements and arthropathy. J Craniomandib Pract 1986;4:75.

52. Montgomery MT, Gordon SM, Van Sickels JE, Harms SE: Changes in signs and symptoms following temporomandibular joint disc repositioning surgery. J Oral Maxillofac Surg 1992;50:320.

53. Montgomery MT, Van Sickels JE, Harms SE: Success of temporomandibular joint arthroscopy in disk displacement with and without reduction. Oral Surg Oral Med Oral Pathol 1991;71:651.

54. McCain JP, Podrasky AE, Zabiegalski NA: Arthroscopic disc repositioning and suturing: A preliminary report. J Oral Maxillofac Surg 1992;50:568.

55. Tarro AW: A fully visualized arthroscopic disc suturing technique. J Oral Maxillofac Surg 1994;52:362.

56. Ogilvie-Harris DJ, Basinski A: Arthroscopic synovectomy of the knee for rheumatoid arthritis. Arthroscopy 1991;7:91.

57. Quinn JH: Arthroscopic management of temporomandibular joint disc perforations and associated advanced chondromalacia by discoplasty and abrasion arthroplasty: Preliminary results. J Oral Maxillofac Surg 1994;52:800.

58. Merrill RG: Arthroscopy of the temporomandibular joint. In Keith DA (ed): Surgery of the Temporomandibular Joint, ed 2. Boston, Blackwell Scientific, 1992, p 70.

59. McCain JP, Morales OJ: Mandibular dislocation. In McCain JP (ed): Principles and Practice of Temporomandibular Joint Arthroscopy. St. Louis, Mosby, 1996, p 246.

60. Ohnishi M: Arthroscopic surgery for hypermobility and recurrent mandibular dislocation. Oral Maxillofac Surg Clin North Am 1989;1:153.

61. Kopp S, Carlsson GE, Haraldsson T, Wenneberg B: Long-term effect of intra-articular injections of sodium hyaluronate and corticosteroid on temporomandibular joint arthritis. J Oral Maxillofac Surg 1987;45:929.

62. Bertolami CN, Gay T, Clark GT, et al: Use of sodium hyaluronate in treating temporomandibular joint disorders: A randomized, double-blind, placebo-controlled clinical trial. J Oral Maxillofac Surg 1993;51:232.

63. Holmlund A: Criteria for temporomandibular joint treatment outcome. In Stegenga B, de Bont LGM (eds): Management of Temporomandibular Joint Degenerative Disease: Biologic Basis and Treatment Outcome. Basel, Birkhauser, 1996, p 63.

CHAPTER

15

Surgery for Internal Derangement

Robert A. Bays

The surgical management of a collection of signs and symptoms without a clear definition of the pathology is risky at best.[1, 2] Temporomandibular disorders (TMDs) are such a collection, in that the responsible pathology is not clearly understood or identified. The National Institutes of Health Conference on Management of TMDs has determined that scientifically based guidelines for the diagnosis and management of TMDs are still unavailable.[3] Consequently, most attempts to document the rationale for diagnosis or management are fraught with subjectivity—a subjectivity biased by clinical experience. Additionally, TMDs are often self-limited, so clinical experience may be overly optimistic in assessing the influence of a particular treatment on patient outcome. With these limitations in mind, this chapter defines both internal derangement and a rationale for surgical treatment that minimizes the risk to the patient and assists in the overall management of the signs and symptoms.

Implicit in this discussion is the concept that surgery is not the first or the only endeavor in the management of patients with TMDs. On the contrary, the clinical management of TMDs is often convoluted in its intertwining of medical, occlusal, physical therapeutic, and sometimes psychological methods. The contribution of each of these factors differs in each patient, and treatment must therefore be tailored to the individual. It is widely acknowledged that TMDs are nearly always multifactorial,[3] although the mix of predisposing, precipitating, and perpetuating factors varies. Even if surgery is indicated, ignorance of these contributing factors—however minor—may lead to clinical failure; thus the surgeon must weigh and investigate all these factors when deciding whether surgery is necessary. Before surgery is undertaken, the surgeon must consider all these factors, maximize their management, and ensure that the necessary resources—human and otherwise—are available to optimize the patient's postoperative course. Failure to do so may diminish the patient's chances for a successful outcome and may lead to the erroneous conclusion that the surgical procedure has failed on its own merits.

Over the last 20 years, many surgical procedures that were initially advocated and supported with clinical follow-up studies have fallen from favor and become obsolete.[1, 4–13] These techniques were often discontinued on the basis of clinical experience and hearsay long before any documentation of failures or complications was published, if indeed such literature ever appeared. A detailed discussion of the worst of these failed procedures can be found elsewhere in this text (Volume 4, Chapters 16–18). However, for those procedures that have not been proved harmful but seem to succeed in some hands and not in others, one must wonder whether the difference between clinical success and failure is neglect of the contributing factors.

Surgery for the treatment of temporomandibular joint (TMJ) internal derangement (ID) can be successful if the following tenets are observed:

1. The pathology to be corrected by surgery (i.e., ID) is clearly defined.
2. The patient is shown to suffer from this pathologic process by history, physical examination, and, often, imaging studies.
3. Concomitant signs and symptoms of TMD that are not ID related are investigated for their contribution to the patient's total problem. This may be the most important consideration, because the presence of ID in a patient with head and neck pain does not establish that ID is causative.
4. If ID is a major contributor to the patient's suffering, the other aspects of TMD must be clinically managed preoperatively and postoperatively.
5. A surgical procedure that specifically addresses ID is used.

ID was first described by Hey and Davies[14] in 1814 as localized mechanical fault interfering with the smooth action of a joint and more recently has been defined as "a disturbance in the normal anatomic relationship between the disc and condyle that interferes with smooth movement of the joint and causes momentary catching, clicking, popping or locking."[15] ID requiring clinical attention can be further defined as a condition that produces pain and significant limited range of motion. For purposes of this discussion, ID is classified according the Wilkes system[16]:

Stage I   Early reducing disk displacement
Stage II   Late reducing disk displacement
Stage III   Nonreducing disk displacement—acute/subacute
Stage IV   Nonreducing disk displacement—chronic
Stage V   Nonreducing disk displacement—chronic with osteoarthrosis

This chapter considers surgery for ID stages I–IV (and mild stage V), except for those cases requiring major joint reconstruction, which is discussed elsewhere in this volume. This includes situations in which a perforated or partially degenerated disk has enough diskal and retrodiskal tis-

sue remaining to perform the bilaminar flap repair or temporalis muscle fascia flap reconstruction as described later.

Excluding trauma, congenital deformities, and neoplasia, pain and severe limitation of motion (LOM) are generally the only reasons that intracapsular TMJ surgery should be considered. There are also rare occasions when the noise produced by ID may be sufficiently embarrassing to a patient to compel treatment, although the patient must be educated as to the possibility of postoperative complications—pain being the most notable—before proceeding.

The most crucial issue regarding ID is not that it exists but rather whether it is the source of the pain. It is widely accepted that painless ID exists frequently in the general population without consequence.[17] It therefore follows that ID may coexist with other elements of TMD and not contribute greatly to pain or LOM.

History, Physical Examination, and Imaging

The complete work-up of TMD patients is covered elsewhere (Volume 4, Chapters 7 and 8). The subjective and objective patient information discussed here is limited to that which is relevant to the surgical management of ID.

Historical information that is helpful in identifying surgically correctable ID includes:

1. Pain with function. ID pain is usually immediate upon loading of the joint and is localized to the joint at the time of loading. Myofascial pain as a result of loading is usually more gradual and builds to a crescendo over time. Patients who do not experience pain in the affected joint at the time of chewing or biting probably will not respond to TMJ surgery. Diagnostic local anesthesia to the joint may be helpful in localizing the source of pain. However, soreness in the joint is not pathognomonic for ID and may not be correctable by TMJ surgery.
2. Presence or history of joint noise associated with pain. If clicking or popping is (or was) present, it is important to

ascertain whether the noise is (was) coincident with pain. This is often difficult to determine, because many TMD patients have been totally indoctrinated as to the pathology of joint noises. Careful, instructive questioning is required to make it clear to the patient that joint noises need not be associated with pain or even with pathology. If joint noises are not present, it is important to know whether they ever existed and, if so, whether pain was associated with the noises. Also, at the time the noises ceased, was there pain, deviation, and LOM? The absence of these factors casts doubt on the probability that ID is the primary source of pain.

Physical findings that may indicate ID are:

1. Opening and reciprocal clicking that do not occur at exactly the same condylar position (stage I or II).
2. Joint tenderness to palpation, especially with function.
3. Deviation to the affected side until clicking occurs. If bilateral clicking is present, deviation may occur to one side until it clicks, and then to the other side until it clicks.
4. Deviation of opening (in unilateral cases) with lack of significant palpable translation (stages III–V).
5. Pain in the affected joint while biting on a wooden tongue depressor.
6. Crepitus, which is often associated with chronic disk displacement, perforation, and degenerative changes (stage V).
7. Elimination of pain following local anesthesia of the affected joint.

The need for imaging confirmation of ID is controversial.[1–3, 18–23] Panographic imaging is the standard for screening of the jaws, including the general morphology of the condyles. Legal and insurance documentation aside, in most cases a skilled clinician does not need additional imaging to make a diagnosis of ID.[1, 20–23] The disk-condyle relationship is often obvious from the history and physical examination, especially in stages I and II disease. Of course, this does not mean that the disk-condyle relationship is the source of the patient's pain. Stages III, IV, and V may be more difficult to diagnose from history and physical examination alone. The absence of an imaging study may also make it more difficult to identify the disk position in the more chronic cases of stages IV and V, primarily because the mandibular opening is often nearly normal, with minimal deviation or lack of lateral excursions.

Experienced clinicians often use imaging to confirm their belief that the disk is *not* displaced so that the patient and referring clinician will abandon the idea of surgery. However, it is noted that magnetic resonance imaging (MRI) and arthrography tend to overdiagnose disk displacement.[22] Therefore, the clinical diagnosis should be the ultimate determining factor in the decision to perform surgery.

Concomitant Myofascial Pain and Internal Derangement

Perhaps the most confusing patients are those who present with clear evidence of ID in combination with other TMJ complaints that are usually consistent with myofascial pain (MP). ID can contribute to or cause MP, and MP can cause painful joints with or without ID. If both are present, how can one determine which came first? First, one must determine that ID is truly present. Imaging may be helpful in such situations. Second, the physical findings listed earlier can help.

Management of Myofascial Pain

It is recognized that nonsurgical methods such as physical therapy, occlusal control, medical management, and psychological counseling are all recommended modalities for the management of TMDs, and these same methods are appropriate pre- and postoperatively to ensure the successful surgical treatment of ID. Acute changes in the occlusion such as a "high" restoration are known to precipitate MP signs and symptoms in nonpatient populations. Therefore, acute changes in the occlusion of a TMJ surgery patient may also provoke an MP reaction. Control of the occlusion during the immediate postoperative period is necessary, especially because most TMJ surgeries create—at least temporarily—some minor but significant alteration in the occlusion. Many surgeons who have abandoned conservative TMJ surgery because of poor success have also derided the use of preoperative and especially postoperative splints. In contrast, our experience with splints is that they can carry a significant percentage of TMJ surgery patients through the first 6 postoperative weeks or so, at which point sufficient healing has occurred to permit a decrease in occlusal management. In concomitant MP-ID patients, splints may be necessary for much longer periods—even permanently at night. If it is useful, postoperative nighttime splint wear does not signal failure, especially if the patient was in pain preoperatively with full-time splint use.

The primary goals of treatment should always be the relief of pain, followed by the elimination of other treatment needs, such as splints, physical therapy, psychological help, or medicines, which can inconvenience the patient's life. However, the temporary or long-term use of physical therapy, nonsteroidal anti-inflammatory drugs (NSAIDs), and psychological counseling may be useful in conjunction with TMJ surgery. The TMJ surgeon will be most successful if the surgical management of ID is approached as an adjunct to the overall treatment of the TMD patient. Because only a portion of TMD patients have pure ID without some other TMJ problems, to address ID in isolation is to invite failure.

Sequencing of Intracapsular and Orthognathic Surgery

Patients who need surgery for both ID and malocclusion represent a special group. No strict rules can be made regarding which problem to address first, but some general guidelines may be helpful. Correcting a malocclusion in the hope of solving a TMJ problem is precarious and unpredictable. If malocclusion is a major contributor to TMD, it is more likely an MP problem than ID.[24] A centric relation splint, properly made and adjusted, usually alleviates MP that is occlusally related. If it does not, this is valuable information, because orthognathic correction of the occlusion will probably not improve the MP either. Conversely, if a centric splint provides major improvement and removal of the splint leads to return of symptoms, one can usually conclude that malocclusion is important to the pain process. This line of thinking is tempered by the knowledge that many treatments are successful for awhile in many MP patients, so short-term improvement may be capricious owing to the cyclic nature of MP. Splint treatment before presurgical orthodontics will allow sufficient time to diagnose the etiology of pain complaints. Centric splints may also be helpful immediately before orthognathic surgery, especially in patients who have shown a propensity toward MP during the treatment course (see Volume 4, Chapter 12).

Orthognathic surgery has little or no place in the treatment of pure ID, but it may be necessary to correct malocclusion in patients with ID. Although some emerging information exists that connects ID with mandibular retrognathism developmentally (see Volume 4, Chapter 11), there is no indication that correcting ID before orthognathic surgery adds to the stability or success of the procedure.[25, 26] It is advised that ID be addressed first—either conservatively or surgically, depending on the case—if a patient's primary complaints are related to ID. Those patients with mild, intermittent ID complaints, although being prime candidates for orthognathic surgery, are highly problematic; close consultation is required between the patient and family and the orthodontist and surgeon. Usually it is best to initiate presurgical orthognathic treatment with the understanding that the possible return of ID afterward will not be due to the orthognathic treatment per se. Experience has taught us that in such cases the orthognathic surgeon must be careful not to "posteriorize" the condyles during the orthognathic surgery or create an occlusion that will require class III elastics in the postoperative phase. Either of these situations may increase the possibility of postoperative ID stage I, II, or III.

Finally, among patients with TMDs who require orthognathic surgery, some have both ID and MP. If pain is the primary complaint, there are true indications for intracapsular surgery (as outlined elsewhere in this chapter), and nonsurgical treatment has failed, preorthognathic TMJ surgery seems reasonable. It is probably best to treat this patient without regard to future orthodontics or surgery until the ID and MP complaints are resolved. Our studies generally showed that orthognathic correction of class II malocclusions causes a slight improvement in the signs and symptoms of MP in normal orthognathic patients.[25, 26] The craniomandibular index[27, 28] was used to evaluate the TMD signs and symptoms in these patients. However, these were not TMD patients but routine orthognathic class II patients. Additionally, there was no improvement in ID in these studies. Therefore, if TMD signs and symptoms are the chief complaints, they should be addressed separately and independently.

Surgical Procedures

Many techniques have been suggested for the treatment of ID. It is generally accepted that Annandale in 1887 was the first to describe surgery for the correction of internal derangement,[29] although it is said that the Aztecs may have used thorns to perform arthrocentesis as long as 500 years ago.[30] Since that time, many surgical procedures have been elaborated, without a distinct winner. These include:

1. Arthrocentesis and lavage (see Volume 4, Chapter 14)
2. Arthroscopy (see Volume 4, Chapter 14)
3. Arthrotomy with disk repair[6, 20, 29, 31–40]
   a. Plication[6, 20, 29, 31–36, 39, 40]
   b. Bilaminar flap repair[34, 37, 38]
4. Arthrotomy with diskectomy[41–55]
5. Arthrotomy with diskectomy and autologous graft disk replacement[12, 13, 56–58]
   a. Dermis[12, 13, 56, 58]
   b. Auricular cartilage[56, 57]
6. Arthrotomy with diskectomy and autologous flap reconstruction[59]
7. Arthrotomy with diskectomy and alloplastic disk replacement (see Volume 4, Chapter 18)
8. Condylotomy[60–63]

Probably more than other oral and maxillofacial surgeons, TMJ surgeons tend to concentrate on one or two procedures to treat the same diagnosis rather than using the full range of operations. The reasons for their choices are usually based on experience, often negative, with one or more of the techniques. This leads to strong emotional ties (or antagonisms) to specific procedures, frequently with less than firm scientific support.

The TMJ operation chosen for the treatment of ID should:

1. Be the one least likely to result in significant permanent change to the occlusion, damage to the facial nerve, production of degenerative joint disease, relapse of pain and/or joint noises, or limited range of motion (ROM).
2. Be most compatible with the surgeon's skills. Disk repair may be the most technically challenging of all the procedures, but it avoids many of the shortcomings of the other procedures, such as changing the occlusion permanently, producing degenerative joint disease, significantly decreasing the ROM, and requiring other surgical sites.
3. Require the fewest number of surgical sites. All graft procedures require an additional surgical site, with the accompanying potential complications.
4. Require the least amount of postoperative care. Maxillomandibular fixation (MMF) and heavy, prolonged interocclusal elastic wear have been eliminated in orthognathic surgery and are unnecessarily inconvenient. Significant occlusal changes occur in invasive procedures such as condylotomies[1, 7, 61, 64] and diskectomies[10, 41, 42, 45–47, 52–54, 65] at a much higher rate than in other procedures. Significant occlusal changes require additional treatment that is not precipitated by more conservative procedures and may ultimately affect the outcome of the original TMJ surgery.

Regardless of the surgical procedure selected, a thorough knowledge of the anatomy of the TMJ is essential. Numerous texts and articles describe the anatomy.[66–68]

Perioperative Management

PREOPERATIVE

Most authors are not specific regarding what represents conservative or nonsurgical perioperative therapy. I describe in this section the preoperative regimen that has worked for me over the last 20 years. Regardless of which procedure one chooses—disk repair or another—this preparation will enhance the surgical outcome.

If the patient meets the surgical criteria described earlier for consideration of ID surgery, several issues should be resolved. Nonsurgical TMD therapy is described elsewhere in this text, but certain issues deserve reiteration. If a patient has documented ID, every attempt should be made to reduce the disk nonsurgically or relieve pain via medical, physical, or palliative measures. This may include soft diet, NSAIDs, occlusal splints,[69] mandibular manipulation, or a combination of well-known nonsurgical methods. More importantly, MP must be addressed. Splints are often helpful in determining whether the occlusion is a major or minor factor in the overall pain complaint. One principal exception is a stage III case in which a centric splint improves MP but causes severe intracapsular pain, presumably owing to compression of the posterior attachment. Anterior repositioning may improve the intracapsular pain but not relieve the MP or even exacerbate it. In these cases, it may be necessary to continue whichever splint gives the greatest relief until surgery is performed, after which any remaining MP can be addressed with a centric splint and other traditional methods.

After all preoperative, nonsurgical methods have been exhausted and the patient is being managed with the most comfortable combination of splints and other modalities, the referring dental practitioner constructs a centric splint for the purpose of managing postoperative MP. In some cases, this may be the splint that the patient has been wearing during the preoperative attempts to alleviate pain.

POSTOPERATIVE

Because surgery on the TMJs usually results in some temporary alteration in the occlusion, the patient should be seen by the splint therapist within 1 to 2 days postoperatively for a splint adjustment. Commonly, there is a posterior open bite on the side that surgery was done, or bilaterally if the surgery was double sided. In either case, the posterior splint is built up to match the new occlusion, with the realization that this is only a temporary position and will change over the next 6 to 8 weeks. The patient is then seen again at 1, 3, and 6 weeks postoperatively for splint adjustments. These subsequent adjustments usually involve removing posterior height on the splint as the posterior open bite gradually closes. At the 6- to 8-week point, the splint therapist decides whether to continue splint therapy or wean the patient. This is especially important in patients with significant malocclusions that will require subsequent prosthetic, orthodontic, or orthognathic treatment. The splint may prevent trauma to the newly repaired joint until the beginning of the next phase, whatever that may be.

Exercises and physical therapy vary according to the patient's specific needs.[70] Many patients will resume normal ROM within 6 to 8 weeks postoperatively with relatively little organized therapy. Patients are encouraged to begin light, active ROM stretching immediately following surgery. At 3 weeks, the emphasis is increased to include active and passive stretching as well as active lateral and protrusive movements. Also, opening against resistance exercises are begun at this time. With this regimen, most patients will approach their normal opening within the 8-week period.

It is important to note that some legitimate candidates for disk surgery have relatively normal ROM preoperatively, and in others it is significantly decreased. Patients with stage I–II disease usually have relatively normal opening after the disk reduces during opening. Therefore, these patients regain normal opening after surgery with the above-mentioned postoperative exercises. Stage III patients are often the most limited, but their limitation is of short duration. After disk surgery, the effort needed to regain normal opening is not extreme because the myofascial components of the stomatognathic system have not yet shortened.

Some stage IV–V patients may have fairly normal opening because the disk has been out of position for so long that the attachments and other structures are stretched considerably. If the opening is reasonably normal preoperatively, it is generally not difficult to regain that opening within a few weeks postoperatively. Many other stage IV–V patients have long-standing limited opening; these are the most difficult ID patients to return to a relatively normal ROM. If the opening has been limited for many months or years, formal postoperative physical therapy is required to attain an acceptable opening (see Volume 4, Chapter 10).[71]

Arthrotomy with Disk Repair: Plication

This is perhaps the oldest of the various open surgical procedures advocated for the treatment of ID.[29] It may also be the most difficult to perform successfully, which explains the never-ending quest for an easier procedure. This well-intentioned search has led to many other, sometimes disastrous techniques,[1, 2, 5, 7, 9, 12, 48] in spite of positive reports of successful disk repair.[6, 20, 29, 31–36, 38–40, 72] When done well, arthrotomy with disk repair works well and causes few complications. Whether disk position is maintained is controversial[6, 20, 31, 33–36, 73] and may be irrelevant if the patient has a successful outcome. Experience has shown that if clicking does not return and if patients have early relief of pain, they usually do quite well over the long term.[6, 20, 31–36, 40] Even if clicking returns, the result is usually favorable regarding pain relief, although the success rate lessens somewhat; patients need

to be reassured that the return of clicking usually does not signal recurrence of pain and dysfunction. Most importantly, if pain relief does not occur postoperatively, repeat surgery should *not* be attempted.[1, 2, 74] Finally, if relief is obtained for several months after surgery but the patient ultimately relapses, surgery should not be repeated until the routine nonsurgical methods have been retried and the normal surgical criteria are met again. Additionally, the surgeon and the patient should understand that the success rate for repeat surgeries is poorer than that for initial surgeries. If a second surgery is ultimately unsuccessful, rarely should any further surgery be attempted for the treatment of pain.

SURGICAL TECHNIQUE

A preauricular, endaural approach is used because it has proved to be extremely safe and free from permanent complications.[34, 36, 75, 76] The incision is divided into three parts (Fig. 15–1): (1) the curvilinear superior aspect from the top of the pinna to the top of the tragus; (2) the prelobular section in the most convenient crease from the inferior aspect of the tragus to the lowest level of the lobe; and (3) the endaural portion, which connects the first two incisions from the skin crease just above the tragus to the skin crease just below it (Fig. 15–2). The crease in front of the lobe either descends directly inferiorly or curves toward a pierced hole in the lobe; either one may be followed.

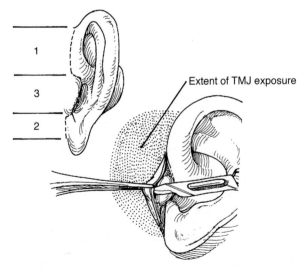

Extent of TMJ exposure

FIGURE 15–1. Preauricular, endaural incision divided into three parts: (1) superoanterior to the pinna; (2) inferior, just anterior to the lobe in the most convenient crease; and (3) inside the tragus. Although the skin incisions are made in creases to hide them, the deeper dissection hugs the cartilage of the pinna (part 1) or the cartilage of the external auditory canal (parts 2 and 3). The area that is ultimately exposed is shaded.

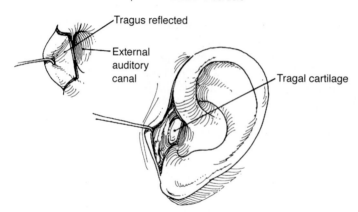

Tragus reflected

External auditory canal

Tragal cartilage

FIGURE 15–2. The skin incision inside the tragus has two sharp angles at the top and bottom. This facilitates reapproximation and closure. The tragus is skinned over the crest of the cartilage, and then a supraperichondrial dissection is continued on the anterior side of the tragal cartilage deep into the wound following contour of the cartilage.

The first incision is made at right angles to the skin surface at the junction of the face and the pinna. Note that the junction of the plane of the face and the skin that curves over the pinna is anterior to the cartilage of the pinna. The skin incision should be made on the facial plane side of this boundary, perpendicular to the facial skin. If the incision is made in the depth of this concave boundary, the scar will form on the convex surface of the skin overlying the cartilage—a location that is more posterior than desired. The second incision is started at the depth of the crease beginning at the base of the tragus and descends to the level of the attachment between the lobe and the face. If a natural crease turns toward a pierced hole in the lobe, it is acceptable to follow that crease in the skin incision only. The tragus is retracted anteriorly, and the third or connecting incision is made about 2 mm inside of the crest of the tragus (see Fig. 15–2). The connections at either end of the endaural incision are made at right angles to facilitate realignment at closure. The skin is carefully dissected free from the tragal cartilage, taking care not to perforate the skin as it is rolled over.

Metzenbaum scissors are used to bluntly dissect the first incision down to the temporalis fascia (Fig. 15–3). If this dissection is kept close to the cartilage of the pinna, even to the point of ducking back under it, the superficial temporal vessels can be avoided. At the level of the temporalis fascia, the wound should be undermined superiorly and anteriorly. Anterior to the tragus, the dissection is deepened at the supraperichondrial level—this cartilage makes up the anterior wall of the external auditory canal (EAC). Care must be taken to follow the

undulations of this cartilage as the dissection deepens. Six or 8 mm deep to the crest of the tragus a curve is found in the cartilage, after which it turns somewhat posteriorly. Staying close to the EAC cartilage at this level avoids bleeding and interruption of the parotid gland. However, attention to the location of the bony postglenoid tubercle, which is just anterior to the EAC cartilage, is crucial. The tympanic membrane

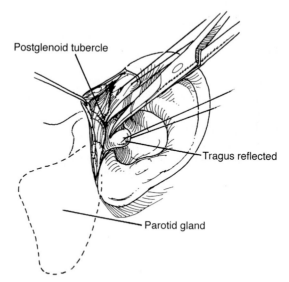

Postglenoid tubercle

Tragus reflected

Parotid gland

FIGURE 15–3. The superior third of the incision is opened down to the temporalis fascia with blunt and sharp dissection directed close to the cartilage of the pinna. If the dissection is too anterior, the superficial temporal vessels are encountered, which is unnecessary. After the temporalis fascia is exposed, the dissection is carried inferiorly along the cartilage of the external auditory canal (EAC) to contact the postglenoid tubercle of the temporal bone and to separate the parotid gland from the EAC cartilage. The dissection around the cartilage inferiorly must stay close to the cartilage and not stray into the parotid gland. Failure to extend far enough in this dissection is often the cause of inadequate exposure. Traction sutures are placed in the tissues inside the superior incision through the tragus.

(TM) attaches to the EAC cartilage approximately at the level where the EAC enters the bony canal. The TM can be damaged if the bony canal is entered; therefore, the dissection along the anterior aspect of the EAC cartilage must stop at the postglenoid tubercle.

The dissection turns around the inferior aspect of the EAC cartilage to separate it from the parotid gland. The surface of the EAC cartilage is followed rather than the line of the skin incision. Following the skin incision would carry the dissection into the parotid gland and endanger the facial nerve. This dissection must be carried around the EAC until it is just under the skin at the lobe. Otherwise, insufficient access is achieved as the joint is spread open later. Traction sutures are placed through the tragal cartilage and inside the superior aspect of the incision, at which point they can be secured to the drapes behind the ear. Anteriorly, the tissue is retracted by an assistant using a Senn's retractor.

At this point, the dissection is nearly at the proper depth, except that there is usually a thickness of tissue overlying the most posterior part of the zygoma. This should be cleaned off down to the supraperiosteal layer so that there is a smooth transition from the temporalis fascia layer to the supraperiosteal layer of the posterior zygoma and postglenoid tubercle. Before proceeding, both ends of the incision should be inspected to ensure that the full skin incision has been used and that the temporalis fascia has been sufficiently undermined anteriorly. The two extremes of the incision are the most likely areas of restriction. The superficial fascia up under the most superior end of the incision should be evaluated and incised if taut. The most inferior end of the incision should also be inspected to appraise the release between EAC cartilage and the parotid gland.

When these inspections have been completed, exposure of the TMJ capsule is performed using the supraperiosteal level over the zygoma as a guide. This layer is developed by splitting the temporalis fascia at a 45-degree angle to the long axis of the zygoma with Metzenbaum scissors (Fig. 15–4). The inferior end of this incision begins at the root of the zygoma and extends 2 cm anterosuperiorly. The dissection continues forward between the superficial and deep

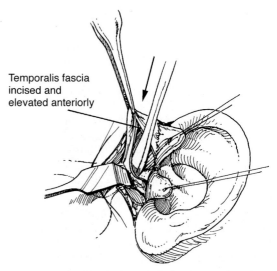

Temporalis fascia incised and elevated anteriorly

FIGURE 15–4. After the temporalis fascia, postglenoid tubercle, and parotid gland have been exposed and identified, the temporalis fascia *(arrow)* is grasped and incised superior to the zygomatic arch. The dissection proceeds below the outer layer of temporalis fascia, but superficial to the deepest layer directly overlying the muscle. This layer can be dissected so that it is continuous with the supraperiosteal layer over the zygoma. Once this layer is found, the dissection proceeds along the zygoma until the articular tubercle is reached, then inferiorly over the lateral aspect of the temporomandibular joint capsule until the inferior extent of the capsule is revealed. At this point, the entire wound should be evaluated to ensure that adequate exposure has been achieved.

layers of temporalis fascia, then connects with the supraperiosteal layer over the zygoma. A sharp No. 9 Molt periosteal elevator is ideal for this dissection because it can be used to cut or push tissue apart while preserving the periosteum over the zygoma. Several small veins are encountered parallel to the zygoma and at least one crossing over them toward the capsule. These should be divided and cauterized so that the dissection can proceed deep to them.

As this dissection approaches the lateral aspect of the articular tubercle, the periosteal elevator is used to descend from the supraperiosteal layer over the TMJ capsule. The capsule can be separated from the overlying tissue to the neck of the condyle using this same elevator. After this dissection is completed, exposure should include the temporalis muscle above the zygoma, with a thin layer of fascia still remaining on the surface; the zygoma, with only periosteum on it from the postglenoid tubercle to the anterior aspect of the articular tubercle; the lateral TMJ capsule; and the neck of the condyle just inferior to the attachment of the lateral TMJ capsule.

The Wilkes spreader (Walter Lorenz Co., Jacksonville, FL) is placed by driving a 0.054-inch Kirschner wire (K-wire) into the zygoma slightly posterior to the articular tubercle (Fig. 15–5A). The spreader is placed over the K-wire so that the knob is anterior to the wound. The neck of the condyle is found, and a second K-wire is placed through the other hole in the spreader and driven into the condylar neck just inferior to the attachment of the lateral capsule. Both K-wires are cut 5 mm above the spreader and bent over so that they are out of the way; at this point, the spreader is opened until the capsule is tight.

Using a needle-point electrocautery, the lateral lip of the glenoid fossa is sounded (see Fig. 15–5B). The cautery is activated to make an incision 1.5 to 2 mm inferior to the lateral lip of the glenoid fossa. The incision is made in several strokes, with each one being aimed more superiorly to travel up under the tissue attached to the lateral lip of the fossa. By doing this, the capsular tissue attached to the fossa is preserved for closure, and the superior joint space is entered without damaging the disk. The spreader is opened with each step to separate the joint as the incisions are made to enter the joint, and the incisions are curved to follow the contour of the lateral fossa lip. The strongest attachment of the capsule is between the lateral pole of the condyle and the articular tubercle. After this tissue has been incised, the joint opens more easily. From here the superior side of the disk can

be inspected, as well as the anterosuperior and posterosuperior recesses.

The lateral aspect of the disk is taken with forceps and retracted superiorly to place tension on the lateral collateral ligament (Fig. 15–6A). Blunt-tipped tenotomy scissors are used to dissect through the lateral disk attachment to expose the inferior joint space. The spreader is opened continuously as this procedure progresses. On completion of this phase, the glenoid fossa, disk, and condyle are visible (see Fig. 15–6B). The condyle-disk-fossa relationship that exists in an awake patient cannot be assessed appropriately with the patient under general anesthesia, the head turned, and the operator moving the jaw; therefore, it is not attempted.

An assessment of the disk integrity is made (Fig. 15–7). If there are no perforations or seriously damaged areas, the amount of tissue to be removed at the posterior junction of the disk and the retrodiskal tissue is determined by holding the disk firmly in place on the anterosuperior contour of the condyle. If the disk has been displaced anteriorly without reduction for a lengthy period, some release anteriorly or medially may be necessary. Medial release is performed with a 90-degree curved Freer's elevator where the medial collateral ligament attaches to the medial pole of the condyle. This dissection must stay close to the bone to prevent penetrating the medial capsule, which usually results in venous bleeding that is difficult to control. For the anterior dissection, release is usually needed where the capsule attaches to the

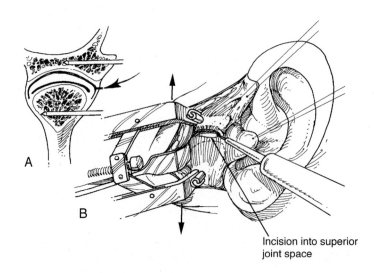

A

B

Incision into superior joint space

FIGURE 15–5. *A,* Following exposure of the temporomandibular joint capsule, the Wilkes spreader is fixed by driving K-wires into the zygoma a few millimeters posterior to the articular tubercle and into the neck of the condyle just inferior to the capsular attachment. *B,* Tension is placed on the capsule by expanding the spreader *(arrows),* and the superior joint space is entered using needle cautery. If the penetration is too deep, the lateral disk or lateral collateral ligament may be damaged.

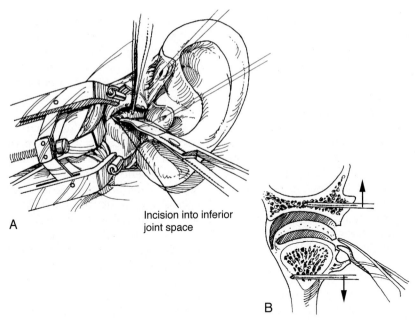

A

Incision into inferior
joint space

B

FIGURE 15–6. *A,* The joint is spread further as the dissection continues. *B,* After the spreader is expanded *(arrows),* the lateral collateral ligament is divided using tenotomy scissors to expose the inferior joint space. The lateral collateral ligament and the lateral capsule are preserved for closure later.

anterior slope of the articular eminence. Once again, it is absolutely necessary to stay close to the bone to prevent penetration of the capsule. If there are worn or traumatized areas, they are usually on the inferior side of the disk attachment to the retrodiskal tissue. In most cases, this area can be excised as the plication is carried out (see Fig. 15–7).

The spreader is closed down somewhat while the amount of tissue to be removed is determined. The disk is held tightly over the condyle, and the posterior tissue is evaluated and then excised with a No. 15 blade or scissors. The first incision is made at the junction of the posterior disk and the retrodiskal tissue, and the second incision is made posterior to the first to facilitate the

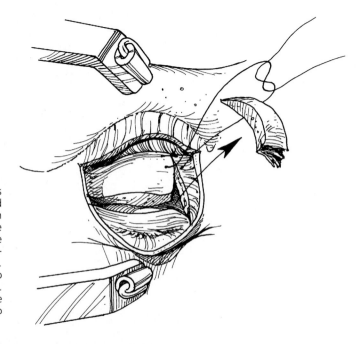

FIGURE 15–7. The joint is spread open as much as feasible. The disk is mobilized and placed in the most anatomically ideal position possible. Tension on the joint from the spreader is relaxed slightly. The excess tissue at the junction of the disk and posterior attachment is excised in wedge fashion *(arrow).* The goal is to leave no loose tissue but to avoid tension that makes closure difficult. Simple 5-0 polyglactin 910 sutures with the knots placed on the superior side are used to achieve the posterior plication.

removal of a pie-shaped wedge. Inexperienced surgeons are advised to remove less tissue than expected at the outset, followed by the removal of additional tissue as needed. The spreader can be opened slightly again to permit access to the medial extent of the excision. The posterior plication is closed with 5-0 polyglactin 910 sutures (see Fig. 15–7). Nonresorbable sutures are not recommended, because slow-resorbing sutures remain in place much longer than it takes for the wound to heal, after which the sutures are only irritants. When large excisions are completed (>6 mm), often the retrodiskal tissue is very thick superoinferiorly, making it difficult to penetrate all the tissue with one pass of a small needle. In such cases, two passes are made through the retrodiskal tissue—one through each lamina, and then one pass through the posterior aspect of the disk, placing the knot on the superior side of the repair. The repair proceeds from medial to lateral until the excision has been closed (see Fig. 15–7).

Occasionally, the lateral pole of the condyle protrudes so far laterally that it is difficult to restore the lateral collateral ligament and cover the lateral surface of the condyle with disk cartilage. A small portion of the lateral pole may be removed carefully with a rongeur or chisel so that the lateral ligamentous portion of the capsule is not disrupted. The articular covering of the condyle should not be removed except when the bone was removed laterally. The superior articulating surface of the condyle is preserved in all cases. It is rare to see significant irregularities on the condylar surface in the absence of perforations. However, the condyle may show some irregular proliferation of the articular cartilage and bone if there is damage to the inferior side of the disk without full perforation, producing surface irregularities that can be shaved down with a No. 15 blade.

The final and perhaps most important feature of the surgery is the lateral plication (Fig. 15–8). This is done with 4-0 polyglactin 910 sutures placed in a horizontal mattress fashion. The spreader is closed to remove tension from the disk. The first pass is made up through the capsule and lateral collateral ligament, staying as close to the capsular attachment to the bone as possible. The next pass is made through the lateral edge of the disk, and the third pass is made back

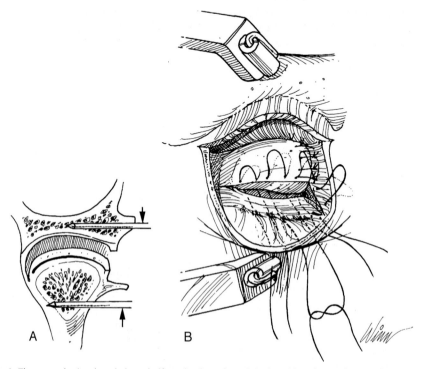

FIGURE 15–8. *A,* The spreader is relaxed about halfway back to the original position *(arrows). B,* Perhaps the most important phase of the repair is the lateral plication. This is achieved using horizontal mattress sutures of 4-0 polyglactin 910. Four or five of these are placed with a slight posterolateral direction to cinch the disk snugly against the condyle.

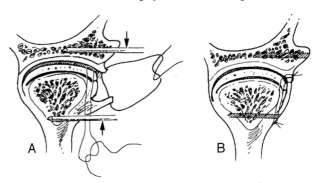

FIGURE 15–9. *A,* The spreader is closed completely to hold the disk-condyle complex snugly against the glenoid fossa *(arrows). B,* The capsule is then closed with the same 4-0 suture. These sutures are placed with a slight posterior pull on the inferior edge of the capsular incision.

down through the edge of the disk in a mattress fashion. Finally, the last pass is the reverse of the first one, down through the capsular attachment at the neck of the condyle (Fig. 15–9). The four passes are made so that the disk is pulled laterally and slightly posterior. The objective is to pull the lateral edge of the disk into the sulcus between the condyle and the lateral capsule (see Fig. 15–9). The purpose of this maneuver is to restore the lateral collateral ligamentous attachment of the disk to the condyle. It is often beneficial to place one of these sutures at the lateral edge of the posterior plication closure so that the second pass goes through the disk and the third through the retrodiskal tissue. The first and fourth passes are the same as for the other lateral mattress sutures, thereby joining the posterior and lateral plication closures. The lateral capsule is rarely inadequate (<1% of cases) to hold the mattress sutures, although in such cases a hole can be drilled in the posterior lateral neck of the condyle to provide a place to secure these sutures.[77] In most cases, however, the lateral capsule is not the weakest link in the lateral plication; rather, the disk is more likely to pull through.

The spreader is now closed until the condyle and disk complex is seated superiorly in the glenoid fossa (see Fig. 15–9). This permits tension-free closure of the lateral capsule with the same 4-0 resorbable sutures in an interrupted fashion. These interrupted sutures are directed in a slightly posterior orientation on the superior wound edge to help resist anterior pull on the condyle. The remainder of the closure is carried out in layers. Before closing the skin, a suture is placed through the subcutaneous tissue of the skin that lies on the anterior aspect of the tragal cartilage and is then attached to the anterior tragal perichondrium. This is to prevent tenting of the skin over the tragus, without the proper depression in front of the tragus, which is seen so often following rhytidectomy (Fig. 15–10).

SKIN CLOSURE

Skin closure is achieved with 5-0 nylon sutures (see Fig. 15–10). First, the corners where the connecting endaural incision was made are approximated with two simple interrupted sutures (see Fig. 15–2). Then one additional interrupted suture is placed between the two initial sutures, followed by two or three interrupted sutures to close the inferior lobular incision. Finally, the remaining superior skin is closed with a running subcuticular suture that ends endaur-

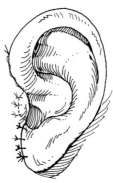

FIGURE 15–10. The wound is closed in layers with 4-0 polyglactin 910 acid suture. The tissue immediately anterior to the tragal cartilage should be sutured down before skin closure to prevent tenting of the skin over the tragal cartilage, obliterating the natural depression in the face anterior to the tragus. The skin is closed by placing simple, interrupted sutures at the corners and in the middle of the endaural skin incision with 5-0 monofilament nylon. The inferior aspect of the incision is closed with simple sutures, and finally the superior part is closed with a continuous, subcuticular "pullout" suture, all with 5-0 monofilament nylon.

ally (see Fig. 15–10). The gauze placed in the EAC preoperatively is removed, and the EAC is irrigated copiously. A new gauze is then placed, followed by a pressure dressing over the entire area. The pressure dressing and gauze are removed the next morning, and the wound is left open thereafter.

Arthrotomy with Disk Repair: Bilaminar Flap Repair

If one is dedicated to disk repair whenever possible, bilaminar flap repair offers an alternative to diskectomy or other more invasive procedures.[34, 37, 38] The technique is based on the understanding gleaned from animal studies, specifically those in which the healing process was observed following the creation of disk perforations in monkey TMJs.[78] Although most perforations did not heal spontaneously (only one did), there was gross and histologic evidence that an exuberant synovial response resulted in reparative tissue surrounding the injured area.[78] Additional studies of human cadaver material confirmed that a strong synovial reaction could form numerous bridges along the margins of the perforations.[79] Because soft tissue flaps are used all over the body to close defects that are traumatically induced, the bilaminar flap was developed to take advantage of this strong synovial response.[34, 37, 38] The technique involves standard soft tissue principles of tissue elevation and advancement without tension,[34] although it must be stressed that the procedure as described here is technically difficult and should not be tried without specific hands-on training.

SURGICAL TECHNIQUE (STAGES IV AND V WITH DISK PERFORATIONS)

Degenerative joint disease, or osteoarthritis (OA), results in the development of lesions—such as erosions and irregularities on articular surfaces—and disk alterations with or without perforations. OA may involve the articular eminence, condyle, or disk, especially when perforations are present; however, localized OA may develop with an intact but deformed disk. In addition, radiographic changes observed in the

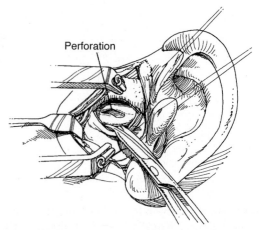

FIGURE 15–11. All aspects of surgery to repair perforated disk are the same as those described for simple disk repositioning, except that the incision through the lateral collateral ligament is made lateral to the perforation, even if the perforation is more lateral than usual. This preserves any disk tissue that remains in front of or behind the perforation on the lateral side.

TMJ have been associated with OA, such as roughening of the condyle, narrowing of the joint space, flattening of the condyle and eminence, and osteophytosis.

ID and OA are thought by some to represent a continuum of the same disease process.[80] Prolonged joint loading with an anteriorly displaced disk without reduction may lead to condylar and articular eminence remodeling and disk deformation. Subsequent disk perforation may develop, thereby exacerbating the degenerative condyle and fossa changes. Conversely, disk perforation leads to osteoarthritic changes on the condylar and fossa surfaces.[78, 79, 81]

The surgical technique to repair perforated and badly damaged disk uses the same preauricular, endaural approach described previously to expose the TMJ capsule and to enter the joint space (see Figs. 15–1 to 15–6). The lateral collateral ligament is generally intact on the outer edge of even the most lateral perforations. The lateral aspect of the disk near the perforation is grasped, and the collateral ligament is divided using blunt-tipped tenotomy scissors (Fig. 15–11). Enough ligamentous tissue should be left lateral to the perforation to allow the perforation to be encircled completely by the disk, bilaminar tissue, and medial and lateral collateral ligaments once the inferior joint space is fully exposed. The spreader is opened until adequate exposure is achieved.

If exposure is insufficient, it is often because the anterior aspect of the capsule is inadequately incised, which can be rectified by carrying the incision slightly further forward.

Traction sutures are placed in three sites for orientation and retraction (Fig. 15–12). One is placed through the lateral edge of the disk just anterior to the perforation. The other two are placed posterior to the perforation—one in the superior lamina, and the other in the inferior lamina of the retrodiskal tissue (bilaminar zone). The bridge of tissue that is lateral to the perforation between the anterior and the two posterior traction sutures is then divided, thereby opening the lateral aspect of the perforation (see Fig. 15–12).

The remaining anterior portion of the disk, which is often biconvex, must be mobilized as much as possible so that it can be repositioned posteriorly (Fig. 15–13). Posterior tension is placed on the disk with forceps while a sharp periosteal elevator disrupts the junction of the anterior capsule and the periosteum of the anterior slope of the articular eminence. Care is taken to avoid penetrating the vascular tissue ante-

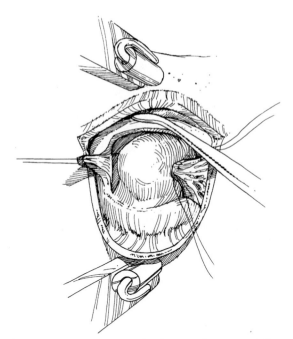

FIGURE 15–13. The spreader is opened more, and the edges of the perforation are freshened. Remaining disk cartilage is mobilized as much as possible to achieve maximal condylar coverage from these anterior tissues.

rior to the capsule, which can cause annoying but controllable bleeding. This same procedure may be necessary at the junction of the inferior aspect of the capsule and the condylar neck. The disk usually does not mobilize nearly as much as the bilaminar flaps.

The bilaminar flaps are raised by placing light tension on the two posterior traction sutures to separate the laminae, at which point the laminae are divided with tenotomy scissors (Fig. 15–14). Hemostasis is achieved by the use of the bipolar cautery. The superior lamina is dissected posteriorly to its attachment at the tympanic plate of the temporal bone. In large perforation repairs, this dissection may extend so far medially that the petrotympanic fissure is exposed. The superior lamina should be kept as thick as possible to avoid creating a dehiscence. In order for the division of the laminae to extend medially to the perforation, the posterior rim of the perforation is divided equally between the superior and inferior laminae from a lateral to medial direction.

The inferior lamina is mobilized ending at its point of attachment to the posterior condylar neck. This flap should also be kept

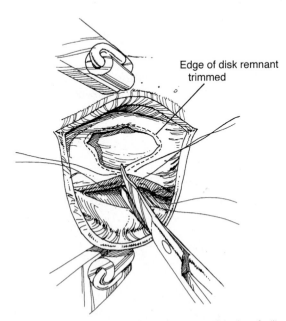

Edge of disk remnant trimmed

FIGURE 15–12. Three traction sutures are placed to facilitate exposure. One is placed anterior to the thinnest lateral wall of the perforation. Two are placed just posterior to this. One of these is placed in the superior layer of the retrodiskal attachment, and the other in the inferior layer. As the lateral wall of the perforation is incised, these stay sutures maintain proper orientation for the repair.

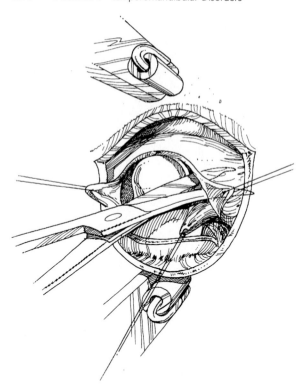

FIGURE 15–14. The upper and lower portions of the retrodiskal attachment are divided to create a bilaminar zone. The amount of mobilization varies with the size of the defect to be closed after the anterior disk tissue has been mobilized. In severe cases, the upper lamina can be separated from the lower one until the tympanic plate of the temporal bone is contacted. Separating the two layers affords significant freedom to each of them by eliminating the tethering effect of the connective tissue that normally limits mobility.

as thick as possible and should not be completely detached from the condyle. Because the dissection is open and under direct vision, bleeding is easily controlled with the bipolar cautery.

The question might be asked, why is this division necessary? Considerable mobility is achieved with the division of the laminae because numerous multidirectional fibrous connections between them are incised concomitantly. In addition, the superior lamina is separated from half of its attachment to the lateral inferior section of the tympanic plate in a subperiosteal fashion. The superior laminar flap therefore tends to be more mobile than the inferior one.

The most medial edge of the perforation is also divided equally, so that the division is continuous with the separation between the laminae (Fig. 15–15). If the disk edge of the perforation is sharp or feather-edged, it is blunted. A No. 15 blade is used to fillet this disk edge, which facilitates suturing of the two laminae to the disk.

Mobilization at all areas is continued until the bilaminar flaps and disk can be approximated without tension (see Fig. 15–15). A double-layer closure is achieved with a 5-0 polyglactin 910 suture (Fig. 15–16). The least accessible layer is closed first from

a medial to lateral direction, with the knots buried away from the synovial surfaces. Releasing the tension on the spreader may facilitate the closure. If the inferior surface of the disk is too convex where it contacts the condyle, it can be reshaped on the surface with a No. 15 blade.

Following completion of the repair (Fig. 15–17A), a lateral plication is achieved just as it would be in the case of a routine plica-

Posterior

Anterior

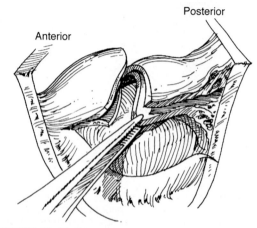

FIGURE 15–15. The anterior edge of the perforation, after it is freshened, is "filleted" to facilitate closure. This facilitates a double-layered closure similar to closure of an oroantral fistula.

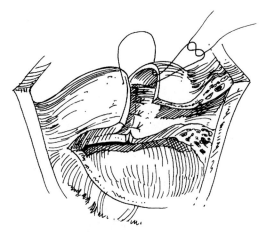

FIGURE 15–16. The two layers are closed simultaneously so that the sutures are buried in the middle. Usually the lower layer is more difficult to close, so it is done first.

tion procedure (see Fig. 15–17B). The remainder of the closure is also the same as described previously.

Arthrotomy with Diskectomy

In spite of several long-term studies supporting its use, diskectomy in the treatment of ID remains controversial.[41–46, 50, 53, 54] As with most of the literature on TMJ surgery, these studies are not randomized clinical trials and generally follow only a small portion of the patients treated from the outset. The inability to follow an entire group of consecutively treated patients raises concerns about the inherent bias toward an overly optimistic report of success. This is true not only of diskectomy but of all the literature regarding TMJ surgery.[82] Reports dissuading the use of diskectomy are also based primarily on the surgeon's experience, either good or bad, with this and other procedures to treat ID.[47, 48, 51, 52] The concern of these and many other surgeons is that in most cases of ID the disk can be saved and repaired.

Degenerative changes of the bony parts of the joint are more severe with diskectomy than with disk repair.[43, 52–55, 65] However, some surgeons have found relapse of symptoms to be greater with disk repair.[42] Perhaps the most sensible approach is to save the disk if possible and to remove it if not.[32, 45, 52] This calls for staging the severity of disk deterioration, if not preoperatively then at least postoperatively. Although many procedures have been advocated for the replacement of the enucleated disk (see elsewhere in this volume), none has been shown to be superior to removal without replacement.[44, 45] Although this author

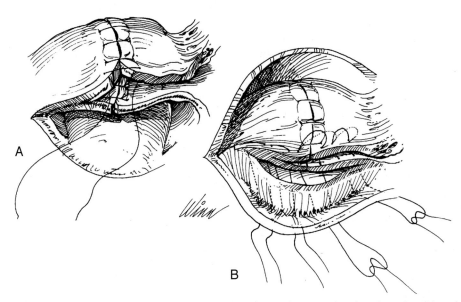

FIGURE 15–17. *A,* After both layers are closed, the lateral mattress sutures are placed to draw the disk and retrodiskal tissues posterolaterally. The first suture is placed so that it crosses the posterior plication of both layers. *B,* The remainder are placed to draw the disk tissues posterolaterally and to close the two layers together. The remaining closure is as described previously for simple plication.

makes every effort to save and repair disks, an alternative procedure that has significant long-term support is the diskectomy.

SURGICAL TECHNIQUE

The most attractive feature of diskectomy is the ease with which it can be performed. Technically, little skill is required to successfully complete the procedure. The same exposure described earlier (see Figs. 15–1 to 15–6) suffices for diskectomy. Most authors recommend removing only the disk fibrocartilage, leaving the synovial tissue surrounding the disk intact. Additionally, any gross irregularities on the condylar or fossa surfaces should be smoothed. Postoperative therapy may be no different from that for other intracapsular procedures.

Arthrotomy with Diskectomy and Autologous Graft Disk Replacement

Autologous grafting to replace the TMJ disk has been done with many materials, but auricular cartilage and dermis have been the most widely used.[12, 13, 56–58, 83] As stated earlier, there is little evidence that free graft replacement of the disk is superior to no replacement at all.[44, 45] The rationale for disk replacement seems to be more aesthetic, probably owing to surgeons' fastidious nature and their desire to fix things. Hypothetically, the graft provides a scaffold for the ingrowth of tissue from the surrounding synovium. Animal and human studies reveal that, to some extent, this does happen.[57, 84, 85] Another hope is that these materials may help prevent the degeneration that follows diskectomy, a downside that has been reported by even the most enthusiastic supporters of diskectomy.[42, 44–46] However, to date, there are no data to support this hope.

A disadvantage of autologous grafting is the need for a separate donor site. Dermal grafts require either a full-thickness excision of tissue with primary closure or a split-thickness harvest with replacement of the epidermis. Auricular cartilage harvest potentially weakens the external ear,[56] but few complications have been reported. Dermal grafts have been associated with at

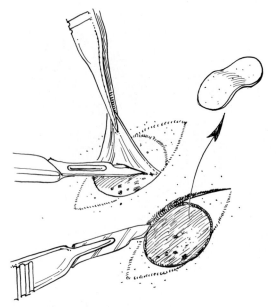

FIGURE 15–18. Dermal harvest includes removal of the epidermis over an ovoid area of skin, usually the lateral thigh. The epidermis is discarded.

least four cases of epidermoid cysts occurring in the TMJ following implantation for disk replacement,[10–12, 86] one of which resulted in invasion of the middle cranial fossa.[12] This should not be surprising, as the occurrence of similar cysts after dermal implantation in extraoral sites has been reported for many years.[72, 87]

SURGICAL TECHNIQUE

The procedure for removal of the disk does not differ from the simple diskectomy

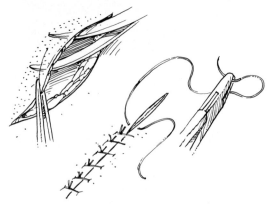

FIGURE 15–19. The oval is converted to a full-thickness fusiform shape that is at least three times longer than it is wide. This split-thickness oval, along with the rest of the fusiform, is removed down to the subcutaneous fat. The full-thickness corners are excised. The wound is then undermined and closed primarily.

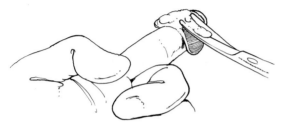

FIGURE 15–20. The oval dermal graft is de-fatted by hand using a No. 15 blade.

as described earlier. Dermal graft harvesting may be performed using one of two methods. The full-thickness method is preferred, because it leaves a less visible scar and results in a thicker removal of epidermis, thereby theoretically reducing the potential for cyst formation. The technique is begun with a fusiform outline on the skin (Fig. 15–18). A circular area in the middle of the outlined area is de-epithelialized freehand (see Fig. 15–18), leaving a circular area of dermis with triangular areas of skin on each end of the fusiform. The entire outlined tissue is removed, and the remaining area is undermined and closed primarily (Fig. 15–19). The full-thickness skin ends

are excised from the dermal graft, and the dermal graft is de-fatted via the freehand method (Fig. 15–20).

The second method for dermal graft harvest requires the removal of a split-thickness skin graft with a dermatome and then the removal of the dermis, followed by replacement of the epidermis over the wound. Although this technique may be somewhat faster, it leaves a more unsightly scar and may result in a greater tendency to include epithelial elements in the graft.

Dermal grafts may result in adhesions between the graft and the glenoid fossa, stimulating some surgeons to place a temporary Silastic sheet between the graft and the fossa for 8 to 10 weeks; however, this practice is discouraged. It is generally recommended that dermal grafts be cut larger than the defect they are to fill, thus providing an overlap, especially on the medial side, where suturing is difficult (Fig. 15–21). In addition, it is believed that dermal grafts are better for repair of disk perforations because vertical restoration is usually not necessary in such cases. To achieve this type of repair, the graft is either sutured into place using a few horizontal mattress sutures or

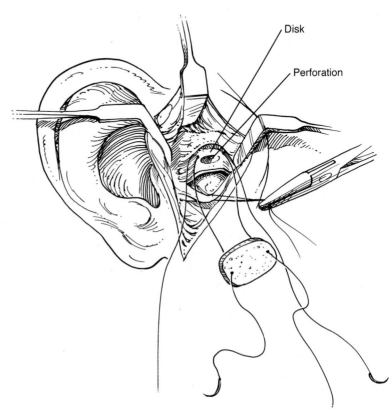

Disk

Perforation

FIGURE 15–21. The graft is fashioned to overlap the perforation by 2 mm in all dimensions and is then sutured in place.

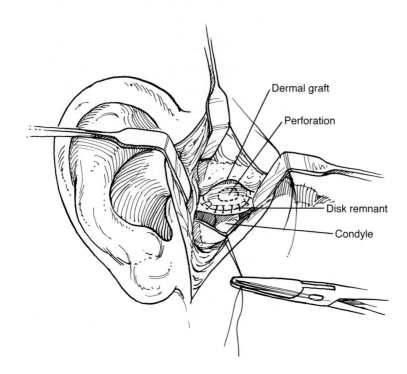

FIGURE 15–22. The dermal graft sutured into place.

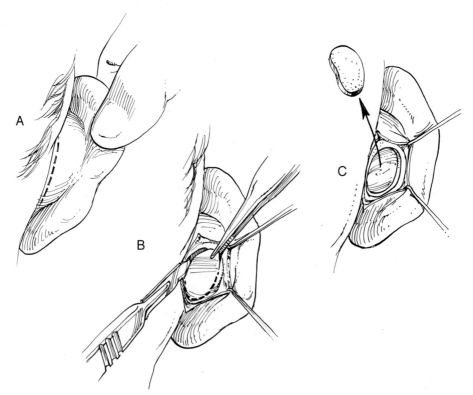

FIGURE 15–23. *A,* Auricular cartilage is harvested via a vertical incision on the posterior aspect of the concha. *B,* The cartilage is exposed, and the amount needed is outlined. The perichondrium is left on the convex surface of the cartilage. *C,* The outlined portion is excised and removed so that the perichondrium is not taken with the graft. The graft now has perichondrium on the convex side and none on the concave side.

wired to the lateral lip of the glenoid fossa (Fig. 15–22).

Harvesting of auricular cartilage can be performed from an anterior or posterior approach. The posterior approach is most common and is described here (Fig. 15–23). Regardless of the method used, it is important that the perichondrium remain on the convex side of the cartilage—a position that is said to preserve cell viability and promote revascularization. It is also considered important to remove the perichondrium from the concave side to prevent adhesions between the graft and the condyle.[56]

The posterior approach involves a vertical, linear incision on the posterior side of the conchal bowl and a supraperichondrial dissection over the convex surface of the cartilage (see Fig. 15–23). The cartilage is incised parallel to the helix, leaving sufficient cartilage behind to support the ear. A subperichondrial dissection is carried out on the concave surface, the graft is removed, and the skin incision is closed primarily.

The placement technique depends on the size and shape of the remaining joint defect.

Auricular cartilage grafts are preferred over dermis when complete diskectomy or removal of a failed implant is performed. If only a single thickness is required, the cartilage graft can be sutured into place—as the dermal graft was—using a few horizontal mattress sutures, or it can be wired to the lateral lip of the glenoid fossa (Fig. 15–24). Medial placement is stressed to extend the graft beyond the medial pole of the condyle. In cases of a very steep eminence, the graft may be placed more posteriorly to avoid overly augmenting the eminence (Fig. 15–25). If vertical height has been lost, several thicknesses of cartilage can be placed either in the fossa or on the condylar surface, as well as in the fossa (Fig. 15–26).

Arthrotomy with Diskectomy and Autologous Flap Reconstruction

Insertion of tissue from outside the TMJ capsule may be required when the disk is too severely perforated for bilaminar flap

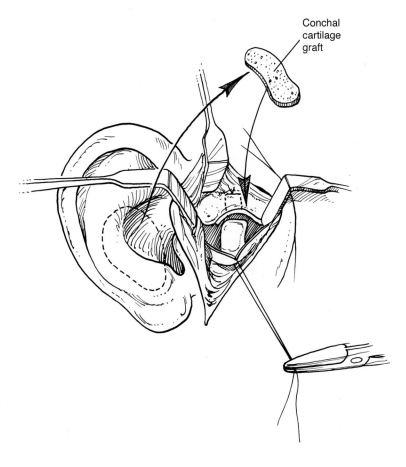

Conchal cartilage graft

FIGURE 15–24. Cartilage graft is sutured with wires or heavy sutures to the fossa, including the posterior slope of the eminence.

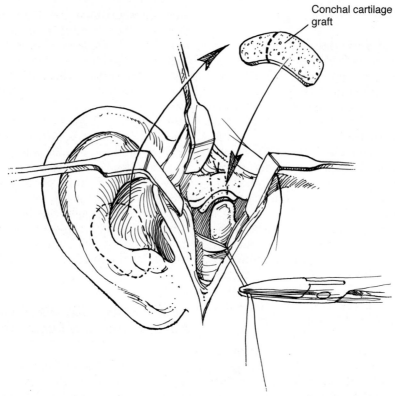

Conchal cartilage graft

FIGURE 15–25. If the eminence is very steep or the fossa deep, the cartilage graft may be placed more posteriorly.

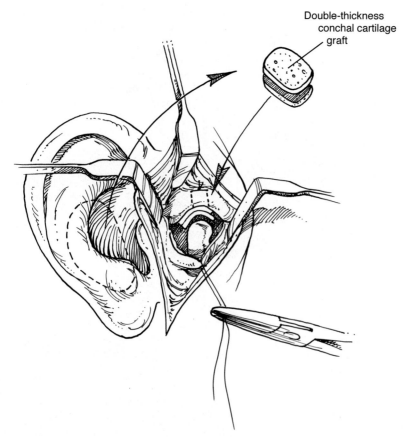

Double-thickness conchal cartilage graft

FIGURE 15–26. If vertical height has been lost, two layers of cartilage can be layered.

repair (see Figs. 15–11 to 15–17) or too degenerated. The temporalis muscle–fascia flap is a viable choice for surgeons who are uncomfortable leaving the joint without a disk replacement and also wish to avoid a separate donor site.[59, 88] As noted in volume 4, Chapter 18, this flap has been used mostly in cases of failed alloplastic implants (see that chapter for a description of the procedure). It should be noted, however, that the temporalis muscle–fascia flap is a vascularized flap, not a free graft. If done properly, this flap brings a blood supply that may be lacking in the degenerated joint. Studies have revealed that the muscle tissue provided by this technique remains viable at 15 months, with some fibrosis.[59, 88]

Condylotomy

Condylotomy has an interesting and troubled history. Although the procedure was first described for the treatment of dentofacial deformities in 1898,[89] it became popular in the United States in the 1950s as a method for reducing mandibular prognathism by using a blind Gigli saw technique through the condylar neck.[90] Several British oral surgeons subsequently noticed a decrease in TMD signs and symptoms in two patients following accidental fracture of the mandibular condyle. These patients had been treated successfully with anterior repositioning oral appliances before their fractures. A few other patients with previous TMD signs and symptoms without appliance therapy also seemed to have fewer problems after condylar fractures. Finally, it was frequently reported that patients with condylar fractures did not develop TMD complaints after closed reduction of the fractures. Based on these clinical observations, Ward and colleagues published the technique of blind condylotomy as a treatment for ID.[62] The blind procedure was used for nearly 20 years by Ward and his disciples, culminating in the oft-quoted paper by Banks and Mackenzie in which they reported on 211 cases with a 91% cure rate.[8] In one of the more remarkable recantations in the TMD literature, Banks in 1997 paraphrased the venerable 18th-century poet and essayist Samuel Johnson: "the operation of condylotomy is like the dog walking on its hinder legs; whether or not it is done well, we are surprised to see it done at all."[7] After many years' experience with the procedure, Banks proceeded to build a case against condylotomy that was based on its unpredictable results and the lack of evidence that either the condylotomy or the so-called modified condylotomy had been tested under acceptable scientific clinical control.[7]

Nevertheless, the condylotomy has strong support in some circles.[60, 61, 63, 91] Its development seems to have paralleled refinement of the intraoral vertical ramus osteotomy (IVRO),[92, 93] a procedure that many orthognathic surgeons have abandoned owing to poor predictability and the need for MMF. As with the arthroplasty mentioned earlier, condylotomy is predicated on the belief that the condyle-disk relationship is important and achievable. The procedure is advocated for early/intermediate and intermediate (Wilkes stages I–III) categories of ID.[16] One rationale for the technique is based on the goal of using anterior repositioning splints to advance the condyle to catch up to an anteriorly displaced disk. Anterior repositioning splint techniques are numerous, but they usually advance the mandible to recapture the disk and then, after a period of time, attempt to either seat the condyle with a centric splint or, more radically, rebuild the patient's occlusion prosthetically to the anterior position. If all the patients with these clinical criteria (Wilkes stages I–III) were treated with anterior repositioning splints followed by centric splints, probably 90% would not need surgery at all.[36, 69]

The modified condylotomy has been purported to involve less postoperative management,[60] but the 3 to 6 weeks of MMF followed by more weeks of "training" elastics and outpatient arch bar removal is much more extensive than the normal postsurgical management required for the procedures discussed earlier.[6, 94] The contention that only minor alterations in occlusion occur is in opposition to the experience of most orthognathic surgeons, including this author. There is no doubt that many patients can be "trained" to bite in maximal intercuspation during the postoperative period, but there are also some who cannot, and this unpredictability is a concern.

Perhaps the most compelling argument in favor of the modified condylotomy is that there is no surgical invasion of the TMJ capsule; it cannot be denied that arthrotomy results in scarring of the capsule and occasionally adhesions in the joint. But with the success of such procedures as nonsurgical disk recapturing, arthrotomy, and arthrocentesis with lavage, condylotomy—despite some interesting qualities—has not garnered wide support among TMJ surgeons.

Summary

Ultimately, the treatment of TMDs is more of an art than a science, but that does not sanction the abandonment of what science there is to support therapeutic rationale. Evidence suggests that findings such as joint noises, malocclusion, and muscle pain and imaging evidence of disk displacement should play only secondary roles in the decision to undertake surgery. The clear diagnostic indicators for ID surgery are pain in the joint upon palpation, with function, and associated with joint noises that is consistent with a history, imaging findings, and physical findings of ID.

ID surgery can and does work when the proper diagnostic criteria are met, but it is technically difficult and requires the judicious use of pre- and postoperative care. Repeat surgery is rarely indicated, has a poor success rate, and carries a high risk of causing a permanent deterioration in the patient's condition.

REFERENCES

1. Goss A: Toward an international consensus on temporomandibular joint surgery: Report of the second international consensus meeting, April 1992, Buenos Aires, Argentina. Int J Oral Maxillofac Surg 1993;22:78–81.
2. Goss A: The opinions of 100 international experts on temporomandibular joint surgery, a postal questionnaire. Int J Oral Maxillofac Surg 1993;22:66–70.
3. Albino J (ed): National Institutes of Health Technology Assessment Conference on Management of Temporomandibular Disorders. Bethesda, MD, 1996.
4. Ericksson L, Westesson P: Temporomandibular joint diskectomy. Oral Surg Oral Med Oral Pathol 1992;74:259–272.
5. Feinerman D, Piecuch J: Long-term retrospective analysis of twenty-three Proplast-Teflon temporomandibular joint interpositional implants. Int J Oral Maxillofac Surg 1993;22:11–16.
6. Bronstein S: Modified condylotomy for treatment of the painful temporomandibular joint with a reducing disc: Discussion. J Oral Maxillofac Surg 1993;51:143–144.
7. Banks P: The case against mandibular condylotomy in the treatment of the painful, deranged temporomandibular joint. J Oral Maxillofac Surg 1997;55:70–74.
8. Banks P, Mackenzie I: Condylotomy: A clinical and experimental appraisal of a surgical technique. J Maxillofac Surg 1975;3:170–181.
9. Estabrooks L, Fairbanks C, Collet R, Miller L: A retrospective evaluation of 301 TMJ Proplast-Teflon implants. Oral Surg 1990;70:381–386.
10. Muto T, Tomioka K, Michiya H, Kanazawa M: Epidermoid cyst in the temporomandibular joint after a dermal graft. J Craniomaxillofac Surg 1992; 20:270–272.
11. Bonnington G, Langan M, Joy E: Epithelial inclusion cyst in the temporomandibular joint after a dermal graft. J Oral Maxillofac Surg 1987;45:705–707.
12. MacIntosh B: A current spectrum of costochondral and dermal grafting. In Bell W (ed): Modern Practice in Orthognathic and Reconstructive Surgery. Philadelphia, WB Saunders, 1992, pp 872–949.
13. MacIntosh R: Fat and dermis grafting in oral and maxillofacial surgery. In MacIntosh R (ed): Oral and Maxillofacial Surgery Clinics of North America. Philadelphia, WB Saunders, 1993, pp 579–598.
14. Hey W, Davies C (eds): Practical Observations in Surgery, Illustrated by Cases, ed 3. London, T. Cadell and W. Davies, 1814.
15. Laskin DM: Etiology and pathogenesis of internal derangements of the temporomandibular joint. In Laskin DM (ed): Oral and Maxillofacial Surgery Clinics of North America: Current Controversies in Surgery for Internal Derangements of the Temporomandibular Joint. Philadelphia, WB Saunders, 1994, pp 217–222.
16. Wilkes C: Internal derangements of the temporomandibular joint: Pathological variations. Arch Otolaryngol Head Neck Surg 1989;115:469–477.
17. Solberg W, Woo M, Houston J: Prevalence of mandibular dysfunction in young adults. J Am Dent Assoc 1979;98:25.
18. Delfino J, Eppley B: Radiographic and surgical evaluation of internal derangements of the temporomandibular joint. J Oral Maxillofac Surg 1986;44:260–267.
19. Westesson P: Diagnostic imaging of internal derangements of the temporomandibular joint. In Laskin DM (ed): Current Controversies in Surgery for Internal Derangements of the Temporomandibular Joint. Philadelphia, WB Saunders, 1994, pp 227–244.
20. Dolwick MF, Nitzan DW: The role of disc-repositioning surgery for internal derangements of the temporomandibular joint. In Laskin DM (ed): Current Controversies in Surgery for Internal Derangements of the Temporomandibular Joint. Philadelphia, WB Saunders, 1994, pp 271–275.
21. Mongini F, Ibertis F, Manfredi A: Long-term results in patients with disc displacement without reduction treated conservatively. J Cranio Pract 1996;14:301–305.
22. Watt-Smith S, Sadler A, Baddeley H, Renton P: Comparison of arthrotomographic and magnetic resonance images of 50 temporomandibular joints with operative findings. Br J Oral Maxillofac Surg 1993;31:139–143.

23. Donlon W, Moon K: Comparison of magnetic resonance imaging, arthrotomography and clinical and surgical findings in temporomandibular joint internal derangements. Oral Surg 1987;64:2.

24. Schiffman E, Fricton J: The relationship of occlusion, parafunctional habits and recent life events to mandibular dysfunction in a non-patient population. J Oral Rehabil 1992;19:201–223.

25. DeBoever A, Bays RA, Keeling S, et al: Influence of mandibular advancement surgery on TM signs and symptoms [abstract]. J Dent Res 1994;73:439.

26. Rodrigues Garcia R, Nemeth D, Hatch J, et al: Effects of mandibular advancement surgery on temporomandibular signs and symptoms in class II patients. J Orofacial Pain (in press).

27. Fricton J, Schiffman E: The craniomandibular index: Validity. J Prosthet Dent 1987;58:222–228.

28. Fricton J, Schiffman E: Reliability of a craniomandibular index. J Dent Res 1986;65:1359–1364.

29. Annandale T: On displacement of the interarticular cartilage of the lower jaw and its treatment by operation. Lancet 1887;1:411.

30. Nitzan DW: Arthrocentesis for management of severe closed lock of the temporomandibular joint. In Laskin DM (ed): Current Controversies in Surgery for Internal Derangements of the Temporomandibular Joint. Philadelphia, WB Saunders, 1994, pp 245–257.

31. Kuwahara T, Bessette R, Maruyama T: A retrospective study on the clinical results of temporomandibular joint surgery. J Craniomandib Pract 1994;12:179–183.

32. Gundlach K: Long-term results following surgical treatment of internal derangement of the temporomandibular joint. J Craniomaxillofac Surg 1990;18:206–209.

33. Mercuri LG, Laskin DM: Indications for the surgical treatment of internal derangements of the temporomandibular joint. In Laskin DM (ed): Current Controversies in Surgery for Internal Derangements of the Temporomandibular Joint. Philadelphia, WB Saunders, 1994, pp 223–226.

34. Bays R: Temporomandibular joint disc preservation. In Frost D (ed): Joint Preservation Procedures. Philadelphia, WB Saunders, 1996, pp 33–50.

35. Swift J, Schiffman E, Look J, et al: TMJ disc displacement without reduction: A randomized clinical trial [abstract]. J Oral Maxillofac Surg 1997;55:116.

36. Bays R: Temporomandibular joint meniscus repair surgery: A follow-up study. Fac Orthop Temporomandib Arthr 1985;2:11.

37. Sharawy M, Helmy E, Bays R, et al: Repair of TMJ disc perforation using synovial membrane flap in *Macaca fascicularis* monkey: Light and electron microscopic studies. J Oral Maxillofac Surg 1994;52:259.

38. Bays R, Helmy E, Sharawy M: The synovial membrane flap for repair of TMJ disc perforations in *Macaca fascicularis*: A stereoscopic study [abstract]. AAOMS national meeting, Washington, DC, 1985.

39. McCarty W, Farrar W: Surgery for internal derangements of the temporomandibular joint. J Prosthet Dent 1979;42:191.

40. Dolwick M, Nitzan D: TMJ disk surgery: 8-year follow-up evaluation. Fortschr Kiefer Gesichtschir 1990;35:162.

41. Widmark G, Kahnberg K, Haraldson T, Lindstrom J: Evaluation of TMJ surgery in cases not responding to conservative treatment. J Craniomandib Pract 1995;13:44–49.

42. Trumpy I, Lyberg T: Surgical treatment of the internal derangement of the temporomandibular joint: Long term evaluation of three techniques. J Oral Maxillofac Surg 1995;53:740–746.

43. Wilkes C: Surgical treatment of internal derangements of the temporomandibular joint. Arch Otolaryngol Head Neck Surg 1991;117:64–72.

44. Holmlund A, Gynter G, Axelsson S: Diskectomy in the treatment of internal derangement of the temporomandibular joint: Follow-up at 1, 3, and 5 years. Oral Surg 1993;76:266–271.

45. Eriksson L: Surgical treatment of internal derangement of the temporomandibular joint: Long-term evaluation of three techniques: Discussion. J Oral Maxillofac Surg 1995;53:746–747.

46. Widmark G, Dahlstrom L, Kahnberg K, Lindvall A: Diskectomy in temporomandibular joints with internal derangement: A follow-up study. Oral Surg 1997;83:314–320.

47. Poswillo D: Surgery of the temporomandibular joint. In Temporomandibular Joint: Function and Dysfunction. Copenhagen, Munksgaard, 1979, p 397.

48. Troller P: Temporomandibular arthropathy [abstract]. Proc R Soc Med 1974;67:153.

49. Bowman K: Temporomandibular joint arthrosis and its treatment by extirpation of the disc. Acta Chir Scand 1947;95:1.

50. Dingman R: Meniscectomy in the treatment of lesions of the temporomandibular joint. J Oral Surg 1951;9:214.

51. Dingman R, Constant E: A fifteen year experience with temporomandibular joint disorders. Plast Reconstr Surg 1969;44:119.

52. Dingman R, Dingman D, Lawrence R: Surgical correction of lesions of the temporomandibular joints. Plast Reconstr Surg 1975;55:335.

53. Widmark G, Grondahl H, Kahnberg K, Haraldson T: Radiographic morphology in the temporomandibular joint after discectomy. Cranio 1996;14:37.

54. Widmark G: On surgical intervention in the temporomandibular joint. Swed Dent J 1997;123:1.

55. Yaillen D, Shapiro P, Luschei E, Feldman G: Temporomandibular joint meniscectomy—effects on joint structure and masticatory function in *Macaca fascicularis*. J Maxillofac Surg 1979;7:255.

56. Tucker M, Spagnoli D: Autologous dermal and auricular cartilage grafts for temporomandibular joint repair. In Frost D (ed): Atlas of the Oral and Maxillofacial Surgery Clinics of North America. Philadelphia, WB Saunders, 1996, pp 75–92.

57. Tucker M, Kennady M, Jacoway J: Autologous auricular cartilage implantation following discectomy in the temporomandibular joint. J Oral Maxillofac Surg 1990;48:38.

58. Georgiade N: The surgical correction of TMJ dysfunction by means of autologenous dermal grafts. Plast Reconstr Surg 1962;30:68.

59. Feinberg S, Larsen P: Reconstruction of the temporomandibular joint with pedicled temporalis muscle flaps. In Bell W (ed): Modern Practice in Orthognathic and Reconstructive Surgery. Philadelphia, WB Saunders, 1992, p 733.

60. Hall H, Nickerson J, McKenna S: Modified condylotomy for treatment of the painful temporomandibular joint with a reducing disc. J Oral Maxillofac Surg 1993;51:133–142.

61. Upton LG: The case for mandibular condylotomy in the treatment of the painful, deranged temporo-

mandibular joint. J Oral Maxillofac Surg 1997;55:64–69.

62. Ward T, Smith D, Sommar M: Condylotomy for mandibular joints. Br Dent J 1957;103:147.

63. Tasanen A, Lamberg M: Closed condylotomy in the treatment of recurrent dislocation of the mandibular condyle. Int J Oral Maxillofac Surg 1978;7:1.

64. Shevel E: Intra-oral condylotomy for the treatment of temporomandibular joint derangement. Int J Oral Maxillofac Surg 1991;20:360–361.

65. Takaku S, Toyoda T: Long-term evaluation of discectomy of the temporomandibular joint. J Oral Maxillofac Surg 1994;52:722–726.

66. Boyer C, Williams T, Stevens F: Blood supply of the temporomandibular joint. J Dent Res 1964;43:224.

67. Sharawy M: Anatomy of the temporomandibular joint. In Bays R, Quinn P (eds): Oral and Maxillofacial Surgery. Philadelphia, WB Saunders, 1999, p 1.

68. Al-Kayat A, Bramley P: A modified pre-auricular approach to the temporomandibular joint and malar arch. Br J Oral Surg 1998;17:91.

69. Williamson E, Sheffield J: The treatment of internal derangement of the temporomandibular joint: A survey of 300 cases. J Craniomandib Pract 1987;5:19.

70. Bays R: Arthrotomy and orthognathic surgery for TMD. In Kraus S (ed): Temporomandibular Disorders, ed 2. New York, Churchill Livingstone, 1994, p 237.

71. Keith T: Postoperative physical therapy protocol. In Kraus S (ed): Temporomandibular Disorders, ed 2. New York, Churchill Livingstone, 1994, p 298.

72. Peer L, Paddock R: Histologic studies on the fate of deeply implanted dermal grafts: Observations on sections of implants buried from one week to one year. Arch Surg 1937;34:268.

73. Montgomery M, Gordon S, Van Sickles J, Harms S: Changes in signs and symptoms following temporomandibular joint disc repositioning surgery. J Oral Maxillofac Surg 1992;50:320–328.

74. Van Sickles J, Dolezal J: Clinical outcome of arthrotomy after failed arthroscopy. Oral Surg Oral Med Oral Pathol 1994;78:142–145.

75. Nellestam P, Eriksson L: Preauricular approach to the temporomandibular joint: A postoperative follow-up on nerve function, hemorrhage and esthetics. Swed Dent J 1997;21:19–24.

76. Weinberg S, Kryshtalskyj B: Facial nerve function following temporomandibular joint surgery using the preauricular approach. J Oral Maxillofac Surg 1992;50:1048–1051.

77. Walker R, Kalamchi S: A surgical technique for management of internal derangements of the temporomandibular joint. J Oral Maxillofac Surg 1987;45:299.

78. Helmy E, Bays R, Sharawy M: Osteoarthrosis of the temporomandibular joint following experimental disc perforation in *Macaca fascicularis*. J Oral Maxillofac Surg 1988;46:979.

79. Helmy E, Bays R, Sharawy M: Histopathological study of human TMJ perforated discs with emphasis on synovial membrane response. J Oral Maxillofac Surg 1989;47:1048.

80. de Bont L, Stegenga B: Pathology of temporomandibular joint derangement and osteoarthrosis. Int J Oral Maxillofac Surg 1993;22:71–74.

81. Oberg T, Carlsson G, Fajers C: The temporomandibular joint: A morphologic study on human autopsy material. Acta Odontol Scand 1971;29:349.

82. Holmlund A: Surgery for TMJ internal derangement: Evaluation of treatment outcome and criteria for success. Int J Oral Maxillofac Surg 1993;22:75–77.

83. Witsenburg B, Gfeihofer P: Replacement of the pathologic temporomandibular articular disc using autogenous cartilage of the external ear. Int J Oral Surg 1984;13:401.

84. Stewart H, Hahn J, DeTomasi D, et al: Histologic fate of dermal grafts following implantation for temporomandibular joint meniscal perforation: A preliminary study. Oral Surg 1986;62:481.

85. Yih W, Zysset M, Merrill R: Histologic study of the fate of autogenous auricular cartilage grafts in the human temporomandibular joint. J Oral Maxillofac Surg 1992;50:964.

86. Weinberg S, Kryshtalskyj B: Epidermoid cyst in a temporomandibular joint dermal graft. J Oral Maxillofac Surg 1995;53:330–332.

87. Ruffer A: Cyst formation seven years after a cutis graft repair of hernia. BMJ 1955;4919:951.

88. Umeda H, Kaban L, Pogrel M, Stern M: Long-term viability of the temporalis muscle/fascia flap used for temporomandibular joint reconstruction. J Oral Maxillofac Surg 1993;51:530–533.

89. Caldwell J, Gerhard R, Lowry R: Orthognathic surgery. In Kruger G (ed): Textbook of Oral and Maxillofacial Surgery, ed 6. St Louis, Mosby, 1984, pp 530–531.

90. Reiter E: Surgical correction of mandibular prognathism. Alpha Omegan 1951;45:104.

91. Hall HD: Modification of the modified condylotomy. J Oral Maxillofac Surg 1996;54:548–551.

92. Hall H, Chase D: Evaluation and refinement of the intraoral vertical subcondylar osteotomy. J Oral Surg 975;33:333.

93. Hall H, McKenna S: Further refinement and evaluation of the intraoral vertical ramus osteotomy. J Oral Maxillofac Surg 1987;45:684.

94. Israel H: Modification of the modified condylotomy—discussion. J Oral Maxillofac Surg 1996;54:551–552.

CHAPTER

16

Autogenous Temporomandibular Joint Replacement

Paul Tompach • Thomas B. Dodson
Leonard B. Kaban

Autogenous temporomandibular joint (TMJ) replacement is defined as construction or reconstruction of the mandibular ramus-condyle unit (RCU), glenoid fossa, and TMJ meniscus with the patient's tissue. The TMJ may be constructed to correct congenital deformities, such as hemifacial microsomia, or reconstructed to repair acquired defects, such as TMJ ankylosis, rheumatoid or degenerative arthritis, and failed alloplastic implants.

The goals of total TMJ replacement include restoration of mandibular ramus length and morphology, normal range of motion, and jaw relations and occlusion. In pediatric patients, the constructed or reconstructed RCU must also grow at a rate similar to the opposite side and in concert with the entire maxillofacial skeleton. In this chapter, we discuss the history, available donor sites, techniques, results, complications, and advantages and disadvantages of autogenous total TMJ construction or reconstruction.

History and Background

The use of autogenous tissues has been the traditional standard of care for construction and reconstruction of the TMJ. Early empirical success with autologous human joint transplants was reported by Lexer in 1909.[1] Bardenheuer replaced the mandibular condyle with a patient's fourth metatarsal in 1909, and in 1920, Gillies first described the use of the costochondral graft (CCG) to reconstruct the human RCU.[2]

Early investigations documented the biologic basis for autogenous bone and cartilage transplantation. Laskin and Sarnat studied the metabolism of autogenous cartilage transplants in rabbits.[3] They demonstrated that chondrocyte metabolism decreased by 50% during the first week after transplantation. However, chondrocytes within the cartilage transplants remained viable and showed little tendency to resorb. Peer transplanted autogenous human rib cartilage into the abdominal wall in children and observed continued cartilage growth and cell division.[4] He postulated that initial graft survival was dependent on diffusion of nutrients until graft circulation was established. Graft circulation was reestablished within approximately 3 days, primarily by anastomosis of existing vascular channels. Kluzak and Musil studied autogenous cartilage transplants using radiolabeled phosphate compounds.[5] They found that autogenous cartilage transplants survive and that their metabolism rapidly integrates with that of the adjacent host tissue within hours of transplantation.

Donor Site Alternatives

RAMUS-CONDYLE UNIT

Costochondral Graft

Early experimental studies demonstrating cartilage viability and chondrocyte proliferation led to the thought that condylar cartilage proliferation was essential for growth of the entire mandible. Using histologic and autoradiographic techniques, Ware and Taylor demonstrated the growth potential of mandibular condylar cartilage after replanting excised condyles in rhesus monkeys.[6] The replanted condyles retained vitality, and the cartilage continued to proliferate 1 year after replantation. Based on the concept that condylar cartilage was the major growth center of the mandible, autogenous CCGs gained popularity for replacing the RCU in growing patients. In another animal study, Ware and Taylor demonstrated the feasibility of growth center transplantation.[7] They compared mandibular and facial growth in rhesus monkeys following unilateral condylotomy without replacement to RCU reconstruction using CCG or fourth metatarsal head (MH). The results indicated that both the CCG and MH could serve as a substitute condylar growth center, but growth was variable and unpredictable.

Poswillo hypothesized that the CCG was not an autogenous growth center but rather was adaptive to the environment and function.[8] Using a primate model, he replaced excised mandibular condyles with either sliding ramus grafts or CCGs. After 2 years, both techniques produced functional condyles. The CCGs, however, demonstrated radiologic and histologic features consistent with remodeling and adaptation; they were similar to the unoperated side. These studies demonstrated the capacity of a CCG to remodel into functional condyle-like structure. Poswillo further hypothesized that the ability of the transplant to adapt and respond to forces of the functional matrix might permit further mandibular growth and development.

In an animal study, Perrott and coworkers replaced the RCU in nongrowing monkeys with a CCG.[9] With function, the reconstructed RCU decreased in height and settled superiorly, with a progressive widening of the articulating surface. The occlusion remained stable despite this small decrease in length. Morphologically and histologically, the transplanted graft appeared to function well. New bone and cartilage progressively surrounded the transplanted cartilage, and the reconstructed RCU remodeled to a size and shape morphologically and histologically similar to the native condyle.

Metatarsal Head Graft

MH transplants have been used to reconstruct the RCU based on their morphologic similarity to the mandibular condyle. Dingman and Grabb replaced the deformed mandibular condyles of five growing children with first and second branchial arch syndrome using autogenous MH transplants.[10] They reported successful results based on physiologic hinge action of the joints and radiographic evidence of graft retention. However, the authors recorded progressive facial asymmetry during the 5-year follow-up period. The asymmetry was attributed to inadequate transplant growth. Ware and Taylor performed unilateral condylectomy in young rhesus monkeys and replaced the missing condyle with autogenous fourth MH.[7] Mandibular function was adequate, but transplant growth was variable and unpredictable.

Sternoclavicular Joint Graft

Transplantation of autogenous sternoclavicular joints (SCJs) to replace the TMJ in growing monkeys has been accomplished with satisfactory functional results.[11] Snyder and associates reported construction of the TMJ with whole SCJ transplantation in five monkeys.[11] They favored the SCJ because it is functionally and morphologically similar to the TMJ, it can function as a growth center, and donor site morbidity is acceptable. The investigators encountered problems with graft fixation and jaw immobilization, but the transplants united with the native mandible; the animals achieved good range of motion and a stable occlusion.

Similarity between the SCJ and the monkey TMJ at all stages of postnatal development has been demonstrated histologically.

After replacement of the mandibular condyle with the autogenous sternal head of the clavicle, the similarity persists.[12–13] High success rates have been reported with the use of autogenous SCJ grafts for TMJ reconstruction in patients with failed alloplasts and inflammatory and noninflammatory TMJ pathology. Wolford and colleagues reported the results in 38 patients who received sagittally split SCJ transplants to reconstruct the RCU.[14] The noninflammatory, nonalloplast patients had the best results, with a 90% overall success rate. Donor site morbidity included five clavicle fractures in four patients with no pneumothorax or branchial plexus injuries.

Calvarial Bone Graft

The skull may prove to be a promising donor site for reconstructing the RCU.[15–16] Calvarial bone is commonly used for reconstruction of the facial skeleton in the form of onlay or interpositional grafts.[17–21] An important advantage of calvarial bone grafts is minimal donor site morbidity.[17, 19–23] The calvarial donor site is often in the same operative field as the recipient site, and the graft can be harvested with a straight or convex contour.[17, 20, 21, 24, 25] The grafts consolidate and mature in a time frame comparable to rib or ileum.[19] When used as an onlay or interpositional graft, cranial bone exhibits an increased volume of graft survival when compared with ileum or rib.[19–23, 25, 26] In addition, cranial bone is more structurally rigid than other autogenous grafts and may allow earlier function with a decreased risk of failure.

Based on these material advantages, Bays and coworkers hypothesized that cranial bone grafts may provide a more predictable result than other autogenous or alloplastic materials when used to reconstruct the RCU.[15] To test this hypothesis, an animal study was conducted in a nonhuman primate model.[16] When compared with CCG in a similar model, the calvarial bone graft was more resistant to loss of vertical height.[9]

AUTOGENOUS DISK REPLACEMENT (GLENOID FOSSA LINING)

In the normal TMJ, a dense collagenous disk separates the joint space into upper and lower compartments, allowing rotation to occur in the lower compartment and translation in the upper.[27] An interpositional TMJ lining structure may also absorb shock and distribute force during function, improve the fit between bony surfaces, facilitate multidirectional jaw motion, and spread lubricating synovial fluid over the articular surfaces.[28, 29] Although there is controversy regarding the need to replace the disk after meniscectomy, disk preservation or autogenous disk replacement is often advocated during TMJ construction or reconstruction.

Dermis Graft

Autogenous dermis has been used both for the repair of disk perforation and as an interpositional soft tissue material in TMJ reconstruction.[30, 31] Animal studies suggest that dermis may be effective for disk replacement. Collagen and elastic fibers were preserved, but skin appendages atrophied in the transplanted dermis.[32] The ability of a dermal graft to survive and function as a disk replacement may be related to mesodermal metaplasia within the graft.[33] This hypothesis is supported by the similar collagen and elastic tissue content noted in both the recipient site tissues and the grafted autogenous dermis 5 years after subcutaneous transplantation.[34] When used to line the glenoid fossa, dermal graft survival has been documented up to 7 years postoperatively.[35] A reported complication of dermal grafting is the development of cysts due to inadvertent inclusion of surface epithelium or the cystic potential of the hair follicles and secretory glands present in properly harvested dermis.[36]

Auricular Cartilage Graft

Autogenous auricular cartilage has been used as glenoid fossa lining materials after diskectomy and for total TMJ reconstruction.[37] Cartilage grafts survive by virtue of their low metabolic rate and decreased vascular demands compared with other tissues.[3, 38] Furthermore, the presence of attached perichondrium is not necessary for the survival of an autogenous cartilage graft.[39] Auricular cartilage offers the advantage of regional proximity to the TMJ, but when reconstructing deformities such as hemifacial microsomia, loss of auricular structures in many cases may prohibit the use of ipsilateral ear cartilage.

TMJ disk replacement by auricular cartilage in primates results in fewer degenerative changes in the osseous TMJ components of the grafted versus the nongrafted side.[40] A transient decrease in protein synthetic capacity has been noted in autogenous auricular cartilage grafts in a guinea pig model.[37]

Clinical studies have confirmed the experimental work showing that auricular cartilage grafts retain their viability years after implantation.[41] Reports on the use of autogenous auricular cartilage for human TMJ disk replacement indicate favorable results.[42, 43] Auricular cartilage is an autogenous material that remains viable and biologically inert; the donor site is close to the surgical site, and the harvest results in little morbidity or deformity; the graft is easily shaped to fit the anatomy of the glenoid fossa; the graft resists pressure; and its smooth surface allows unimpeded mandibular function. However, other studies describe a predilection for adhesion between the cartilage graft and the mandibular condyle, leading to pain and hypomobility.[44] The experience of some investigators reveals that previous TMJ procedures may decrease the probability of success with the use of autogenous auricular cartilage grafts to line the glenoid fossa.[45]

Temporalis Myofascial Flap

Temporalis muscle and fascia, as an axial pedicled flap, has been used to provide soft tissue lining for TMJ reconstruction.[46] In addition, the flap has been used as an interpositional tissue for the gap arthroplasty procedure for ankylosis.[47, 48] The temporalis flap is commonly based inferiorly on the deep temporal artery and rotated over the zygomatic arch into the joint, with the muscle facing the condylar surface. Other investigators describe an anteriorly and inferiorly based temporalis myofascial flap rotated beneath the zygomatic arch and also positioned so that the fascia lines the glenoid fossa and the muscle faces the condyle.[49] Still others recommend that the flap

be posteriorly based and passed under the arch.[50]

The blood supply to the temporalis muscle is derived mainly from the anterior and posterior deep temporal arteries, terminal branches of the maxillary artery.[51] The vessels enter from the deep surface of the temporalis muscle in its inferior third. There is an additional blood supply derived from the middle temporal artery, a branch of the superficial temporal artery. This vessel runs lateral to the surface of the muscle to supply the temporal fascia, and a few branches enter the temporalis muscle. The middle temporal branch is not essential for vascularity of the temporalis muscle and is normally lost during harvesting of the flap.[52] Because the vessels usually enter the muscle inferiorly and run longitudinally, safe longitudinal sectioning can be performed toward the superior aspect of the muscle. The intramuscular vessel network is concentrated on the lateral and medial side of the muscle, with significantly lower vascular density in the middle.[53] This vascular pattern provides support for splitting the muscle in the sagittal plane to obtain a thinner flap if desired.[54] Barium angiogram studies of temporalis muscle flaps in primates showed patency of the deep temporal arteries after rotation and surgical repositioning into the oral cavity. These findings were confirmed by histology demonstrating viability in the flap tissue.[51]

The temporalis muscle is innervated by the anterior and posterior deep temporal and middle temporal nerves. These are branches of the anterior portion of the mandibular division of the trigeminal nerve. Like the vascular supply, the nerves enter the muscle and fascia from an inferior, medial, and posterior direction. These anatomic relationships support the use of inferior and posterior based flaps.[55]

GLENOID FOSSA

The articulating surfaces of the glenoid fossa and articular eminence are formed by the squamous portion of the temporal bone. The posterior nonarticulating portion of the glenoid fossa is the tympanic portion of the temporal bone. The glenoid fossa is composed of a thin layer of cortical bone separating the TMJ from the middle cranial fossa. The normal glenoid fossa is smooth and concave, wider mediolaterally than anteroposteriorly. The articular eminence is composed of cancellous bone with a thin cortical bone surface that is convex anteroposteriorly and concave mediolaterally. The articulating surfaces of the glenoid fossa, including the articular eminence and the anterior fossa, are lined by fibrocartilage. The nonarticular surfaces of the fossa are covered by fibrous connective tissue identical to periosteum.[56] Construction of a glenoid fossa may be necessary to correct conditions that result in an abnormally positioned, malformed, or absent fossa.

Technique

RCU RECONSTRUCTION

Rib

The patient is placed in a supine position, and the ipsilateral chest is elevated with a blanket roll. The incision is in the inframammary crease. In children, the incision is placed approximately 2.5 cm from the nipple-areola complex to avoid nipple retraction. The dissection proceeds through skin and subcutaneous tissue until the lower fibers of the pectoralis major muscle are encountered as they originate from the sixth rib. The white vertical fibers of the rectus fascia will also be noted as they insert on the same rib. The periosteum is incised along the convex anterior surface of the rib cortex. The rib is exposed using an Alexander elevator to reflect the periosteum. Careful dissection is the key to harvesting a rib without a pleural tear and resultant pneumothorax. As the dissection progresses posteriorly from the costochondral junction, muscle fibers from the serratus anterior are transected; the limitation of rib length is the lateral border of the latissimus dorsi muscle. When the superior and inferior surfaces of the rib are reached, an Overholt elevator is used to dissect over the edges to the pleural side posteriorly. Next, a Doyen elevator is used to strip the remaining periosteum from the pleural cortex on the deep surface of the rib. When a costochondral junction is required, a sleeve of perichondrium is left intact across the

junction on the superficial surface of the graft to prevent separation of junctional cartilage.

After an appropriate length of rib and costochondral junction is exposed, the rib is harvested by transecting the cartilage at the costochondral junction with a straight rib cutter or a No. 15 scalpel blade. Once the anterior end of the rib is separated from the sternum, the rib is elevated and the pleural surface is protected. An angled rib cutter is used to make the posterior osteotomy, and the donor end is smoothed with a bone file. If a second rib is needed, one may harvest the adjacent rib. Alternatively, one may preserve the adjacent rib and harvest the next rib (i.e., the fifth or seventh rib). CCGs may be harvested from either side of the chest and used to reconstruct either the right or left RCU. The chest wound is irrigated, and positive pressure ventilation is performed by the anesthesiologist while the surgeon examines the field for an air leak indicative of pleural tear. The wound is closed in layers.

If a pleural tear is detected during the rib harvest, a small red rubber catheter is placed in the pleural cavity through the opening. A pursestring suture is placed around the tube. While the anesthesiologist administers positive pressure ventilation, the tube is placed on suction and withdrawn while tying the suture. If this is not successful in reinflating the lung, a chest tube is placed.

A chest radiograph is obtained postoperatively. If a pneumothorax greater than 10% is detected, a chest tube is inserted and suction is placed. The tube is removed when no leak is observed for 24 to 48 hours after suction has been discontinued.

After harvesting the rib, attention is redirected to the preauricular region to complete the reconstruction of the condyle. The cartilage component of the CCG is contoured to be 2 to 4 mm thick and round (Fig. 16–1). The superior (cartilaginous) surface of the graft is placed against the joint lining, and the graft is rigidly secured to the mandible with two or three 2- or 2.7-mm pretapped bone screws. Alternatively, the graft may be stabilized by using 2-mm screws and a plate that serves as a washer. Maxillomandibular fixation (MMF) is maintained for 3 to 10 days, depending on the thickness and rigidity of the CCG.

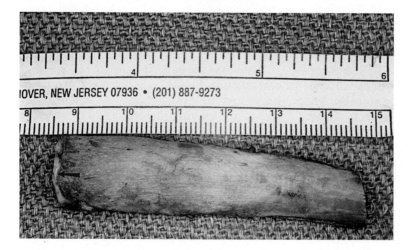

FIGURE 16–1. Harvested costochondral graft prepared for reconstruction of the mandibular condyle. Note the residual 2- to 3-mm cartilaginous cap (*arrow*) after trimming off the excess cartilage.

Metatarsal Head

The short length of available metatarsal donor tissue restricts its use to pediatric patients requiring condylar replacement. The distal second, third, or fourth metatarsal bones are most suitable for reconstruction of the mandibular condyle. The metatarsal bones are excised distal to the cuboid-metatarsal joint through a dorsal approach. Case reports describe wire osteosynthesis of the graft to the condylar neck and several weeks of jaw immobilization for graft consolidation.[10] Currently, the graft may be stabilized using a rigid technique.

Sternoclavicular Joint

The SCJ is approached through a longitudinal incision approximately 1 cm above and parallel to the clavicle. The incision is extended from the manubrium approximately 6 to 8 cm laterally to allow harvest of the medial one third of the clavicle. The dissection is carried inferiorly toward the clavicle in a subcutaneous plane. The muscle attachments on the medial one third of the clavicle are released, exposing the joint capsule. The articular disk and approximately 1 cm of ligamentous attachments of the SCJ capsule are preserved at the head of the clavicle. Once the clavicle is exposed and the sternoclavicular junction is preserved, an osteotomy is designed to include the superior portion of the clavicle and a portion of the articular disk. The superior half of the clavicular head is easily adapted to fit the glenoid fossa, and maintaining the integrity of the lower half of the clavicle ensures arm and shoulder support. A reciprocating saw is used to complete the osteotomy through the anterior and posterior cortical plates of the clavicle. A broad malleable retractor is used to protect the soft tissues adjacent to the posterior cortical plate. A gradual upward curve is created with the reciprocating saw as the osteotomy is completed. The osteotomy is extended medially through the head of the condyle near

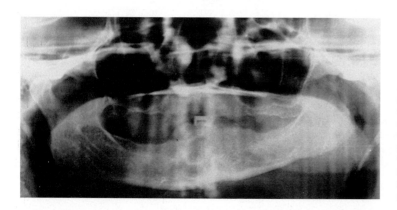

FIGURE 16–2. Preoperative panoramic radiograph of a 42-year-old white woman illustrating loss of left mandibular posterior ramus height following failure of a costochondral graft due to unanticipated resorption of the graft. We elected to reconstruct the mandibular condyle and restore posterior ramus height using an autogenous cranial bone graft.

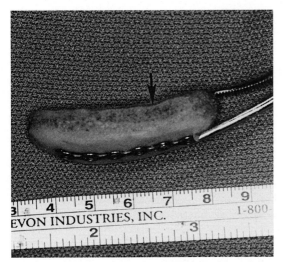

FIGURE 16–3. This photograph illustrates a typical cranial bone graft prepared for mandibular condyle reconstruction. It may be necessary to reduce graft width by removing or recontouring the inner cortical table of the cranial bone graft where it contacts the native mandible (*arrow*). The bone plate was stabilized to the lateral aspect (outer table) of the graft with two monocortical bone screws (2 mm).

its midpoint, with care taken to preserve the articular disk. The articular disk is sectioned with a scalpel to preserve the portion overlying the harvested clavicular head. The donor site is irrigated and closed in layers to maintain a periosteal sleeve to facilitate bone regeneration.

Calvaria

The parietal bone is approached using a hemicoronal flap for unilateral reconstruction or a complete coronal flap for bilateral TMJ reconstruction. A template is prepared preoperatively from developed radiographic film to estimate the appropriate size of the graft. A full-thickness cranial bone graft is harvested with the assistance of a neurosurgeon. The template is positioned over the donor site so that most of the graft is harvested from the flattest part of the parietal bone, except for the most superior portion, which includes the more curved aspect of the bone. The curved aspect of the graft is directed into the glenoid fossa above the ramus and remains a bicortical graft. The inferior aspect of the graft is thinned and shaped to facilitate its adaptation to the lateral surface of the ramus. If necessary, flair of bone at the gonial angle is reduced to improve contact between the graft and the ramus. For bilateral reconstructions, a larger graft is harvested and divided longitudinally. The donor site defect can be repaired with methyl methacrylate. Bone substitutes can also be considered to repair the donor site defect. Alternatively, a second full-thickness graft may be harvested and then split to repair both donor site defects. A TMJ arthroplasty is performed in the standard fashion to correct the underlying deformity. The graft is inserted and positioned using both the preauricular incision and a small retromandibular incision to allow access for positioning and stabilizing the inferior aspect of the graft. The graft is fixed to the native mandible using bone screws and a plate, which functions as a washer (Figs. 16–2 to 16–4).

GLENOID FOSSA LINING

Dermis

The most common donor sites for harvesting dermal grafts are the ipsilateral buttock, upper lateral thigh, and groin. A split-thickness skin flap is elevated with a

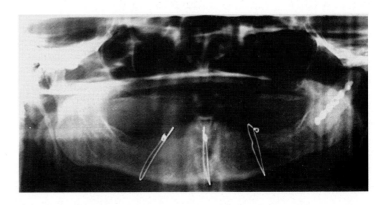

FIGURE 16–4. Postoperative panoramic radiograph documenting graft position and restoration of posterior ramus height.

dermatome set at 0.015 to 0.020 inches. The skin is left attached at its distal end and turned away from the donor bed. The underlying dermis is then removed with a second pass of the dermatome set at 0.020 inches or with a free-hand technique using a scalpel and scissors. The graft is at least twice the diameter of the recipient site to compensate for contraction of the elastic fibers in the dermis after it is excised. After obtaining adequate hemostasis, the superficial skin flap is fenestrated to allow the escape of fluid and sutured to cover the underlying harvest site. The wound is covered with a semipermeable membrane and a pressure dressing for 7 days to ensure revascularization of the skin. The skin sutures are removed in 7 days, and the patient is instructed to protect the donor site from sunlight for 6 months to prevent hyperpigmentation. The dermal graft is defatted and trimmed to fit the size and shape of the recipient area. The dermis at the upper and outer quadrant of the buttock is approximately 0.8 to 1.2 mm thick and, when folded on itself, is usually of sufficient bulk to line the glenoid fossa. The dermal graft is sutured anteriorly to the lateral pterygoid muscle, and posteriorly and medially to tissue remnants. Additional stabilization through fascia over the lateral rim of the glenoid fossa may be placed during closure.

Auricular Cartilage

The technique most commonly used for harvesting auricular cartilage grafts involves a linear incision on the posterior aspect of the helix of the ear. The postauricular skin over the concha auriculae is elevated in the supraperichondrial plane. The perichondrium and cartilage are lightly scored with a scalpel to outline the graft, with the most distal cut just proximal to the antihelix. A small elevator is used to dissect the anterior perichondrial layer from the cartilage, and the graft is delivered. Perichondrium is left attached to the convex surface to maintain graft integrity and maximize graft revascularization and cell viability. The convex surface, which is covered by perichondrium, is placed against the glenoid fossa along the anterior slope of the articular eminence. The concave portion of the graft is against the mandibular condyle;

this surface is free of the perichondrial cover to decrease the likelihood of developing fibrous connective tissue adhesions. The lateral aspect of the graft is sutured to the joint capsule or to the edge of the temporal fascia overlying the zygomatic arch. A small drain is placed in the ear wound, and the skin incision is closed in the standard fashion. A light pressure dressing is placed at the auricular donor site for 24 hours to prevent hematoma formation. Cotton rolls wrapped in petrolatum gauze are secured to the anterior and posterior concha with a horizontal mattress suture.

Temporalis Myofascial Flap

The TMJ procedure is completed in the usual manner selected by the surgeon, and attention is redirected to the temporal region. The flap is outlined on the fascia with a skin marker or methylene blue. It extends as far superiorly as necessary to give proper length for lining the joint, remembering that it contracts as it is raised (Fig. 16–5). The dissection is carried to the proper depth, including fascia only or muscle and fascia. When required, only the superficial portion of the muscle is harvested. This provides adequate thickness for a joint lining and minimizes the contour defect in the temporal region. The flap is extended only to the level of the zygomatic arch. Occasionally the zygomatic arch has to be reduced in thickness to permit rotation of the flap without producing excessive contour. The flap is secured with six sutures (5-0 resorbable suture such as polyglycolic acid)—two in the medial capsule region, two in the anterior attachment, and two in the posterior attachment. Hemostasis is achieved in the donor area with electrocautery. A suction drain is used for 24 to 48 hours.

For disk replacement, the medial attachment of the disk should be retained whenever possible so that the temporalis flap can be sutured medially. When the medial attachment cannot be retained, the flap is secured only to the anterior and posterior attachments. The capsule is then repaired and sutured to the lateral aspect of the flap.

GLENOID FOSSA CONSTRUCTION

Selection of the site for glenoid fossa construction may be difficult in the absence

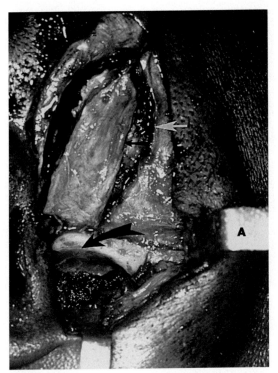

FIGURE 16–5. Intraoperative photograph of a right temporalis fascia flap demonstrating contraction of the flap after it has been raised. The anterior aspect of the patient is noted by *A*, the white arrow points to the original incision, the small black arrow points to the edge of the flap, and the curved black arrow points to the empty glenoid fossa following resection of ankylotic bone.

of normal anatomic landmarks. The glenoid fossa should be constructed in the best possible three-dimensional location relative to the contralateral joint. A preoperative guide to the proper position of the fossa is obtained on an anteroposterior cephalogram by drawing a vertical line from the crista galli through the nasal septum. A horizontal line is drawn perpendicularly at the level of the normal glenoid fossa. The site for the new TMJ can be selected by measurements on the radiographs.[57]

Glenoid fossa and zygomatic construction is accomplished through a coronal incision. A zygomatic arch is constructed with full-thickness calvarial bone. A cortical graft of autogenous ileum, rib, or calvaria is anchored medial to the constructed zygoma to create a concave surface into which the mandibular condyle can fit.[58] The constructed glenoid fossa is lined with a suitable joint lining material such as dermis, cartilage, or temporalis fascia.

Correction of Mandibular Hypomobility

Successful treatment of mandibular hypomobility requires a thorough understanding of the underlying disorder. Ankylosis of the TMJ may be classified according to location (intraarticular or extraarticular), type of tissue involved (bony, fibrous, or fibroosseous), or extent of fusion (complete, incomplete).[49] Unlike true ankylosis, pseudoankylosis may involve extraarticular structures, muscle hyperactivity or spasm, coronoid hyperplasia, or a depressed zygomatic arch fracture.

Ankylosis is most commonly associated with trauma (31% to 98% of cases), local or systemic infection (10% to 49%), systemic disease (10%), or neoplasm. In the case of trauma, it is hypothesized that intraarticular hematoma, with scarring and excessive bone formation, leads to hypomobility. Infection of the TMJ is most commonly the result of contiguous spread from otitis media or mastoiditis but may also result from hematogenous spread, including tuberculosis, gonorrhea, and scarlet fever. Systemic causes of TMJ ankylosis include ankylosing spondylitis, rheumatoid arthritis, and psoriasis.

Restoration of normal motion and function in patients with TMJ ankylosis has been difficult. Many operative techniques have been described in the literature, but results have been variable and often less than satisfactory. A common mistake made by inexperienced surgeons is to focus on the reconstruction and inadequately treat the primary disease. For example, CCGS or total joint prostheses are not the treatment but rather potential reconstructive methods for patients with TMJ ankylosis. A seven-step protocol has been developed for the treatment of TMJ ankylosis, achieving an average long-term postoperative maximal incisal opening (MIO) of 32.6 ± 8.3 mm (range 25 to 51 mm).[59]

Step one in this approach consists of aggressive resection of the bony or fibrous ankylotic segment (Figs. 16–6 to 16–11). Recurrent ankylosis is most commonly caused by incomplete removal of the bony or fibrous mass, especially from the medial aspect of the joint. A preoperative computed tomogra-

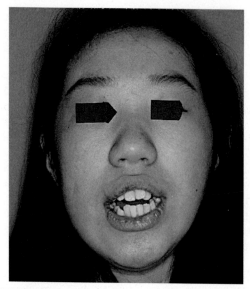

FIGURE 16–6. This photograph demonstrates the patient's preoperative maximal incisal opening (MIO) with recurrent bilateral temporomandibular joint ankylosis. The patient had an anterior open bite, and her preoperative MIO was 0 mm.

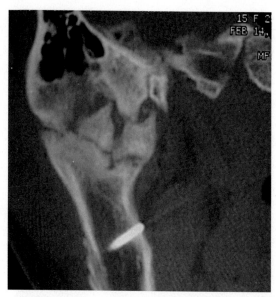

FIGURE 16–8. Preoperative coronal computed tomography scan of the right temporomandibular joint illustrating the ankylotic mass.

phy scan is helpful to delineate the boundaries of the ankylotic segment. In some cases of TMJ ankylosis following a condylar fracture, the proximal stump is identified medial and anterior to the joint and is fused to the posterior maxilla.

Step two consists of dissection and stripping of the temporalis, masseter, and medial pterygoid muscles; scar release from the ramus; and ipsilateral coronoidectomy. Longstanding ankylosis may result in temporalis muscle atrophy and fibrosis. Ipsilateral cor-

onoidectomy has been recommended to facilitate intraoperative interincisal opening.[60, 61]

Following step two, the MIO is evaluated. It should be at least 35 mm without force, and in unilateral cases, the opening should be accompanied by translation of the opposite normal condyle. If this is not achieved, the third step consists of contralateral coronoidectomy and stripping of the masseter, medial pterygoid, and temporalis muscles. Exploration of the contralateral TMJ may

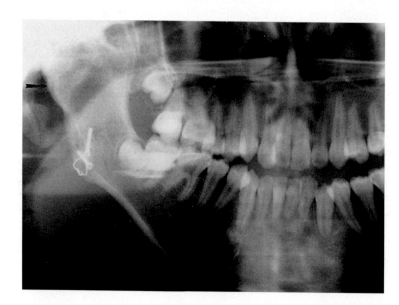

FIGURE 16–7. Preoperative panoramic radiograph demonstrating ankylosis of the right temporomandibular joint (*arrow*). The hardware visible in this radiograph stabilized a costochondral graft used to reconstruct the mandibular condyle in a previous attempt to treat the ankylosis.

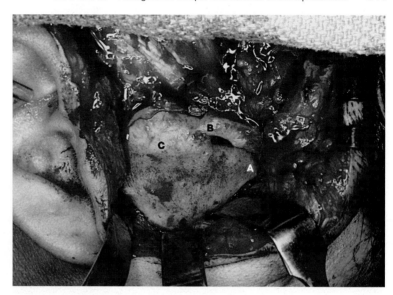

FIGURE 16–9. Intraoperative view of the right temporomandibular joint demonstrating the ankylotic mass ('C') and fusion of the previously reconstructed condyle to the zygomatic arch ('B'). 'A,' anterior aspect of the patient.

be required when preoperative evaluation reveals decreased joint space or condylar irregularity on the contralateral side.

In step four, a new joint lining is constructed. Failure to replace the disk allows direct contact between the reconstructed condyle and the bony glenoid fossa, increasing the risk of recurrent ankylosis. If an intact disk is identified during the proce-

dure, it is maintained to line the glenoid fossa.

Steps five and six consist of reconstruction of the condyle with a CCG and rigid fixation of the graft (Figs. 16–11 and 16–12). The seventh step is early mobilization and

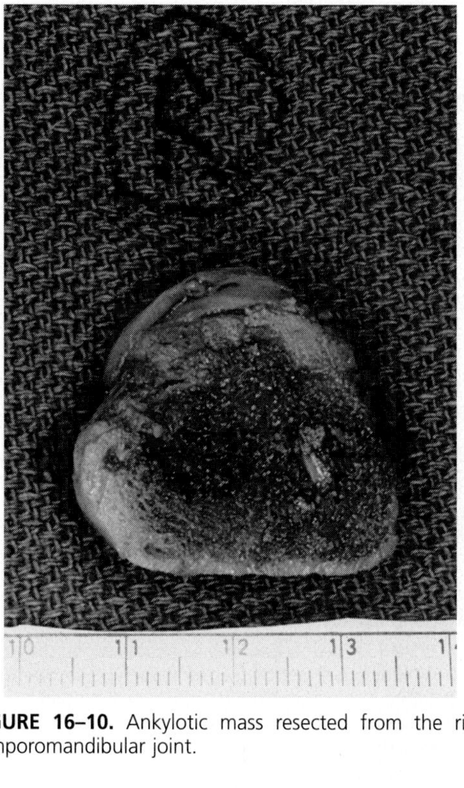

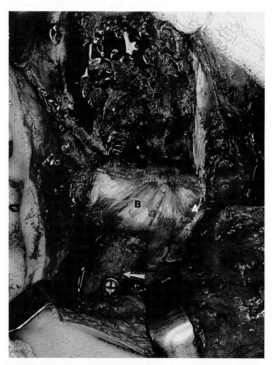

FIGURE 16–11. This photograph illustrates the reconstructed ramus-condyle unit. The glenoid fossa of the right temporomandibular joint was lined with a temporalis fascia flap rotated over the zygomatic arch ('B'), and the mandibular condyle was reconstructed with a costochondral graft (*white arrow*). 'A,' anterior aspect of the patient.

FIGURE 16–10. Ankylotic mass resected from the right temporomandibular joint.

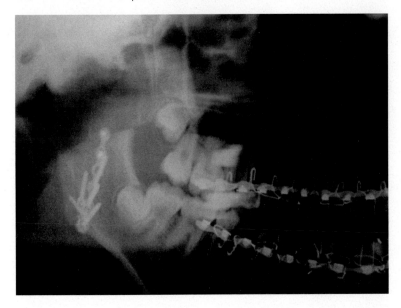

FIGURE 16–12. Postoperative panoramic radiograph illustrating the reconstructed right ramus-condyle unit.

aggressive physiotherapy. After release of MMF (usually 3 to 10 days), patients begin a soft diet and jaw-opening exercises. These exercises consist of active range of motion, lateral excursive motion, and passive range of motion by manual finger stretching in front of a mirror. During the next 3 to 4 weeks, the diet is advanced to a solid consistency. Our physical therapy program consists of heat, massage, ultrasonography, gum chewing, range-of-motion exercises, and the use of a passive jaw motion device (Therabite, Therabite Corp., Newtown Square, PA) four to five times daily for 20 minutes. Six weeks after surgery, if the patient is not able to achieve the documented intraoperative MIO or if the MIO shows no signs of improvement, the tissues are stretched under general anesthesia. Patients are followed monthly for at least 1 year (Fig. 16–13).

Using this protocol, 14 patients (18 joints) were treated.[59] For this study, we defined normal function as an MIO greater than 30 mm, the ability to make lateral excursive mandibular movements, minimal to no pain during function, and resumption of normal diet. All patients were followed postoperatively for at least 1 year. The mean preoperative MIO was 16.6 ± 9.06 mm (range 2 to 32 mm). After resection and coronoidectomy, the glenoid fossa was lined with temporalis fascia (n = 12), native disk (n = 3), or perichondrium (n = 1). The RCU was reconstructed with a CCG in 16 joints.

In one patient, two prosthetic condyles were placed.

Three months postoperatively, all facial asymmetry remained corrected. The mean MIO was 31 ± 6.13 mm (range 20 to 40 mm), with lateral excursions present in 16 of 18 joints. This represented an average MIO increase of 231.4%. Deviation to the affected side was present in 6 of 10 unilateral cases and absent in all bilateral cases.

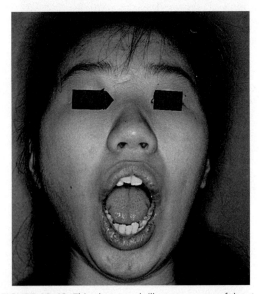

FIGURE 16–13. This photograph illustrates successful restoration of functional mandibular movement. The open bite was closed during reconstruction of the ramus-condyle unit, and the maximal incisal opening 1 year after the procedure was 39 mm.

Pain with function was present in 2 of 18 joints. One patient required manipulation under general anesthesia to increase MIO 6 weeks postoperatively.

Six months postoperatively, no facial asymmetry was noted. The mean MIO was 34.57 ± 5.23 mm (range 27 to 42 mm), with a mean increase of 254.14%. Lateral excursions remained present in 15 of 18 joints. Mandibular deviation was present in 5 of 10 unilateral joints and absent in all bilateral cases. Pain with function was still present in 2 of 18 joints.

Periodic panoramic radiographs were obtained and demonstrated progressive incorporation of the grafts into the ramus of the native mandible. With time, the grafts became increasingly calcified and more closely resembled the shape of the normal condyle.

With the use of autogenous materials and this approach to the treatment of TMJ ankylosis, the incidence of complications, including recurrent ankylosis, has been minimized, and long-term satisfactory motion has been achieved.

Long-Term Results of Autogenous TMJ Replacement

A long-term follow-up of 26 patients (33 CCGs) who underwent construction or reconstruction of the RCU has been completed.[62] Indications for construction or reconstruction included ankylosis, condylar resorption, degenerative joint disease, or congenital absence of a condyle. Growing patients and nongrowing patients were followed for an average of 48.6 months (range 24 to 72 months) and 46.4 months (range 14 to 40 months), respectively. Patients were evaluated by history, physical examination, and measurements made on serial standardized panoramic radiographs. Evaluation parameters included facial appearance, MIO, occlusion, and contour changes of the operated and unoperated RCUs.

All patients underwent the same operative procedure for reconstruction of the RCU and lining of the glenoid fossa. The TMJ was approached through a curvilinear preauricular incision that extended 3 cm into the temporal region for exposure of the temporal fascia. In patients with anklyosis, degenerative joint disease, tumor, or idio-

pathic condylar resorption, an ostectomy was done from the sigmoid notch to the posterior border of the ascending ramus. If an intact disk was identified during joint exploration, it was maintained to line the glenoid fossa (n = 10 joints). In other cases, the glenoid fossa was lined with a temporalis myofascial flap.[55] The occlusion was established by placing the patient into MMF in a prefabricated occlusal splint. A 2- to 3-mm posterior open bite was created on the operated side to compensate for remodeling of the CCG. The CCG was then inserted to reconstruct the condyle and stabilized as described earlier.

Long-term follow-up of seven growing patients (eight joints) revealed no signs of linear overgrowth of the constructed or reconstructed RCUs. Two growing patients developed lateral contour overgrowth with an abnormal increase in mass of the graft in the region of the costochondral junction. The long-term MIO was 36 mm (range 27 to 51 mm). This long-term change in the MIO was statistically significant ($P < 0.05$), as compared with preoperative measurements.

In the 19 nongrowing patients, 4 had a clinically visible mandibular asymmetry. Two asymmetries were the result of contralateral (unoperated) condylar resorption, and two were the result of remodeling (decrease in length) of the reconstructed RCU. No patients showed signs of linear overgrowth, but one patient did develop lateral contour overgrowth in the region of the costochondral junction. Of the 12 patients with preoperative pain, 6 had resolution of the pain, and 6 had improved or manageable pain. Three patients developed unstable occlusion as a result of ramus-condyle shortening (n = 2) and contralateral ramus-condyle resorption (n = 1). The mean long-term MIO was 33.9 mm (range 25 to 49 mm). This change in MIO was statistically significant ($P < 0.05$), as compared with the preoperative measurements.

By radiographic analysis, most of the constructed or reconstructed RCUs in growing patients (n = 5) decreased in length. The mean change in the operated RCU was −2.8 mm, and for the unoperated side it was +3.2 mm. Three constructed or reconstructed RCUs in two patients increased in length, equal to the growth on the unoperated side. In nongrowing patients, the mean change in the reconstructed RCU length was -5.7 mm, and on the unoperated side it was -0.1 mm. In 22 of 25 reconstructed RCUs, there was an overall decrease in the reconstructed RCU length as a result of settling and remodeling.

Summary

Experimental and clinical studies have established a foundation for the use of autogenous materials to reconstruct the TMJ. Use of autogenous tissues decreases the likelihood of foreign-body reaction; the constructed RCU can be fashioned to include a cartilaginous articulating surface; and a permanent bony union occurs at the new RCU which may undergo biologic remodeling in response to function. Finally, autogenous CCG transplants may retain their growth potential when used for constructing or reconstructing the RCU in growing patients. Further laboratory and clinical studies are necessary to optimize fully the use of autogenous materials for TMJ replacement.

REFERENCES

1. Lexer E: Ueber gelenktransplantation. Arch Klin Chir 1909;90:264.
2. Gillies HD: Plastic Surgery of the Face. London, Oxford University Press, 1920.
3. Laskin DM, Sarnat GB: Respiration and anaerobic glycolysis of transplanted cartilage. Proc Soc Exp Biol Med 1952;79:474.
4. Peer LA: Cell survival theory versus replacement theory. Plast Reconstr Surg 1955;16:161.
5. Kluzak R, Musil J: The use of labelled phosphorus in the study of the metabolism of cartilage grafts. Acta Chir Plast 1960;2:150.
6. Ware WH, Taylor RC: Replantation of growing mandibular condyles in rhesus monkeys. Oral Surg Oral Med Oral Pathol 1965;19:669.
7. Ware WH, Taylor RC: Cartilaginous growth centers transplanted to replace mandibular condyles in monkeys. J Oral Surg 1966;24:33.
8. Poswillo D: Experimental reconstruction of the mandibular joint. Int J Oral Surg 1974;3:400.
9. Perrott DH, Vargervik K, Kaban LB: Costochondral reconstruction of mandibular condyles in nongrowing primates. J Craniofac Surg 1995;6:227.
10. Dingman RO, Grabb WC: Reconstruction of both mandibular condyles with metatarsal bone grafts. Plast Reconstr Surg 1964;34:441.
11. Snyder CC, Benson AR, Slater PV: Construction of the temporomandibular joint by transplanting the autogenous sternoclavicular joint. South Med J 1971;64:807.
12. Ellis E, Carlson DS: Histologic comparison of the costochondral, sternoclavicular, and temporoman-
13. Daniels S, Ellis E, Carlson DS: Histologic analysis of the costochondral and sternoclavicular grafts in the temporomandibular joint of the juvenile monkey. J Oral Maxillofac Surg 1987;45:675.
14. Wolford LM, Cottrell DA, Henry C: Sternoclavicular grafts for temporomandibular joint reconstruction. J Oral Maxillofac Surg 1994;52:119.
15. Bays RA, Dodson TB, Pfeffle RC, et al: Cranial bone graft to reconstruct the mandibular condyle in *Macaca mulatta*. J Oral Maxillofac Surg 1995;53 (suppl 4):94.
16. Dodson TB, Bays RA, Pfeffle RC, Barrow DL: Cranial bone graft to reconstruct the mandibular condyle in *Macaca mulatta*. J Oral Maxillofac Surg 1997;55:260–267.
17. Tessier P: Autogenous bone grafts taken from the calvarium for facial and cranial applications. Clin Plast Surg 1982;9:531–538.
18. Wolfe SA, Berkowitz S: The use of cranial bone grafts in the closure of alveolar and anterior palatal clefts. Plast Reconstr Surg 1983;72:659–668.
19. Harsha BC, Turvey TA, Powers SK: Use of autogenous cranial bone grafts in maxillofacial surgery: A preliminary report. J Oral Maxillofac Surg 1986;44:11–15.
20. Jackson IT, Helden G, Marx R: Skull bone grafts in maxillofacial and craniofacial surgery. J Oral Maxillofac Surg 1986;44:949–955.
21. Maves MD, Matt BH: Calvarial bone grafting of facial defects. Otolaryngol Head Neck Surg 1986;95:464–470.
22. Jackson IT, Adham M, Bite U, Marx R: Update on cranial bone grafts in craniofacial surgery. Ann Plast Surg 1987;18:37–40.
23. Petroff MA, Burgess LPA, Anonsen CK, et al: Cranial bone grafts for post-traumatic facial defects. Laryngoscope 1987;97:1249–1253.
24. Powell NB, Riley RW: Cranial bone grafting in facial aesthetic and reconstructive contouring. Arch Otolaryngol Head Neck Surg 1987;113:713–719.
25. Markowitz RN: Cranial bone grafting in oral and maxillofacial surgery. J Am Dent Assoc 1992;123:207–211.
26. Zins JE, Whitaker LA: Membranous versus endochondral bone: Implications for craniofacial reconstruction. Plast Reconstr Surg 1983;72:778.
27. Rees LA: The structure and function of the mandibular joint. Br Dent J 1954;96:125.
28. Williams PL, Warwick R: Gray's Anatomy. Edinburgh, Churchill Livingstone, 1980.
29. Osborn JW: The disc of the human temporomandibular joint: Design, function, and failure. J Oral Rehabil 1985;12:279.
30. Zetz MR, Irby WB: Repair of the adult temporomandibular joint meniscus with autogenous dermal graft. J Oral Maxillofac Surg 1984;42:167.
31. MacIntosh RB: Costochondral and dermal grafts in temporomandibular joint reconstruction. Oral Maxillofac Clin North Am 1989;1:363.
32. Georgiade N, Altany F, Pickrell K: An experimental and clinical evaluation of autogenous dermal grafts used in treatment of temporomandibular joint ankylosis. Plast Reconstr Surg 1957;19:321.
33. Georgiade N: The surgical correction of temporomandibular joint dysfunction by means of autogenous dermal grafts. Plast Reconstr Surg 1962;30:68.
34. Thompson N: The subcutaneous dermis graft. Plast Reconstr Surg 1960;26:1.

35. MacIntosh RB: Costochondral and dermal grafts in temporomandibular joint reconstruction. Oral Maxillofac Clin North Am 1993;5:579.

36. Bonnington G, Langan M, Joy ED: Epithelial inclusion cyst in the temporomandibular joint after a dermal graft. J Oral Maxillofac Surg 1987; 45:705–707.

37. Ioannides C, Maltha JC: Replacement of the interarticular disc of the craniomandibular joint with fresh autogenous sternal or articular cartilage. J Craniomaxillofac Surg 1988;16:343.

38. Davidson M: A study of the fate of autogenous cartilage grafts. Laryngoscope 1959;69:1259.

39. Dupertuis SM: Growth of young human autogenous auricular cartilage grafts. Plast Reconstr Surg 1950;5:486.

40. Tucker MR, Kennady MC, Jacoway JR: Autogenous auricular cartilage implantation following discectomy in the temporomandibular joint. J Oral Maxillofac Surg 1990;48:38.

41. Yih WY, Zysset M, Merrill R: Histologic study of the fate of autogenous auricular cartilage grafts in the human temporomandibular joint. J Oral Maxillofac Surg 1992;50:964.

42. Witsenburg B, Freihofer HPM: Replacement of the pathological temporomandibular joint discs using autogenous cartilage of the external ear. Int J Oral Surg 1984;13:401.

43. Ioannides C, Freihofer HPM: Replacement of the damaged interarticular disc of the temporomandibular joint. J Craniomaxillofac Surg 1988;16:273.

44. Hall HD, Link JJ: Discectomy alone and with ear cartilage interposition grafts in joint reconstruction. Oral Maxillofac Clin North Am 1989;1:329.

45. Freihoffer HPM: Discussion of auricular cartilage grafting after discectomy of the temporomandibular joint. J Oral Maxillofac Surg 1993;51:260.

46. Verneuil AAS: De la creation d'une fausse articulation par section on resection partielle de l'os maxillaire inferieur. Arch Gen Med V Serie 1872;15:284.

47. Murphy JB: Ankylosis of the temporomandibular joints. Surg Clin 1912;1:905.

48. Murphy JB: Bony ankylosis of the jaw with interposition of flaps from the temporal fascia. Surg Clin 1913;2:659.

49. Rowe NL: Ankylosis of the temporomandibular joint, part 3. J R Coll Surg Edinb 1982;27:209.

50. Toller PA: Temporomandibular capsular rearrangement. Br J Oral Surg 1974;11:207.

51. Bradley P, Brockbank J: The temporalis muscle flap in oral reconstruction—a cadaveric, animal and clinical study. J Maxillofac Surg 1981;9:139.

52. Abdul-Hassan Ascher GVD, Acland RD: Surgical anatomy and blood supply of the fascial layers of the temporal region. Plast Reconstr Surg 1986;77:17.

53. Habel G, Hensher R: The versatility of the temporalis muscle flap in reconstructive surgery. Br J Oral Maxillofac Surg 1986;24:96.

54. Cheung LK: The vascular anatomy of the human temporalis muscle: Implications for surgical splitting techniques. Int J Oral Maxillofac Surg 1996;25:414.

55. Pogrel MA, Kaban LB: The role of the temporalis fascia and muscle flap in temporomandibular joint surgery. J Oral Maxillofac Surg 1990;48:14.

56. Boering G: Anatomical and physiological considerations regarding the temporomandibular joint. Int Dent J 1979;29:245.

57. Kaban LB, Mulliken JB, Murray JB: Three-dimensional approach to analysis and treatment of hemifacial microsomia. Cleft Palate J 1981;18:90.

58. Mulliken JB, Kaban LB: Analysis and treatment of hemifacial microsomia in childhood. Clin Plast Surg 1987;14:91.

59. Kaban LB, Perrott DH, Fisher K: A protocol for management of temporomandibular joint ankylosis. J Oral Maxillofac Surg 1990;48:1145.

60. Guralnick WC, Kaban LB: Surgical treatment of mandibular hypomobility. J Oral Surg 1976; 34:343.

61. Kent JN, Misiek DJ, Shen RK, et al: Temporomandibular joint condylar prosthesis: A ten-year report. J Oral Maxillofac Surg 1983;41:245.

62. Perrott DH, Umeda H, Kaban LB: Costochondral graft construction/reconstruction of the ramus/condyle unit: Long-term follow-up. Int J Oral Maxillofac Surg 1994;23:321.

CHAPTER

17

Alloplastic Reconstruction of the Temporomandibular Joint

Peter D. Quinn

Reconstruction of the temporomandibular joint (TMJ) with alloplastic materials can be a difficult challenge for oral and maxillofacial surgeons.[1–3] Clearly, a predictably successful autogenous joint replacement would be the procedure of choice, because it would obviate the need for inevitable revision surgeries with prosthetic implants. The history of alloplastic reconstruction procedures has, unfortunately, been characterized by multiple failures based on inappropriate design, lack of attention to biomechanical principles, and ignorance of what had already been documented in the orthopedic literature. In addition, because the TMJ is the only ginglymoarthrodial joint in the body and its function is intimately related to occlusal harmony, a prosthetic TMJ implant necessitates characteristics not considered in orthopedic implants. The premise of this chapter is that all nonsurgical, conservative treatment has been exhausted, and all conservative surgical methodologies have been used in a patient before alloplastic joint replacement is considered. Currently accepted indications for joint reconstruction are as follows:

- Ankylosed, degenerated, or resorbed joints with severe anatomic discrepancies
- Failed autogenous bone grafts resulting in a scarred, poorly vascularized tissue bed
- Destruction of an autogenous bone graft by preexisting foreign body reactions (e.g., Proplast–Teflon giant-cell reactions)
- Severe polyarticular inflammatory joint disease affecting the TMJs
- Recurrent ankylosis with a history of excessive heterotopic bone formation

Other indications for joint replacement may include irreparable condylar fractures, avascular necrosis, neoplasia requiring extensive joint resection, and congenital disorders such as hemifacial microsomia. Clearly, autogenous grafting (e.g., costochondral grafts) should be considered the procedure of choice in most patients with these disorders.[4–11]

The chief disadvantages associated with autogenous grafts are donor site morbidity and the variability of the biologic behavior of the graft (i.e., resorption, ankylosis, or excessive growth). Theoretically, a prosthetic joint prosthesis would afford:

- Lack of donor site morbidity
- Reduced surgical time
- Potential for decreased hospitalization
- Immediate function and no need for prolonged intermaxillary fixation
- Ability to maintain stable occlusion postsurgically because of lack of dimensional change in implant, as opposed to potential resorption of autogenous graft
- Opportunity to manipulate prosthesis design to discourage heterotopic bone formation

The major disadvantages of joint prostheses are the potential for wear debris with associated pathologic responses, the unpredictable need for revision surgery, the fit limitations of a stock prosthesis, and the cost of the prosthesis itself. It is an unfortunate fact that a percentage of patients requiring total joint alloplastic reconstruction could be classified as iatrogenic cases because multiple, inappropriate surgeries were performed or alloplastic materials were used that caused extensive, destructive foreign body reactions. This fact does not obviate the need for a safe and effective prosthesis in those patients with acquired or congenital disorders necessitating joint reconstruction.

History of TMJ Alloplastic Reconstruction

John Nobel once said, "The purpose of medicine is to prevent significant disease, to decrease pain, and to postpone death when it is meaningful to do so. Technology has to support these goals, if not, it may even be counterproductive." Our past failures with alloplastic material should not lead to an abandonment of research in this area but should guide us to exercise caution when introducing new alloplastic materials. We are still bound by the principle of "Primum non nocere" (First do no harm).

According to Mercuri,[1] New York surgeon John Murray Carnochan documented the first instance of interposing a prosthetic material between surfaces of a joint.[12] In 1840, he treated an ankylosed TMJ by placing a small block of wood between the base of the skull and the osteotomized condyle.

In more recent history, interpositional joint materials were described in 1933, when Risdon[13] used gold foil as an interpositional material after gap arthroplasty. Eggers[14] in 1946 and Goodsell[15] in 1947 reported using tantalum foil for the same purpose.

These early attempts at a form of hemiarthroplasty also included fossa prostheses such as those designed by Robinson (1960),[16] Christensen (1963 and 1971),[17, 18] and Morgan (1971).[19] These metallic "fossa liners" were usually secured to the zygomatic arch.

In an excellent review article, van Loon and colleagues[3] summarized the alloplastic implant design, methods of fixation, and literature review up to 1995. The authors separated fossa prostheses, condylar prostheses (Fig. 17–1), and total joint prostheses. Tables 17–1 to 17–3 show the results of their literature review. We review the total joint systems used extensively in the United States, including the Kent-Vitek, Synthes, Christensen, and Tech-Medica (TMJ Concepts).

The first total joint system that was extensively used in the United States was the Kent-Vitek prosthesis (Fig. 17–2) in the early 1970s. Kent and colleagues developed a glenoid fossa implant (VK-1) that originally consisted of a bilaminate fossa with a polyaramid fabric–reinforced ultra-high-molecular-weight, polyethylene articular surface.[20] The inner layer of the prosthesis was composed of Proplast-hydroxyapatite, which could be contoured to fit against the base of the skull. This Proplast layer originally came in thicknesses of 2.5 and 4.5 mm, which allowed the surgeon to move the articulating surface inferiorly if the fossa were to articulate against a natural condyle that had lost vertical height secondary to degenerative disease. The flange of the prosthesis was secured to the zygomatic arch with screws.

The condylar prosthesis was constructed of chromium-cobalt with a layer of Proplast on the inner surface of the ramal flange to encourage rapid ingrowth of both hard and soft tissues. Also, an L-shaped flange was incorporated into the posterior and inferior edge of the ramal surface as an antirotational groove. The original VK-1 fossa had an articulating surface composed of polytetrafluoroethylene (PTFE). The fossa was re-

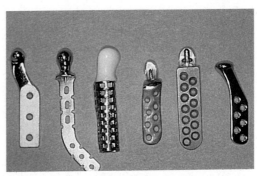

FIGURE 17–1. Various designs for alloplastic condylar prostheses. Left to right: Kent-Vitek, Synthes, Delrin-TiMesh, Christensen type I, Christensen type II, Lorenz.

TABLE 17–1. | Survey of Temporomandibular Joint Fossa-Eminence Prosthesis Designs

Design	Period of Use	Materials Used	Method of Fitting	Method of Fixation	No. of Evaluated Prostheses (Patients)	Follow-up Period (Years)	Evaluation
Eggers[14]	Before 1946	Tantalum foil	Material adapts itself	None	1 (1)	1	Good result
Smith & Robinson[58]	1947–1957	Stainless steel	Adapt skull	Screws	12 (?)	1–10?	Good results?
Robinson[16]	Before 1960	Stainless steel	Adapt skull	Screws	1 (1)	2	Good result
Christensen[18]	1960 and later	Cr-Co	Different shapes	Screws	100 (?)	1–11	2 reoperations
Morgan,[19] follow-up by House et al[59]	1965–?	Cr-Co	Different shapes + adapt skull	Screws	167 (103)	1–12	71% good / 14% fair / 15% poor

From van Loon J, DeBont LGM, Boering G, et al: Evaluation of temporomandibular joint prostheses. J Oral Maxillofac Surg 1995;53:984–996.

TABLE 17–2. | Survey of Temporomandibular Joint Condylar Prosthesis Designs

Design	Period of Use	Materials Used	Method of Fitting	Method of Fixation	No. of Evaluated Prostheses (Patients)	Follow-up Period (Years)	Evaluation
Kent et al[22] Flat design:	1972–1975	Cr-Co + Proplast	Bending and different sizes	Screws and coating; grooves in jaw	(80 patients)	Average = 2 (1–10)	Success rate 60%
Box design:	1975–1983				35 (?)		Success rate 90%
Spiessl[60]	1976 and later	Ti	Bending and different sizes	Screws	74 (?)	?	Good results in 73% of joints; bone resorption of skull
Follow-up by Lindquist et al[61]	1984–1990				11 (8)	1–6	
Silver et al[62]	Before 1977	Cr-Co	PMMA	Stem + PMMA	3 (3)	4–5	2 slightly protrusive; mobility, 1 hinge joint
Raveh et al[63]	1982 and later	Ti	Bending	Screws	3 (3)	?	Good results
Flot et al[64]	1984–1987	Stainless steel + PE	Not applicable	Screwed stem	Total: 62 (?)	1–7	13 removed because of inaccurate position of stem
Follow-up by Chassagne et al[65]	1987 and later	Ti alloy + PE + Al_2O_3					
Westermark et al[32]	1990 and later	Ti mesh + POM head	Bending	Screws	1 (1)	2	Not removed
MacAfee & Quinn[33]	1992		Ti mesh	Screws	4 (4)	4	Good results

PE, polyethylene; PMMA, polymethyl methacrylate; POM, polyoxymethylene.
From van Loon J, DeBont LGM, Boering G, et al: Evaluation of temporomandibular joint prostheses. J Oral Maxillofac Surg 1995;53:984–996.

TABLE 17–3.	Survey of Temporomandibular Joint Total Joint Prosthesis Designs							
Design	**Period of Use**	**Materials Used**	**Method of Fitting Fossa Part**	**Method of Fitting Condylar Part**	**Method of Fixation**	**No. of Evaluated Prostheses (Patients)**	**Follow-up Period (Years)**	**Evaluation**
Christensen[18]	1965 and later	Cr-Co + PMMA head	Different shapes	Different sizes	Screws	No information	No information	No information
Kiehn et al[23]	1974–1979	Cr-Co + PMMA head	Glued with PMMA	Bending	Glued with PMMA	27 (27)	1–4	2 removed, 1 recemented
Morgan[66]	1976 and later	Cr-Co + PMMA head	Different shapes	Different sizes	Screws	24 (?)	?–16	No reoperations
Momma[67]	1976–1978	Cr-Co	Adapt skull	PMMA	Screws	15 (?)	0–2	None removed
Kummoona[68]	Before 1978	Cr-Co	Adapt skull	PMMA	Screws/PMMA	3 (3)	1–4	None removed
Kent et al[20, 69] Articulating surface: Teflon (T) Polyethylene (PE)	1982–1986 1986–1990	Cr-Co condyle + T + PE	Adapt prosthesis	Different sizes	Screws and coating	Articulating surface: T:110 (66) T:96 (?) T:96 (?) PE:118 (?)	1–4 1–4 1–9 1–6	Cumulative success rate: 90% 55% 20% 80%
Sonnenburg & Sonnenburg[50, 70]	1978–1982 1983 and later	Cr-Co Ti alloy + PE	PMMA	Bending	Screws	9 (6) 16 (12)	2–6 1–5	1 removed No complications
McBride[2]	1990 and later	Ti + Cr-Co head + PE fossa	PMMA	Bending	Screws	No information	No information	No information
Wolford et al[52] (Tech-Medica)	1990 and later	Ti/Ti alloy + Cr-Co head + PE	Custom-made from CT scans	Custom-made from CT scans	Screws	100 (56)	1–4	58% good, 26% fair, 16% poor
Falkenström[56] prototype	1993	Ti alloy/Cr-Co/ Al_2O_3	Custom-made or PMMA	Different sizes	Special screws	—	—	—

CT, computed tomography; PMMA, polymethyl methacrylate.
From van Loon J, DeBont LGM, Boering G, et al: Evaluation of temporomandibular joint prostheses. J Oral Maxillofac Surg 1995;53:984–996.

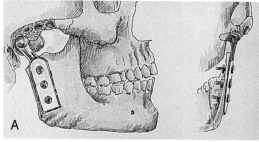

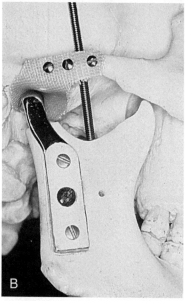

FIGURE 17–2. *A,* Kent-Vitek total joint prosthesis. *B,* Kent-Vitek total joint prosthesis with VK-1 fossa implant.

vised and called the VK-2 fossa, and its articulating surface was composed of ultra-high-molecular-weight polyethylene (UHM-WPE).

Kent and Misiek reported a series of 170 patients who had received 182 joints for partial or total joint reconstruction between 1982 and 1988.[21] There was a higher success rate in the patients reconstructed with the VK-2 fossa (94%) than the VK-1 fossa (75%). In a 10-year retrospective by Kent and colleagues in 1983,[22] a success rate of 87% was reported. Complications included glenoid fossa resorption, especially in patients who had undergone ramal lengthening. Several authors, including Kiehn and associates,[23] reported successful joint reconstruction with the use of a VK fossa and a Synthes condyle. The spherical head of the Synthes condyle may have provided better mating for the condylar-fossa components and decreased the occurrence of "variable point" loading, which over a long period could in-

duce mobility in the fossa prosthesis and fragmentation of the PTFE.

The PTFE was clearly the problematic material in this design, and it is covered in detail elsewhere in this text. Sir John Charnley, an orthopedic surgeon, stopped using PTFE in orthopedic implants in 1963 because of the tissue reaction to wear debris, which caused loosening of the acetabular component secondary to bony erosion.[24] These findings were confirmed by Leidholt and Gorman in 1963,[25] who placed hip prostheses with PTFE in dogs. They reported both an acute and a chronic inflammatory reaction to PTFE particles characterized by giant cells. A U.S. Food and Drug Administration (FDA) safety alert appeared in December 1990 advising oral and maxillofacial surgeons against the use of PTFE-coated disk implants.

In 1986, Kent and colleagues reported a retrospective study of 59 glenoid fossa implants in 49 patients.[20] These included both the trilaminate VK-1 before 1982 and the bilaminate VK-2 after 1982. The success rate for the 29 joints reconstructed with the VK-1 fossa was 62.2%, and removal of the fossa prosthesis was necessitated in 10 joints because of infection, erosion, or implant displacement (Fig. 17–3). The success rate for the VK-2 fossa was 90%. We have followed 16 patients who had total joint reconstructions with a Kent fossa and a Synthes condyle. The mean follow-up for these patients was 12.2 years, and 12 of the prostheses are currently functional; four have been revised with the Lorenz prosthesis.

One of the issues that is generic to all alloplastic joint systems is the necessity for proper surgical access for placement of both a fossa and a condylar prosthesis (Fig. 17–4). We currently use a combination of an endaural incision, which is a modified rhytidectomy incision, and a posterior mandibular incision (see Fig. 17–4). The rhytidectomy incision is carried from the lobular attachment of the ear superiorly, inside the tragal cartilage, with a 45-degree release into the temporal hairline. Great care is taken not to incise the perichondrium on the tragal cartilage during the initial incision. An attempt is made to dissect along the tragal cartilage to the root of the zygoma and establish a single plane of dissection in order to protect the branches of the

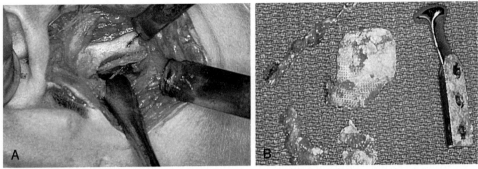

FIGURE 17–3. *A,* Interpositional polytetrafluoroethylene (PTFE) meniscal implant at time of removal, secondary to chronic inflammatory foreign body reaction. *B,* Kent-Vitek total joint prosthesis after removal of components was necessitated by foreign body reaction to fragmented PTFE.

facial nerve. Based on the classic work by Al-Kayat and Bramley,[26] we know that the upper trunk of the facial nerve can cross the root of the zygoma anywhere from 8 to 35 mm anterior to the most anterior portion of the bony auditory canal.[27–29]

The posterior mandibular incision for a retromandibular approach is useful for

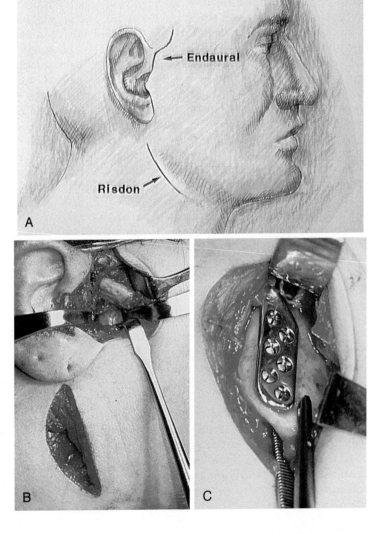

FIGURE 17–4. *A,* Combination of endaural and rhytidectomy-type incision for preauricular approach combined with posterior mandibular incisions. This incision is a modification of the Risdon incision, in that it is placed more posterior and superior relative to the posterior ramal border. *B,* Proper placement of endaural and posterior mandibular incisions for prosthetic joint replacement. *C,* Relatively tension-free exposure of the entire ramal height from angle to condylar neck to facilitate proper screw placement for condylar prosthesis.

gaining access for tumor resection, costochondral grafting, access to condylar fractures, and total alloplastic joint reconstruction. The incision is made on a curvilinear line approximately 5 cm long and 2 cm distal to the most inferior point of the mandibular angle where its midpoint is situated. The surgeon must avoid the marginal mandibular branch of the facial nerve, which, according to Dingman and Grabb,[30] passes above the inferior border of the mandible in 81% of cadaver dissections. Even in light of this, care must be exercised, because it can run as much as 3 cm below the inferior border of the mandible deep to the platysma muscle. The nerve does run superficial to the facial vein, which is why it is recommended to ligate the facial vein and retract it superiorly as part of the normal dissection. After dissecting deep to the platysma, the anterior border of the sternocleidomastoid muscle is identified and dissected in a plane between the anterior border of the sternocleidomastoid and the capsule of the submandibular gland. Once the inferior border of the mandible can be identified, the aponeurosis between the masseter muscle and the medial pterygoid is incised with a No. 15 blade. This allows the surgeon to cleanly strip off the masseter muscle and establish communication with the endaural incision. Anterosuperior traction of the retromandibular incision should now allow for wide access to the ramus for placement of the condylar prosthesis.

In 1987, Boyne and coworkers reported the use of a condylar prosthesis that was secured by screws to a titanium mesh plate.[31] The condylar head was constructed of Delrin (polyoxyethylene). There was no fossa prosthesis used in conjunction with the condyle, because the Delrin had a modulus of elasticity that was closer to bone than any metallic condylar head and could theoretically function against a natural glenoid fossa. Westermark and associates[32] reported the use of this prosthesis for bilateral ankylosis. MacAfee and Quinn published their results with this prosthesis in 1992.[33] The prosthesis did not attract widespread use because Delrin was reported to induce bone formation, which could result in deposition of heterotopic bone. In addition, the mechanical design, which required the use of self-tapping screws to secure the Delrin to the titanium mesh, did not lend itself to long-term stability. The Delrin head necessitated an ostectomy at the superior-posterior aspect of the ramus to allow for insetting of the condylar prosthesis. This was technically difficult and could lead to an increased risk of facial nerve palsy.

Currently, the most widely used system for alloplastic total joint reconstruction is the Christensen prosthesis marketed by TMJ, Inc. In the early 1960s, Christensen[17] initially reported the use of a cast Vitallium glenoid fossa against a natural condyle for treatment of mandibular ankylosis. In 1965, he devised a condylar prosthesis to complement the fossa eminence prosthesis (Fig. 17–5). The original cast cobalt-chromium fossa was available in 20 different sizes based on anatomic variations in human adult skulls. Currently, there are more than 45 preshaped sizes for both the right and the left sides. Template "sizers" are used to select the proper fossa.

Originally, the highly polished articulating surface of the fossa was designed to articulate directly with a natural condyle. The fossa was ultimately extended to be used not only after meniscectomy and ankylosis surgery but also in the presence of a meniscus to avoid formation of adhesions between the superior surface of the meniscus and the glenoid fossa itself. With regard to the glenoid fossa used alone in a hemiarthroplasty, Chase and coworkers[34] published the results of using the fossa prosthesis in 40 joints (22 patients) in which the disk was retained. The indication was for use in "internal derangement with associated pain and dysfunction that did not respond to non-surgical treatment." The mean follow-up time was 2.2 years. Although the majority of patients had an increase in their

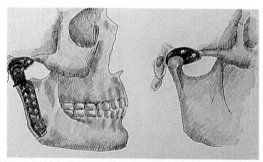

FIGURE 17–5. Christensen total joint prosthesis and Christensen fossa prosthesis articulating with the natural condyle.

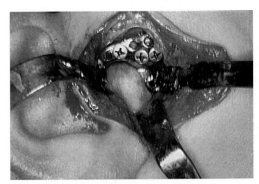

FIGURE 17–6. Christensen fossa prosthesis placed against natural condyle after meniscectomy.

functional abilities and a decrease in pain, 36% of the joints underwent another surgical procedure an average of 13 months after the initial surgery to remove the meniscus.

In another group of patients (26 patients and 49 joints), a fossa prosthesis was placed at the time of the meniscectomy (Fig. 17–6). In this group, only two patients required reoperation during the mean follow-up time of 5.1 years.

With respect to placement of the fossa, it is extremely important to gain maximal extended coverage of the articular eminence so that during the range of motion of either the natural or the prosthetic condyle, the condylar head does not traverse the actual edge of the fossa prosthesis. This can result in "lipping" of the natural condyle and potential mechanical obstruction with the prosthetic condyle. In addition, it is sometimes necessary to use judicious bone contouring, even with all the precast sizes available, to achieve a stable fit of the prosthesis. The prosthesis is secured to the zygo-

matic arch with a minimum of four self-tapping screws.

In our own series of hemiarthroplasties in which the fossa prosthesis alone was placed against a natural condyle after meniscectomy, 55% of the patients ultimately underwent revision surgery for placement of a Christensen condylar prosthesis. There were 23 joints in 16 patients with an average follow-up of 6.3 years. In a retrospective analysis of this group, it was our conclusion that when there were significant signs of degenerative joint disease at the time of placement of the glenoid fossa implant, continued pain, dysfunction, and condylar degeneration could be expected. In no way should this be construed as a failure of the implant, but rather a confirmation of the orthopedic literature in which hemiarthroplasty is generally not advised. This is especially true in a multiply operated patient with a poorly vascularized tissue bed secondary to scarring. It is also not advisable to use a fossa prosthesis in the face of vertical bone loss from condylar degeneration, because the fossa cannot restore ramal height and correct laterognathia.

The original condylar prosthesis was a cobalt-chromium ramal component with a polymethyl-methacrylate (PMMA) head (Fig. 17–7). In the study by Chase and co-workers[34] they followed 21 patients with 34 joints. Follow-up in this group ran from 1 to 10 years, with a mean of 2.4 years. Ninety-five percent of the patients showed a significant decrease in pain, and 86% showed a significant improvement in ability to eat. All prostheses in this group were functioning at the time of publication. This first

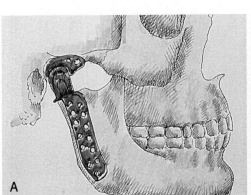
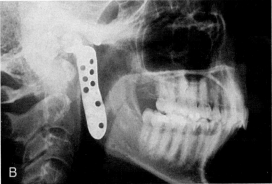

FIGURE 17–7. *A,* Christensen total joint prosthesis with type I Christensen condylar prosthesis using a methyl methacrylate head. *B,* Lateral skull film showing Christensen total joint prosthesis (Christensen type I condylar prosthesis).

iteration of the Christensen prosthesis is referred to as the Christensen type I prosthesis.

Methyl methacrylate is a high-molecular-weight acrylic material that can undergo the polymerization process at room temperature (cold cure) or as a result of a thermoplastic reaction (heat cure).[35] In its solid form, PMMA is quite strong and relatively biocompatible. It is eventually covered by a thin fibrous tissue envelope if it remains in its solid form. The reaction to particulate debris from PMMA cement has been extensively discussed in the orthopedic literature.[36-40] Osteolysis at the implant-bone interface in hip prostheses can be multifactorial and is secondary to foreign body reactions to polyethylene and PMMA. Regardless of the initiating event, the final common pathway in implant loosening is bone resorption at the implant-bone interface secondary to osteoclastic activity. Clearly, motion and particulate debris can result in formation of a "pseudomembrane" that is sometimes seen with aseptic loosening of orthopedic implants.

In addition to the PMMA head, the original type I condylar prostheses were structurally weaker than the type II prostheses, and the screw hole placement was not always optimally controlled. The condylar prosthesis was available in lengths of 45, 50, and 55 mm. The recommended surgical technique was to complete the arthroplasty with condylectomy and removal of all adhesions and heterotopic bone. The glenoid fossa prosthesis was placed, and the patient was placed in intermaxillary fixation in an optimal occlusion. Condylar sizers were used to select the proper vertical length of the prosthesis. The condylar prosthesis was secured with self-tapping bicortical screws. We recommended that two screws be placed initially and then the mandible be manipulated to ensure that there was an intercisal opening of at least 30 mm with no evidence of subluxation or dislocation. Because there is no lateral pterygoid function with an alloplastic condylar prosthesis, 30 to 35 mm of pure rotational movement would be a reasonable expectation. It was also important that the prosthesis be angled approximately 18 to 20 degrees, with the condyle head angled posteriorly so that the head of the condyle began its rotation in the posterior portion of the prosthetic fossa. If the prosthesis was positioned vertically straight or with the condylar head angled anteriorly, the ultimate range of motion of the prosthesis would be limited. Six to eight ramal screws were recommended, and it was important to ensure that the screw placement did not violate the inferior alveolar canal. In cases in which there was significant destruction of the ramus of the mandible, which would preclude the use of adequate bone to stabilize the prosthesis, there was a condylar prosthesis available in an L shape (Chase modification). This was very useful in post-tumor reconstruction or where there had been significant resorption of the lateral ramal cortical bone secondary to previous attempts at autogenous joint reconstruction.

In multiply operated patients who have restricted range of motion before alloplastic joint replacement, it is extremely important to remove all the heterotopic bone and scarring within the joint itself, especially on the medial surface of the glenoid fossa. In addition, it may be necessary to strip the foreshortened attachments of the masseter and pterygoid muscles and perform coronoidectomies, if necessary.

The first revision of the Christensen condyle was a reinforced version that retained the PMMA head but used a thicker cobalt-chromium ramal strut with computer-designed offset screw holes (Fig. 17–8). In our experience, this completely solved the

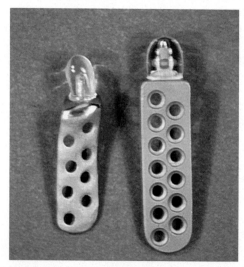

FIGURE 17–8. Comparison of Christensen type I and type II prostheses. Note the reinforced structural design of the ramal component, as well as the increased number of offset screw holes.

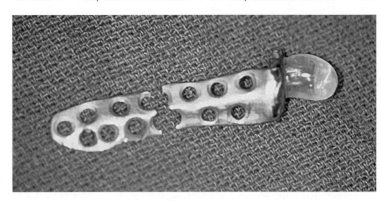

FIGURE 17–9. Fractured type I Christensen prosthesis.

problem we had encountered with condylar prosthesis fracture.

We have followed a series of 90 patients with a total of 109 total joint reconstructions with Christensen prostheses. There were 71 unilateral and 19 bilateral cases. The follow-up ranged from 36 to 108 months, with a mean follow-up of 73.1 months. In that series, there were nine fractures of the condylar prosthesis, and all these occurred in the type I Christensen prosthesis. We have not encountered any fractures in the type II condylar prosthesis. The fractures tended to occur at the point superior to the most superior ramal screw and often in the area of two screw holes that were not offset by design (Fig. 17–9). Theoretically, metal fatigue occurred at the junction of the "screw-fixated" component and the nonfixated components of the condylar prosthesis.

It is critical to have reasonable expectations of alloplastic prostheses, especially because this is the most complicated joint in the body. The fractures that occurred in the type I prostheses were functioning for an average of 5.8 years and were highly correlated with parafunctional habits such as bruxing. Although we do not have good long-term data on the TMJ alloplastic implant as compared to the orthopedic experience, it is our belief that 8 to 11 years is a reasonable expectation for an alloplastic prosthesis at this time, given the lack of long-term data.

The second area of concern was wear in the PMMA head, which was readily apparent in the majority of the explanted condylar prostheses. Fortunately, tissue samples taken at the time showed no evidence of significant inflammatory tissue responses to acrylic wear débridement. There was evi-

dence of some fibrous encapsulation of PMMA particles.

In the Christensen total joints that continue in follow-up, we have seen significant reduction in pain from an average of 9.2 on a digital analog scale of 0 to 10 to a mean of 2.6. The average interincisal opening increased from 13.9 to 28.7 mm.

Recently, TMJ Inc. has marketed a metal-to-metal total joint prosthesis (Fig. 17–10). In orthopedics, there is a renewed interest in metal-to-metal joint implants. This is of

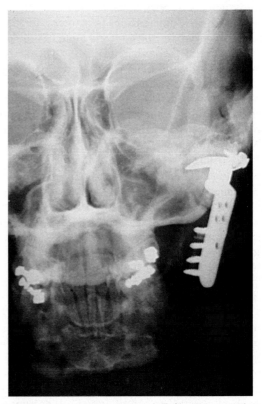

FIGURE 17–10. Posteroanterior skull film showing Christensen metal-to-metal prosthesis in position.

special import because of the concern about polyethylene wear debris and aseptic loosening. Metal-to-metal hips were reported by McKee and Chen[41] in 1973 as well as by Breck,[42] Muller,[43] and Wilson and Scales.[44] Potential problems with metal-to-metal prostheses include the high frictional torque, which could result in loosening, and the potential for wear debris, which, with cobalt-chromium, could be more toxic than with polyethylene.[45] In addition, the wear particles are smaller and therefore more numerous for a given wear volume. The incidence of metal sensitivity has been proved to be greatest in metal-to-metal joint prostheses with high wear rates.[46, 47] Many researchers in the orthopedics field now believe that the poor clinical results in the 1960s and 1970s with metal-to-metal prostheses may have been attributable to poor stem and cup design and inconsistent manufacturing of the metals themselves.

Lippincott and colleagues recently reported on the TMJ Inc. metal-to-metal TMJ prosthesis.[48] In vitro testing of the metal-to-metal device showed "no adverse wear, no fatigue failure of the test devices, no loosening of the implants from the synthetic bone substitute, no gross material removal or device failure–deformation is shown, only a slight blemish on the condyle head. Analysis of the cyclic fatigue tests under these extreme conditions at the five million cycles shows a survivorship calculation of the implant device well over sixty years of duration." Metallic wear debris (particle sizes 40 to 200 μm) was injected into the TMJs of New Zealand white rabbits. "There was a mild inflammatory reaction in the early time period sacrifice of one to three months, but no sign of foreign body reaction or large infiltration of inflammatory cells."

In Lippincott's study, 23 patients with metal-to-metal TMJ prostheses were followed for a mean period of 26 months (follow-up time ranged from 3.5 to 50 months). There was significant pain reduction and increase in interincisal opening.

In our own series of 9 patients with 11 metal-to-metal Christensen joints, our mean follow-up time to date is 4.1 years. We have had no overt implant failures but will need a much longer follow-up to judge the efficacy of these metal-to-metal systems.

In the metal-to-metal group of patients, the preoperative range of motion averaged 11.2 mm; postoperatively, at 1 year it was 26.8 mm. Pain scales, on a visual analog scale of 0 to 10, averaged 8.8 preoperatively and 2.9 postoperatively (1 year).

TMJ Inc. also has the ability to construct custom cobalt-chromium, metal-to-metal joints from computed tomography (CT)–generated data (Fig. 17–11). A CT scan performed according to a defined protocol can be used to generate a three-dimensional computer-assisted design–computer-assisted manufacture (CAD-CAM) model for custom joint construction. These joints are especially useful in multiply operated patients with gross anatomic discrepancies.

In 1995, Mercuri and colleagues reported their results with the Tech-Medica system.[49] The system was developed in 1988 and used a CAD-CAM total TMJ reconstruction prosthesis that was designed as a custom prosthesis for each patient (Fig. 17–12). The fossa was constructed of a commercially pure titanium custom-formed sheet with a welded mesh that interfaces with the bone of the residual fossa and is mechanically bonded to a dense UHMWPE articulating surface. The condylar prosthesis was composed of a chromium-cobalt-molybdenum condyle mechanically attached to a titanium alloy ramus component. The prosthesis was placed in 215 patients in a well-designed multicenter study. The preliminary report detailed the results of 48 months' follow-up. The CAD-CAM design necessitated, at times, that patients undergo a "phase I" surgery to remove failed autogenous grafts or failed alloplastic grafts and thorough dé-

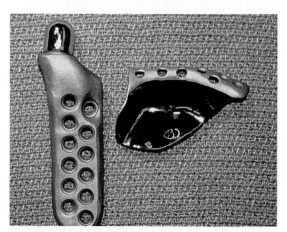

FIGURE 17–11. Custom Christensen metal-to-metal prosthesis fabricated from three-dimensional computed tomography data.

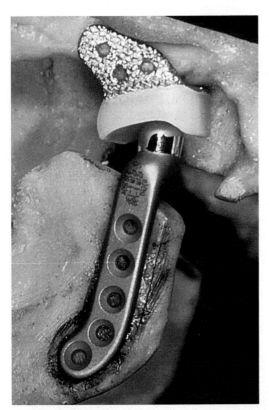

FIGURE 17–12. Custom Tech-Medica CAD-CAM prosthesis (currently marketed by TMJ Concepts).

bridement of the joint, including all metal or foreign materials. The patients were then placed in maxillomandibular fixation, and a CT scan was performed according to protocol. In addition to subjective data regarding pain, interincisal opening, and diet, a life table analysis was done to estimate the proportion of surviving prostheses at the landmark intervals.

There were 363 joints placed—296 bilateral and 67 unilateral. The patients had undergone a mean of 5.4 prior unsuccessful surgeries. The study showed the predictable predominance of females (202 females versus 13 males) with an average age of 40.9 years. "Preliminary analysis of the data reveals a statistically significant decrease in pain, an increase in function, and improvement in diet from the postoperative measurements to one to two years postoperatively."

At the time of publication, there were 19 patients (8.8%) who were defined as failures. According to the authors, "If both design and patient failures are removed which give a truer picture of the long-term safety

and effectiveness of the prosthesis, the corresponding percentages were all 97% (surviving prostheses)." The Tech-Medica prosthesis is now marketed as the TMJ Concepts Inc. prosthesis.

UHMWPE has been used in fossa prostheses designed by Sonnenburg and Sonnenburg, Osteomed, and Tech-Medica.[50–52] It is a linear (unbranched) chain distinguished by its molecular weight of greater than 1 million. Most commercial grades of UHMWPE in use today have an average molecular weight in the range of 3 to 6 million. The wear rate of UHMWPE is considerably lower than that of other polymers that have been used in bearing surfaces (e.g., Delrin, Teflon) (Table 17–4).

In spite of the excellent wear characteristics of polyethylene, it still accounts for the predominant wear particle seen in failed total joint arthroplasties. Polyethylene appears to be a potent stimulator for macrophage activation. Current strategies to improve UHMWPE include improved polymer cross-linking, fiber reinforcement, and alternative sterilization techniques. In spite of its shortcomings, polyethylene remains the "gold standard" for a fixed articulating surface.

Although clearly a custom prosthesis for each patient would be advantageous, the realities of health care economics dictate the need for stock prostheses as well. Several attempts have been made to use UHMWPE prostheses fitted to the base of the skull with PMMA cement (Sonnenburg and Sonnenburg and Osteomed[3]). PMMA was introduced by Charnley[53] and has been used for fixation of total joint prostheses for more than 30 years. Although there is extensive study of

TABLE 17–4.	Wear Rates of Various Orthopedic Bearing Materials Compared with Ram-Extruded Ultra-High-Molecular-Weight Polyethylene (UHMWPE)

Material	Relative Wear Rate
UHMWPE (extruded)	1
UHMWPE (molded)	1
Carbon-filled UHMWPE	1.8–10.3
Polyacetal (Delrin 150)	34
Polytetrafluoroethylene (PTFE)	1510

From Sedel L, Cabanela ME: Hip Surgery. St. Louis, Mosby, 1998.

the cement and bone interface and the potential for aseptic loosening in the cemented hip prosthesis, it is difficult to draw analogies with regard to the TMJ. There has been an association with "thin cement mantel" and failure, which suggests that small loose edges of polymerized cement may be more problematic than a solid, immobile core of cement.[54, 55] Ideally, PMMA cement should not be used as a "loaded" medium to custom fit a stock prosthesis but only as a void filler to avoid potential dead space.

We are currently involved with an FDA-approved clinical study of a TMJ prosthesis designed by Lorenz (Fig. 17–13). The fossa prosthesis is constructed of UHMWPE with a minimum of 4 mm of thickness in the midpoint of the fossa itself. It was designed with exaggerated lipping to protect the condyle from encroachment by heterotopic bone and to avoid dislocation. In the original prototype, the zygomatic extension was patent, and four screw holes were placed at the time of surgery to fixate the prosthesis to the zygomatic arch with four 2-mm self-tapping screws. There are now three stock sizes of the prosthesis available with predrilled holes. The single most important step in reducing the inherent anatomic variability of the articular eminence is flattening of the eminence with a large bur before fossa fitting. Next, with judicious use of bone-contouring diamond burs, the fossa is fitted with tripod stability so that there is a polyethylene-to-bone stability without any rocking motion. At this point, a PMMA orthopedic bone cement reinforced with methyl methacrylate–styrene copolymers (Simplex P) is used to custom fit the prosthesis to the base of the skull. The cement was not

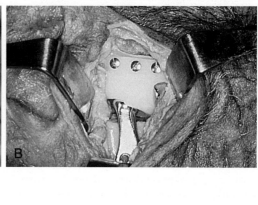

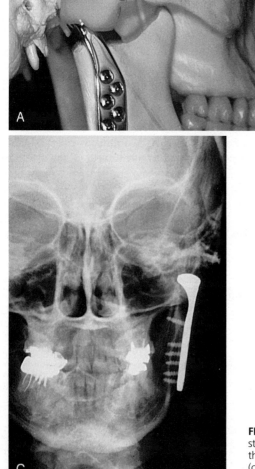

FIGURE 17–13. *A,* Lorenz prosthesis mounted on demonstration skull. *B,* Lorenz prosthesis in cadaver. Note how the design of the prosthesis moves the point of rotation (condylion) inferiorly. *C,* Posteroanterior skull film with Lorenz prosthesis in position.

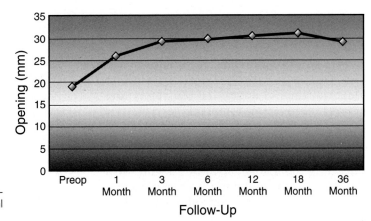

FIGURE 17–14. Lorenz prosthesis: Preoperative and landmark data for interincisal opening (in millimeters).

intended to be used as a "loading medium," and a small dowel is used on the inner surface of the fossa for mechanical locking of the cement. A small amount of cement (average 2 mL) is applied to the inner surface of the fossa, and it is placed against the base of the skull. Before final polymerization takes place, the fossa is removed and all thin edges of the cement are removed. When it is finally polymerized, a specially designed acrylic bur is used to remove any "flashing" to avoid fracture at thin edges. The prosthesis is then reinserted and secured with the zygomatic screws. With continued experience, we have used the PMMA cement less and less and currently utilize it in only 20% to 25% of fossae. The cobalt-chromium condylar prosthesis is available in lengths of 45, 50, and 55 mm and is selected with the patient in intermaxillary fixation. The "swan neck" design of the condylar neck avoids the problem of implant-bone interface obstruction inherent with the right-angle design of most metallic condylar prostheses.

Because the polyethylene thickness displaces the point of rotation (condylion) inferiorly as compared with the natural joints, we have experienced the concept proposed by Falkenström in 1993.[56] He noted that by "placing the point of rotation of the prosthesis substantially inferior to the middle of the natural condyle, translation is imitated when the mouth is opened." This "pseudo-translation" has resulted in a gain of approximately 15% in the interincisal opening with the Lorenz prosthesis.

To date, the results are as follows: 32 patients with 41 implants have been enrolled in this study to date. The mean number of prior surgeries for patients enrolled in the study was 5.7, with a range of 0 to 13. Ninety-one percent of the patients were female and 9% male, with a mean age of 35.8. There has been a statistically significant increase in maximal incisal opening, a decrease in jaw pain intensity, and an increase in functional diet (Figs. 17–14 and 17–15).

We have encountered two complications

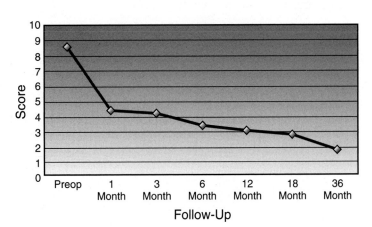

FIGURE 17–15. Lorenz prosthesis: Preoperative and landmark data for patient-reported pain. (Visual Analog Scale: 0 = no pain; 10 = worst pain imaginable.)

to date. Both involve removal of the fossa prosthesis in two multiply operated patients.

This study is still ongoing. It is designed to follow these patients for an appropriate length of time to determine the safety and efficacy of this design implant.

In 1992, the American Association of Oral and Maxillofacial Surgeons convened a workshop to disseminate recommendations regarding the management of patients with TMJ alloplastic implants. The recommendation at that time was that "alloplastic total joint replacement is an option in patients with extensive TMJ disease. However, because the long-term outcomes with currently available total joints have yet to be determined, their application must be considered as compassionate use as of this time." There clearly is a need for safe, effective, and functional total joint alloplastic implants with a reasonable life span. Some of the catastrophic side effects of permanently implanted PTFE and Silastic have clearly made it difficult to find support and funding for advancements in this field. Because past failures should be guideposts to future successes, it is extremely important not to abandon these efforts but to redirect them at well-designed clinical studies.

In *Controversies in Oral and Maxillofacial Surgery*,[57] McBride wrote, "As approved biomaterials and new total joint implant systems become available, and additional experience is gained with total joint implants, the quality of results obtained will continue to improve to the point where total joint reconstruction will become the treatment of choice for severe temporomandibular joint degeneration." Clearly, this can happen only with sound biomaterial science and well-designed clinical studies.

REFERENCES

1. Mercuri LG: Alloplastic temporomandibular joint reconstruction. Oral Surg Oral Med Oral Path 1998;85:631–636.
2. McBride KL: Total temporomandibular joint reconstruction. In Worthington P, Evans JR (eds): Controversies in Oral and Maxillofacial Surgery. Philadelphia, WB Saunders, 1994, pp 381–396.
3. van Loon J, DeBont LGM, Boering G, et al: Evaluation of temporomandibular joint prostheses. J Oral Maxillofac Surg 1995;53:984–996.
4. Braunt KJ (ed): Temporomandibular joint surgery. Part II. Partial and total joint reconstruction and

5. Poswillo D: Biological reconstruction of the mandibular condyle. Br J Oral Maxillofac Surg 1972;25:100.
6. Wolford LM, Cottrell DA, Henry C: Sternoclavicular grafts for temporomandibular joint reconstruction. J Oral Maxillofac Surg 1994;52:119.
7. Worthington P, Evans JR (eds): Controversies in Oral and Maxillofacial Surgery. Philadelphia, WB Saunders, 1994.
8. Lindquist C, Jokinen J, Paukku P, et al: Adaptation of autogenous costochondral grafts used for temporomandibular joint reconstruction: A long-term clinical and radiologic follow-up. J Oral Maxillofac Surg 1988;46:465.
9. Lindquist C, Pihakari A, Tasanen A, et al: Autogenous costochondral grafts in temporomandibular joint arthroplasty: A survey of 66 arthroplasties in 60 patients. J Maxillofac Surg 1986;14:143.
10. MacIntosh RB: Current spectrum of costochondral grafting. In Bell WH, Proffit WR, White RP (eds): Surgical Correction of Dentofacial Deformities. Philadelphia, WB Saunders, 1985.
11. MacIntosh RB: Current spectrum of costochondral grafting. In Bell WH (ed): Modern Practice of Orthognathic and Reconstructive Surgery, vol 2. Philadelphia, WB Saunders, 1992, pp 873–949.
12. Carnochan JM: Mobilizing a patient's ankylosed jaw by placing a block of wood between the raw bony surfaces after resection. Archiv de Medicin 1860;284–286.
13. Risdon F: Ankylosis of the temporomandibular joint. J Am Dent Assoc 1933;21:1933–1937.
14. Eggers GWN: Arthroplasty of the temporomandibular joint in children with interpositional tantalum foil. J Bone Joint Surg 1946;28:603–606.
15. Goodsell JO: Tantalum in temporomandibular joint arthroplasty: Report of case. J Oral Surg 1947;5:41–45.
16. Robinson M: Temporomandibular ankylosis corrected by creating a false stainless steel fossa. J South Calif Dent Assoc 1960;28:186.
17. Christensen RW: The correction of mandibular ankylosis by arthroplasty and the insertion of a cast Vitallium glenoid fossa. J South Calif Dent Assoc 1963;31:117.
18. Christensen RW: The temporomandibular joint prosthesis eleven years later. Oral Implantol 1971;2:125.
19. Morgan DH: Dysfunction, pain, tinnitus, vertigo corrected by mandibular joint surgery. J South Calif Dent Assoc 1971;39:50.
20. Kent JN, Block MS, Homsy CA, et al: Experience with a polymer glenoid fossa prosthesis for partial or total temporomandibular joint reconstruction. J Oral Maxillofac Surg 1986;44:520–533.
21. Kent JN, Misiek DJ: Biomaterials for cranial, facial, mandible and TMJ reconstruction. In Fonseca RJ, Walker RV (eds): Maxillofacial Trauma. Philadelphia, WB Saunders, 1991, pp 1073–1100.
22. Kent JN, Misiek DJ, Akin RK, et al: Temporomandibular joint condylar prosthesis: A ten year report. J Oral Maxillofac Surg 1983;41:245–254.
23. Kiehn CL, DesPrez JD, Converse CF: Total prosthetic replacement of the temporomandibular joint. Ann Plast Surg 1979;2:5–15.
24. Charnley J: Tissue reaction of polytetrafluorethylene. Lancet 1963:1379.
25. Leidholt JD, Gorman HA: Teflon hip prostheses in dogs. J Bone Joint Surg 1965;47(A):1414–1420.

osseous procedures. Selected Readings in Oral and Maxillofacial Surgery 1992;1.

26. Al-Kayat A, Bramley P: A modified pre-auricular approach to the temporomandibular joint and malar arch. Br J Oral Surg 1980;17:91.

27. Debrul EL: The craniomandibular articulation. In Sicher's Oral Anatomy, ed 7. St. Louis, Mosby, 1980, pp 70–79.

28. Dolwick MF, Kretzschmar DP: Morbidity associated with preauricular and perimeatal approaches to the TMJ. J Oral Maxilloac Surg 1982;40:699.

29. Ellis E, Zide MF: Surgical Approaches to the Facial Skeleton. Baltimore, Williams & Wilkins, 1994.

30. Dingman RO, Grabb WC: Surgical anatomy of the mandibular ramus of the facial nerve based on the dissection of 100 facial halves. Plast Reconstr Surg 1962;29:266.

31. Boyne PJ, Matthews FR, Stringer DE: TMJ bone remodeling after polyoxymethylene condylar replacement. Int J Oral Maxillofac Implants 1987;2:29.

32. Westermark AH, Sindet-Pedersen S, Boyne PJ: Bony ankylosis of the temporomandibular joints: Case report of a child treated with Delrin condylar implants. J Oral Maxillofac Surg 1990;48: 861–865.

33. MacAfee KA, Quinn PD: Total temporomandibular joint reconstruction with Delrin titanium implant. J Craniofac Surg 1992;3:160–165.

34. Chase DC, Hudson JW, Gerard D, et al: The Christensen prosthesis—retrospective clinical study. Oral Surg Oral Med Oral Pathol 1995;80:273–278.

35. Kusy RP: Characterization of self-curing acrylic bone cements. J Biomed Mater Res 1978;12:271–305.

36. Miller J, Burke DL, Stachiewicz JW, et al: Pathophysiology of loosening of femoral components in total hip arthroplasty: Clinical and experimental study of cement fracture and loosening of the cement-bone interface. In The Hip: Proceedings of the Sixth Open Scientific Meeting of the Hip Society. St. Louis, CV Mosby, 1978, pp 64–86.

37. Goodman SB, Fornasier VL, Kei J: The effects of bulk versus particulate polymethylmethacrylate on bone. Clin Orthop 1988; 232:255–262.

38. Paiement G, Jasty M, Goldring S, et al: Difference in tissue response to particulate biomaterials (metals vs polymers) in a rabbit wound chamber model. Transactions of the 32nd meeting of the Orthopaedic Research Society, New Orleans, 1986, 11:115.

39. Herman JH, Sowder WG, Anderson D, et al: Polymethylmethacrylate-induced release of bone resorbing factors. J Bone Joint Surg 1989;71A:1530–1541.

40. Macrophage exposure to polymethylmethacrylate leads to mediator release and injury. J Orthop Res 1991;9:406–413.

41. McKee GK, Chen SC: The statistics of the McKee-Farrar method of total hip replacement. Clin Orthop 1973;95:26–33.

42. Breck LW: Metal to metal total hip joint replacement using the Urist socket: An end result study. Clin Orthop 1973;95:38–42.

43. Muller ME: The benefits of the metal-on-metal total hip replacements. Clin Orthop 1995;311:54–59.

44. Wilson JN, Scales JT: The Stanmore metal on metal total hip prosthesis using a three pin type cup: A follow-up of 100 arthroplasties over nine years. Clin Orthop 1973;95:239–249.

45. Haynes DR, Rogers SD, Hay S, et al: The differences in toxicity and release of bone-resorbing mediators induced by titanium and cobalt-chromium alloy wear particles. J Bone Joint Surg 1993; 75A:825–834.

46. Elves MW, Wilson JN, Scales JT, Kemp HB: Incidence of metal sensitivity in patients with total replacements. BMJ 1975;4:376–378.

47. Black J: Biological Performance of Materials: Fundamentals of Biocompatibility. New York, Marcel Dekker, 1992.

48. Lippincott AL, Chase D, Christensen R: Alternative total TMJ arthroplasty: Metal-on-metal for longevity in implant survivorship and patient satisfaction. Surg Technol Int 1998;7:1–10.

49. Mercuri LG, Wolford LM, Sanders B, et al: Custom CAD/CAM total temporomandibular joint reconstruction system: Preliminary multicenter report. J Oral Maxillofac Surg 1995;53:106–115.

50. Sonnenburg M, Sonnenburg I: Development and clinical application of the total temporomandibular joint endoprosthesis. Rev Stomatol Chir Maxillofac 1990;91:165.

51. McBride KL: Total temporomandibular joint reconstruction. In Worthington P, Evans JR (eds): Controversies in Oral and Maxillofacial Surgery. Philadelphia, WB Saunders, 1994, p 381.

52. Wolford LM, Cottrell DA, Henry CH: Temporomandibular joint reconstruction of the complex patient with the Techmedica custom-made total joint prosthesis. J Oral Maxillofac Surg 1994;52:2.

53. Charnley J: An artificial bearing in the hip joint: Implications in biological lubrication. Lubrication and Biomechanics 1966;25:1079–1081.

54. Estok D, Harris WH: Factors affecting cement strains near the tip of a cemented femoral component. J Arthroplasty 1997;12:40–48.

55. Lee IY, Skinner HB, Keyak JH: Effects of variation of prosthesis size on cement stress tip of a femoral implant. J Biomed Mater Res 1994;28:1055–1060.

56. Falkenström CA: Biomedical design of a total temporomandibular joint replacement. Thesis, University of Groningen, 1993.

57. Worthington P, Evans JR (eds): Controversies in Oral and Maxillofacial Surgery. Philadelphia, WB Saunders, 1994.

58. Smith AE, Robinson M: A new surgical procedure for the creation of a false temporomandibular joint in cases of ankylosis by means of a non-electrolytic metal. Am J Surg 1957;94:837.

59. House LR, Morgan DH, Wall WP: Temporomandibular joint surgery: Results of a 14-year joint implant study. Laryngoscope 1984;94:534.

60. Spiessl B: Erste Erfahrungen mit einer Kiefergelenkprothese. Fortschr Kiefer Gesichtschir 1976; 21:119.

61. Lindquist C, Soderholm AL, Hallikainen D, et al: Erosion and heterotopic bone formation after alloplastic temporomandibular joint reconstruction. J Oral Maxillofac Surg 1992;50:942.

62. Silver CM, Motamed M, Carlotti AE Jr: Arthroplasty of the temporomandibular joint with use of a Vitallium condyle prosthesis: Report of three cases. J Oral Surg 1977;35:909.

63. Raveh J, Geering AH, Sutter F, et al: Erste Erfahrungen mit einer neuen Kiefergelenkprothese, Vorläufige Resultate. SSO Schweiz Monatsschr Zahnheilkd 1982;92:681.

64. Flot F, Stricker M, Chassagne JF: Place de la prothèse intermédiaire a cupule non scellée dans la chirurgie reconstructive de l'articulation temporomandibulaire. Ann Chir Plast Esthet 1984;29:253.

65. Chassagne JF, Flot F, Stricker M, et al: Prothèse totale intermédiaire de l'articulation temporo-

mandibulaire: bilan apres 6 ans. Rev Stomatol Chir Maxillofac 1990;91:423.

66. Morgan DH: Development of alloplastic materials for temporomandibular joint prosthesis: A historical perspective with clinical illustrations. J Craniomandib Pract 1992;10:192.

67. Momma WG: Kombinierte autoplastisch-alloplastische Rekonstruction des Unterkiefers nach Hemimandibulektomie mit Exarticulation. Fortschr Kiefer Gesichtschir 1978;23:141.

68. Kummoona R: Functional rehabilitation of ankylosed temporomandibular joints. Oral Surg Oral Med Oral Pathol 1978;46:495.

69. Kent JN, Block MS, Halpern J, et al: Update on the Vitek partial and total temporomandibular joint systems. J Oral Maxillofac Surg 1993;51:408.

70. Sonnenburg I, Sonnenburg M: Total condylar prosthesis for alloplastic jaw articulation replacement. J Oral Maxillofac Surg 1985;13:131.

CHAPTER

18

Management of Failed Alloplastic Implants: Immunologic Considerations

Doran Ryan

The exact function of the articular disk of the temporomandibular joint is not known. It is thought that the disk itself functions as a shock absorber system and distributes forces over the head of the condyle and the articular eminence.[1, 2] The displacement or loss of this disk is associated with morphologic changes involving the mandibular condyle and the temporal bone. These can be as minor as flattening and broadening of the articular surfaces or as severe as loss of a major portion of a mandibular condyle. Along with the hard tissue changes, scarring of the joint with limited range of motion and even ankylosis can occur.[3–11] In order to prevent these changes and/or to replace lost bony structure, alloplastic materials, many of which have been used to replace other parts of the body, were designed or modified for use in the temporomandibular joint. Softer material such as silicone and Proplast/Teflon (P/T) was believed to function as a shock absorber system that could prevent remodeling or degenerative changes of the condyle and prevent adhesion formation that could limit range of motion.[4, 12–15] Advantages over autogenous tissues include ease of placement, lack of donor site morbidity, and decreased operating time.

The first alloplastic material placed in the temporomandibular joint was by Eggers in 1946.[16] He placed tantalum foil at the base of the skull and over the mandibular stump after a gap arthroplasty to try to prevent recurrent ankylosis. In 1957, Smith and Robinson[17] placed a curved steel plate between the temporal bone and the former mandibular condyle to prevent recurrence of bony ankylosis. This was the precursor to the temporomandibular joint fossa and eminence prostheses of Christenson and Morgan,[18, 19] which are still in use today. The history of partial and total joint replacement materials is not discussed in this chapter. Several of the individual alloplasts, including stainless steel, cobalt chrome alloy, titanium alloy, high-molecular-weight polyethylene, polymethylmethacrylate, silicone, and Proplast/Teflon (P/T), are evaluated as to cellular response and immunologic potential.

History of Alloplastic Usage in the Temporomandibular Joint

Table 18–1 gives a chronologic account of the history of silicone and Proplast/Teflon implant usage in the temporomandibular joint. The first report in the literature of silicone use in the temporomandibular joint is that of Robinson in 1969,[20] when he created a false joint using a silicone sponge fossa. First mention of the use of silicone as a disk substitute also occurred in 1969, when Henny[21] recommended that silicone

TABLE 18–1.	Chronologic History of Temporomandibular Silicone and Proplast/Teflon Implants

1960s	Silicone used in the TMJ		Aug. 1988	AAOMS position paper "Temporomandibular Joint Surgery"
1973	Vitek I Laminates first distributed		Mar. 1990	Vitek, Inc., voluntarily withdraws products
1976	Medical Device Amendment Required medical devices to be shown to be safe and effective; silicone was the standard for TMJ devices		Dec. 1990	FDA "Safety Alert" for Proplast implants
			Sept. 1991	FDA Public Health Advisory for all Vitek TMJ products
1978	FDA classified Proplast products as safe and effective		Oct. 1991	AAOMS Digest summary of FDA recommendations
1982	Vitek Kent I total joint placed; Proplast/Teflon II IPI manufactured		June 1992	Congressional hearings on TMJ implants
1983	Proplast/Teflon IPI classified as safe and effective		July 1992	"Parameters of Care for Oral and Maxillofacial Surgery," published by AAOMS
1984	"Criteria for TMJ Meniscus Surgery" published by AAOMS		Aug. 1992	AAOMS TMJ implant advisory; summary of FDA recommendations
1984	Silastic sheeting changed to high-performance sheeting; contrast added		Nov. 1992	AAOMS sponsored workshop on TMJ implants
1985	Wilkes temporary silicone implant produced		Jan. 1993	Dow Corning removes silicone sheeting from market
1988	Vitek Kent II total joint marketed		Oct. 1993	Published consensus report of workshop in JOMS "Recommendations for the Management of Patients with Temporomandibular Joint Implants"
			Sept. 1995	Second version of "Parameters of Care for Oral and Maxillofacial Surgery," published by AAOMS

sheets be used after condylectomy if the perforation of the meniscus were extensive. Dr. Henny[22] had been using silicone for this purpose for several years before the report. The first documented clinical and radiographic follow-up of interpositional silicone implants also appeared in 1969.[23] In that study, four patients, one with bilateral procedures, were followed after the implantation of a silicone sponge 3 to 4 mm thick, which was sewn to the capsular soft tissue structures after disk removal. At 3 years all patients demonstrated normal joint space with a slight decrease in motion of the condyle but without pain.

In 1970, Habbi and associates[24] described the creation of surgical fractures below the condyle in rabbits and placement of either silicone or Supramid as an interpositional material. The materials produced similar histologic results, with chronic inflammation the first week and then diminution with time such that minimal reaction was noted at 6 weeks. A fibrous connective tissue lining was observed around the pseudoarticulation. Detailed histologic information was not available. A follow-up study by Murnane and Doku[25] using the same rabbit population found capsular formation around the pseudoarticulation lined with synovial tissue and the presence of synovial fluid. A slight foreign body giant cell reaction was also noted.

In 1981, Sanders[26] presented a large series of silicone implants wired to the glenoid fossa. The early results were excellent. In 1984, Bessette[27] reported the results of polymeric silicone (Silastic) block implants sutured to the soft tissue of the temporomandibular joint after partial meniscectomy in humans and monkeys. Of the 62 patients treated, 87% obtained relief of symptoms and 62% had increased range of motion. In 4 of the 10 animals, only a mild tissue reaction was demonstrated. In the other 6 animals, mild to moderate chronic inflammation was seen only immediately adjacent to the implants. No adverse effects on condylar growth were noted. Ryan,[28] at the 1984 American Association of Oral and Maxillofacial Surgeons (AAOMS) Clinical Congress, reported an 89% success rate in 150 patients (185 joints) after meniscectomy and replacement with Dacron-reinforced silicone, which was wired or sutured to the glenoid fossa and articular eminence. The average follow-up was 1.5 years.

Criteria for temporomandibular joint (TMJ) meniscus surgery were published by AAOMS in 1984.[29] In that publication, the use of alloplasts as interpositional implants (IPIs) was recognized as an acceptable treatment. Around that same time, Dow Corning changed their Silastic sheeting to a high-performance material to prevent tearing of the implant under function. Contrast medium was also added to the material to improve visibility on plain film imaging. Merrill in 1986[4] reviewed 69 patients who had meniscectomy and Dacron-reinforced silicone sutured to the fossa and eminence and reported a 91% success rate. Dolwick and Aufdemorte[30] found a foreign body giant cell reaction around fragments of failed silicone implants dispersed throughout the tissues of eight patients. Furthermore, they identified the presence of cervical lymphadenopathy on the ipsilateral side of a silicone implant in the temporomandibular joint. A biopsy specimen showed a silicone-induced foreign body giant cell reaction in the lymph node. Wilkes,[31] as early as 1982, was using temporary silicone implants in the temporomandibular joint to help prevent postoperative adhesions after diskectomy or disk repair. This method was reported by Hall in 1985.[12] The Wilkes design of a high-performance silicone TMJ implant was marketed by Dow Corning in 1985. The

recommendation for that implant was as a temporary implant with removal 2 months postoperatively in disk repair procedures and after diskectomy. In a 1991 radiographic and clinical follow-up study, Wilkes[32] pointed out that the use of temporary silicone implants does not result in further joint damage over the long term. These findings differ from those of Ericksson and Westesson,[33] who found no positive clinical or radiographic effects of temporary silicone implants and questioned their use. Unfortunately, the Wilkes protocol of early removal was not followed in their study; the time from surgery until removal of the implant ranged from 1 to 25 months. High-performance silicone was used in only 3 of 22 joints.

By 1985, many surgeons had given up using permanent silicone and had gone to Proplast/Teflon laminates. Of the 47 surgeons surveyed,[34] only 5 surgeons were using permanent silicone implants, 2 others were using thin silicone sheets as a temporary implant, and 17 surgeons were using P/T IPIs after diskectomy. In 1985, Timmis and coworkers[35] compared silicone and P/T implants in the temporomandibular joints of rabbits. Many of the silicone implants became dislodged and wear particles were found throughout the soft tissue of the joint. The bone reaction was mild to moderate compared with the moderate to severe reaction secondary to the P/T implants.

Ryan[36] (1989) examined the results of the use of 1-mm Dacron-reinforced silicone implants (Fig. 18–1) or 1.3-mm P/T II (Figs.

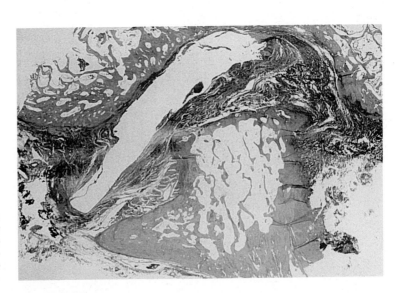

FIGURE 18–1. Sagittal section through the left TMJ of a monkey 15 months after diskectomy, silicone implant, and condylar shave. A connective tissue capsule surrounds the space occupied by the silicone.

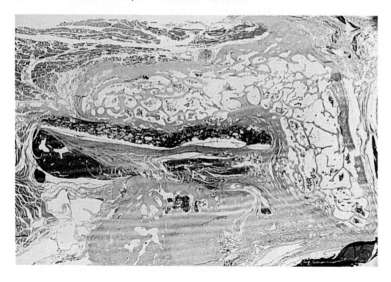

FIGURE 18–2. Sagittal section through the left TMJ of a monkey 15 months after diskectomy, P/T implant, and condylar shave. Note foreign body giant cell lesion anterior to condyle.

18–2 and 18–3) as disk replacement material in the joint of the *Macaca mulatta* monkeys. The joints were evaluated histologically at 15 months. A well-defined connective tissue capsule was found to surround all implants. All implants except one that was made from silicone were torn, and all showed varying degrees of wear. Microscopic fragments of the implants were found throughout the fibrous tissue capsule in all joints and in the marrow of the condyle of the two joints with silicone implants and one with a P/T implant. The fragments were surrounded by giant cells. In general, the foreign body giant cell reaction and bone destruction were much less intense with the silicone implants than the P/T II implants.

Tucker and Burke[37] evaluated the tempo-

rary use of 0.020-inch-thick silicone sheeting as a replacement after diskectomy and high condylar shave of the temporomandibular joint of four *Macaca fascicularis* monkeys. All implants were removed at 3 months and the animals were killed at 0, 1, 2, and 3 months after the removal. A fibrous connective tissue capsule around the silicone implant was found at all intervals. At 3 months after implant removal, no significant presence of inflammatory cell infiltrate was seen. These researchers found less bony degenerative change on the silicone side than on the controlled side. Bosanquet and coworkers[38] placed 2-mm-thick nonreinforced silicone sheeting as a disk replacement material in the temporomandibular joint of four merino sheep 20 weeks after

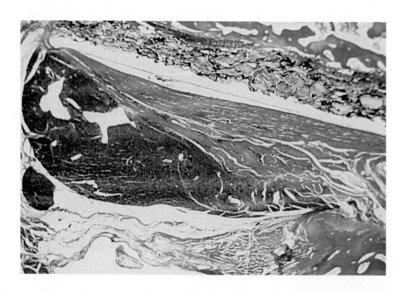

FIGURE 18–3. Higher magnification of same giant cell lesion seen in Figure 18–2. Also note temporal bone changes developing.

creation of a disk perforation. The implants were left for 40 weeks, then the animals were killed and the joints evaluated. All four joints exhibited a foreign body giant cell reaction; two joints had a severe destructive response and two had a less severe reaction. Silicone particles were found within the condyles of two animals. The author recommended reevaluation of the use of silicone as a long-term implant.

Clinical and radiographic evaluation of 20 silicone implants was undertaken by Bronstein.[39] Patients were generally pleased with the function although in many cases his criteria for success were not satisfied. Radiographic examination showed less disturbing bone erosion response than that seen with the P/T implants. He also pointed out that bony apposition and osteophyte formation may be seen in joints in which silicone implants have been placed. Regular and high-performance Silastic, with and without Dacron reinforcement, and Wilkes implants were removed from the market by Dow Corning in January 1993. Other companies continue to manufacture silicone sheeting. It was the consensus of the workshop on temporomandibular joint implant surgery, conducted by AAOMS in November 1992, that permanent placement of silicone as an interpositional material of the temporomandibular joint should no longer be done except when used to prevent recurrence of ankylosis. There was a diversity of opinion concerning the use of temporary silicone after discectomy. This 2 1/2-day workshop involved 21 experienced surgeons and 2 clinicians experienced in nonsurgical management of TMJ disorder. In addition, 6 experts in various aspects of biomaterials, orthopedics, TMJ radiography, and meta-analysis presented papers and attended as observers. The National Institute of Dental Research was also represented.

Proplast/Teflon

Proplast is the porous form of Teflon (polytetrafluoroethylene [PTFE]) and has been fused with either vitreous carbon (Proplast I) or aluminum oxide (Proplast II) and then laminated with Teflon. Teflon, a dense nonporous material, was used in 1960 by Charnley for total and partial hip replacements.[40] He measured the coefficient of friction between bone and substances commonly used in arthroplasty and concluded that the only solid that remotely approached articular cartilage was PTFE. Calnan, in 1963,[41] attempted to establish standards of quality for the use of foreign materials in reconstructive surgery. He pointed out that movement can be a problem and can ultimately lead to failure. He also evaluated tissue reactions to different materials, looking at macrophages, giant cells, and the fibrous reaction, including capsule formation around the implant. The PTFE was the least reactive. In fact, the smooth form was without giant cell reaction. Although PTFE produced less fibrous reaction than other materials, a complete capsule was formed. Calnan concluded that the "tissue reaction to PTFE is less than with any other material. For this reason it is recommended that the use of all less satisfactory materials be discontinued." The PTFE used in this study was not medical grade; it had been obtained from the Crain Packing Company.

In 1963, Leidholt and Gorman[42] conducted experiments on dogs having hip prosthesis with PTFE parts. The PTFE cup showed wear and deformation after an average of 8.7 months. The surrounding capsule and synovium were grossly thickened, and all animals showed acute and chronic inflammation of the joint tissues in which were found PTFE particles. Giant cells were frequent, indicating a foreign body reaction. Those investigators could not determine whether particle size or some characteristics of the local tissue were the principal factors in the reaction. Similar results were observed in an implant taken from a patient of one of these authors. Leidholt and Gorman thought PTFE should not be used in weight-bearing joints. Charnley and Kamangar[43] stopped using PTFE for hip sockets in 1963 and reported on the results in 1969. They stated that the most serious aspect of failure of PTFE was the production of tissue reactions by wear debris, which caused loosening of the socket by erosion of the bone. They believed the particles were produced too fast to be disposed of by the tissue. By 1972, Homsy[44] had developed Proplast; he believed that the pore size of the Proplast encouraged tissue ingrowth and therefore stability of the implant (Fig.

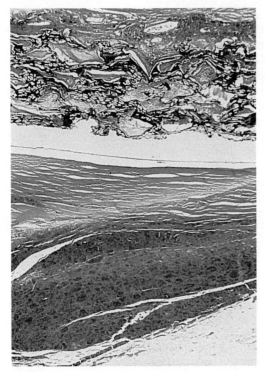

FIGURE 18–4. Same section as Figure 18–2 demonstrating fibrous growth into the Proplast and surrounding giant cell lesion.

18–4). The Proplast I was fused to the Teflon and used as an augmentation material as early as 1973. In 1975, Farrell and Kent[45] described its use as an interpositional material in the temporomandibular joint. Initially it was used after a high condylectomy sutured to the disk and/or condyle to maintain vertical stability and prevent adhesions. In 1982, Gallagher and Wolford[46] reported good results using 10 implants in the temporomandibular joint over the previous 4 years. These implants were placed between the condyle and the meniscus after condylectomy and wired to the condyle. Silicone was also used in the same manner in 9 joints, with 3 failures secondary to breakage of the ligature wire and herniation of the implant through the capsule. These authors felt that P/T was a better implant because of ingrowth of fibrous tissue, which led to better stability.

Clinical success of P/T IPI was highly touted in the early 1980s. Kiersch,[15] using P/T I and II as an interpositional material for both disk repair and disk replacement, reported a 93% success rate over 9 years for 250 implants. Carter,[47] at the 1983 national meeting of the AAOMS, reported an 87% success rate on 52 patients over a 3-year period using P/T as a meniscus replacement. In 1982, Proplast II replaced Proplast I as the material available. In 1986, Vitek, Inc. conducted a written survey[48] among oral and maxillofacial surgeons who perform TMJ surgery, to compare techniques and results. Among those 259 surgeons who used P/T, 5070 implants were placed with a 91.5% rate of satisfactory results. No guidelines for defining success were discussed. Moriconi and colleagues[49] identified P/T as "a more predictable mode of temporomandibular joint reconstruction." They pointed out that the ingrowth of tissue was of utmost importance. No results were presented.

Problems with P/T were first identified in writing by this author in a temporomandibular joint newsletter from the Medical College of Wisconsin in 1985.[50] On recall examination, the development of an anterior open bite was noted in 20% of the patients, as was occasional continued degeneration of the condyles. The cause of this problem was not identified. Timmis and coworkers[35] reported at the AAOMS annual meeting in 1985 an animal study that showed when the meniscus was replaced with P/T II, there was marked osteoclastic activity with resorption and severe degenerative changes in both the condyles and the glenoid fossa. Implant tearing was seen in 46% of the joints. Lagotteria and colleagues, in 1986,[51] reported regional lymph node involvement with collection of Teflon particles, multinucleated giant cells, histocytes, and granulation tissue (Fig. 18–5). Breakdown of a Proplast I implant with perforation and extensive giant cell reaction was found in the ipsilateral temporomandibular joint. The largest particle found in the node was a carbon fiber of 42 μm. P/T fragments were only a few microns in diameter. Bony changes were noted in 11 of 12 joints examined by Heffez and colleagues.[52] Despite these signs of failure, few symptoms of failure were noted. In 1988, Florine and coworkers[53] followed up 55 PTFE and 18 discoplasty treated joints for 20 months and 48 months, respectively. More than 60% of the joints of P/T implants showed severe destructive osseous changes, whereas none of the joints managed by discoplasty showed any changes. The authors speculated that when the size and number of particles exceed the capacity

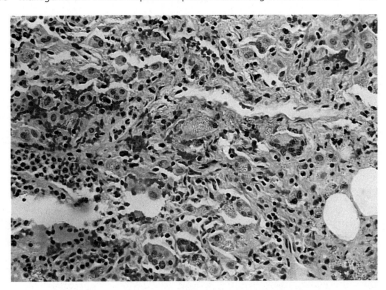

FIGURE 18–5. Multiple fragments of P/T particles found in histiocytes and foreign body giant cells of an ipsilateral preauricular lymph node in a patient with a failed P/T IPI. (Courtesy of Scott N. Levin, D.D.S., Milwaukee, Wisconsin.)

of the lymphatic system to remove them, the reaction in the joints themselves would be one of destructive arthritis. The patient's comfort, function, and satisfaction were high and did not correlate with the condyle degeneration. Schelhas and associates[54] reported two cases of failed P/T implants with erosion through the temporal bone to the dura of the middle cranial fossa. Others have reported similar findings with dura perforation possible.[55–60] In 1990, Estabrooks and coworkers[61] reported on a retrospective review of 301 diskectomies with P/T IPI replacements. The overall success was 88.7% with an average follow-up of 33 months. These results were much better than those reported by others. The authors believed that the results were improved by wiring the implants in place and preventing early function of the joint. The follow-up and radiographic techniques used were not standardized. Vitek, Inc. voluntarily withdrew the P/T products from the market in March 1990.[62] In December, the U.S. Food and Drug Administration (FDA) issued a "Safety Alert" for the Vitek IPI, followed by a Public Health Advisory for all Vitek TMJ products in September 1991.[63] In 1992, a multicenter retrospective evaluation conducted via survey was published.[64] Of 680 P/T IPIs, 86% were still in place an average of 33 months later. However, 249 of the 584 joints with implants still in place showed some degree of condyle resorption, whereas only 24 of those patients had symptoms of failure. In 1992, Fontenot and Kent[65] investigated the in vitro wear performance of 1.3-mm P/T IPIs used in a mechanical TMJ simulator. The joints were loaded with a 20-pound force. Implant failure was categorized into three phases: thinning, deformation, and cold flow with thinning leading to fracture and accelerated wear with fracture fragmentation and particulation of the underlying Proplast. The authors predicted an in vivo service life of 757 days. They suggested that this short service life could be further reduced by parafunctional habits and overuse of the jaw. With load, the Proplast was found to collapse, reducing the porosity from 80% to less than 50%, a detriment to stabilization. Feinerman and Piecuch[66] followed up 23 P/T IPIs in a 1993 study in which there were 18 failures with an average removal time of 4 years and 9 months. The other 5 implants also had clinical and radiographic evidence of failure. They recommended removal of all P/T IPIs. Ryan,[67] in a letter to the editor, made the same recommendations. The 1992 workshop did not reach consensus on prophylactic removal of P/T IPIs but did recommend removal if the patient had progressive signs and symptoms of implant failure.

Review of Immunology

The human immune system is extremely complex. Elements of the immune system include not only the contributions of the humoral response of B lymphocytes and cell mediated response of the T lymphocytes, but also the acute and chronic inflammatory responses, the actions of complement, and the pervasive role of macrophages in each of the components (Fig. 18–6). Separate elements of immunity are interdependent on one another in terms of activation, potentiation, and modulation of their roles in host immunity through direct interaction and by remote control via secretion of cytokines. The immune system must be able to distinguish between self and nonself and mount the appropriate attack against the nonself antigens. An aberrant immune system reacts against self antigens and is believed to play a critical role in such autoimmune disorders as rheumatoid arthritis and systemic lupus erythematosus or other connective tissue diseases. How the immune system reacts to a particular alloplast determines its biocompatibility. Once the alloplast particulates, the response mustered by the immune system determines whether it is then a local reaction or systemic reaction that could lead to autoimmune disease.

Cell Types

Macrophages that are derived from monocytes are found throughout the body in normal tissues, not in response to inflammation, but to phagocytizing (ingesting) of bacteria or dead cells. Histiocytes are macrophages in connective tissue. Osteoclasts are also derived from circulating monocytes and are generally associated with bone resorption. Macrophages may also play a direct and an indirect role in

bone resorption. Contact between wandering macrophages and a foreign substance may occur by chance or by chemotaxis. When the macrophages make contact with a foreign material, they try to ingest the substance. At the same time, the substance is presented to the lymphocytes for possible initiation of an immune response. If the macrophages cannot ingest the material because of size, they fuse together, forming multinucleated giant cells, which then surround the particles. The macrophage can also release lysosome enzymes, which include acid hydrolases, natural proteases, and mediators of inflammation, including prostaglandin, complement lymphocyte activating factor, and fibroblast stimulating activity.

B cell lymphocytes mediate the humoral immunity by differentiating into plasma cells that secrete antigen specific antibodies (immunoglobulins) (Fig. 18–7). The immunoglobulins activate the complement system, which facilitates recognition of foreign materials and signals, stimulates, and mediates other components of the immune system. B cells can also present antigens directly to the T cells.

T cells are the major circulating lymphocytes. In the cell mediated immunity response (Fig. 18–8), T lymphocytes differentiate and proliferate in response to contact with an antigen and subsequently attack and kill the invading pathogens. A T lymphocyte may encounter the antigen directly or through interaction with a macrophage that has phagocytized the pathogen and acts as an antigen presenting cell. The first step in T-cell activation by an antigen is the appropriate processing of the antigen by the antigen presenting cells. Soluble antigens

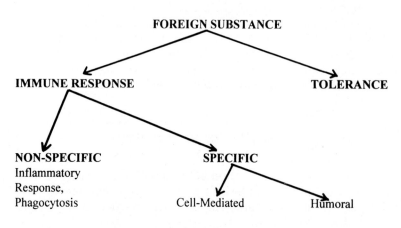

FIGURE 18–6. The body's response to the introduction of a foreign substance.

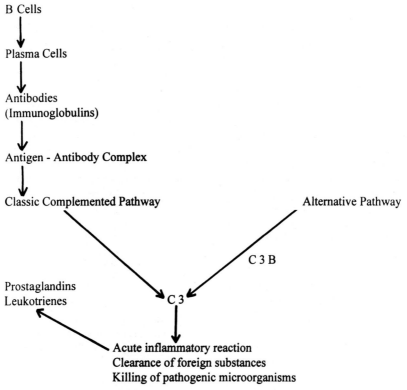

FIGURE 18–7. The humoral immune response to a foreign substance.

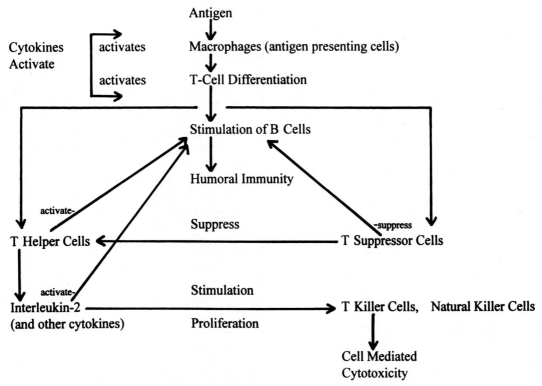

FIGURE 18–8. The cell mediated immune response to a foreign substance.

are physically taken up by the specialized antigen presenting cells, which include the macrophages and B lymphocytes. The antigens are degraded and a portion of the degraded antigen is then expressed on the cell surface. T cells, through secretion of lymphokines (i.e., interleukins and interferons), also modulate the inflammatory response. Three types of T cells are important to the immune reaction. The T killer cells are involved in direct cell destruction. T suppressor cells are available to suppress B-cell formation and therefore decrease immunoglobulin production. T helper cells stimulate B-cell production, increasing the immunoglobulin production, and stimulate production of interleukin-2, which stimulates proliferation of T killer cells. Another component of the cell mediated response is manifested in the role of natural killer cells. These are distinct lymphocytic cell lines that function to lyse host cells that exhibit nonself-membrane labeling. They constitute 5% to 20% of circulating lymphocytes in adults and may form the first line of defense. Interleukin-2 can cause proliferation of natural killer cells in the absence of other stimuli. Natural killer cells are believed to develop in the bone marrow similarly to B cells, whereas the T cells are formed in the thymus. Immunoglobulins, antibodies formed in the response to antigens, fix complement and initiate the enzymatic complement cascade. The importance of each immunoglobulin is outlined in Table 18–2.

T cells, B cells, macrophages, and fibroblasts can produce a variety of immunologically active substances called *cytokines*. Cytokines are glucoproteins that are active in very low concentrations that have the ability to influence the production, proliferation, and differentiation of numerous classes of lymphocytes including T cells and B cells. These cytokines are thought to be important in the regulation of immunity and chronic inflammation. These include the interleukins, of which there are at least eight; necrosis factors alpha and beta; interferons; and others that play either an unknown or a smaller role in the immunologic response.

Tissue Response to Implant Materials

The most common materials used recently within the temporomandibular joint

TABLE 18–2.	**Major Immunoglobulins and Their Function**

IgG

Most predominant immunoglobulin
Responsible for secondary (recall) immune response
Attaches to macrophages and B-cell receptors to facilitate phagocytosis

IgM

Responsible for primary immune response
Rapidly replaced by IgG
Most efficient Ig for activation of complement system

IgA

Ig for all mucosal surfaces
20% of circulating serum immunoglobulins
Found in body secretions

IgD

Receptor on B lymphocytes
Trace amounts in serum; actual function unknown
May help stimulate B lymphocytes to produce antibodies

IgE

Elevated level in immediate hypersensitivity reactions
Binds to receptors on mast cells and basophils
Causes release of histamines and other vasoactive substances
Response is amnestic: i.e., repeat exposure to antigen causes increasing reaction

include the solid form of silicone, P/T, chrome cobalt alloy, titanium alloy, high-molecular-weight polyethylene, polymethylmethacrylate, and stainless steel. All of these products were thought to be biocompatible in the body in the preformed design. Particulation of these materials stimulates a different tissue response. How the body manages this particulation appears to be the key to the length of success of the individual alloplasts. All known alloplasts used in joint reconstruction have a wear rate that can be adversely affected by the coefficient of friction of the particular material, excessive stress of overloading, lack of lubrication, damage to the surface of the implants during surgical implantation, movement of the implant against the irregular bony surface, and contamination of the surface of the implant during production or during preparation for placement. Aging of material and absorption of proteins, lipids, and other organic compounds onto the surface or into the body of the implant also alter the physical and chemical properties of the implant immediately and over time.[68]

After implantation of an alloplast, the normal healing process consists of acute inflammation followed by an ingrowth of fibroblasts and blood vessels. Next comes phagocytosis of surgical tissue debris by histiocytes (macrophages found in connective tissue), polymorphonuclear leukocytes, macrophages, and their aggregate foreign body giant cells. Finally, reorganization of the normal tissues of the joint takes place. In addition to the normal healing process, the body must cope with the implant and the chemical components left over from the manufacturing techniques, sterilization residue, and handling of the implant during surgery. The tissue response to these components consists of a foreign body reaction with the development of a fibrous encapsulation of the implant and the continued appearance of foreign body giant cells until the phagocytosis is completed.[69–71] Normal healing time in a human is around 8 to 10 weeks. As wear particles develop, the tissue responds by the activation of histiocytes. The histiocytes attempt to reduce and digest these particles. If the particles cannot be eliminated or digested, the process of healing recurs around each particle, causing encapsulation or proliferation of granulation tissue. Wear particles are digested by histiocytes if the diameter is 5 μm or less.[68] The larger particles are surrounded by foreign body giant cells.[72] Transportation of particles away from the site of formation can occur through lymphatic vessels. Particles as large as 80 μm have been transported in this fashion. Filtration occurs in the lymph nodes, where storage of particles takes place[30, 73, 74] (see Fig. 18–5). The largest particle from a TMJ implant found in a lymph node is 42 μm.[75] If a state of stability occurs, that is, particles are encapsulated, digested, or transported as fast as they are formed, damage to surrounding tissue is minimal.

However, if the body is unable to maintain the status quo, acute and chronic inflammation develops. Macrophages release prostaglandins, complement, lymphocyte activating factor, and degradative enzymes such as acid hydrolases and neutral proteinases that activate osteoclasts to resorb bone.[76–81] This reaction continues until the implant fails and is finally removed. The severity of the inflammatory response is influenced by many factors, including the characteristics of the particles, the number of particles, the rate of production, and the clearance of particles. The principal characteristics of the particles involved are their chemical composition, size, shape, and solubility. Other factors such as hypersensitivity or immunologic status of the patient also influence the tissue response. Milam and colleagues[81] demonstrated that implant particles are rapidly coated with proteins. How the cells perceive these distorted proteins on the surface of the particles determines the extent of the inflammatory response. If this hypothesis is true, then again size and shape of the particle determine the intensity of the reaction.

Immunologic Response to Synthetic Material

HYPERSENSITIVITY REACTIONS

The common sensitizers nickel, cobalt, chromium, and acrylics and the potential sensitizers titanium, aluminum, and polyethylene are all used in the development of alloplastic materials for the TMJ. The most common sensitivity is to nickel, caused by corrosion or leaching of ions from metals in direct skin contact.[82] Nickel sensitivity is more common in females than in males and is attributed to the metals used in jewelry such as earrings, watches, snaps, and fasteners. Sensitivity to chrome is very common in the general population and usually results from contact with stainless steel, which is 18% to 20% chromium.[83] Chromium is also found in cleaning fluids and cements.[84] Sensitivity to titanium is uncommon because contact with titanium ions or corroding titanium is uncommon.[85] Sensitivity to polyethylene is unlikely because polyethylene is composed only of carbon, hydrogen, and oxygen; however, in the process of manufacturing these materials, metal catalysts are used that could trigger a reaction. With particulation of the polyethylene, these metal ions could be released and initiate sensitivity reactions.[86]

Polymethylmethacrylate (PMMA), especially the monomer methylmethacrylate, is a known sensitizer to dentists; sensitivity in the general population results from the use of glues and adhesives that contain PMMA.[87] Allergies to denture materials do occur. Aluminum has been documented in the literature as a sensitizing agent.[88, 89] Since the titanium alloys contain 6% aluminum, sensitivity to this material is a possibility. Sensitivity to metals was a major issue in the orthopedic community around 1970. Most total joints at the time were metal on metal. Many orthopedic surgeons switched to metal against polyethylene because of concern about allergic reactions to the metals, secondary to metallosis.[90–92] The first total hips were made of 316 stainless steel; they were corrosion resistant and contained approximately 12% to 14% nickel. It was evident that nickel was released but in small amounts.[93] Eventually cobalt chromium alloys with a nickel content of only 1% replaced the stainless steel. The cobalt chrome alloy contains 18% to 20% chromium, which can also initiate a sensitivity reaction. Even though cobalt chrome alloys are corrosion resistant, leaching of the metals does occur with wear. There is no question a patient can exhibit a sensitivity response to an implant device.[94–96] But what is the clinical significance?

In investigating the magnitude of the problem, Merritt and Brown,[97] using blood tests to document sensitivity, came to several conclusions. A sensitivity to one or more of the metals can develop during use of the total joint replacement. Rashes and allergy symptoms may have been associated with the presence of the allergy but were not the actual cause of implant failure. There was no correlation between sensitivity and the reason for removal. Pain was the primary reason for removal of all devices; there was no higher incidence in the allergic group. In a few cases in which the symptoms of sensitivity were thought to be the reason for removal of the device, analysis of the peri-implant tissue revealed the presence of lymphocytes and metal debris. Titanium and chromium were the most prevalent. The recommendation from this study is that there is no reason to deviate from a normal surgical decision because the patient is known to be allergic to metal. However, patients who have reactions to previous implants are more likely to have problems with other implants than nonallergic patients are. Manifestations of allergic reactions did not occur for 6 months to 1 year. Nickel and chromium were the most frequent sensitizers.

In a study by Merritt and Rodrigo,[98] blood cell migration tests were used to determine the immune sensitivity. These tests were accomplished preoperatively and 3 to 12 months later. Of the patients, 26% experienced a positive response after placement of the implants. In seven patients, there were four sensitivities to titanium, two to cobalt, four to chromium, and one to nickel. The investigators concluded that there are documented instances in which sensitivity reactions have necessitated premature removal of implants, but the best that they could determine is that the incidence is small, probably less than 1%. Those data suggested that a positive immune response is not a significant predictor of a total joint survivorship. They believe that cobalt chrome alloys are safe in nickel sensitive patients and the likelihood of a reaction is very small. A patient who has had a reaction to a previous implant runs a higher but still small risk of having a sensitivity reaction that would necessitate premature removal of the total joint system. Patients who have symptoms of sensitivity reaction to an interpositional implant need to base their decision on removal on the degree and the discomfort of the reaction. They should also consult a dermatologist or allergist to see whether some possible therapeutic agents could be used to minimize the symptoms. If the implant is removed, using an implant of different materials may be a possibility. Rooker and Wilkinson[99] patch tested their patients before and after hip replacement with stainless steel high-density polyethylene prostheses. Of the six patients who had a positive reaction to nickel, chromium, or cobalt, five had a negative reaction to these metals after the operation. Induction of immunologic tolerance may thus be a possible additional benefit of alloplastic implants. Trumpy and Lyberg,[100] having found aluminum in the microfragments of P/T IPIs, suggested that there may be toxic and hypersensitive reactions to aluminum involved in the pathogenesis of bone destruction with these implants. Hypersensitivity reactions to elements of any TMJ implant have not been investigated as of this date.

TISSUE RESPONSE TO SILICONE

There are a wide variety of silicones available for implantation. Silicones are a family of silicon dioxide polymers that differ in the addition of organic side chains, polymer length, use of fillers, and degree of cross-linking.

The siloxane polymer backbone combines silicon and oxygen (SiO) in a flexible molecular linkage. Curing is undertaken with catalysts (i.e., platinum) to form cross-linking of the polymer chains, resulting in solid silicone rubbers or elastomers. Fumed amorphous silica is added to increase tensile strength. Silicones have been chosen as materials for implantable devices because they are chemically inert and were previously thought to be biologically inert. Several recent review articles have addressed the biocreativity of silicones, and it is clear that they do not completely fulfill the requirements of ideal synthetic soft tissue substitutes.[101]

The speculated causal association between implanted dimethylpolysiloxane, in the form of mammary silicone gel filled implants (SGFIs), and autoimmune disorders has triggered numerous scientific and clinical studies in an attempt to clarify this issue. As yet, there is no evidence to suggest that a chemically induced autoimmune disease occurs.[102] However, there are reports in the literature, both experimental and clinical, that suggest that some individuals may experience an exaggerated local or systemic response to implanted SGFIs.[103] The outer envelope of these implants is composed of silicone elastomer. Silicone elastomer implantable joint prostheses were introduced at about the same time as SGFIs.

Because there is no clear clinical evidence supporting an association of any of these substances with immune reactions, and since it has been previously suggested that the shorter polymer length forms are nonimmunogenic and chemically nonreactive,[104] it is important to be specific regarding these issues. Conclusions drawn regarding observations of one form of silicone may not be directly applicable to other forms. Of most interest to oral and maxillofacial surgeons are the results obtained when silicone elastomers are used in TMJ or facial reconstructive surgery. However, it is useful to review studies including the various forms of silicone to obtain a better understanding of the host response.

The local tissue reactions to various silicones have been studied and are remarkably similar. Andrews[105] described the following reaction to injected silicone fluid in mice: A mild exudative phase is seen in the first 3 days, consisting of polymorphonuclear cells, a few plasma cells, and macrophages surrounding empty spaces thought to contain silicone. This then changes to a predominance of lymphocytes, fibroblasts, and plasma cells. Intracellular silicone was also described in polymorphonuclear cells, monocytes, and macrophages, and the persistence of microparticles of silicone leads to the development of a foreign body granulomatous reaction characterized by silicon-containing giant cells (Fig. 18–9). The interaction of macrophages containing silicon and lymphocytes was demonstrated by electron microscopy.[106] This study also showed evidence of an in vivo cellular immune response to silicone gel in sensitized guinea pigs, using a macrophage migration inhibition model. Histologic observation of the cortex of lymph nodes showed a pronounced interaction between lymphocytes and macrophages with silicon containing vacuoles at the terminals of the cytoplasmic bridges. The histologic reaction at the silicone site was characterized by chronic inflammatory reaction (consisting of polymorphonuclear cells, some lymphocytes, and foreign body giant cells) and a more striking collection of lymphocytes, plasma cells, and giant cells with ingested silicone.

The encapsulation by a foreign body reaction leading to "capsule" or "pseudocapsule" formation, although detrimental in breast surgery, can be of benefit in patients requiring TMJ meniscectomy. These capsules are mostly acellular and well vascularized, with a predominance of type III collagen.[107] Temporary silicone elastomer sheeting prevents direct scarring between the fossa and condyle. This is necessary for the preservation of both rotational and translatory movements and can give stable postoperative results for many years.[108]

If silicones gain access to the reticuloendothelial system, there is potential for an immune response. The transportation of silicones can occur via the lymphatic system or phagocytic cells. Although there is no direct evidence documenting the migration of silicone polymers through the lymphatics, the presence of silicon-like and silicone-like particles in lymph nodes has been documented after mammoplasty, silicone rubber

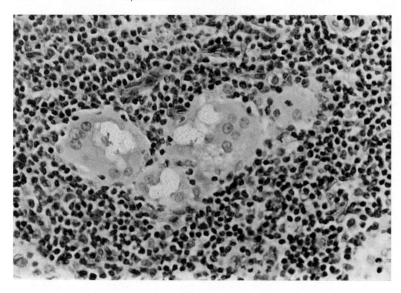

FIGURE 18–9. Foreign body giant cells containing silicone particles.

temporomandibular joint meniscal replacement, and various other joint arthroplasties.[30, 108] Implants for use in small joint arthroplasties were introduced by Swanson in the mid-1960s. Khoo[109] reviewed the role of silicone elastomer implants in small joint reconstruction of the upper extremity. Silicone synovitis is a recognized complication of these implants and is characterized by pain, stiffness, and swelling at the site of silicone joint replacement arthroplasty after initial relief of symptoms. Similar reactions have been described for silicone sheeting used as a TMJ interposition and for orbital reconstruction with similar complications.[110, 111] In his review, Khoo[109] states that immunologic reactivity and development of soft tissue autoantibodies have not been causally linked to the presence of silicone implants, and that it is much more likely that the silicone synovitis is a nonspecific reaction (see Fig. 18–6) to particulate material. There is no reported incidence of connective tissue disease following the implantation of silicone elastomer devices (including finger joints, ventriculoperitoneal shunts, and intraocular lenses). Although it has been stated that "the polymeric and hydrophobic characteristics of silicone and the presence of electrostatic charges and organic side groups make it a potentially ideal immunogen,"[101] there is experimental evidence to suggest that the host response to silicones is a nonspecific response (see Fig. 18–6) without an immune component.[107] There are also clinical and experimental

data to suggest that the response is antigen specific, has immunologic memory, and is cell mediated (see Fig. 18–8). Clinical data that are supportive of an antigen specific immune response have been found in the immunohistochemical analysis of periprosthetic capsular tissues from patients with SGFIs.[112] Antibody staining was present in tissue from 96% of the patients. The cellular infiltrate in the capsular tissue was relatively constant, consisting primarily of macrophages and T helper cells. The authors state that this suggests that silicone gel implants incite an antigen specific immune response rather than a nonspecific foreign body reaction. Experimentally, silicone gel was shown to induce an in vitro T-cell proliferative response in certain strains of inbred mice.[113] In sheep previously exposed to silicone gel, an in vivo antigen specific, lymphocyte mediated response to silicone gel, suggestive of delayed hypersensitivity, was demonstrated.[114] Both genetic and environmental factors may play a significant role in the magnitude of these responses.[103]

In summary, the present state of knowledge suggests that silicones can obtain access to the reticuloendothelial system, immune responses to various forms of silicone may occur, and these responses may occur in a subset of patients subject to environmental factors. A well defined foreign body response occurs, leading to encapsulation of silicone elastomer implants with development of a progressive synovitis with bone and implant degradation. Only anecdotal evidence supporting adverse immune responses in patients with silicone gel implants without evidence of autoimmune disease compared to patients with silicone elastomer implants is documented. Silicones are not ideal alloplasts but provide the most useful, if only temporary, IPIs available for TMJ surgery.

Tissue Response to Proplast/Teflon

All studies to date have shown a different reaction to the particulation of P/T than to the other alloplasts used in the temporomandibular joint. The particle size appears to vary greatly, and the shape exposes more surface area than with other materials (Fig. 18–10). Zardeneta and coworkers[81] have demonstrated a protein interaction with the surface of the particulate Teflon. This coating of protein onto these particles happens very rapidly, and the protein can be structurally distorted. They speculate that cells such as macrophages respond to this distortion of the proteins and release cytokines, enzymes, and free radicals, which may well amplify the inflammatory response. There is the possibility that these distorted proteins on the P/T particles may be recognized as foreign or nonself, thus provoking an immune response. Bonfield and coworkers[115] evaluated this macrophage response to proteins absorbed onto the surface of the poly-

mers in vitro. These proteins influence the interaction of monocytes and macrophages with the polymer surface. Different proteins appear to elicit different responses in terms of cytokine production. Therefore, not only do different proteins elicit different monocyte and macrophage responses, but different cytokines are produced in response to a specific combination of proteins and polymers. Again, because of the unusual shapes of the P/T particles, they allow more total surface area to be exposed. Kulber and colleagues[116] in 1995 reported on a severe cutaneous foreign body giant cell reaction that had spread from the temporomandibular joint from a fragmented P/T IPI. The reaction eventually encompassed the entire cheek; foreign material that appeared to be Proplast was found in the subcutaneous fat and dermis. This required a radical resection of the soft tissue over the cheek and a skin graft to cover the defect. Because of the presence of particles of Proplast in the 50- to 100-μm range, this reaction was not considered an immunologic reaction but a severe foreign body giant cell inflammatory reaction that had spread from the TMJ.[117] To this date, Proplast has been identified in the regional lymph nodes, parotid gland, and subcutaneous dermis and epidermis surrounding the temporomandibular joint. But no particles have been found beyond this area.

Trumpy and associates[118] in 1996 investigated the cellular tissue response to P/T IPI by morphologic and immunohistochemical

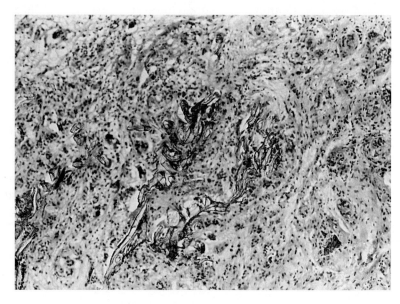

FIGURE 18–10. Irregular shards of Proplast/Teflon of various sizes surrounded by macrophages, foreign body giant cells, and fibrous tissue.

means. Using a panel of leukocyte antibodies, both monoclonal and polyclonal, they found that CD68 positive monoclonal derived cells dominated the reactive infiltrate, indicating that the reaction was a histocytic macrophage and giant cell reaction with release of lysosomes. The lymphocytic infiltrate contained no B cells. They concluded that the P/T IPI induced tissue reaction gave no indication of a toxic or an immunologic pathogenesis. Namey and coworkers[119] looked at the possible relationship between certain arthropathies and increased incidence of specific human leukocyte antigen (HLA). They performed HLA typing on patients with TMJ dysfunction and failed P/T implants. Working on the hypothesis that an increased incidence of HLA markers could be associated with a predisposition to connective tissue and autoimmune diseases, he found that his patient population showed an increase in the number of HLA markers as compared to those of a control subject group. These were markers to psoriasis and psoriatic arthritis, juvenile rheumatoid arthritis, sarcoidosis, ankylosing spondylitis, Reiter's syndrome, Sjögren's syndrome, scleroderma, Still's disease, and systemic lupus erythematosus, among other conditions. The authors suggested that a predisposition to connective tissue and autoimmune diseases may lead to immune dysfunction and treatment failure. Wolford and colleagues[120] did a preliminary study evaluating the human immunologic response to P/T implants in 12 patients. Total lymphocyte count was calculated and an immune response assessed by immunophenotyping peripheral blood lymphocytes. The 1A subset was below that of controls, and 73% of patients had CD4:CD5 ratios that were significantly below the normal range. The CD56 subset was elevated in 60% of the patients. They also found lymphocytic activity consisting of activated T-cell response in 4 of 6 patients evaluated. The immunologic consequence of the activated T-cell response remains to be investigated. T-cell lymphocytes represent a recognition response to the immunogen whether the latter is silicone or P/T particles, a denatured protein in association with these particles, or some other unknown substance. Suggestive evidence for this concept is the presence of a significant population of helper T cells in association with antigen processing macrophages. However, the presence of T-cell lymphocytes alone is not evidence that an active immune response is ongoing because of the possibility that large numbers of suppressor T cells also may be present. Yih and Merrill[55] found few lymphocytes in the tissue surrounding silicone or P/T failed implants.

In a continuing investigation at the Medical College of Wisconsin, the humoral and cellular-mediated tissue response in humans is being studied by obtaining tissue from either the capsule surrounding the silicone implant or the granulomas formed in response to the breakdown of P/T implants.[121] The patients being studied are those who have undergone placement of permanent silicone or P/T implants into the temporomandibular joint and who have experienced symptoms requiring their removal. A portion of the specimen is routinely processed and stained with hematoxylin and eosin. The remainder of the tissue is used for immunologic studies. Humoral response is assessed with use of fluorochrome-labeled monochromal antibodies against immunoglobulin G (IgG), IgM, IgA, fibron, and C3 complement. The presence of these proteins in these tissues is recorded. Cell mediated response is assessed with use of monoclonal antibodies to determine lymphocyte lineage. B-cell lineage is determined by a positive L26 marker, and T-cell lineage is assessed with MT1 and UCHL-1 markers in serial sections. Histologic and immunologic evaluation of the tissue surrounding 12 silicone implants and 32 P/T implants has been completed. All antibody studies of these tissues had negative results; no immunologically related proteins were found. The cell mediated response has been more difficult to evaluate. Small numbers of B cells and T-cell lymphocytes along with suppressor and helper T cells were found, but because of the low numbers of these lymphocytes no consistent ratios could be established. The low numbers of lymphocytes suggest that no cell-mediated immunity occurs. The tissue deposition of the immunoglobulins expected to be present if the humoral immunity response had been mounted against the materials was not present. Similarly, no deposits of C3 were demonstrated. The absence of activated complement is further evidence against humoral immunity activity since antibody-antigen complexes are the most potent initiators of the classic pathway of complement. If humoral immunity played a role in the formation of chronic and foreign body giant cells, granuloma deposition of both immunoglobulins and complement would be expected to be demonstrable in the peri-implant tissues. The fact that these were not present suggests that some process other than humoral immunity is responsible for the clinical manifestations caused by the breakdown of these implants under function in the temporomandibular joint. At present, no cause-and-effect relationship between associated immune disorders and these implants appears to exist. Sex hormones are known to affect the immune response. The influence of sex hormones, such as estrogen and prolactin, on the foreign body response to particle disease may be important.[122–126] In a paper presented by Milam,[127] a rat-pouch model was used in which 50 mg of 50- to 300-μm sized particles of PTFE were placed. The cellular response to particulated P/T was similar to the human reaction, but observers found significantly greater numbers of multinucleated giant cells in the female as compared to the male rats.

Tissue Response to Other Alloplasts

The other alloplasts used in the TMJ are components of total joint systems studied for many years by the orthopedic community. Pandey and associates[128] evaluated the tissue response to particulates of titanium, stainless steel, chrome cobalt, high-density polyethylene (HDP), and PMMA. The subcutaneous lesions produced by the particles were partially or completely surrounded by fibrous tissue that was thicker around implanted PMMA and HDP particles than around metal particles. The heaviest macrophage and giant cell response was seen in granulomas formed in response to implanted PMMA and HDP (Figs. 18–11 and 18–12). Looking at the resorptive activities of the granulomas around the different types of particulation, they were able to show that the greatest percentage of bone resorption was associated with macrophages in the granuloma of the PMMA and, in descending order, HPD, titanium, chrome cobalt, and then stainless steel. Resorption associated with PMMA granuloma derived macrophages was significantly greater than that of macrophages associated with HDP, titanium, chrome cobalt, and stainless steel granulomas. Resorptive association with HPD and titanium granuloma–derived macrophages was also significantly greater than that of macrophages derived from chrome cobalt and stainless steel granulomas. Irrespective of the type of biomaterial implanted, the mononuclear phagocytes elicited in this foreign body response were all capable of differentiating into cells capable of extensive bone resorption. Thus, wear particles shed from all biomaterials commonly used in joint replacement surgery must be regarded as having the potential to form the focus of a macrophage response

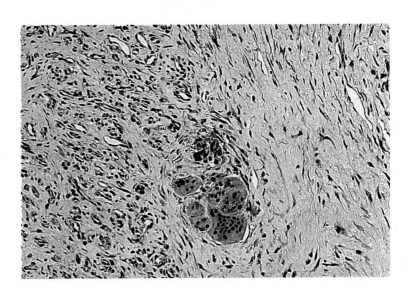

FIGURE 18–11. Foreign body giant cell reaction to PMMA from a Christensen total joint implant. (Courtesy of David Datillo, D.D.S., Pittsburgh, Pennsylvania.)

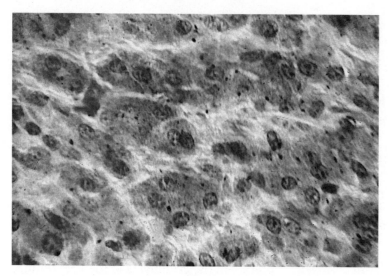

FIGURE 18–12. Many small HDP particles imparting a pink, granular appearance to the cytoplasm of the macrophages and foreign body giant cells. (Courtesy of Jeffrey Toth, Ph.D., Director of Biomaterials Research, Medical College of Wisconsin, Milwaukee, Wisconsin.)

from which aseptic loosening can result. Others[129–131] found a difference between the high-density polyethylene particles and the cobalt chrome particles. Polyethylene debris appeared to stimulate osteoclastic bone resorption, whereas the cobalt chrome debris showed evidence of hyalodegeneration and cell necrosis, suggesting a toxic effect.

The inertness of titanium alloy is greatly enhanced by the in vivo formation of a stable oxide surface layer, usually to a depth of 10 nm.[132] This has improved the wear resistance and hardness. The process of implanting nitrogen ions on the surface of titanium alloys further improves the resistance to wear and fatigue properties and enhances the resistance to corrosion.[132] Particles are still released from the titanium implants that can elicit a histiocytosis and giant cell tissue response around the prosthesis, leading to a dark stain on the peri-implant soft tissues (Figs. 18–13 and 18–14). This staining is seen with all metal implants, giving rise to the term *metallosis*.

Gonzales and associates[133] looked at the role of titanium in aseptic loosening of total joint systems. The study concluded that titanium particles were capable of stimulating an inflammatory response at the prosthetic interface via macrophages and osteoblasts. This effect involves tumor necrosis factor release from macrophages and

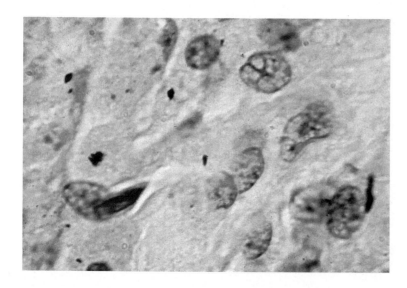

FIGURE 18–13. Higher magnification of intracellular metal fragments in macrophages. (Courtesy of Jeffrey Toth, Ph.D., Director of Biomaterials Research, Medical College of Wisconsin, Milwaukee, Wisconsin.)

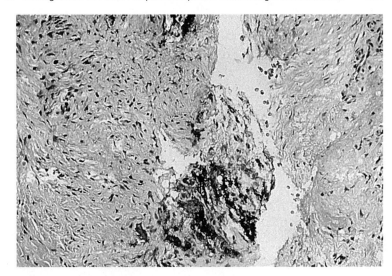

FIGURE 18–14. Metallosis from a cobalt chrome condyle of an Osteomed total joint system. (Courtesy of Louis G. Mercuri, D.D.S., M.S., Loyola University Medical Center, Maywood, Illinois.)

prostaglandin E2 release from osteoblasts. Although the mediator profile of the titanium is similar to that of PMMA, PMMA appears to stimulate mediator release to a greater extent and to lead to bone resorption, which was not observed with titanium particles. This study was done with commercially pure titanium with particle size 1 to 3 μm. Malloney and colleagues,[134] looking at retrieved titanium alloy particles from failed human total joint implants, found no evidence of cellular necrosis on histologic examination. They also found that the titanium alloy particles stimulated macrophages, which generated factors noted to have a role in bone resorption, i.e., prostaglandin E2, interleukin-1β, interleukin-6, and tumor necrosis factor alpha. Haynes and colleagues[135] showed that macrophages respond to titanium alloy wear particles by producing a variety of bone resorbing mediators. They also noted that cobalt chrome alloy particles were very toxic to these cells. Haynes and associates in 1996[136] showed that when these metal particles were phagocytized, the pH of the surrounding tissue dropped to as low as 5, causing corrosion of the metal wear particles, which released soluble products and also caused the release of cytokines, causing bone resorption.

Apart from biomaterial composition, there are numerous other biomaterial factors such as particle size, shape, surface irregularity, and surface area that are known to influence the number of macrophage responses including bone resorption. Particle size in particular is believed to be an important determinant of the macrophage response–associated aseptic loosening. Small, irregularly shaped, and sharp-edged polyethylene particles induce the formation of bone-resorbing granulomas, whereas larger and smooth-surfaced polyethylene pieces are enclosed within a thin layer of hypocellular fibrous tissue[137] (Figs. 18–12 and 18–15). Eventually the quantity of the small irregular deposited particulates intensifies the reaction to a point that the body can no longer control, leading to the release of mediates of inflammation, which partake in the destruction and resorption of the neighboring structures. Maloney and colleagues[134] found titanium alloy particles that were globular and rod shaped and ranged from 0.1 to 10 μm. The particles were titanium, aluminum, and vanadium. Others[138, 139] measured metal particles in the range of 0.1 to 5 μm with 83% measured at less than 1.13 μm. The shapes were quite irregular, with sharp edges, corners, and points. Others were oval and round. There was no predominant shape.

The process of osteolysis secondary to alloplastic particles is a complex continuum involving soluble mediator cells and mechanical aspects. Polymeric wear debris is of more concern than metallic wear debris in tissue breakdowns, most likely because of relative volume of particulate generated (Figs. 18–16 and 18–17). The surface area exposed to protein binding is determined by particle size and shape. Therefore, the

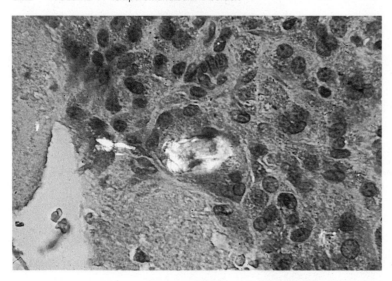

FIGURE 18–15. A large HDP fragment completely phagocytized by a foreign body giant cell. (Courtesy of Jeffrey Toth, Ph.D., Director of Biomaterials Research, Medical College of Wisconsin, Milwaukee, Wisconsin.)

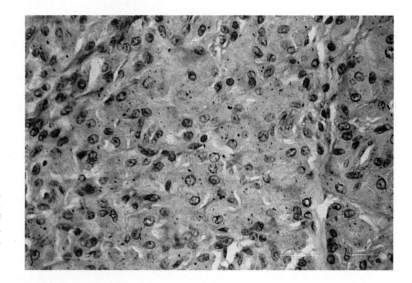

FIGURE 18–16. Metal debris surrounded by macrophages and foreign body giant cells. (Courtesy of Jeffrey Toth, Ph.D., Director of Biomaterials Research, Medical College of Wisconsin, Milwaukee, Wisconsin.)

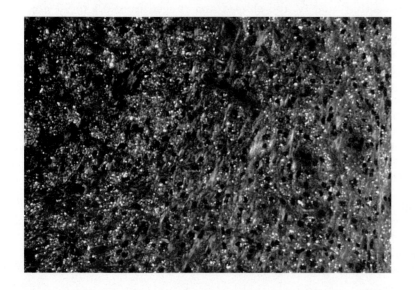

FIGURE 18–17. Same photograph as Figure 18–16 using polarized light to show all the very small HDP particles not visible in Figure 18–16. (Courtesy of Jeffrey Toth, Ph.D., Director of Biomaterials Research, Medical College of Wisconsin, Milwaukee, Wisconsin.)

volume of particles produced appears to be a major contributor to the overall reaction.

Diagnosis of Failed Alloplastic Implants

All alloplastic implants fail in time; their lifespan depends on many factors. Overloading of the joint secondary to parafunctional habits, muscle hyperactivity or fibrosis, micromovement of the implants after placement caused by poor fixation or loosening of the fixation devices, shedding of alloplastic particles leading to chronic inflammatory response and osteolysis, and hypersensitivity reactions to the materials can all lead to failure. The subjective symptoms of implant failure include the following:

1. Swelling with or without visual confirmation and increased tightness in and around the joint(s)
2. Decreased hearing or fullness in the ears without abnormal otologic findings
3. Increased pain in the joint with function and/or increased headaches in the temple area
4. Decreasing ability to masticate food

Clinical signs of implant failure include the following:

1. Decreasing range of mandibular motion
2. Increasing noise in the joint
3. Posterior open bite caused by acute swelling in the joint or more likely a progressive anterior open bite secondary to either loss of alloplastic mass or bone degeneration

The radiographic evaluation of interpositional implants can include panoramic radiography, tomography, coronal or axial computed tomography (CT), or magnetic resonance imaging (MRI). Generalized hard tissue changes of the condyle are usually well visualized on a panoramic radiograph. The more recent silicone sheeting implants contain a contrast agent that makes these implants highly visible with plain films. However, the temporal bone is not always clearly visualized with this technique. If temporal bone resorption is suspected, coronal CT is preferred for demonstration of

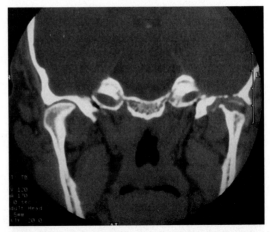

FIGURE 18–18. Coronal CT of left condyle and temporal bone showing fractured P/T implant, condylar and temporal bone erosion, and perforation into the middle fossa.

bone loss in both the condyle and the temporal bone (Fig. 18–18). Perforations of the temporal bone into the middle cranial fossa can also be depicted by CT and MRI (Figs. 18–18 and 18–19). The presence of increased soft tissue formation around either silicone or P/T IPIs is best seen on an MRI (Figs. 18–19 and 18–20), although if the implants were fixed with some type of metal device, the images are too distorted to allow diagnosis. Large defects in the implant can be seen on CT scans, but smaller defects are best seen with MR imaging.

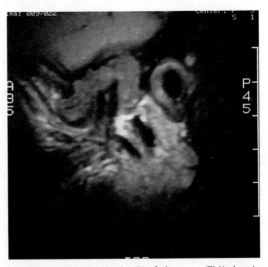

FIGURE 18–19. A sagittal MRI of the same TMJ showing not only the condylar and temporal bone erosion and perforation but also a large soft tissue mass surrounding a fragmented P/T implant.

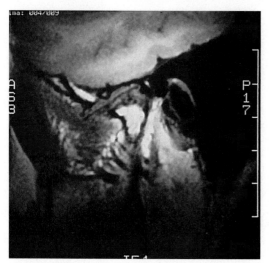

FIGURE 18–20. A sagittal MRI of a TMJ with a silicone implant in place between the condyle and temporal bone. The soft tissue reaction to the silicone is seen, as are mild to moderate bone changes.

Treatment Options after Failed Implants

The chance of success of a temporomandibular joint surgery decreases with each operation. When an alloplastic implant fails, the surgeon could face three separate problems: pain, poor function of the joint, and malocclusion secondary to loss of condylar or temporal bone height. Each problem should be treated separately, and ideally the treatments dovetail. Unfortunately several treatments and/or surgeries may be necessary.

The AAOMS has adopted the position of the 1992 workshop on temporomandibular joint implant surgery as to whether and when interpositional implants of silicone or P/T should be removed.[140] Once the implant has been removed, the guidelines become cloudy, leaving the ultimate decision to the surgeon and the patient.

Silicone

At this date, even though particles have been found in the TMJ years after initial removal, no recurrent foreign body giant cell reaction has been demonstrated after removal of a silicone interpositional implant. Particles stimulate three cell types:

macrophages, multinucleated giant cells, and fibroblasts. Which cell type dominates is one of the factors determining the type of reaction that occurs. Fibroblasts, which cause encapsulation, tend to limit the reaction. Fibroblasts appear to dominate in response to the silicone particles. Silicone particles can be found in the soft tissue interface between the condyle and the temporal bone. Silicone particles have also been identified in the condyle. Fortunately, the body encapsulates these particles, limiting the extent of the reaction. Therefore, the general consensus is that the soft tissue surrounding the implant can act as a soft tissue barrier between the condyle and the temporal bone. By leaving this barrier in place, further degenerative changes or fibrous adhesions may be prevented.[12, 37, 140, 141] This capsule should appear as a dense white connective tissue.[107] If granulation tissue is present, it should be removed. If minimal bone changes are present, replacement may not be necessary. Orthodontic appliances, arch bars, or Oliver loops along with functional elastics plus aggressive range of motion constitute appropriate postoperative therapy. If ankylosis is feared, a temporary silicone implant may be placed[22, 37, 108] (Fig. 18–21). This temporary implant can be designed by tracing the shape of the original implant and then slipping the new implant into the connective tissue pouch.

If there are moderate to severe bony changes, several approaches can be tried. The implant can be removed and the joint treated with functional elastics and aggressive range-of-motion therapy. After healing, the occlusion is reevaluated and reconstruction of any malocclusion becomes a secondary procedure. This treatment may consist of crown and bridge restorations, orthodontics, orthognathic surgery, occlusal adjustment, or permanent splint therapy. The second alternative is placement of an autogenous graft material to fill in the defect and then use of fixation appliances and functional elastics plus aggressive range of motion to try to stabilize the occlusion while returning function to the joint.[55, 142] With severe bone changes, a more aggressive option is removal of the implant, followed by placement of either a costochondral rib graft or a total joint system for which safety and efficacy have been established by a recognized regulatory agency.[143, 144]

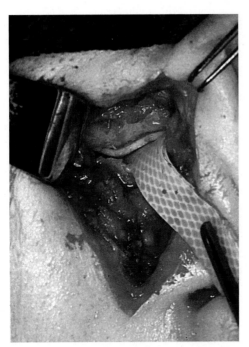

FIGURE 18–21. A temporary 1-mm Dacron reinforced silicone implant with retrieval tab placed between an auricular cartilage graft and the condyle. The implant is held in place with resorbable sutures tied to the temporal bone.

Proplast/Teflon

The failed Proplast/Teflon interpositional implant is treated more aggressively. The implant and surrounding affected soft tissues should be removed. Meticulous débridement including possible burring of bone tissue should be accomplished. Frozen sections of the peripheral soft tissues may help determine the margins. Chances of removal of all particles approach zero. One study found foreign body giant cell granuloma (FBGCG) still present in the joint an average of 40 months after implant removal and after an average of 4.5 additional surgeries.[145] The treatment recommendations for P/T IPIs that have not failed or demonstrated signs and symptoms of failure but for which the patient refuses removal are reported in the October 1993 *Journal of Oral and Maxillofacial Surgery*.[140] Others[66, 67] have recommended removal of all P/T IPI implants as soon as possible. With minimal bony changes, no replacement may be necessary and the implant may have a good chance of success.[146] Temporary silicone can also be used.[66] Fat grafts have been suggested to reduce fibrosis.[147] If vertical height has been

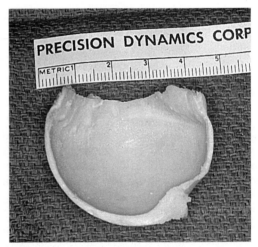

FIGURE 18–22. Bone has been removed from the articular cartilage of a fresh frozen femoral head.

altered by loss of either condyle or temporal bone, the choices are the same as described for silicone. Either establish function of the joint first and then, after healing of the joint, treat the occlusal problems or immediately replace the lost bone structure with autologous or banked tissues. If bone loss is mild to moderate, replacement with dermis, temporalis fascia muscle flap, costocartilage, auricular cartilage, or fresh frozen femoral head cartilage (Figs. 18–22 and 18–23) has been utilized.[55, 66, 142, 145, 148] If the bone loss is severe, placement of a costo-

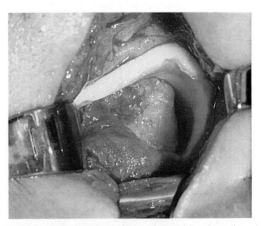

FIGURE 18–23. The fresh frozen femoral head cartilage is turned inside out so the articular side of the femoral cartilage is against the condyle. The cartilage is flexible, is easily formed around the medial and posterior of the condylar head, and still conforms to the shape of the fossa and articular eminence. The cartilage is secured to the temporal bone with nonresorbable sutures. The cartilage can be stacked to replace lost bone in the joint.

chondral rib graft or a total joint system is acceptable.[143, 144]

Secondary Problems

Temporal bone perforations[55, 57–60, 151] and recurrent FBGCG formation[66, 67, 116, 149–151] can result from P/T IPIs. Fortunately, temporal bone perforations are rarely located in the area of articulation but are usually found in the medial, superior, or posterior aspect of the glenoid fossa. The majority of perforations do not need repair (Fig. 18–24). Occasionally the defect may be large and include the lateral one third of the glenoid fossa, the articular eminence, and part of the zygomatic arch. Bony repair is based on the need for support for the condyle or any replacement material. Any bone or cartilage source can be used for repair of the defect, including freeze-dried bone (Fig. 18–25). For the smaller defects, the autogenous or allogeneic soft tissue used as an interpositional material adequately covers the perforation. Cerebrospinal fluid (CSF) leaks have been noted, necessitating dural repair by primary closure or a patch graft of temporal fascia or fasciculata.[59] Fibrin glue can be helpful in holding the graft in place. It can be made from autodonated or donated blood products.

A further complication of a failed P/T IPI is recurrent reactions caused by remaining particles. The recurrent FBGCG is a much bigger problem. This recurrent giant cell lesion has been noted as early as 1 year and

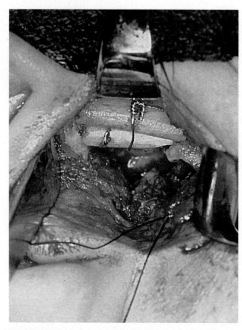

FIGURE 18–25. A large loss of bone including the lateral third of the glenoid fossa and the articular eminence. A bone graft is placed to establish contour and a stable base for further reconstruction.

as late as 6 years after implant removal.[116, 145] In the majority of the cases, the recurrence is found during surgical evaluation of a failed secondary repair.[55, 145] Whether the failure of the secondary surgery was caused by the recurrent FBGCG or by failure of the graft material is difficult to determine. In many cases, the FBGCG appears to be progressive, as particle disease is found in and around the grafted materials[55] (Fig. 18–26). Occasionally, this reaction occurs outside the joint capsule and can be severe. This reaction has been found in the parotid gland; soft tissues surrounding the joint, including the dermis and skin; as well as regional lymph nodes.[116] Grafted tissues that maintain viability may offer the best results in resisting destruction by the FBGCG. Auricular cartilage, costocartilage, and temporalis muscle flaps have given the best results.[55, 142] Cartilage, with a low metabolic rate and largely anaerobic metabolism, can survive the hypoxic state that occurs during the early period of transplantation[152] (Figs. 18–21, 18–27, and 18–28). Overloading of the joint can be detrimental by interfering with the diffusion of nutrient fluid through the intercellular substance of the cartilage.[153] The temporalis muscle fascia flap based on the anterior branch of the deep

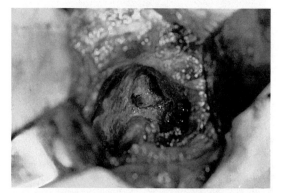

FIGURE 18–24. A perforation in the posterior medial glenoid fossa with exposed dura. A perforation of this size does not need a graft as function in this area is minimal.

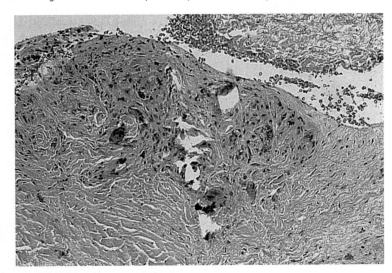

FIGURE 18–26. Foreign body giant cell reaction to P/T particles in and around a dermal graft that failed. (Courtesy of Dr. Wei Yung, Oregon Autogenous Health Science University, Portland, Oregon.)

temporal artery and coronoid process has been reported to maintain vascularity[142, 154, 155] (Fig. 18–29). The success of this procedure has been promising. When the vascularity has been compromised, the success rate declines considerably.[145]

Trying to prevent the recurrent FBGCG is most important. The critical mass of particles needed to stimulate recurrence is unknown and appears to vary among patients. Age and sex of the patient can alter the response. Other factors including vascularity, previous surgery of the TMJ, medications, overloading of the joint, and systemic disease may exacerbate this recurrent reaction. Extensive débridement of the joint done microscopically, along with burring of irregular bony surfaces, should greatly reduce the

chance of recurrent foreign body giant cell reaction.[117, 142, 149] Unfortunately, burring of the bony surfaces can open up marrow spaces, increase bleeding in the joint, and lead to increased fibrosis. The most common causes of failure after P/T removal are fibrosis and bony ankylosis.[55, 145] The degree of hard and soft tissue removal becomes a judgment call for which scientific guidance is lacking. McIntosh[143] and Kulber and coworkers[116] recommended waiting 1 year be-

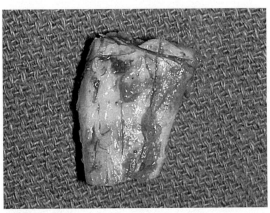

FIGURE 18–27. Cartilage harvested from the confluence of the sixth, seventh, and eighth ribs at the anterior medial border. The thickness is excellent, but the length and width can be limiting factors.

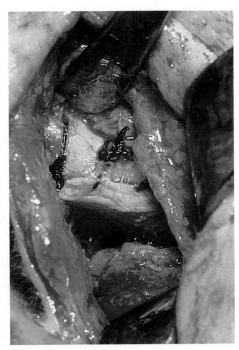

FIGURE 18–28. The rib cartilage in place in the TMJ secured to the temporal bone with nonresorbable sutures.

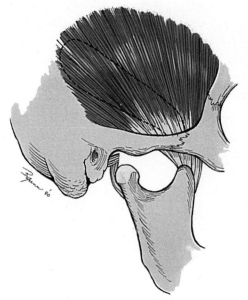

FIGURE 18–29. Anterior based temporalis muscle flap, which can maintain vascularity from the anterior branch of the deep temporal artery.

fore reconstruction, followed by biopsy of the joint until no FBGCG is found. Then and only then should reconstruction of the joint take place.

Summary

The body appears to tolerate alloplastic materials in the form of implants. Only with particulation (particle disease) does the immune system respond by attempting to remove the foreign substance. Neither the cell mediated immune response nor the humoral immune response have been found to be activated against any of the commonly used TMJ alloplasts. A cause-and-effect relationship has not been identified between particle disease and autoimmune disorders. A nonspecific immune reaction does occur in the form of an inflammatory response mediated by macrophages. The severity of the inflammatory response is determined by characteristics of the particles, including chemical composition, size, shape, and solubility. Along with the number of particles and rate of production, the response of the immune system differs among patients and is the deciding factor as to the extent of the inflammatory reaction. Hypersensitivity

reactions to alloplasts are rare and seldom are the reason for removal of the material.

Proplast/Teflon particles are the most reactive of all the alloplastic materials utilized and are more likely to cause a severe nonspecific reaction leading to hard and soft tissue damage, usually confined to the TMJ structures. Temporal bone perforations and local spread of the particle disease outside the capsule of the joint are well documented. Spread beyond the regional lymph nodes has not been shown to occur. Recurrent giant cell granuloma formation secondary to P/T particles occurs without time constraints even after thorough removal of all visible particles. Meticulous débridement at the time of implant removal diminishes the chance of recurrence. The reaction to silicone particles is much milder than that seen with P/T and rarely leads to temporal bone destruction or recurrent reactive disease. Silicone may still have a use as a temporary spacer in the prevention of fibrous or bony ankylosis.

Ultimately, the reconstruction of the TMJ after implant failure is based on the application of present scientific knowledge, past experience, and clinical judgment.

REFERENCES

1. Williams PL, Warwick R: Gray's Anatomy. Edinburgh, Churchill, Livingstone, 1980.
2. Osborn JW: The disc of the human temporomandibular joint: Design, function and failure. J Oral Rehabil 1985;12:279.
3. Yaillen DM, Shapiro PA, Luschei ES, Feldman GR: Temporomandibular joint meniscectomy: Effects on joint structure and masticatory function in *Macaca fascicularis*. J Maxillofac Surg 1979;7:255–264.
4. Merrill RG: Historical perspectives and comparisons of TMJ surgery for internal derangements and arthropathy. J Craniomandibul Pract 1986;4:74.
5. Helmy E, Bays R, Sharawy M: Osteoarthrosis of the temporomandibular joint following experimental disc perforation in *Macaca fascicularis*. J Oral Maxillofac Surg 1988;46:979–990.
6. Block MS, Bouvier M: Adaptive remodeling of the rabbit temporomandibular joint following discectomy and dietary variations. J Oral Maxillofac Surg 1990;48:482–486.
7. Axelsson S, Holmlund A, Hjerpe A: An experimental model of osteoarthrosis in the temporomandibular joint of the rabbit. Acta Odontol Scand 1992;50:273–280.
8. Hinton RJ: Alterations in rat condylar cartilage following discectomy. J Dent Res 1992;71:1292–1297.
9. Macher DJ, Westesson PL, Brooks SL, et al: Temporomandibular joint: Surgically created disc dis-

placement causes arthrosis in the rabbit. Oral Surg Oral Med Oral Pathol 1992;73:645–649.

10. Axelsson S: Human and experimental osteoarthrosis of the temporomandibular joint: morphological and biochemical studies. Swed Dent J Suppl 1993;92:1–45.

11. Lang TC, Zimny ML, Vijayagopal P: Experimental temporomandibular joint disc perforation in the rabbit: A gross morphologic, biochemical, and ultrastructural analysis. J Oral Maxillofac Surg 1993;51:1115–1128.

12. Hall HD: Meniscectomy for damaged discs of the temporomandibular joint. South Med J 1985; 75(5):569.

13. Hansen WC, Deshazo BW: Silastic reconstruction of the temporomandibular joint meniscus. Plast Reconstr Surg 1969;43:4.

14. Gallagher DMW: Comparison of Silastic and Proplast implants in the temporomandibular joint after condylectomy for osteoarthritis. J Oral Maxillofac Surg 1982;40:627.

15. Kiersch TA: The use of Proplast-Teflon implants for meniscectomy and disc repair in the temporomandibular joint. Clinical Congress on Reconstruction with Biomaterials. San Diego, 1984.

16. Eggers GWN: Arthroplasty of the temporomandibular joint in children with interposition of tantalum foil. J Bone Joint Surg 1946;28:603.

17. Smith AE, Robinson M: A new surgical procedure for the creation of a false temporomandibular joint in cases of ankylosis by means of a non-electrolytic metal. Am J Surg 1957;94:837.

18. Christenson RW: Mandibular joint arthrosis corrected by the insertion of a cast vitallium glenoid fossa prosthesis: A new technique. Oral Surg Oral Med Oral Pathol 1964;17:712.

19. Morgan DH, Hall WP, House LR, et al: Temporomandibular joint surgery: Results of a 14-year joint implant study. Laryngoscope 1984;94:534.

20. Robinson M: Temporomandibular ankylosis corrected by creating a false Silastic sponge fossa. J South Calif Dent Assoc 1968;36:14–16.

21. Henny FA: Surgical treatment of the painful temporomandibular joint. J Am Dent Assoc 1969; 79:171–177.

22. Wilkes C: Personal communication. 1985.

23. Hansen WC, Deshaza BW: Silastic reconstruction of temporomandibular joint meniscus. Plast Reconstr Surg 1969;43:388–391.

24. Habbi I, Murnane TW, Doku HC: Silastic and Supramid in arthroplasty of the temporomandibular joint in the rabbit. J Oral Surg 1970;28:267.

25. Murnane TW, Doku NC: Non-interpositional intercapsular arthroplasty of rabbit TMJ's. J Oral Surg 1971;29:268.

26. Sanders B: Surgical Treatment of the TMJ. Abstracts of the Clinical Congress of the American Association of Oral and Maxillofacial Surgeons, Philadelphia, 1981.

27. Bessette RW: Surgical management: Silastic implants. Presented at the Third Annual Meeting on Temporomandibular Joint Pain and Dysfunction. Philadelphia, November 1984.

28. Ryan DE: Meniscectomy with Silastic Implants. Abstracts of the Clinical Congress of the American Association of Oral and Maxillofacial Surgeons, San Diego, 1984.

29. Criteria for TMJ meniscus surgery. Published by American Association of Oral and Maxillofacial Surgeons, November, 1984.

30. Dolwick MF, Aufdemorte TB: Silicone-induced foreign body reaction and lymphadenopathy after temporomandibular joint arthroplasty. Oral Surg 1985;59:449–452.

31. Wilkes C: Personal communication. 1996.

32. Wilkes CH: Surgical treatment of internal derangement of the temporomandibular joint. Arch Otolaryngol Head Neck Surg 1991;117:64–72.

33. Eriksson L, Westesson PL: Temporomandibular joint discectomy: No positive effect of temporary silicone implant in a 5 year follow-up. Oral Surg Oral Med Oral Pathol 1992;74:259–272.

34. Merrill RG: A survey of preferred implant after TMJ discectomy. Presented at Western Society of Oral and Maxillofacial Surgeons Annual Meeting. Lake Tahoe, Nevada, June 1986.

35. Timmis DP, Aragon SB, Van Sickels JE, et al: A comparative study of alloplastic TMJ meniscal replacement in rabbits. Case Reports and Outlines of Scientific Sessions, 67th Annual Meeting, American Association of Oral and Maxillofacial Surgeons, Washington, DC, 1985, p 40.

36. Ryan DE: Alloplastic implants in the temporomandibular joint. Oral Maxillofac Surg Clin North Am 1989;1:429.

37. Tucker MR, Burke EJ: Temporary Silastic implantation following discectomy in the primate temporomandibular joint. J Oral Maxillofac Surg 1989;47:1290.

38. Bosanquet AG, Ishimaru J, Goss AN: The effect of Silastic replacement following discectomy in sheep temporomandibular joints. J Oral Maxillofac Surg 1991;49:1204–1209.

39. Bronstein SL: Retained alloplastic temporomandibular joint disc implants: A retrospective study. Oral Surg 1987;64:135–145.

40. Charnley J: Surgery of the hip-joint: Present and future developments. Br Med J 1960;1:821–826.

41. Calnan J: The use of inert plastic materials in reconstructive surgery. Br J Plastic Surg 1963; 16:1–22.

42. Leidholt JD, Gorman HA: Teflon hip prostheses in dogs. J Bone Joint Surg 1965;47(A):1414–1420.

43. Charnley J, Kamangar A: The optimum size of prosthetic heads in relation to the wear of plastic sockets in total replacement of the hip. Med Biol Eng 1969;7:31–39.

44. Homsy CA, Cain TE, Kessler FB, et al: Porous implant systems for prosthesis stabilization. Clin Orthop 1972;89:220–235.

45. Farrell CD, Kent JN: Clinical applications of Proplast in oral and maxillofacial surgery. Alpha Omegan 1975;68:21–26.

46. Gallagher DM, Wolford LM: Comparison of Silastic and Proplast implants in the temporomandibular joint after condylectomy for osteoarthritis. J Oral Maxillofac Surg 1982;40:627–630.

47. Carter JB: Meniscectomy in the management of chronic internal derangements of the TMJ. Abstracts of the Scientific Sessions, Annual Meeting of the American Association of Oral and Maxillofacial Surgeons, Las Vegas, 1983.

48. Vitek, Inc: Survey of TMJ Surgical Results. Houston, Vitek, 1986.

49. Moriconi ES, Popowich LD, Guernsey LH: Alloplastic reconstruction of the temporomandibular joint. Dent Clin North Am 1986;30:307–325.

50. Ryan DE: Temporomandibular Joint Newsletter. Milwaukee, WI, Medical College of Wisconsin, 1985, p 3.

51. Lagotteria L, Scapino R, Granston AS: Patient with lymphadenopathy following temporomandib-

ular joint arthroplasty with Proplast. J Craniomandib Pract 1986;4:172.

52. Heffez L, Mafee MF, Rosenberg H, Langer B: CT
evaluation of TMJ disc replacement with a Proplast-Teflon laminate. J Oral Maxillofac Surg
1987;45:657–665.

53. Florine BL, Gatto DJ, Wade ML, Waite DE: Tomographic evaluation of temporomandibular joints
following discoplasty or placement of polytetrafluoroethylene implants. J Oral Maxillofac Surg
1988;48:183–188.

54. Schelhas KP, Wilkes CH, El-Deeb M, et al: Permanent Proplast temporomandibular joint implants: MR imaging of destructive complication.
AJR 1988;151:731.

55. Yih WY, Merrill RG: Pathology of alloplastic interpositional implants in the temporomandibular
joint. Oral Maxillofac Surg Clin North Am
1989;1:415.

56. Ryan DE: The Proplast/Teflon dilemma. J Oral
Maxillofac Surg 1989;47:319–320.

57. Berarducci JP, Thompson DA, Scheffer RB: Perforation into middle cranial fossa as a sequel to use
of a Proplast-Teflon implant for temporomandibular joint reconstruction. J Oral Maxillofac Surg
1990;48:496–498.

58. Spagnoli D, Kent JN: Multicenter evaluation of
temporomandibular joint Proplast-Teflon disc implant. Oral Surg Oral Med Oral Pathol
1992;74:411–421.

59. Chuong R, Piper MA: Cerebrospinal fluid leak
associated with Proplast implant removal from
the temporomandibular joint. Oral Surg Oral
Med Oral Pathol 1992;74:422.

60. Smith RM, Goldwasser MS, Sabol SR: Erosion of
a Teflon-Proplast implant into the middle cranial
fossa. J Oral Maxillofac Surg 1993;51:1268–1271.

61. Estabrooks LN, Fairbanks CE, Collett RJ, et al:
A retrospective evaluation of 301 TMJ Proplast-
Teflon implants. Oral Surg Oral Med Oral Pathol
1990;70:381.

62. FDA: Serious Problems with Proplast Coated
TMJ Implant. Rockville, MD, Department of
Health and Human Services, 1990.

63. FDA: Vitek Proplast Temporomandibular Joint
Implants. Rockville, MD, Department of Health
and Human Services, 1991.

64. Spagnoli D, Kent JN: Multicenter evaluation of
temporomandibular joint Proplast/Teflon disc implant. Oral Surg Oral Med Oral Pathol 1992;
74:411.

65. Fontenot MG, Kent JN: In vitro wear performance of Proplast TMJ disc implants. J Oral
Maxillofac Surg 1992;50:133–139.

66. Feinerman DM, Piecuch JF: Long-term retrospective analysis of twenty-three Proplast-Teflon temporomandibular joint interpositional implants.
Int J Oral Maxillofac Surg 1993;22:11–16.

67. Ryan DE: The Proplast-Teflon dilemma. J Oral
Maxillofac Surg 1989;47:222.

68. Buchhorn GH, Willert HG: Effects of plastic wear
particles on tissue in biocompatibility of orthopaedic implants. In Williams DF (ed): Biocompatibility of Clinical Implant Materials, vol II. Boca
Raton, FL, CRC Press, 1982, pp 249–266.

69. Revell PA, Weightman B, Freeman MAR, et al:
The production and biology of polyethylene wear
debris. Arch Orthop Trauma Surg 1978;91:167.

70. Smahel J, Meyer V: Structure of capsules around
silicone implants in hand surgery. Hand
1983;15:47–52.

71. Swanson AB: Fingerjoint replacement by silicone
rubber implants and the concept of implant fixation by encapsulation. Ann Rheum Dis 1969;
28(suppl):47–55.

72. Chambers TJ: Multinucleate giant cells. J Pathol
1978;126:125.

73. Benjamin E, Ahmed H, Rashid ATMF, et al: Silicone lymphadenopathy: A report of two cases, one
with concomitant malignant lymphoma. Diagn
Histopathol 1982;5:133–141.

74. Christie A, Wienberger K, Dietrich M: Silicone
lymphadenopathy and synovitis. JAMA 1977;
237:1463–1464.

75. Lagrotteria L, Scapino R, Granston AS, et al:
Patient with lymphadenopathy following tempo-
romandibular joint arthroplasty with Proplast. J
Craniomandibul Pract 1986;4:172–178.

76. Chambers TJ: The pathobiology of the osteoclast.
J Clin Pathol 1985;38:241.

77. Holtrop ME, King GJ: The ultrastructure of the
osteoclast and its functional implications. Clin
Orthop 1977;123:177.

78. Pazzaglia UE, Pringle JAS: Bone resorption in
vitro: Macrophages and giant cells from failed
total hip replacement versus osteoclasts. Biomaterials 1989;10:286–288.

79. Pazzaglia UE, Pringle JAS: The rate of macrophages and giant cells in loosening of joint replacements. Arch Orthop Trauma Surg 1988;
107:20–26.

80. Rae T: The macrophage response to implant
materials—with special reference to those used
in orthopedics. CRC Crit Rev Biocompatability
1986;2:97.

81. Zardeneta G, Mukai H, Marker V, Milam SB:
Protein interactions with particulate Teflon: Im-
plications for the foreign body response. J Oral
Maxillofac Surg 1996;54:873–878.

82. Peltonen L: Nickel sensitivity in the general population. Contact Dermatitis 1979;5:27–32.

83. Goh CL: Prevalence of contact allergy by sex, race
and age. Contact Dermatitis 1986;14:237–240.

84. Gammelgaard X, Fullerton A, Avnstorp C, Menne
T: Permeation of chromium salts through human
skin in vitro. Contact Dermatitis 1992;27:302–
310.

85. Maurer AM, Merritt K, Brown SA: Cellular uptake of titanium and vanadium from addition of
salts or fretting corrosion in vitro. J Biomed
Mater Res 1994;28:241–246.

86. Meldrum RD, Bloebaum RD, Dorr LD: Metal ion
concentrations in retrieved polyethylene total hip
inserts and implications for artifactually high
readings in tissue. J Biomed Mater Res 1993;
27:1349–1356.

87. Maloney WJ: Biological reaction to surgical bone
cement. Technol Orthop 1993;8:237–244.

88. McFadden N, Lyberg T, Hensten-Pettersen A:
Aluminum induced granulomas in a tattoo. J Am
Acad Dermatol 1992;20:903–908.

89. Meding B, Augustsson A, Hansson C: Patch test
reactions to aluminum. Contact Dermatitis
1984;10:107.

90. Benson MKD, Goodum PG, Boostoff J: Metal sensitivity in patients with joint replacement
arthroplasties. Br Med J 1975;4:374–377.

91. Elves MW, Wilson JN, Scales JT, Kemp HBS:
Incidence of metal sensitivity in patients with
total joint replacements. Br Med J 1975;4:376–
378.

92. Evans EM, Freeman MAR, Miller AJ, Vernon-

Roberts B: Metal sensitivity as a cause of bone necrosis and loosening of prostheses in total joint replacements. J Bone Joint Surg 1974;56B:626–629.

93. Brown SA, Merritt K, Farnsworth LJ, Crowe TD: Bilogical Significance of Metal Ion Release. In Lemons J (ed): Quantitative Characteristics and Performance of Porous Implants, STP 953. Philadelphia, ASTM, 1987; pp 163–181.

94. Merritt K, Brown SA: Metal sensitivity reactions to orthopedic implants. Int J Dermatol 1981; 20:89–94.

95. Merritt K, Brown SA: Effects of metal particles and ions on the biological system. Technol Orthop 1993;8:228–236.

96. Merritt K, Brown SA: Particulate metals: Experimental studies. In Morrey BF (ed): Biological, Material, and Mechanical Considerations of Joint Replacement. New York, Raven Press, pp 1993;147–160.

97. Merritt K, Brown SA: Tissue reaction and metal sensitivity: An animal study. Acta Orthop Scand 1980;51:403–411.

98. Merritt K, Rodrigo JJ: Immune response to synthetic materials: Clin Orthop 1996;326:71–79.

99. Rooker GD, Wilkinson JD: Metal sensitivity in patients undergoing hip replacement. J Bone Joint Surg Br 1980;62:502–505.

100. Trumpy IG, Lyberg T: Aluminum toxicity failure of implant. J Oral Maxillofac Surg 1993; 51(6):624–629.

101. Sanchez-Guerro J, Schur PH, Sergent JS, Liang MH: Silicone breast implants and rheumatic disease. Arthritis Rheum 1994;37(2):158–168.

102. Hochberg MC: Invited discussion: Antibodies and silicone gel implants. Ann Plast Surg 1994; 32:5–7.

103. Bridges AJ, Conley C, Wang G, et al: A clinical and immunologic evaluation of women with silicone breast implants and symptoms of rheumatic disease. Ann Intern Med 1993;118:929–936.

104. Boyce GB, Toriumi DM: Considerations in the use of biologic grafts and alloplastic implants in facial plastic and reconstructive surgery. J Long-Term Effects Med Implants, 1992;2:199.

105. Andrews JM: Cellular behaviour of injected silicone fluid: A preliminary report. Plast Reconstr Surg 1966;38:581.

106. Heggers JP, Kossovsky N, Parsons RW, et al: Biocompatibility of silicone implants. Ann Plast Surg 1983;11:38.

107. DeHeer DH, Owens SR, Swanson AB: The host response to silicone elastomer implants for small joint arthroplasty. J Hand Surg [Am] 1995; 20A(3):S101–S109.

108. Hartman LC, Bessette RW, Baier RE, et al: Silicone rubber temporomandibular joint meniscal replacement: Post-implant histopathologic and material evaluation. J Biomed Mater Res 1988; 22(6):475–484.

109. Khoo CTK: Silicone synovitis: The current role of silicone elastomer implants in joint reconstruction. J Hand Surg [Br] 1993;18B(6):679–686.

110. Acton C, Hoffman G, McKenna H, Moloney F: Silicone-induced foreign body reaction after temporomandibular joint arthroplasty: Case report. Aust Dent J 1989;34(3):228–232.

111. Morrison AD, Sandeson RC, Moos KF: The use of silastic as an orbital wall defects: Review of 311 cases treated over 20 years. J Oral Maxillofac Surg 1995;53(4):412–417.

112. Young VL, Nemecek JR, Gilliam C, et al: Immunohistochemical analysis of periprosthetic capsular tissue from breast implant patients. Plastic Surgical Forum, 62nd Annual Scientific Meeting. New Orleans, September, 1993.

113. McDonald AH, Weir K, Sanger JR: Silicone induced T-Cell proliferation in mice. Curr Top Microbiol Immunol 1996;210:189–198.

114. Narini PP, Hay JB, Semple JL: Repeat exposure to silicone gel can induce delayed hypersensitivity. Plast Reconstr Surg 1995;96(2):371–380.

115. Bonfield TL, Colton LE, Marchant E, Anderson JM: Cytokine and growth factor production by monocytes/macrophages on proteins preabsorbed polymers. J Biomed Mater Res 1992;26:837–850.

116. Kulber DA, Davos I, Aronowitz JA: Severe cutaneous foreign body giant cell reaction after temporomandibular joint reconstruction with Proplast-Teflon. J Oral Maxillofac Surg 1995;53:719–722.

117. Ryan DE: Discussion. J Oral Maxillofac Surg 1995;53:722–723.

118. Trumpy IG, Roald B, Lyberg T: Morphologic and immunohistochemical observation of explanted Proplast-Teflon temporomandibular joint interpositional implants. J Oral Maxillofac Surg 1996;54:63–68.

119. Namey T, Henry CH, Nikaein A, Wolford LM: HLA-B loci associated with connective tissue diseases and TMD (abstract). J Oral Maxillofac Surg 1994;52(suppl):131.

120. Wolford LM, Henry CH, Nikaein A, et al: The temporomandibular joint alloplastic implant problem. In Sessle BJ, Bryant PS, Dionne RA (eds): Progress in Pain Research and Management, vol 4. Seattle: IASP Press, 1995; pp 443–447.

121. Ryan DE, Sanger JR, Komorowski R: Milwaukee, WI, Medical College of Wisconsin, 1993. Unpublished data.

122. Berczi I, Nagy E, Kovacs K, Horvath E: Regulation of humoral immunity in rats by pituitary hormones. Acta Endocrinol 1981;98:506–513.

123. Berczi I, Nagy E: A possible role of prolactin in adjuvant arthritis. Arthritis Rheum 1982;25:591–594.

124. Amara RA, Itallie CV, Dannies PS: Regulation of prolactin production and cell growth by estradiol: Difference in sensitivity to estradiol occurs at level of messenger ribonucleic acid accumulation. Endocrinology 1987;120:264–271.

125. Ahmed SA, Aufdemorte TB, Chen JR, et al: Estrogen induces the development of autoantibodies and promotes salivary gland lymphoid infiltrates in normal mice. J Autoimmun 1989;2:543–552.

126. Ansar AS, Talal N: Sex hormones and autoimmune rheumatic disorders. Scand J Rheumatol 1989;18:69–76.

127. Milam SB: Failed implants and multiple operations. Oral Surg Oral Med Oral Pathol Oral Radiol Endod 1997;83:156–162.

128. Pandey R, Quinn J, Joyner C, et al: Arthroplasty implant biomaterial particle associated macrophages differentiate into lacunar bone resorbing cells. Ann Rheum Dis 1996;55(6)388–395.

129. Howie DW, Manthey B, Hay S, Vernon-Roberts B: The synovial response to intra-articular injection in rats of polyethylene wear particles. Clin Orthop 1993;292:352–357. (Published erratum appears in Clin Orthop 1994;298:249.)

130. Howie DW, Vernon-Roberts B: The synovial response to intra-articular cobalt-chrome wear particles. Clin Orthop 1988;232:244.

131. Vernon-Roberts B, Freeman MAR: The tissue response to total joint replacement prostheses. In Swanson SAU, Freeman MAR (eds): The Scientific Basis of Joint Replacement. Tunbridge Wells, Kent Pitman Medical Publishing, 1977, p 86.

132. Buchanan RA, Rigney ED Jr, Williams JM: Ion implantation of surgical Ti-6A1-4V for improved resistance to wear-accelerated corrosion. J Biomed Mater Res 1987;21:355–366.

133. Gonzales JB, Purdon MA, Horowitz SM: In vitro studies on the role of titanium in aseptic loosening. Clin Orthop 1996;(330):240–250.

134. Maloney WJ, James RE, Smith RL: Human macrophage response to retrieved titanium alloy particles in vitro. Clin Orthop 1996;322:268–278.

135. Haynes DR, Rogers SD, Hay S, et al: The differences in toxicity and release of bone resorbing mediators induced by titanium and cobalt chrome alloy wear particles. J Bone Joint Surg 1993; 75A:825–834.

136. Haynes DR, Rogers SD, Howie DW, et al: Drug inhibition of the macrophage response to metal wear particles in vitro. Clin Orthop 1996; 323:316–326.

137. Boss JH, Shajrawi I, Aunullah J, Mendes DG: The relativity of biocompatibility: A critique of the concept of biocompatibility. Isr J Med Sci 1995;31(4):203–209.

138. Willert HG, Buchhorn GH, Semlitsch M: Particle disease due to wear of metal alloys. Morrey BF (ed): Biological, Material, and Mechanical Considerations of Joint Replacement, New York, Raven Press, 1993.

139. Lee JM, Salvati EA, Betts F, et al: Size of metallic and polyethylene debris particles in failed cemented total hip replacements. J Bone Joint Surg 1992;74B:380–384.

140. Recommendations for management of patients with temporomandibular joint implants. J Oral Maxillofac Surg 1993;51:1164–1172.

141. Wilkes CH: Surgical treatment of internal derangement of the temporomandibular joint. Arch Otolaryngol Head Neck Surg 1991;117:64–72.

142. Kearns GJ, Perrott DH, Kaban LB: A protocol for the management of failed alloplastic temporomandibular joint disc implaants. J Oral Maxillofac Surg, 1995;53:1240–1247.

143. McIntosh RB: Costochondral and dermal grafts in temporomandbibular joint reconstruction. Oral Maxillofac Surg Clin North Am 1989;1:363–397.

144. Wolford LM, Cottrell DA, Henry CH: Temporomandibular joint reconstruction of the complex patient with the Techmedia custom made total joint prosthesis. J Oral Maxillofac Surg 1994; 53:2–10.

145. Henry CH, Wolford LM: Treatment outcomes for temporomandibular joint reconstruction after Proplast/Teflon implant failure. J Oral Maxillofac Surg 1993;51:352–358.

146. Lorge PS, Swift JQ, Diehl RL: Removal of temporomandibular joint (TMJ) Proplast implants without reconstruction-results of 24 patients. J Oral Maxillofac Surg 1993;51(3):134.

147. Wolford LM, Karras SC: Autologous fat transplantation around temporomandibular joint total joint prosthesis: preliminary treatment outcomes. J Oral Maxillofac Surg 1997;55:245–250.

148. Ryan DE, Indresano AT: Department of Oral Maxillofacial Surgery, Medical College of Wisconsin, Milwaukee, WI, 1998. Unpublished data.

149. Chuong R, Piper MA, Boland TJ: Recurrent giant cell reaction to residual Proplast in the temporomandibular joint. Oral Surg Oral Med Oral Pathol 1993;76(1):16–19.

150. Ryan DE: Alloplastic disc replacement. Oral Maxillofac Surg Clin North Am 1994;6:307–321.

151. Piecuch JF: Recurrent giant cell reaction to residual Proplast in the temporomandibular joint (letter). Oral Surg Oral Med Oral Pathol 1994; 77(1):3–4.

152. Laskin DM, Sarnot BG: The metabolism of fresh transplanted and preserved cartilage. Surg Gynecol Obstet 1953;96:493.

153. Ioannides C, Freihoter PM: Replacement of the damaged intra-articular disc of the TMJ. J Craniomaxillofac Surg 1981;16:273–278.

154. Feinberg SF: Use of composite temporalis muscle flaps for disc replacement. Oral Maxillofac Surg Clin North Am 1994;6(2):335–348.

155. Albert TW, Merrill RG: Temporalis myofascial flap for the reconstruction of the temporomandibular joint. Oral Maxillofac Surg Clin North Am 1989;1:341.

CHAPTER

Tumors of the Temporomandibular Joint

David C. Stanton • Jeffery C. B. Stewart

Benign and malignant processes can affect the structures of the temporomandibular joint (TMJ). Even though the incidence of tumors is low when compared with the prevalence of osteoarthritis and internal derangement, surgeons must be cognizant of the signs of neoplasia. Space-occupying lesions of the TMJ may present with preauricular swelling, pain, trismus, deviation of mandibular motion, and malocclusion. When clinical and radiographic examinations suggest the presence of a tumor, arthroscopy or open arthrotomy is warranted to obtain tissue for diagnosis. All the component tissues of the TMJ region can become a source of neoplastic proliferation. Although they are rare, consideration should also be given to locally invasive proliferations of parotid, middle ear, or lymphocytic origin, as well as metastatic lesions.

When formulating a differential diagnosis for any jaw lesion, it is helpful to organize the pathologic entities into several categories and then compare the characteristics of the presenting lesions with those of lesions in each category. We and others[1] have organized jaw lesions into the following six categories:

1. Developmental cysts
2. Odontogenic cysts
3. Benign odontogenic tumors and lesions
4. Benign nonodontogenic tumors and lesions
5. Inflammatory, metabolic, and genetic disorders
6. Malignant and locally invasive lesions

The presence of developmental cysts, odontogenic cysts, and benign odontogenic tumors in the condyle or TMJ is rare and generally represents an extension of a process that initiated in the tooth-bearing segments of the mandible. Diagnosis and management of those lesions are covered elsewhere and are not discussed here.

Benign Nonodontogenic Tumors and Lesions

When evaluating TMJ pathology, the category of benign nonodontogenic tumors and lesions is the most comprehensive and includes processes with origins from all the component tissues of the TMJ.

ARTERIOVENOUS MALFORMATION

Facial vascular anomalies are not an uncommon finding in maxillofacial surgical patients. Many of these vascular anomalies, such as port wine stains, have a benign course. However, the subset of anomalies classified as arteriovenous malformations (AVMs) has significant morbidity and mortality. Intraosseous AVMs are particularly difficult to diagnose, may not present until adolescence or early adulthood, and often present with symptoms that mimic periodontal disease. Mandibular AVMs account for approximately 1% of all facial AVMs. A small percentage of these present in the TMJ (Fig. 19–1). Death secondary to intractable hemorrhage occurs in approximately 8% of patients.

Treatment of these malformations continues to provide a clinical challenge. Because of the poor prognosis of untreated AVMs, radical cure is mandatory. Treatment modalities used in the past have included radiation therapy, sclerosant therapy, cryosurgery, selective embolization, and surgical resection. Resection of the malformation and the surrounding bone is considered the optimal treatment to prevent recurrence. However, profound surgical hemorrhage and significant postoperative deformity have prompted clinicians to pursue alternative treatments that may have a lower morbidity and mortality. A major advance in the treatment of these malformations has been the development of selective embolization. Selective embolization can serve as the only treatment but is often used as a surgical adjunct to provide preoperative devascularization. Reznik and colleagues[2] and Flandroy and Provo[3] described a technique for the treatment of mandibular AVMs in which embolization is performed through direct transosseous puncture. Surgeons and radiologists at the University of Pennsylvania have further modified the technique to perform the embolization with microcatheters that are introduced transosseously.

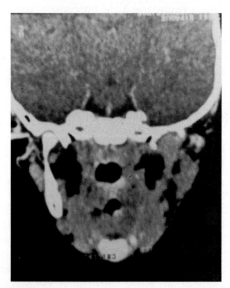

FIGURE 19–1. Magnetic resonance imaging scan of an 8-year-old boy with a large arteriovenous malformation of the right mandible. Note that the entire right condyle and ramus have been replaced with the malformation.

Histologically, AVMs consist of numerous medium- to large-caliber arteries and veins that are directly connected without intervening capillary-size vessels. These vessels are supported by a variably collagenous stroma.

CHONDROBLASTOMA

Chondroblastoma is a distinct entity that usually involves the long bones but sometimes occurs in the cranial bones and in the mandibular condyle. This benign central bone tumor occurs predominantly in young people. The incidence in males is roughly double that in females.[1] Conservative surgical excision is generally acceptable treatment.

Chondroblastomas consist of a proliferation of immature cartilage cells with focal production of a variably differentiated cartilaginous matrix. The lesion consists of a sheetlike proliferation of mononuclear cells resembling chondroblasts, often seen with focal collections of multinucleated giant cells. Calcification is typically present in the form of thin, delicate streaks that outline individual chondroblastic cells, producing a so-called chicken-wire pattern.

CHONDROMA

This neoplasm demonstrates no sex predilection and may develop at any age. Chondroma generally presents as a painless, slowly enlarging swelling. The radiographic appearance is that of an irregular radiolucent or mottled region of the bone.[1]

Chondromas consist of well-defined lobules of mature hyaline cartilage that may contain areas of calcification. Although the degree of cellularity may vary within individual lesions, chondrocytes are typically small, with single, uniform nuclei. Chondrocytes are often arranged in clusters within the chondroid lobules. The histopathologic distinction between a chondroma and a well-differentiated low-grade chondrosarcoma of the TMJ is often difficult. Many pathologists suggest that any chondroma of the jaws should be regarded as potentially a low-grade chondrosarcoma.

CONDYLAR HYPERPLASIA

Although space-occupying benign or malignant lesions can displace the condyle from the fossa and cause asymmetry with malocclusion, condylar hyperplasia can have similar presenting symptoms. The etiology of this disorder is not well understood. Histologic sections demonstrate the abnormal presence of hyaline cartilage that undergoes ossification and results in abnormal growth. The articular surface of a normal condyle is composed of fibrocartilage that exhibits appositional growth in contrast to endochondral ossification.

Condylar hyperplasia has been categorized into two types. The type I deformity, or hemimandibular elongation, is the most common variant. The mandible is asymmetric, with deviation of the chin to the contralateral side and a concomitant dental crossbite (Fig. 19–2). In patients with the type II deformity, or hemimandibular hypertrophy, deviation of the chin is not a prominent feature, but a marked vertical open bite is present on the ipsilateral side of the hyperplasia (Fig. 19–3).[4, 5] Condylar hyperplasia is not a truly neoplastic process but actually a self-limited disorder. Radionuclide bone scans with technetium 99m can be useful in differentiating between active and inactive disorders. Some surgeons favor the use of a high condylar shave to remove the zone of abnormal tissue if the disorder is diagnosed early in its active stage. Removal of only 5 or 6 mm of the most superior condylar surface is usually adequate, and condylectomy is unnecessarily aggressive.[6, 7]

Recontouring of the inferior border and angle of the mandible is sometimes necessary to correct the inferior component of the asymmetry. When a bone scan indicates that the process is inactive, orthognathic procedures, such as a vertical subsigmoid osteotomy, can be useful in correcting an open bite while maintaining a functional joint articulation (Fig. 19–4).[6, 7]

FIBROUS DYSPLASIA

Fibrous dysplasia most commonly presents as an asymptomatic, slow enlarge-

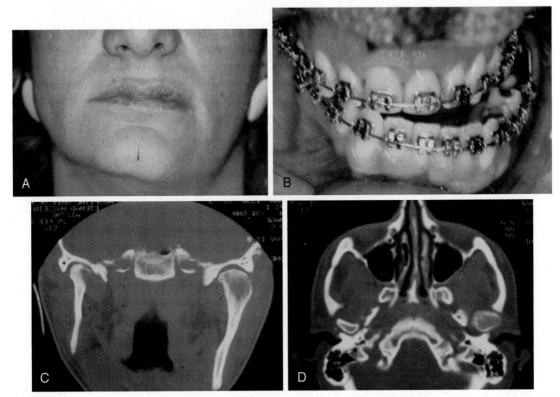

FIGURE 19–2. *A*, Type I condylar hyperplasia (hemimandibular elongation). This patient demonstrates the characteristic facial asymmetry, with deviation of the chin to the contralateral side. *B*, The same patient exhibiting the concomitant dental crossbite. *C* and *D*, Computed tomography scans of the enlarged condylar process and head.

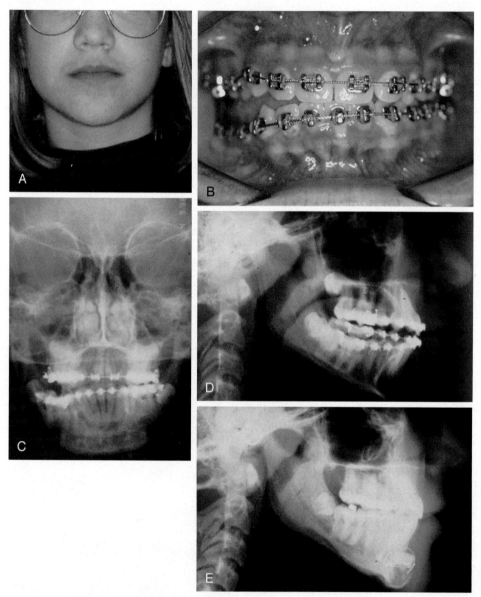

FIGURE 19–3. *A*, This patient demonstrates the characteristic findings of type II condylar hyperplasia (hemimandibular hypertrophy). Deviation of the chin is not a prominent feature when viewed from the front. *B*, The characteristic vertical open bite of a patient with type II condylar hyperplasia. *C* and *D*, Posteroanterior and lateral cephalograms of a patient with type II condylar hyperplasia. Note the relative facial symmetry and the presence of a marked vertical open bite on the ipsilateral side of the hyperplasia. *E*, Postoperative lateral cephalogram depicting closure of the posterior open bite with a vertical ramus osteotomy and correction of the profile with a genioplasty.

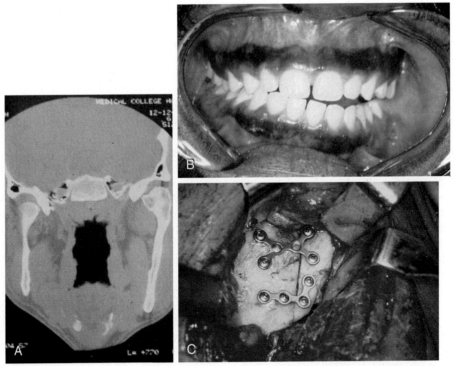

FIGURE 19–4. *A*, Computed tomography scan of a patient with type I condylar hyperplasia. *B*, Occlusion of a patient with type I condylar hyperplasia. *C*, Intraoperative photograph of treatment of condylar hyperplasia with an extraoral vertical ramus osteotomy and rigid fixation.

ment of the involved bone. Monostotic fibrous dysplasia accounts for up to 80% of cases. Jaw involvement is common in this form of the disease. The entire ramus-condyle complex can be involved and present as facial asymmetry.[1] Often the clinical presentation is difficult to distinguish from that of condylar hyperplasia. The radiographic presentation is sometimes similar to that of Garré's osteomyelitis (Fig. 19–5, also see Fig. 19–16).

Following a variable period of growth, fibrous dysplasia frequently stabilizes, or growth slows significantly after the onset of

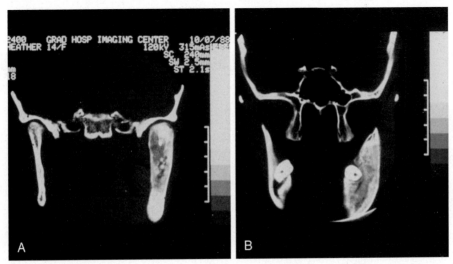

FIGURE 19–5. *A* and *B*, Axial computed tomography scans of a patient with fibrous dysplasia of the left mandibular body and ramus involving the entire condylar process and head.

puberty. Once pathologic diagnosis is confirmed by biopsy, the only treatment required may be periodic follow-up. However, if significant cosmetic or functional deformity has occurred, surgical intervention with osseous recontouring may be undertaken.

The histologic findings in fibrous dysplasia consist of a cellular, fibrous connective tissue proliferation that contains foci of irregularly shaped trabeculae of immature bone. A relatively constant ratio of fibrous tissue to bone throughout a given lesion has been described as characteristic. The collagen fibers may completely lack orientation or, alternatively, may be arranged in a storiform pattern of interlacing collagen bundles. The fibroblasts exhibit uniform spindle- to star-shaped nuclei. The bony trabeculae assume bizarre, irregular shapes, likened to Chinese characters. These trabeculae do not display any apparent functional orientation. The bone is predominantly woven bone that appears to arise directly from the collagenous stroma without prominent osteoblastic activity. In a mature fibrous dysplasia lesion, lamellar bone may be found. Aneurysmal bone cysts have been reported in association with fibrous dysplasia. It should be noted that fibrous dysplasia shares many microscopic features with ossifying fibroma.

GANGLION CYST

Ganglion cysts usually measure 1.5 to 2.5 cm in diameter. They frequently present as unilocular or multilocular masses in the connective tissue of a joint capsule or tendon sheath of a wrist. A female predominance is noted, and the age range of occurrence is 30 to 50 years of age. Computed tomography (CT) or magnetic resonance imaging (MRI) scans are useful in the diagnosis. Excision of the cyst is appropriate treatment.

Ganglion cysts of the TMJ are very rare, with only eight cases having been reported in the literature.[8] In approximately half of the cases, the lesions were associated with dysfunction, and patients reported tenderness or pain.

Intraosseous ganglion cysts are pseudocysts that consist of a central cavity lined by fibrous connective tissue often displaying areas of myxoid change. Scattered inflammatory cells, including macrophages containing mucinous material, may be seen. Although an epithelial lining is not evident, the central cavity typically contains acellular, mucinous, or myxoid deposits.

GIANT CELL GRANULOMA

Giant cell granuloma is found predominantly in children and young adults, with 75% of cases presenting before age 30. Females are affected approximately twice as frequently as males. These lesions occur more frequently in the mandible than the maxilla. Giant cell granuloma typically presents as a painless expansion or swelling of the affected jaw.[1] The radiographic appearance is frequently a unilocular or multilocular radiolucency (Fig. 19–6).

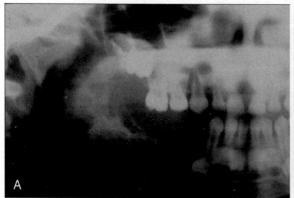
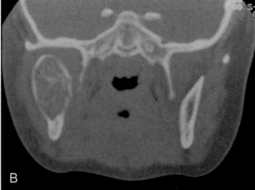

FIGURE 19–6. *A,* Panorex radiograph depicting a recurrent giant cell granuloma in a 4-year-old boy. The granuloma involves the entire right ramus and extends into the condylar process. *B,* Coronal computed tomography scan depicting extension of the giant cell granuloma into the condylar process, involving the entire condylar head.

The clinical behavior of central giant cell lesions is widely variable. Some may progress slowly with only minimal destruction of bone. The more aggressive variety may progress rapidly and result in massive bone loss and cortical perforation. The histopathologic appearance may not correlate with the clinical behavior.[1] Consequently, the treatment may vary from simple enucleation of small, slowly enlarging lesions to condylectomy or wide resection of aggressive, rapidly enlarging lesions.

Giant cell granulomas consist of a proliferation of spindled and ovoid fibroblasts in a vascular stroma containing variable amounts of collagen. Multinucleated giant cells are typically aggregated in richly vascular areas where hemorrhage and hemosiderin-laden macrophages are often present. Inflammatory cells are not prominent, although some lesions may contain foci of new, reactive bone trabeculae. Giant cell granulomas associated with foreign body reactions differ histologically only by the presence of the foreign material causing the reaction (Fig. 19–7).

GIANT CELL TUMOR

Giant cell tumors represent a true neoplasm that occurs most frequently in the long bones. Considerable controversy exists as to the relationship of this entity to giant cell granuloma and whether it actually occurs in the facial bones. If a clinician is presented with a clinicopathologic diagnosis of giant cell tumor of the TMJ, condylectomy is probably warranted (Fig. 19–8).[6]

Giant cell tumors consist of a richly cellular proliferation of oval to round mononuclear stromal cells with numerous, evenly dispersed, multinucleated giant cells. The nuclear characteristics of both the mononuclear and the multinucleated elements are generally similar, consisting of round, regular contours, evenly distributed chromatin, and prominent nucleoli. In contrast to giant cell granulomas, collagen production is minimal, and production of osteoid is rarely noted.

HEMANGIOMA

The maxilla and mandible are the most common sites of occurrence of hemangioma of bones after the vertebrae and skull. The posterior mandible is the most frequent site of incidence in the jaws.[1] The lesion commonly presents as a firm, slowly enlarging, expansile swelling of the bone. Spontaneous intraoral bleeding may occur. Bruits and pulsation of large hemangiomas may be detected with careful auscultation or palpation of the thinned cortical plates. The common radiographic presentation is that of a multilocular radiolucency (Fig. 19–9). The most significant feature of hemangioma of bone is the life-threatening hemorrhage that may occur if these lesions are improperly managed. Management may include embolization, sclerosing agents, and surgery.

Hemangiomas consist of a proliferation of mature blood vessels of varying calibers supported by a fibrous connective tissue stroma. Cavernous hemangiomas display numerous dilated, thin-walled vascular spaces lined by a single layer of benign endothelial cells. Some hemangiomas are composed of smaller capillary-size vascular channels. Frequently, a mixture of both cavernous and capillary-size vascular elements is present in a single lesion.

LANGERHANS' CELL DISEASE

Langerhans' cell disease, formerly known as histiocytosis X, is characterized by proliferation of cells exhibiting phenotypic characteristics of Langerhans' cells. This disease may manifest as solitary or multiple bone lesions or as disseminated visceral, skin, and bone lesions.

Generally, Langerhans' cell disease is a childhood disease and has been reported by some authors to have a male predilection. It generally presents as a painful swelling. Radiographically, it presents as sharply circumscribed, punched-out radiolucencies. In the condylar region, generalized bone destruction may be present and may be confused with other entities, such as phantom bone disease. Diagnosis of a jaw lesion mandates a skeletal survey and a thorough physical examination and history to determine the extent of systemic involvement.

Treatment varies with the severity of the disease dissemination. Treatment of an isolated lesion may consist of curettage only. Adjuvant chemotherapy and radiation ther-

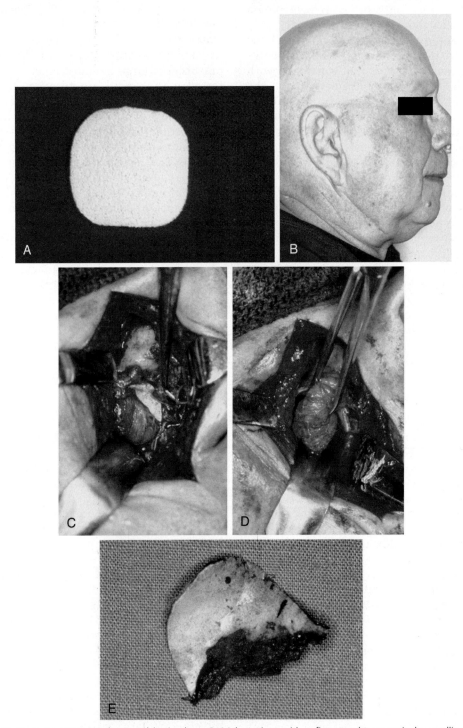

FIGURE 19–7. *A*, An intact Proplast condylar implant. *B*, Male patient with a firm, tender preauricular swelling overlying the site of a previous temporomandibular joint arthroplasty during which a Proplast implant was placed. *C*, Exposure of the preauricular mass and Proplast implant. *D*, Delivery of the preauricular mass, which later was interpreted to be infiltration of giant cells reacting to the Proplast foreign body. *E*, The fragmented Proplast implant.

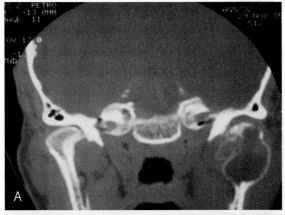

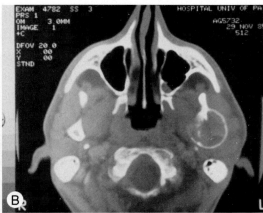

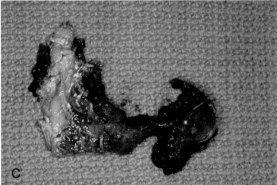

FIGURE 19–8. *A*, Coronal computed tomography (CT) scan depicting a multilocular radiolucency that was subsequently found to be a giant cell tumor. *B*, Axial CT scan depicting marked expansion of the bony cortices of the mandible and the condyle from the giant cell tumor. *C*, The tumor was removed in total with a condylectomy.

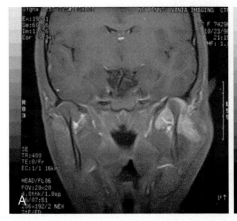

apy may be used when more disseminated disease is present.

Langerhans' cell disease consists of a diffuse proliferation of large mononuclear cells with abundant cytoplasm and pale-staining oval to reniform nuclei. Some cells exhibit nuclei with prominent nuclear grooves. These proliferative cells have been shown by electron microscopic and immunohistochemical studies to be derived from Langerhans' cells. The proliferative cells are often admixed with relatively dense aggregates of eosinophils. Other inflammatory cells, including macrophages, as well as multinucleated giant cells and foci of necrosis may be evident.

NEUROFIBROMA

Neurofibroma may appear as isolated lesions or as multiple lesions as part of the

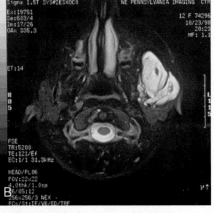

FIGURE 19–9. *A* and *B*, Coronal and axial magnetic resonance imaging scans of a large compressible preauricular mass in a child. Note the enhancement, consistent with the vascularity of a hemangioma.

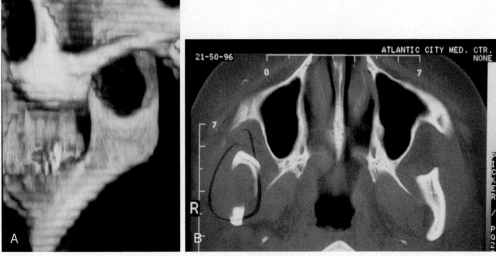

FIGURE 19–10. *A,* Three-dimensional reconstruction of a patient with a firm swelling in the region of the temporomandibular joint. Note the destruction of the condyle and ramus from the external compressive force of the neurofibroma. *B,* Axial computed tomography scan depicting destruction of the condyle and ramus from external compression by a neurofibroma.

syndrome of neurofibromatosis.[1] Bone changes can be seen in patients with neurofibromatosis in the form of cortical erosion from adjacent soft tissue tumors or medullary resorption from intraosseous lesions (Figs. 19–10 and 19–11). Appropriate treatment is surgical excision or debulking of large lesions if they are symptomatic.

Neurofibromas consist of a proliferation of spindle-shaped cells that characteristically exhibit elongated, wavy nuclei. These uniform cells are often arranged in a haphazard fashion, although interlacing fascicles of cells may be observed in some areas.

The component cells of neurofibromas are primarily perineural fibroblasts mixed with some Schwann cells. The cellular elements are typically present in a delicate, collagenous matrix that may exhibit foci of myxoid change.

OSTEOCHONDROMA AND OSTEOMA

Perhaps the two most common benign tumors of the TMJ are osteoma and osteochondroma. Radiographic studies fre-

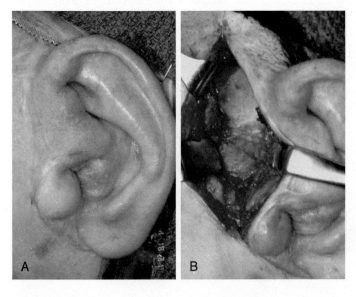

FIGURE 19–11. *A* and *B,* Cutaneous preauricular mass that extended to involve the temporomandibular joint capsule. The mass was subsequently determined to be a neurofibroma.

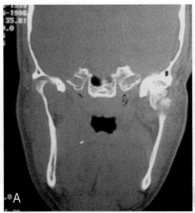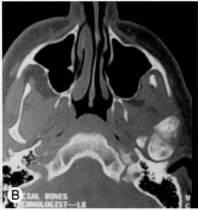

FIGURE 19–12. *A* and *B,* Coronal and axial computed tomography scans depicting the characteristic radiographic findings of an osteochondroma of the temporomandibular joint. Note the irregularly shaped mass in the region of the condylar head and the normal length of the ramus and condyle.

quently reveal an abnormally shaped condyle or a tumor mass attached to an abnormally shaped condyle (Fig. 19–12). In contrast to condylar hyperplasia, the condylar neck is generally of normal length. Also, the growth rate is usually slower than that of condylar hyperplasia. The anatomic location and size of most benign tumors of the condyles are such that a condylectomy is usually warranted to ensure complete removal.

Osteochondromas consist of a stalk or nodule of trabecular, cancellous bone that is surfaced by a cap of hyaline cartilage. A zone of endochondral ossification is evident between the cartilaginous cap and the underlying cancellous bone. Osteomas consist primarily of mature, lamellar bone. Two histologic variants involving the mandibular bone have been described. Compact osteomas are composed of relatively dense, cortical-type bone with osteons, haversian canals, and only minimal marrow tissue. Cancellous osteomas consist of trabeculae of mature bone with abundant fibrofatty or fibrovascular marrow tissue. Osteoblastic activity is variable but may be prominent in some osteomas.

PIGMENTED VILLONODULAR SYNOVITIS

Villonodular synovitis is a rare condition of unknown etiology that occurs more often at the knee than at the hip and rarely presents in the TMJ. Monoarticular involvement is the rule, although a few cases affecting both hips have been reported. Clinical manifestations are often subtle, in contrast to dramatic radiographic changes. Pain is often intermittent and may be triggered by excessive use. Even when pain is continuous, attacks of excruciating acute or subacute pain with limitation of joint motion are present. Joint swelling is rarely the initial presentation.[1]

Radiographs are consistently abnormal at presentation. The most suggestive radiographic findings are radiolucencies consistent with a cystic change, which can develop in the condylar head or neck located within the synovial area. Wide communication between the radiolucencies and the joint space is seen on CT scan. Invasion of the erosions by synovial proliferation may also be delineated (Fig. 19–13A). A frequent MRI finding is hypertrophy of the synovial membrane with nodules that generate very low-intensity signals on T1 and T2 images, denoting the presence of hemosiderin (Fig. 19–13B and *C*). Surgical synovectomy, with filling of any bone cavity, if needed, is the conventional treatment in other joints. However, in the TMJ, condylectomy may be more practical[6] (Fig. 19–13D and *E*).

Pigmented villonodular synovitis consists of irregular villous and nodular proliferations of synovial membranes into the joint space, associated with destruction of adjacent cartilage and bone. The thickened synovial membrane surface tissue is diffusely infiltrated by large cells with abundant cytoplasm that are derived from monocytes and macrophages. Scattered multinucleated giant cells and hemosiderin-laden macrophages are also consistently evident.

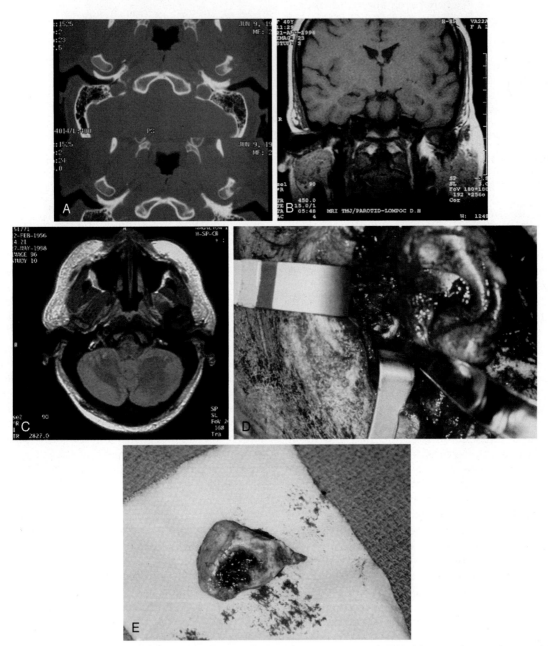

FIGURE 19–13. *A*, Axial computed tomography images demonstrating erosion of a condyle secondary to the synovial proliferation of pigmented villonodular synovitis. *B* and *C*, Axial and coronal magnetic resonance images demonstrating the synovial proliferation and low-intensity nodules of pigmented villonodular synovitis. *D* and *E*, Approach to the capsule of the left temporomandibular joint through a preauricular parotidectomy-type incision. Note the erosion of the condylar head by the proliferation of synovium and the darkly pigmented character of the tissue in the erosion secondary to hemosiderin deposits. (Courtesy of Dr. Anthony Pitrowski, Santa Maria, CA.)

SYNOVIAL CHONDROMATOSIS

Synovial chondromatosis is a rare benign arthropathy. Usually monoarthritic, it is characterized by the development of metaplastic, highly cellular cartilaginous foci in the synovial membrane. It has been reported under other names such as synovial osteochondromatosis, synovial chondrosis, articular chondrosis, synovial metaplasia, synovialoma, synovial chondrometaplasia, and periarticular tenosynovial chondrometaplasia.

The characteristic clinical presentation is periarticular swelling, pain, and limitation of joint movement, but it has been reported without these symptoms. The condition is manifested radiographically as a widened joint space (Fig. 19–14), limitation of motion, irregularity of the joint surfaces, presence of calcified loose bodies, and sclerosis or hyperostosis of the glenoid fossa.[9] The absence of radiopaque bodies on radiographs does not preclude the diagnosis of synovial chondromatosis, because the appearance of loose bodies varies with the degree of calcification of the cartilaginous nodules. CT and MRI scans are useful for diagnosis and to delineate the extent of the lesion.

Treatment consists of removal of the loose bodies and/or associated mass. A con-

dylectomy or more extensive resection may be necessary, depending on the size and extension of the mass. Intracranial extension has been reported with advanced lesions. McCain[9] reported a case that was diagnosed and treated arthroscopically, although he maintains that open arthrotomy may be necessary if particles larger than 3 mm are present (Fig. 19–15).

Synovial chondromatosis is a rare metaplastic condition involving articulator synovial membranes in which nodules of cartilage are produced. The cartilaginous nodules may be present within the synovial membrane or as detached, loose bodies within the joint space. The cellular elements are either arranged in clusters or more uniformly distributed within hyaline and myxoid chondroid matrix that may focally calcify. Individual cells may exhibit mild to moderate cytologic atypia, which should not be interpreted as representing features of malignancy. Clinical and radiographic correlation is often important in the diagnosis of synovial chondromatosis.

Inflammatory, Metabolic, and Genetic Disorders

The inflammatory-metabolic-genetic category accounts for a small percentage of

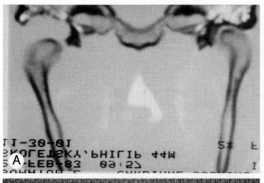
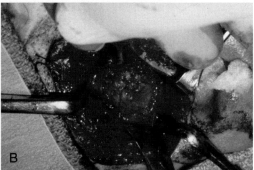
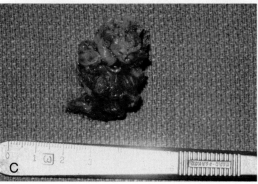

FIGURE 19–14. *A,* Coronal computed tomography scan depicting the characteristic widened joint space of a patient with synovial chondromatosis. *B,* Surgical exploration found a large, firm mass involving the right temporomandibular joint capsule and condyle. *C,* Treatment of synovial chondromatosis with a condylectomy.

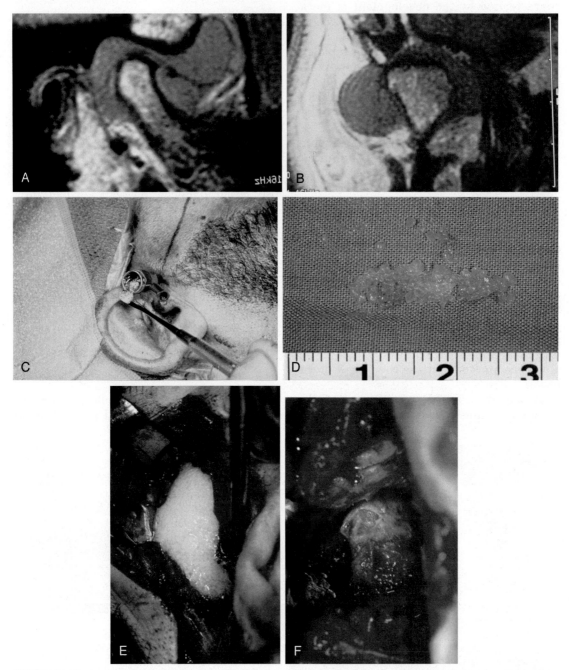

FIGURE 19–15. *A* and *B*, Coronal and axial magnetic resonance images of a patient with synovial chondromatosis of the temporomandibular joint. Note the enlarged joint space with the outpouching of synovium anteriorly and laterally. *C*, Extrusion of loose bodies from the joint space. *D*, Close-up of multiple loose cartilaginous bodies of synovial chondromatosis. *E*, Initial appearance at open arthrotomy of the patient depicted in *A*. Note the multiple small, loose cartilaginous bodies. *F*, Postoperative appearance after removal of all the loose cartilaginous bodies.

TMJ pathology and includes acromegaly, Garré's osteomyelitis, hemifacial hypertrophy, hemifacial microsomia, heterotopic bone formation, phantom bone disease, and septic arthritis. The characteristics of hemifacial microsomia, hemifacial hypertrophy, and acromegaly are well outlined elsewhere in this text and are not discussed in this chapter.

GARRÉ'S OSTEOMYELITIS

Garré's osteomyelitis can be considered a variant of chronic osteomyelitis with a concomitant prominent periosteal inflammatory reaction. This type of osteomyelitis is uncommon. It has been described in the tibia and in the maxillofacial region. In the mandible, it most commonly results from a periapical abscess associated with a molar. It has also been associated with pericoronal infections and infections following tooth extraction.[1] Rarely, this process may involve bone in the area of the TMJ. Patients typically present with a bony hard swelling of the posterior mandible. The overlying skin and mucosa characteristically appear normal. Occasionally the swelling may be tender.

The radiographic appearance is that of a centrally mottled radiolucency similar to chronic osteomyelitis. The peripheral periosteal reaction provides a distinctive radiographic appearance. The mandibular cortex is expanded, with concentric opaque layers (onion skin) noted on occlusal radiographs or CT scans. The clinician must differentiate Garré's osteomyelitis from benign mandibular neoplasms (Fig. 19–16). Radiographs are helpful to rule out certain neoplasms, but the radiographic presentation of fibrous dysplasia is often similar. Biopsy for histopathologic examination and bone culture is useful.

Removal of the etiologic agent is of paramount importance in the treatment of Garré's osteomyelitis. Some surgeons advocate additional treatment with antibiotic therapy. Others advocate wide exposure of the affected area with perforation of the mandibular cortex to allow for capillary ingrowth.

HETEROTOPIC BONE FORMATION

Heterotopic ossification is a condition in which mature lamellar bone is formed in tissues that do not normally ossify. Heterotopic ossification is considered to occur in three basic forms: traumatic, neurogenic, and myositis ossificans progressiva. It has also been described, although rarely, following tetanus, burns, poliomyelitis, and some forms of carcinoma. It is a well-recognized entity following injuries such as total hip arthroplasty and internal fixation of acetabular fractures.[10–12] It rarely occurs in the TMJ (Fig. 19–17).

The onset of heterotopic bone formation usually occurs approximately 2 weeks after injury, although symptoms may not present until 8 to 10 weeks later. A diminished range of motion of the joint is a hallmark characteristic and is often the earliest sign. Patients may also complain of pain, swelling, and local tenderness. Management includes arthroplasty and physiotherapy. Radiotherapy and pharmacologic therapy with

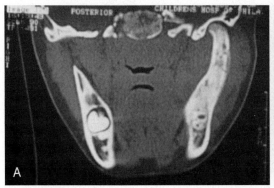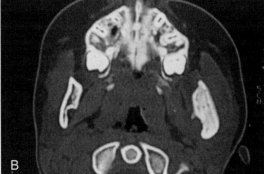

FIGURE 19–16. *A* and *B,* Coronal and axial computed tomography scans of a child with Garré's osteomyelitis involving the left mandibular ramus and condyle. Note the expansion of the mandibular cortex when compared with the normal side.

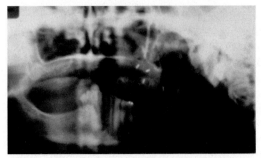

FIGURE 19–17. Panorex radiograph of the left temporomandibular joint depicting a firm, heterogeneous opaque mass involving the left condyle. This was subsequently diagnosed as a heterotopic bone formation. The formation of bone was induced by facial animation surgery to treat a facial nerve palsy.

agents such as bisphosphonates and non-steroidal anti-inflammatory drugs have been advocated as prophylaxis to prevent heterotopic bone formation.

PHANTOM BONE DISEASE

Phantom bone disease, also known as vanishing bone disease or massive osteolysis, is a rare clinical entity, with approximately 70 cases reported since its initial description in 1838. Only 15 cases have been reported in the maxillofacial region. The clinical course is characterized by a slowly progressive localized destruction of bone. Although the disease is progressive, its course can vary. With time, the bone destruction may spontaneously abate, or the bone may gradually disappear. No effective treatment is known for phantom bone disease.[1] Recently, controversy has developed as to whether this process represents a distinct entity or is a misinterpretation of other pathologic processes. Practitioners are encouraged to consider other pathologic entities when presented with a condition diagnosed as "phantom bone disease."

SEPTIC ARTHRITIS

Infections in the TMJ are extremely rare, even in cases of trauma or surgical intervention in this region. In underdeveloped countries, where prompt antibiotic treatment of middle ear infections is not available, direct extension of infections to the TMJ may occur. Prompt surgical drainage or arthroscopic lavage is appropriate management[6] (Fig. 19–18).

Malignant and Locally Invasive Lesions

The category of malignant and locally invasive lesions includes malignant tumors with cell origins from the component structures of the TMJ, metastatic tumors, and tumors with cell origins from tissues near the TMJ that are locally aggressive or malignant.

MALIGNANT TUMORS OF TMJ ORIGIN

Chondrosarcoma

It is paramount to distinguish chondrosarcoma from synovial chondromatosis of

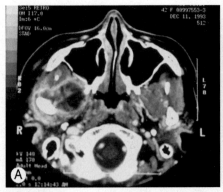
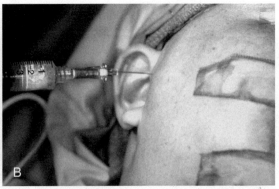

FIGURE 19–18. *A,* Axial computed tomography scan depicting a ring-enhancing lesion involving the right temporomandibular joint (TMJ) of a febrile patient. *B,* Aspiration of the right TMJ produced purulent material that subsequently led to a diagnosis of gonococcal arthritis.

the TMJ, as the treatment protocols of the two entities differ markedly. Additionally, the clinician should be cognizant that chondroid areas of pleomorphic adenomas arising in the parotid gland over the TMJ may mimic cartilaginous tumors of the bone. Integration of the pathologic, clinical, and radiographic presentations aids in the diagnosis.

Chondrosarcoma of the mandible and maxilla is extremely rare, accounting for approximately 1% of all chondrosarcomas. Most mandibular chondrosarcomas present in the mandibular body, with an occasional occurrence in the condylar process. No gender predilection has been noted, and it is present predominantly in adulthood. Although the mean age of occurrence is 60 years, almost half of cases arise in the third and fourth decades of life.[1]

The most common presentation is that of a painless swelling, with expansion of the underlying bone. The radiographic appearance varies from moth-eaten radiolucencies that are solitary or multilocular to diffusely radiopaque lesions. Because chondrosarcomas are radioresistant neoplasms, wide local or radical surgical excision is the treatment of choice. The 5-year survival rate for chondrosarcoma of the mandible is 17%.

Chondrosarcomas consist of a proliferation of malignant mesenchymal cells that produce a chondroid matrix in the absence of osteoid matrix production. The neoplastic cartilage cells are present within lacunar spaces of lobulated hyaline cartilage exhibiting variable degrees of calcification. Well-differentiated or grade I chondrosarcomas exhibit minimal cellularity and cells that appear to be relatively mature or display only minimal cytologic atypia. Grade II chondrosarcomas consist of tumors with a greater density of neoplastic cartilage cells that also exhibit larger, hyperchromatic, atypical nuclei. Grade III chondrosarcomas, rare in the jaws, are highly cellular with a high mitotic rate and individual cells that display significant nuclear atypia.

Multiple Myeloma

Plasma cell neoplasms are derived from bone marrow stem cells of B lymphocyte lineage. Multiple myeloma occurs after the fifth decade, with a mean age of occurrence of 63 years. Involvement of the jaws may be asymptomatic or may produce pain, swelling, expansion, numbness, and pathologic fracture.[1] The radiographic appearance is typically that of multiple punched-out but noncorticated radiolucent areas of bone destruction. Occasionally, the lesions may be expansile or radiographically sclerotic. Treatment usually consists of chemotherapy with radiation directed at painful lesions.

Multiple myeloma consists of a proliferation of malignant plasma cells forming broad sheets. The neoplastic plasma cells that infiltrate medullary bone vary from those that resemble normal plasma cells to those that are greatly enlarged and exhibit marked cytologic atypia and multinucleated forms. The neoplastic plasma cells are recognized by ample eosinophilic cytoplasm, eccentric nuclei, clumped chromatin at the nuclear membrane, and prominent nucleoli.

Osteosarcoma

Approximately 5% of osteosarcomas occur in the jaws. Osteosarcomas are reportedly associated with several preexisting bone abnormalities, including Paget's disease, fibrous dysplasia, giant cell tumor, multiple osteochondroma, bone infarct, chronic osteomyelitis, and osteogenesis imperfecta. Other osteosarcomas occur subsequent to radiation therapy to the affected region for unrelated or antecedent disease.

The peak incidence of osteosarcoma of the jaw is in the third or fourth decade, with a mean age of 34 years. The majority of mandibular osteosarcomas arise in the body (60%), with those arising in the TMJ accounting for a small percentage.[1] Osteosarcomas of the TMJ commonly present as rapidly enlarging, painful localized swelling. Paresthesia may occur secondary to involvement of the trigeminal nerve. Variants of osteosarcoma that may affect the TMJ are osteoblastic, fibroblastic, and chondroblastic osteosarcomas. The typical radiographic appearance is that of a lytic lesion (Figs. 19–19 and 19–20). Treatment generally consists of radical wide excision. Radiotherapy and chemotherapy are reserved for recurrence. The 5-year survival rate for osteosarcoma of the jaws is 25% to 40%. Unfortunately, the recurrence rate is high (40% to 70%), with a metastatic rate of 25% to 50%. The most

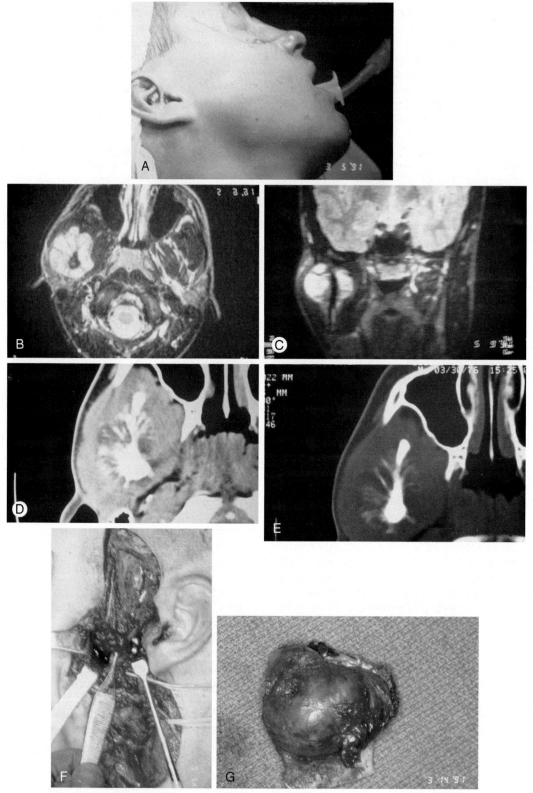

FIGURE 19–19. *A*, A 17-year-old boy with a large, firm, palpable preauricular mass. *B* and *C*, Axial and coronal images depicting a large mass of the right condylar head displacing the pterygoid and masseter muscles. *D* and *E*, Axial computed tomography images disclosing irregular bone spicules radiating from the ramus like the spoke of a wheel. This is characteristic of the so-called sun-ray appearance of osteosarcoma. *F* and *G*, Surgical wide excision of osteosarcoma through a preauricular parotidectomy-type incision; 2-cm bony margins were obtained.

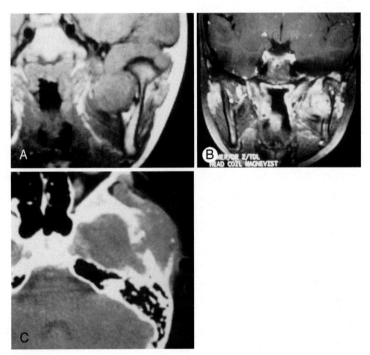

FIGURE 19–20. *A* and *B,* Coronal magnetic resonance images of a large soft tissue mass involving the left temporomandibular joint. Note the erosion of the mass through the base of skull and the extension into the deep and superficial temporal spaces, as well as the medial pterygoid space. *C,* The same left preauricular mass was seen eroding through the zygomatic arch on the computed tomography scan. This mass was an osteosarcoma.

common sites of metastases are the lung and brain, with extremely rare involvement of regional lymph nodes.[6]

Osteosarcoma consists of a proliferation of malignant mesenchymal cells that produce an osteoid matrix. In some cases of osteosarcoma, the malignant cells are also capable of producing a cartilaginous matrix or collagenous connective tissue. The chondroblastic form of osteosarcoma constitutes a greater percentage of total cases in the jaws than at other skeletal sites. The neoplastic mesenchymal cells are often quite pleomorphic, demonstrating variably sized hyperchromatic nuclei with irregular, angular contours. Some osteosarcomas are characterized by malignant cells that assume a spindle shape. Difficulties in diagnosis include lesions that exhibit osteoid production by cells exhibiting only minimal cytologic atypia and lesions in which osteoid matrix production is nearly absent.

Synovial Sarcoma

Synovial sarcoma of the head and neck area is predominantly a disease of young people, the median age being 19 years. A painless, deep-seated swelling is commonly the presenting complaint.[1] Early radical excision is probably the best treatment for synovial sarcoma of the head and neck. In other sites, the 5-year survival rate varies between 25% and 50%.

Synovial sarcoma consists of a proliferation of predominantly spindle-shaped cells that form broad sheets or fascicles. Biphasic synovial sarcoma also contains clusters of columnar or cuboidal epithelial cells, which may form small nests or line pseudoductal spaces. Monophasic forms of synovial sarcoma consist only of the spindle cell component.

INVASIVE TUMORS NOT OF TMJ ORIGIN

Aggressive Fibromatosis

Aggressive fibromatosis is classified as histologically benign but is extremely aggressive clinically, with a tendency to recur. The lesion is also known as extra-abdominal desmoid and desmoplastic fibroma. It presents in children and young adults with an approximately equal gender distribution. Approximately 10% of cases occur in the head and neck, with the mandible and perimandibular tissues the most frequently involved site in the region.[1] In some cases the presenting symptom is trismus, secondary to infiltration into the masseteric space (Fig. 19–21).

Recurrence after conservative surgical excision has been reported to be as high as 60%. Consequently, the lesion should be approached surgically as a malignancy. Adjuvant chemotherapy has been used in recurrent cases.[6]

Fibromatosis consists of a moderately cellular proliferation of uniform fibroblastic cells, which characteristically demonstrate ill-defined borders and a highly infiltrative periphery. The proliferating fibroblasts may form haphazardly arranged fascicles. The cells are spindle shaped and exhibit bland nuclei without atypia, hyperchromatism, or mitotic figures. Most examples of fibromatosis produce significant amounts of col-lagen. Diagnosis of aggressive fibromatosis is frequently based on the aggressive clinical behavior rather than on histologic factors.

Cholesteatoma

Cholesteatoma is a benign, locally destructive lesion of the middle ear. Large lesions may erode through the temporal bone to invade the TMJ (Fig. 19–22). Treatment of cholesteatoma generally involves surgical excision through a mastoidectomy approach by an otologist.

Lymphoma

Lymphoma of the head and neck region is a well-documented occurrence. The clinician should consider lymphoma in any patient with a preauricular swelling or swelling in the parotid region. CT scans or MRIs are useful in diagnosis (Figs. 19–23 and 19–24).

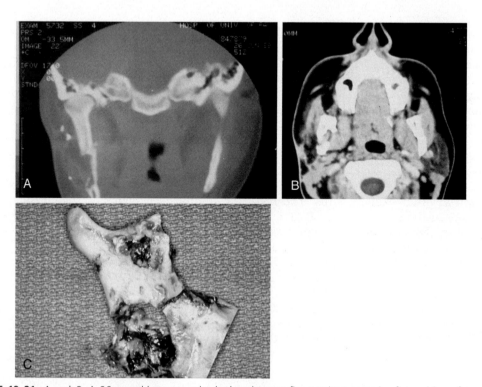

FIGURE 19–21. *A* and *B*, A 26-year-old woman who had undergone five previous surgeries for excision of a recurrent tumor "of the parotid gland." Biopsy of the lesion proved that it was aggressive fibromatosis. These figures demonstrate the extensive bony destruction of the entire right ramus of the mandible. The scans disclosed two distinct lesions: one at the angle of the mandible, and the second skip lesion involving the coronoid and condylar processes. *C*, Treatment entailed a partial mandibulectomy, resecting the entire right mandibular ramus. Note the presence of the two separate lesions in this pathologic specimen.

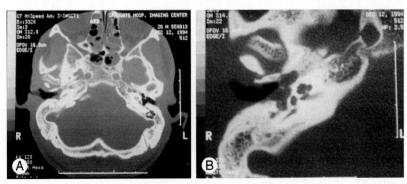

FIGURE 19–22. *A* and *B*, Axial computed tomography scans depicting invasion of the posterior right temporomandibular joint capsule by a lesion that proved to be a cholesteatoma originating in the middle ear.

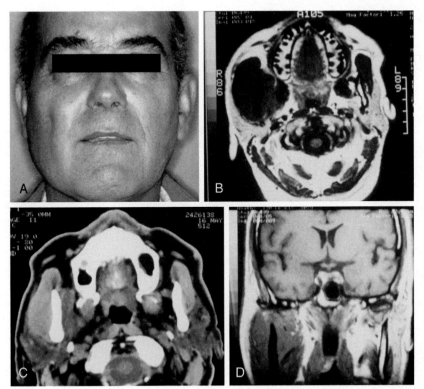

FIGURE 19–23. *A*, A 61-year-old man with painless right facial swelling and masseteric space enlargement. *B*, Magnetic resonance imaging (MRI) discloses diffuse infiltration of the entire masticator space. *C* and *D*, MRI and computed tomography scans depicting diffuse enlargement of the masseter and medial pterygoid muscles, with loss of the fat planes in the entire masticator space. Incisional biopsy subsequently disclosed this to be non-Hodgkin's lymphoma, which was treated with chemotherapy.

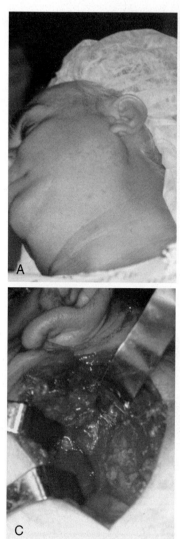

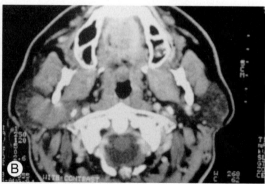

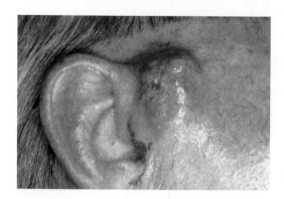

FIGURE 19–24. *A,* A middle-aged man with a firm, painless preauricular swelling. *B,* An axial computed tomography scan disclosed a mass in the right masticator space along the posterior border of the right mandibular ramus. *C,* Exposure of this lesion through the Blair modification of the Risdon incision. Biopsy of this mass proved it to be non-Hodgkin's lymphoma. It was subsequently treated with chemotherapy.

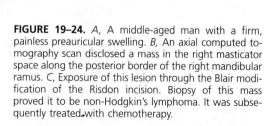

FIGURE 19–25. A firm preauricular mass in an elderly man that subsequently proved to be the initial presentation of metastatic colon carcinoma.

Tissue diagnosis can be obtained by fine-needle aspiration or open biopsy. Treatment frequently involves chemotherapy and radiation therapy.

Metastatic Lesions

A painful, rapidly progressing destructive lesion of the mandibular condyle that may be associated with deficits in trigeminal or facial nerve function should increase the clinician's index of suspicion for a neoplastic process. The presentation of a TMJ mass as a metastatic lesion of unknown origin is uncommon. However, if this does occur, a thorough investigation for the source of the primary tumor is mandatory. Sources of tumors that often metastasize to bone are kidney, ovarian, testicular, lung, prostate, thyroid, and breast. The mnemonic *Kinds Of Tumors Leaping Promptly To Bone* can be helpful in memorizing the possible sources and directing the investigation for the unknown primary tumor (Figs. 19–25 and 19–26).

Parotid Gland Neoplasm

Large parotid gland neoplasms may involve the TMJ. Treatment is dictated by the pathology of the salivary gland tumor and usually involves surgical resection.

REFERENCES

1. Regezi JA, Sciubba JJ: Oral Pathology: Clinical Pathologic Correlations, ed 3. Philadelphia, WB Saunders, 1998.
2. Reznik SA, Russell EJ, Hanson DH, Pecaro BC:

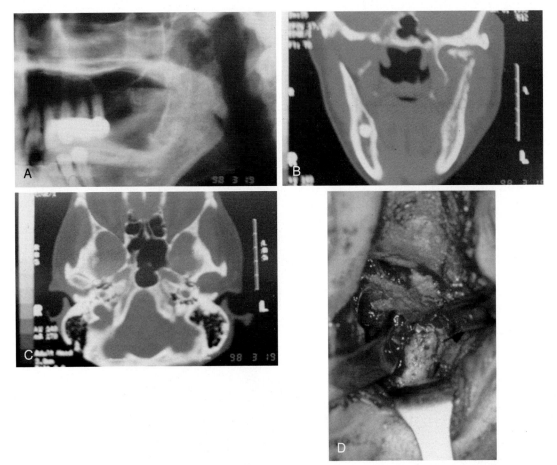

FIGURE 19–26. *A,* Portion of a Panorex radiograph of a 48-year-old woman who presented with trismus, left preauricular pain, and paresthesia of the left inferior alveolar nerve. *B,* Coronal computed tomography (CT) scan depicting erosion and loss of cortical definition of the left temporomandibular joint condyle and ramus. *C,* Axial CT scan depicting loss of the entire left condyle. *D,* Surgical exploration revealed complete erosion and loss of the condylar head. Frozen section pathology and permanent pathology proved this to be metastatic breast carcinoma.

Embolization of a life-threatening mandibular vascular malformation by direct percutaneous puncture. Head Neck 1992;14:372–379.

3. Flandroy P, Pruvo J: Treatment of mandibular arteriovenous malformations by direct transosseous puncture: Report of two cases. Cardiovasc Intervent Radiol 1994;17:222–225.

4. Carlson E: Pathologic facial asymmetries. Atlas Oral Maxillofac Surg Clin 1996;4:28–35.

5. Obwegeser HL, Malek MS: Hemimandibular hyperplasia, hemimandibular elongation. J Maxillofac Surg 1986;14:183–203.

6. Quinn PD: Color Atlas of Temporomandibular Joint Surgery. St. Louis, CV Mosby, 1998, pp 213–224.

7. Epker BN, Fish IC: Unilateral hyperplasia conditions of the mandibular condyle. In Dentofacial Deformities: Integrated Orthodontic Correction, vol 2. St. Louis, CV Mosby, 1986, pp 1108–1179.

8. Chang YM, Chan CP, Kung Wu SF, et al: Ganglion cyst and synovial cyst of the temporomandibular joint: Two case reports. Int J Oral Maxillofac Surg 1997;26:179–181.

9. Quinn PD, Stanton DC, Foote JW: Synovial chondromatosis with cranial extension. Oral Surg Oral Med Oral Pathol 1992;73:398–402.

10. Thomas BJ: Heterotopic bone formation after total hip arthroplasty. Orthop Clin North Am 1992;23:347–358.

11. Singer BR: Heterotopic ossification. Br J Hosp Med 1993;49:247–254.

12. Sedel L, Cabanela M: Hip Surgery Materials and Developments. St. Louis, CV Mosby, 1998.

Nonsurgical Management of Temporomandibular Joint Disorders and Facial Pain

CHAPTER

20

Biobehavioral Assessment and Treatment of Temporomandibular Disorders

Samuel F. Dworkin • Richard Ohrbach

The objectives of this chapter are to provide clinical perspectives, a scientific rationale, and practical methods for assessing and managing the behavioral, psychological, and psychosocial aspects of patients who present to oral and maxillofacial surgeons with temporomandibular disorders (TMD). The term *TMD* has gained widespread use as a label for a broad array of disorders in which the chief complaint is most commonly persistent pain in the masticatory musculature and/or the temporomandibular joint (TMJ) and in which the most important impairment is painful and limited mandibular function. Similarly, the term *biobehavioral* has gained widespread acceptance in the field of behavioral medicine, and it refers to the inevitable integration of biologic, psychological, psychosocial, and behavioral factors that combine to influence both symptom reports and responses to treatment. In this chapter, we refer to TMD broadly, for two reasons: (1) our description of the behavioral and psychosocial assessment and treatment is intended to apply to all persons with TMD, regardless of specific diagnosis, and (2) only a small number of persons have TMD that are limited to the joint structures and that require treatment.

Perspectives on Disease and Illness and Their Treatment

The assessment and management of biobehavioral aspects of a patient presenting with a TMD are crucial to a satisfactory treatment outcome, whether the treatment required is reversible, such as flat-plane occlusal splint therapy, or irreversible, such as a surgical procedure. Surgical management of TMD is not as common as other medical, pharmacologic, and behavioral treatments; nor is it typically recommended as an early treatment for the condition.[1] Nevertheless, surgical interventions are legitimately included in the broad array of treatments available for TMD, notwithstanding the unfortunate sequelae associated with some methods used in the past. This chapter is based on the understanding that almost all surgery for TMD involves surgery of the hard or soft components of the TMJ and that relief from persistent and often refractory TMJ pain is the most compelling and most prevalent reason that surgery is contemplated and undertaken.

In the field of health care, medicine has been greatly influenced by a stream of thinking that suggests that in order to understand the onset, maintenance, and termination of disease, it is necessary to understand that whereas organs get *diseases*, people get *illnesses*; whereas people come seeking *cures* for their *illnesses*, medicine typically offers *treatment* for their *diseases*. There are often critical differences between the facts of a person's disease and the perceptions he or she holds about that disease, that is, the perceived illness. For example, a person who is depressed or agitated over marital conflict and economic pressures may be engaging in stress-related and maladaptive behaviors such as parafunctional jaw activity, experiencing changes in sleep patterns, and seeking consolation or support when exhibiting pain behaviors; the same patient may have a painful joint arthropathy associated with significant abnormalities observed through jaw imaging methods. Although medicines and surgery can correct the *disease*—the joint arthropathy—continuation of the dysfunctional behaviors may be observed unless certain *illness* parameters are also addressed, allowing the person to cope more effectively with psychological stressors and their behavioral consequences that act on the masticatory system. Also, there are often critical differences between what health care providers, whether physicians or dentists (including oral and maxillofacial surgeons), do to treat the organic disease (e.g., surgery for arthropathy) and what the patient wants, expects, or thinks should be done to cure the illness once and for all (e.g., relief from conflicts that manifest as dysfunctional emotions, thoughts, and behaviors). The study of disease and treatment is the scientific study of pathobiology and its scientifically based biomedical applications—principally medicines and surgery. The study of illness and the expectation of cures is the scientific study of behavioral, social, and public health factors that influence whether people get sick or get better. These perspectives concerning an integrated biopsychosocial model are incorporated here because the impact of such a model on dentistry and dental education remains less than optimal.

Relevance of a Biopsychosocial Model

The term *biopsychosocial model*, as its name implies, reflects our growing understanding that illnesses and cures are complex; that to understand how and when we get sick and to understand whether we will respond to treatment, a host of factors in addition to biology must be considered. The biopsychosocial model does not seek to compete with, let alone replace, scientifically derived biologic models or current clinical practices. Rather, the model is an integrative one; it conceives that biologic processes and environmental factors are equipotent for explaining not only illness but also responses to treatment. Thus, no health problem is conceived of as either solely physical or solely mental, as simply biologic or psychological. Instead of trying to force a particular patient onto one end or the other of a single psychological-versus-somatic continuum, the current thinking suggests that at least two axes be conceptualized; that is, that each patient be located on one axis reflecting physical status and on a second axis reflecting psychological, emotional, or behavioral status.

At an operational level, the principles and methods for assessing and managing the thinking, emotions, and health-related behaviors of patients derive from the discipline of behavioral medicine, a specialized branch of clinical psychology. As implied earlier, the term *biobehavioral* refers to the widely accepted and repeatedly documented observation that our personal, psychological, and behavioral repertoire arises from and interacts with our physical health status. Our thoughts, emotions, and behaviors are inexorably intertwined with our biologic processes, so that changes in biology can contribute to changes in thinking, emotions, and behavior, and our psychological life can compel changes in biologic processes.

Temporomandibular Disorder as a Chronic Pain Condition

The most compelling reason for oral and maxillofacial surgeons to consider a biopsychosocial model as clinically relevant derives from the perspective of TMD as a chronic pain condition. Oral surgeons normally do not see TMD patients early in the history of the condition (except perhaps in smaller communities or when managed care plans require triaging new TMD cases from the primary physician directly to the oral and maxillofacial surgeon), and it is fair to say that, for the most part, surgical interventions for TMD are typically attempted only after other so-called conservative methods (e.g., removable splint, physical and behavioral therapies) have failed. Although the most common chronic pain conditions, such as back pain, tension headache, and TMD, differ in their respective anatomic sites, these pain conditions share common behavioral characteristics that have clear implications for both assessment and management.

COMMON BEHAVIORAL CHARACTERISTICS OF TMD AND OTHER CHRONIC PAIN CONDITIONS

- Poor correspondence of pathology with pain and suffering
- Transient psychological distress
- Potential for clinical depression, anxiety, and somatization
- Dysfunctional "chronic pain behaviors," such as interference with daily living and misuse of health care

Fordyce and colleagues[2] were the first to introduce the term *chronic pain behaviors* to emphasize that management of chronic pain involves a *rehabilitation* rather than a *cure* model—that is, the objectives for the management of patients with chronic pain emphasize rehabilitating the patient to return to a useful and productive lifestyle and minimizing depression and other debilitating emotional states, rather than achieving a permanent cure for pain. The concept of rehabilitation as an assessment and treatment approach for chronic pain now constitutes the largest part of all pain clinic programs. The common pain conditions are associated with repeated bouts of treatment that are sometimes initially successful— many reports claim 80% or better "cure" rates[3] for TMD without explaining how such high success rates are paradoxically associated with the need for so much additional treatment.

With regard to TMD surgery specifically, there are few data available that allow dependable prediction of which patients will benefit from any of the TMJ surgical procedures currently available—from arthrocentesis to condylectomy—and those for whom a particular surgical intervention represents only one of a number of diverse attempts to cure the pain. It is now common

practice, when back pain surgery is being contemplated, to include a thorough psychological assessment of the patient as well as the usual physical work-up, in order to determine predictors of successful outcome.[4] The most important predictors of poor outcome for those suffering a chronic pain condition seem to be related to time away from work, depression, somatization, and undue reliance on the health care system for medications or invasive diagnostic and surgical procedures. Physical pathology factors alone often do not adequately predict successful outcome when surgery is attempted solely for the relief of pain.

Behavioral Assessment

The primary reasons for conducting a biobehavioral assessment of TMD patients relate to the potential impact that psychological, emotional, and behavioral factors can have on treatment; to the likelihood of a positive outcome following indicated surgical interventions; or to both. If the outcome of a biobehavioral assessment held no implications for treatment, it would be difficult to justify conducting such an evaluation. In this section, we (1) provide a specific clinical and scientific basis and rationale for conducting a behavioral assessment; (2) describe the content and methods a biobehavioral assessment encompasses; and (3) profile TMD patients based on information derived from current biobehavioral concepts and methods.

CLINICAL BASIS FOR BIOBEHAVIORAL ASSESSMENT

The first application of psychological concepts to the management of chronic pain, by Fordyce,[5] stressed a behavioral approach almost exclusively. Using the term *behavioral* in its historical, narrowest sense is to focus exclusively on observable behavior: the behavior of a pain patient that an independent observer could see, for example, grimacing, limping, and so forth. This narrower behavioral perspective excludes the assessment of emotional or mental states such as anxiety, depression, meaningfulness of symptoms, and expectations for cure. Although the introduction of these narrower concepts of behavioral assessment and associated behavioral management methods had a tremendous impact on and radically altered the management of chronic pain, the term *behavioral assessment* is too narrow to encompass our current concepts about pain; thus the term *biobehavioral assessment* has been introduced to include assessment of the patient's cognitive (i.e., thinking) and affective (i.e., emotional) status, as well as assessment of his or her current level of behavior (i.e., the extent to which behavior in social settings such as home, work, or school, and even when seeking TMD treatment, is adaptive or maladaptive)—in sum, the current level of psychosocial function.

It is equally important to understand that this more broadly defined approach of biobehavioral assessment can take place at many levels, depending on why the assessment is undertaken. Thus, a psychiatrist who must make a decision about the involuntary institutionalization of a suicidal person would need to call on a set of highly specialized biobehavioral assessment and diagnostic skills acquired through a specialized education in biobehavioral science and medicine. In contrast, most doctors—physicians and dentists—can readily acquire the relatively modest skills needed to determine whether caution is needed because a patient is unduly anxious, depressed, or preoccupied with physical symptoms; holds irrational views about his or her condition; is functioning poorly in the world; or any combination.

The concepts and methods advocated in this chapter are intended for nonpsychiatrically trained general dentists and dental specialists such as oral and maxillofacial surgeons. The clinical objective is to obtain a clear working picture of what patients are experiencing by way of pain and other symptoms and their psychological and biobehavioral adaptability to those symptoms. Biobehavioral assessment may point to expanded treatment possibilities that fall within the realm of behavioral and cognitive-behavioral therapies. The data pertaining to current emotional status, when reflected back to the patient by the surgeon, may make a referral for further evaluation of the need for psychologically based adjunctive therapies more palatable to the patient.

Finally, assessment of biobehavioral status facilitates the establishment of a positive and optimistic doctor-patient relationship, or therapeutic alliance, and allows a collaborative set to be formed. A collaborative set refers to surgeon and patient working toward the same objectives: commonly held expectations are developed concerning what is to be done and why. In the process of gathering and reviewing with the patient information pertaining to biobehavioral status, the opportunity naturally presents itself to review the patient's comprehension of alternative treatment plans and his or her willingness and readiness to undertake requisite pre-, intra-, and postoperative regimens.

METHODS FOR BIOBEHAVIORAL ASSESSMENT

Many methods have evolved for the biobehavioral assessment of patients with chronic pain conditions. In general, much more attention has been paid to developing reliable and valid methods for assessing other chronic pain conditions than for assessing TMD. However, from the perspectives discussed earlier, TMD shares many biobehavioral characteristics with other common chronic pain conditions, and it is reasonable to assume that methods applicable to those conditions may be applicable to TMD as well. The four most widely used approaches to the biobehavioral assessment of chronic pain patients are observational, self-report, self-monitoring, and multiaxial. The reader should consult other sources (e.g., Volume 4 Chapter 7; Ohrbach[6, 7]) for elaboration of the physical examination for TMD in general, to provide a complete biobehavioral assessment.

Observational Methods

Direct observation of pain-related physical behaviors was first introduced by Fordyce in the management of chronic back pain; it was then extended and formalized by him into reliable and valid scales for measuring the impact of pain on physical movement.[5] Methods for reliably observing and coding facial behavior for pain have been developed by LeResche and Dworkin[8] and others.[9, 10] Based on a survey of the current literature, it is fair to conclude that direct observational measures of TMD patients for biobehavioral assessment are not as well developed as the widely used self-report measures.[8]

Self-Report Methods

Typically, self-report methods include the use of interview schedules; symptom checklists; psychological and biobehavioral rating scales; and psychological tests assessing mental and emotional status, psychosocial adaptation, coping behaviors, and health care utilization. It is beyond the scope of this chapter to review the many published measures that have received attention from biobehaviorally oriented TMD clinical researchers. The most common self-report measures used for the biobehavioral assessment of chronic pain conditions are summarized.

Minnesota Multiphasic Personality Inventory (MMPI) Perhaps the best known and most widely used instrument for assessing psychological status, the MMPI is not intended as a diagnostic instrument but rather provides a personality profile of psychological function. The test is long and takes highly specialized training to interpret, so its use is not suitable for many clinicians. The clinical value of the MMPI to many non–mental health and biomedical clinicians remains somewhat controversial. Standardization samples used for MMPI scale construction are reported in several independent studies as not being appropriate for chronic pain patients. However, using clustering methods to identify MMPI scale profiles that characterize pain patients, including TMD patients, has proved somewhat more useful. Generally, whether using the MMPI or the more recently revised and restandardized MMPI-2, elevations on scales 1, 2, and 3—hypochondriasis, depression, and hysteria—were associated with perceptions of severe pain, affective disturbance, and maladaptive patterns of psychosocial functioning. When elevations on psychopathic deviancy and schizophrenia scales accompanied elevations on scales 1, 2, and 3, not surprisingly, higher levels of psychopathology and resistance to modification of pain behavior were observed.[11]

Although it was originally anticipated that distinct MMPI profiles would be confirmed for chronic pain patients, these have not emerged clearly, and the use of the MMPI for predicting pain clinic treatment outcome, for example, remains problematic. Nevertheless, the MMPI has been used in many studies of TMD patients, and these studies support the conclusion that clinical psychopathology is present in an appreciable number of TMD patients presenting for treatment.[12] Using the MMPI in a study predicting response to treatment for TMD, McCreary and associates[13] found that somatization was related to jaw function problems at long-term follow-up, but not at early follow-up. They found that "somatization was a significant predictor of outcome" for chronic TMD patients and concluded, "if treatment does not address this somatization process, there is an increased risk there will be no improvement" (p 168). The MMPI may be potentially useful to oral and maxillofacial surgeons if the patient is referred to a psychologist for administration and interpretation of test results.

SCL-90-R The SCL-90-R[14] is a 90-item symptom checklist that yields several scales, the most relevant of which are scales assessing depression, anxiety, and somatization. The SCL-90-R is much briefer than the MMPI, but its overall usefulness with chronic pain patients has not been unequivocally established, and some problems have emerged related to its use in chronic pain populations. For example, there has been difficulty in replicating the original 10-factor structure of the entire SCL-90-R as obtained by Derogatis.[14] Nevertheless, the SCL-90-R has been used extensively to study all types of chronic pain populations, including TMD. When comparing the responses of chronic pain and psychiatric populations, the chronic pain population was distinguished, in studies by Buckelew and colleagues,[15] by reports of psychological distress limited to somatic, as opposed to emotional or cognitive, symptoms of anxiety and depression.

We have used several of the SCL-90-R scales in our own longitudinal research, after developing population norms derived from our own epidemiologic, or population-based, studies for the scales in the assessment instrument we use clinically and for research. The scales include those assessing anxiety, depression, and somatization. We incorporated items of this type into the patient database completed by all TMD patients at the University of Washington Department of Oral Medicine's Orofacial Pain and Dysfunction Clinic and reported extensively on findings derived using these SCL-90-R scales with TMD and other chronic pain patients.[16-18] Findings comparable to ours have been reported using the SCL-90-R in a similar fashion[19] to relate levels of depression and somatization to clinical findings from a TMD physical examination, as well as to examine the relationship between clinical depression and the presence of chronic pain problems. For example, in a study of TMD clinic cases and controls, when TMD was accompanied by multiple somatic pain complaints, the likelihood of a diagnosis of major depression using SCL-90-R algorithms increased dramatically, compared with those with no chronic pain conditions or only a single chronic pain complaint. The risk for depression increased by more than five- or eight-fold, respectively, depending on whether TMD was accompanied by one or more than one coexisting self-reported chronic pain condition such as headache, back pain, chest pain, or stomach pain.

Multidimensional Pain Inventory (MPI) Turk and colleagues[20, 21] developed the MPI, perhaps the most widely used self-report measure, to assess the biobehavioral and cognitive responses of patients with chronic pain. Unlike the IMPATH and TMJ scales (described later), its use is not limited to patients with TMD, and it has been extensively investigated for its psychometric properties, demonstrating acceptable levels of reliability, validity, and predictability of pain response pattern. The measure was developed with pain clinic populations and has been found to yield three distinct patient clusters that appear consistently across diverse chronic pain conditions, including back pain, headache, and TMD.

The chronic pain groups distinguished by the MPI are labeled *adaptive copers, interpersonally stressed,* and *dysfunctional,* and the three types reflect a continuum of increasing disability and pain-related psychosocial dysfunction. Turk and Rudy[20] demonstrated that TMD patients characterized as dysfunctional show significantly elevated depression and report significantly more physical symptoms than those TMD patients that the MPI categorizes as adaptive copers. By contrast, and most important to consider when evaluating patients for TMJ surgery, dysfunctional TMD patients and adaptive copers were not found to differ significantly along physical parameters (e.g., proportion of positive computed tomography [CT] scan findings, objective findings from a TMD clinical examination). More recently, Rudy and colleagues[22] used the MPI to assess the relative efficacy of a cognitive-behavioral treatment intervention compared with physical treatment involving the use of an intraoral occlusal splint. They presented evidence that dysfunctional versus adaptive copers and interpersonally stressed patients responded differentially to these treatments, supporting their conclusion that clinical treatment decisions for TMD patients should include not only assessment of biobehavioral status but also assignment to treatment interventions specifically based on the assessed level of psychosocial function. The MPI is one of the most carefully designed and well-studied self-report measures for assessing biobehavioral and psychosocial functioning in chronic pain patients.

Illness Behavior and Sickness Impact Measures Measures have been developed by Pilowsky—the Illness Behavior Questionnaire (IBQ)[23]—and by Bergner and associates—the Sickness Impact Profile (SIP)[24]—assessing the psychological and biobehavioral impact of illness and illness beliefs. These measures have provided useful information about biobehavioral adaptation to chronic pain, including disability associated with chronic pain conditions (notably, back pain) and differences in beliefs and expectations between pain clinic populations and chronic pain patients seeking treatment elsewhere. The results of these measures have appeared in the TMD literature, supporting the conclusion that for a significant minority of clinic cases, TMD has an appreciable impact on personal functioning, but neither the IBQ nor the SIP is in common use by TMD clinicians or researchers.

Pain Coping Measures Two approaches to assessing how patients cope with chronic pain have received attention. A well-known and widely used measure of pain coping developed by Keefe and Gill[25] indicates that passive coping strategies, particularly catastrophizing and praying, seem to be common among those who respond less well, biobehaviorally and emotionally, to their chronic pain problems. Supporting data come from use of a measure developed by Brown and Nicassio[26] that indicates that those who use active rather than passive pain coping styles and those who perceive themselves as having some control over their pain conditions remain better able to minimize the personal and psychological negative impact.

Numerous additional measures exist that assess diverse dimensions of the chronic pain experience. Some of the more interesting ones that warrant attention from biobehavioral TMD researchers include the Ways of Coping Checklist,[27] which measures coping with stress not specific to chronic pain; measures of daily stress used by Lennon and colleagues[28] to study the psychosocial adaptation of TMD patients; and the Millon Biobehavioral Health Inventory, the Chronic Illness Problem Inventory, the Psychosocial Pain Inventory, and the Pain Beliefs Questionnaire.[11, 29] Reports using these measures, taken together, confirm the extent to which TMD can be disabling for an appreciable segment of TMD sufferers.

TMJ Scale   The TMJ Scale[30–33] was developed as a self-report measure for use in the home or office and assesses three domains: physical, psychosocial, and global. The physical domain includes assessment of pain, and the psychosocial domain assesses psychological factors and stress. The scale, which has reportedly been used quite extensively, requires scoring and interpretation by its developers. It yields information that may be useful for clinicians treating TMD, although some questions about its validity as a psychological assessment tool have been noted by Rugh and coworkers[34] and by Deardorff,[12] as well as by others.[35] Findings from the TMJ Scale indicate that women with TMD report a higher level of severity of all physical and psychological symptoms compared with men, and a relationship between severity of psychological problems and chronicity of TMD has been noted. The authors readily acknowledge that the TMJ Scale has not been the subject of longitudinal studies—that is, cohorts of patients have not been repeatedly assessed with the TMJ Scale over time—but substantial cross-sectional data have been collected over a number of years.

IMPATH Scale   The IMPATH Scale for TMD is an interactive computer-based assessment instrument developed at the University of Minnesota by Fricton and colleagues for use as a screening and personal history instrument.[36] It has the advantage of instantaneous feedback, but unfortunately, the psychometric characteristics of its illness behavior components have not yet been well established. It is mentioned here because, like the TMJ Scale, it may serve as a useful guide for clinicians wishing to obtain a clinical impression of how their patients are doing psychologically and biobehaviorally.

Self-Monitoring Methods

Self-monitoring has been used extensively for decades for a wide variety of clinical problems, and its clinical uses are limited only by the imagination of the clinician and the cooperation of the patient. Its implementation can range from a request from the clinician to observe a simple phenomenon (e.g., whether the TMJ clicks while eating) to a multicolumn table that lists time of day, pain intensity, mood state, cognitions, and behaviors over the preceding 30 minutes, to be completed by the patient after each pain episode for 2 weeks. Self-monitoring was first used for TMD patient assessment to record parafunctional behaviors.[37]

We highly recommend this method to obtain further clinical information, to test specific hypotheses about possible causal relations between behavioral or psychological factors and clinical symptoms or signs, and to involve the patient actively and directly in his or her care. The patient who is "too busy" or who "can't be bothered" by such an activity should be regarded cautiously as a candidate for surgery if uncontrolled lifestyle or behavioral factors could jeopardize the prognosis for a successful surgical outcome. Such refusals to cooperate might serve as a useful indicator for a full behavioral assessment from a psychologist. Caveats to consider in the use of self-monitoring are listed in Table 20–1.

TABLE 20–1.	Guidelines for Patient Self-Monitoring

- Delineate clearly the target sign, symptom, or behavior.
- Have the patient demonstrate understanding of the target (e.g., patient makes jaw click).
- Start with a few simple targets.
- Add other targets or attributes as the patient becomes proficient in self-monitoring.
- Provide written instruction.
- Schedule a short follow-up appointment within 1 week of providing the initial self-monitoring task to check the patient's understanding and enhance his or her motivation.
- Discuss obtained data actively with the patient and use that as a basis for mutual problem solving regarding further self-monitoring targets or specific treatment needs.

Multiaxial Diagnostic and Assessment Methods

Methods that seek to integrate physical and biobehavioral factors into a multiaxial diagnostic and assessment instrument have been developed in recognition of the well-established relationship among physical, behavioral, and psychological factors.

The International Association for the Study of Pain (IASP) Classification of Chronic Pain and Description of Chronic Pain Syndromes[38] uses five axes applicable in the assessment of all chronic pain conditions. Axis I is used to record the body region in which the pain sites occur; axis II designates the physiologic system (e.g., musculoskeletal, cutaneous, nervous) that is functioning abnormally and giving rise to pain; axis III reflects temporal characteristics and patterns of occurrence (e.g., single episode, continuous, fluctuating); axis IV captures the patient's statement of pain intensity and time since onset (e.g., mild, of 1 month or less duration, severe, of more than 6 months' duration); and axis V is reserved for etiology and includes dysfunctional and psychological origin categories as well as designation of the etiology as genetic, inflammatory, and so forth. Although the IASP classification system represents a significant step toward scientifically validating the multidimensional nature of pain, its use has been limited, and it has functioned chiefly in a heuristic fashion to compel the development of multiaxial methods for pain diagnosis and assessment that are both use-ful in clinical research and practical in clinical settings.

Research Diagnostic Criteria for TMD (RDC/TMD) Clinicians and researchers at the University of Washington's Department of Oral Medicine coordinated a National Institute of Dental Research–funded international team in the development of the RDC/TMD, a dual-axis system for diagnosing and classifying TMD patients.[39] Axis I is reserved for physical diagnoses of the most commonly occurring masticatory muscle and/or TMJ disorders. Axis II is used to assess (1) clinically relevant pain status variables; (2) a measure of jaw disability; (3) psychological distress reflected specifically as depression, anxiety, and the presence of nonspecific physical symptoms indicating somatization tendencies; and (4) a graded scale of chronic pain interference and psychosocial dysfunction. The RDC/TMD criteria for axes I and II, operationally defined and at least in part empirically supported, are now available for studies assessing their reliability, validity, and clinical usefulness. Because the RDC/TMD represents a standardized method for assessing both physical and biobehavioral aspects of TMD, it allows comparison of TMD populations across diverse clinical settings. A recent report[19] indicated that comparable prevalence rates were observed for the most common types of TMD appearing at both a major U.S. clinic and a regional TMD public health clinic in Sweden: muscle disorders and joint pain conditions predominated, and disk derangements with limitations in mandibular opening were rare, as were the most advanced forms of degenerative joint disease. The RDC/TMD was offered as a research instrument to the clinical research community for further assessment of reliability and validity, which is an ongoing process. However, it has been used for several years as the major clinical instrument for assessing all new cases at the University of Washington's Orofacial Pain and Dysfunction Clinic. Finally, as an additional limitation, the RDC/TMD was designed to allow dual-axis assessment of both physical and biobehavioral findings for the most commonly occurring TMD conditions, so that operational criteria and examination methods have not been specified for less frequently observed masticatory system disorders such as myositis, focal dyskinesias, dystonia, or other conditions that oral and maxillofacial surgeons may encounter.

PROFILE OF THE TMD PATIENT

The biobehavioral assessment should result in a clinically useful composite picture, or profile, of the TMD patient with regard to pain status, maladaptive or parafunctional jaw behavior, psychological status, and ability to remain free from pain-related interference with usual daily activities. In the section that follows, a practical approach is suggested for arriving at a clinical "working picture" of how the clinical TMD problem in the anatomic structures affects the person's perception of pain, the extent of the patient's psychological distress, and how he or she is coping with the condition's impact on overall and health-related behavior. It would be most helpful if research and shared clinical experience in the biobehavioral aspects of TMD yielded ready-made personality profiles that characterized the typical TMD patient appearing for surgery, or at least usefully categorized TMD patients into a reasonably manageable set of patient "types." However, attempts at profiling TMD patients by personality type—indeed, attempts at personality typing of patients with chronic pain of any kind—have not been rewarding from either theoretical or clinical perspectives. In part, the inability to derive useful personality typologies of pain patients may reflect lingering limitations in the biomedical, as opposed to the biopsychosocial, theories about conditions in which chronic pain is a prominent feature. The biomedical model's implicit stance is to identify the clinical presentation as a problem residing in the patient's physical status or, failing to confirm a disease process coextensive with the presentation, to relegate the condition to a problem in the person—that is, a personality problem. Alternatively, the clinical relevance of the biopsychosocial model is to focus on the person's adaptation to illness, remembering that illness is defined as the self-attribution (not the doctor's) that a disease is present. Two of the assessment methods outlined earlier, the MPI and the dual-axis RDC/TMD approach, both derived from the most current biopsychosocial perspectives, seek to assess how well or how poorly the person

is adapting to his or her perceptions about his or her illness, relegating to the biomedical clinician the management of disease processes in the body.

The MPI accomplishes its biobehavioral assessment objectives by categorizing individuals, as outlined earlier and independent of physical status, into three profiles. The first is a cluster of adaptive responders who report low levels of pain, high levels of social support, low levels of pain interference, and greater amounts of activity; patients in this cluster are coping reasonably well with their clinical condition. The second group, identified as interpersonally stressed, reports lower levels of social support and is less able to maintain adaptive activity levels in response to personal and environmental stressors. The third cluster represents psychosocially dysfunctional patients with chronic pain conditions who perceive the severity of pain to be high, report that pain interferes with much of their daily activities and responsibilities, and experience a high degree of distress. An immediate implication of this trichotomy would be to consider treatment alternatives for these three very different appearing groups (including TMD patients, for whom the taxonomy has been well validated), perhaps recommending for the more dysfunctional group that psychological therapies be integrated into the overall clinical management. In fact, recent evidence confirms the utility of just such an approach, but the conceptual approach is too new to have been adequately tested with randomized clinical trials, as of this writing.

The RDC/TMD seeks to accomplish the same objective of separately considering the physical and the biobehavioral status of the patient, but in a single assessment instrument. The RDC/TMD derives its composite picture of how well or how poorly a TMD patient is currently adapting to his or her clinical condition by measuring separately the intrapersonal subjective experience of the patient through the use of symptom scales to assess anxiety, depression, and somatization. Because the purpose is to derive a clinically useful assessment picture, not a psychiatric diagnosis of mental and emotional pathology, the assessment measures are easy to use and readily interpretable as described by the RDC/TMD.[39] In addition to a reasonably straightforward and intuitive assessment of the extent of anxiety and depression symptoms, the RDC/TMD incorporates a third measure of psychological status, namely, somatization, also in the form of a simple and easy-to-understand checklist comprising the somatization scale of the SCL-90-R.

Somatization has emerged as a relevant factor in chronic pain, and the assessment of somatization is advocated as a useful component of the psychological profile of TMD patients being evaluated for surgery. Somatization may best be understood as a dimension of personal functioning characterized by the tendency to report distress arising from multiple nonspecific physical symptoms. A spectrum of severity has been described for somatization, with one end being occupied by psychiatric disorders recognized in the fourth edition of the *Diagnostic and Statistical Manual of Mental Disorders* (DSM-IV)[40] of the American Psychiatric Association and requiring the presence of at least eight physical symptoms, distributed over multiple organ systems and not explained by a diagnosable medical condition. More relevant to clinicians working with chronic pain problems is that end of the somatization spectrum represented by four to five similarly nonspecific physical symptoms that are perceived as distressful. Table 20–2 shows representative symptoms assessed by the RDC/TMD to evaluate somatization status and includes the items in the RDC/TMD screening assessment for anxiety and depression. It should be noted that the latter scales, intended to assess emotional status, also include many somatic items. Indeed, it is difficult to qualify for a formal affective psychiatric disorder (e.g., major depressive disorder or anxiety disorder) without identifying a number of nonspecific physical symptoms as frequently present and distressing.

Finally, the RDC/TMD also incorporates an easy-to-use Graded Chronic Pain Scale, ranging from Grade 0 to Grade IV (Table 20–3). It is an integrated measure combining pain intensity (rated on a 0–10 visual analog scale) and pain impact (the extent of TMD-related interference with daily activities, measured as a 0–10 visual analog scale number reflecting extent of interference with usual daily activities at home, work, school, or socially, and disability days due to TMD pain). The development of the Graded Chronic Pain Scale and its psychometric properties have been described in detail elsewhere.[41] Because the Graded Chronic Pain Scale was derived from population-based studies of chronic pain in the community (Table 20–4) and not from a pain clinic population, it can be used for data collection under a variety of research designs, ranging from random sample surveys to clinical intervention studies, and has proved to be a useful clinical measure to assess the impact of chronic TMD on our patients.

The Graded Chronic Pain Scale was created not only to provide a meaningful quantitative index of the extent to which pain is perceived as mild or severe in intensity but also to capture the extent to which pain is psychosocially disabling. Disability is measured by the extent of pain-related interference with daily activities and number of lost activity days (e.g., days unable to go to work or school, attend to household responsibilities) attributed to TMD pain. Grade I is

---

TABLE 20–2.	**Physical Symptom Checklists for Assessment of Psychological Status**

Anxiety	Depression	Somatization
Spells of terror or panic	Restless or disturbed sleep	Headaches
Trembling	Trouble falling asleep	Pain in heart or chest
Feeling that something bad is going to happen to you	Early awakening	Pains in lower back
Thoughts or images of a frightening nature	Loss of sexual interest	Nausea or gastric upset
Feeling so restless that you can't sit still	Poor appetite	Muscle soreness
Feeling nervous or shaky inside	Overeating	Faintness or dizziness
Feeling tense or keyed up	Feelings of guilt	Trouble breathing
Suddenly being scared for no reason	Thoughts of death or dying	Hot or cold spells
Heart pounding or racing	Thoughts of ending your life	Numbness or tingling
Feeling fearful		Lump in throat
		Weakness in body
		Heaviness in limbs

TABLE 20–3. Relationship of Chronic Pain Grade to Biobehavioral Variables

Variable	TMD Pain					Headache					Back Pain				
	Grade I	Grade II	Grade III	Grade IV	Total	Grade I	Grade II	Grade III	Grade IV	Total	Grade I	Grade II	Grade III	Grade IV	Total
Graded pain variables															
Average pain intensity	3.4	5.9	5.8	7.4	5.0	4.3	6.3	7.1	7.5	6.0	3.1	5.5	5.4	6.0	4.7
Disability days	0.8	1.7	31.3	114.4	10.4	1.8	2.9	13.9	55.7	10.1	2.9	3.3	23.3	76.8	19.8
Percent high intensity	0.0	100.0	90.2	95.2	58.1	0.0	100.0	91.0	96.1	68.1	0.0	100.0	71.7	89.7	57.6
Selected variables															
Percent 90+ pain days	36.0	59.8	65.0	76.2	51.7	16.9	30.1	20.9	40.8	25.4	24.8	51.9	31.3	58.6	39.4
Days in pain	68.3	104.2	104.4	132.9	91.7	38.1	63.4	45.7	88.8	55.2	52.9	93.9	70.9	111.1	78.5
Years since onset	5.6	6.2	5.4	7.6	6.0	17.1	18.0	16.9	17.4	17.5	11.8	14.0	12.5	10.1	12.3
Elevated depression	16.4	29.4	29.3	57.1	25.6	13.5	30.7	35.9	48.1	28.4	12.1	20.3	24.5	41.7	22.0
Health rated fair to poor	6.9	12.9	14.6	55.0	12.8	6.6	12.3	21.2	24.7	13.7	4.1	9.1	11.8	20.6	9.9
Frequent opioid use	0.0	3.5	4.9	19.1	3.1	0.0	2.6	1.9	9.1	2.3	0.5	4.2	5.1	15.8	5.1
Frequent pain visits	1.3	7.7	22.5	23.8	7.5	1.8	4.6	19.5	29.3	9.2	1.2	5.2	8.0	27.5	8.1
High pain impact	5.1	25.4	63.4	71.4	23.8	14.7	33.1	50.7	75.0	35.4	10.4	25.5	48.5	72.1	32.8
Unemployed	3.9	7.3	12.5	28.6	7.4	1.7	2.4	8.3	21.8	5.2	1.4	0.8	6.3	26.6	6.1

TABLE 20–4.	Prevalence of Chronic Pain Grades in Two Population-Based Studies (1986 and 1992)

	Prevalence (%)	
Chronic Pain Grade	1986	1992
Grade I: low pain, low disability	39	43
Grade II: high pain, low disability	42	35
Grades III and IV: high disability, moderate to severe limitation, typically high pain intensity	19	22

defined as TMD pain of low intensity, averaging less than 5 on a 10-point scale, and associated with little pain-related interference in daily living. Grade II is defined as high-intensity pain, above 5 on a 10-point scale, with moderate amounts of pain-related interference. Grades III and IV are associated with increasing levels of pain-related psychosocial disability regardless of pain level. Data are provided in Table 20–3 to show the relationship between the Graded Chronic Pain Scale and selected biobehavioral variables. For clinical purposes, functional TMD patients (i.e., individuals not significantly disabled by their TMD condition) are defined as grades I and II. Grades III and IV represent those significantly disabled by TMD.

It is important to point out that these demarcations of functional and dysfunctional, although having some empirical support in our data, have not been subject to cross-validation of their clinical utility. Similarly, it is important to note that despite widespread agreement regarding its public health, research, and treatment implications, the concept of dysfunctional chronic pain has only minimally been extended to TMD research and clinical application. Nevertheless, examination of the relationship between chronic pain grade and functional status demonstrates the utility of assessing patients in terms of their profile of psychosocial function. Chronic pain grade over 3 years was compared to levels of depression and somatization. Depression was assessed using the RDC/TMD, which reflects the extent of self-reported subdued mood, feeling blue and sad, and psychomotor and thought retardation, as well as loss of interest in

social activities and work and loss of appetite and libido. Somatization, also measured with the Axis II component of the RDC/TMD, is generally described as having three components: (1) the predisposition to report numerous nonspecific physical symptoms (e.g., pounding heart, sweating, trembling), as well as reporting the presence of pain complaints such as headache, back pain, stomach upset; (2) the tendency to seek medical treatment; and (3) emotional disturbance. Both depression and somatization have been heavily implicated in chronic pain, including TMD.[18, 42]

Functional patients (that is, RDC/TMD Axis II, Grades I and II) show scores for both depression and somatization that are at or near our population mean for these measures. Dysfunctional TMD patients, Grades III and IV, score significantly higher—in the top 15% to 25% on measures of depression and of the presence of nonspecific physical symptoms, including other pains. These are age- and sex-adjusted values where the population mean is zero for these scales. In marked contrast, dysfunctional TMD patients (Grades III and IV), who report high pain intensity together with pain that is frequently present and appreciably limits their daily activities, are indistinguishable from functional (Grades I and II) TMD patients in unassisted vertical range of jaw motion or the total number of joint sounds detected on both vertical and lateral excursions of the jaw. These data indicate that the level of TMD pain-related dysfunction is *not* significantly associated with these commonly assessed TMD signs.

Treatment history data also present challenges to evaluating how best to clinically manage TMD. Most studies of TMD treatment are associated with high rates of reported success, which might indicate that patients typically receive treatment from only one or at most a small number of health care providers, whose treatments are successful. Analysis of baseline RDC/TMD data for TMD patients appearing for clinical care revealed that only about 11% of functional TMD patients had previously sought TMD treatment from five or more providers, whereas about four times as many psychosocially dysfunctional patients, approximately 45%, had seen five or more TMD health care providers. Using RDC/TMD somatization scores with these same patients, it was observed that about 50% of those scoring in the top quartile for somatization level had seen five or more TMD providers, while only about 18% of those in the lowest quartile for somatization had sought care from so many providers. It is important to remember that despite the wide disparity in treatment-seeking patterns between functional and dysfunctional patients as defined through the RDC/TMD Graded Chronic Pain Scale, the clinical signs of TMD are comparable for functional and dysfunctional cases.

In summary, the RDC/TMD Axis II yields potentially useful clinical profiles of the level of psychological and psychosocial function. Patients defined as functional tend to report less severe pain, experience less emotional distress in the form of anxiety and depression symptoms, report fewer nonspecific physical symptoms, seek less treatment for TMD, and report less impact on their daily lives from their TMD. By contrast, dysfunctional patients, constituting about 20% of clinic cases in a population-based study and about 30% of clinic cases observed in a TMD specialty clinic, report more elevated pain levels, have a poorer treatment history, tend to experience more profound psychological upset, and report a significant negative impact on their lives associated with TMD pain.

Finally, virtually every population-based and clinical survey indicates that the modal TMD patient is a woman in her childbearing years. Population-based studies around the world indicate that the prevalence of TMD in women is about twice that for men and that the clinic population favors females in ratios of 4:1 and higher. TMD is a rare condition in older men and drops sharply in prevalence for both genders as advanced middle age approaches.

Evolving a Practical Approach

The concepts and methods just described for the biobehavioral assessment of chronic orofacial pain patients presenting for potential dental, medical, or surgical treatment have been developed over more than a decade and are suited for use in specialty and general dentistry practice. Initially, such methods were limited to research, but both the RDC/TMD Axis I and Axis II assessment methods and measures have become part of the routine evaluation of all patients treated in the clinics of the Department of Oral Medicine at the University of Washington; more recently, the biobehavioral assessment methods have been incorporated into the Department of Oral Medicine's curriculum for dental students in the area of chronic orofacial pain assessment and management and continuing education programs for dentists and dental hygienists.

The content of a biobehavioral assessment for a patient presenting for TMJ surgery or for any other aspect of TMD treatment can be summarized as falling into the four domains in Table 20–5. It is assumed that a thorough clinical examination and history are routine parts of a TMD patient's initial evaluation for surgery. As is readily apparent, most of the content for a biobehavioral assessment is familiar to medical and dental specialists, and the only specialized assessment instruments needed beyond those reasonably expected to be incorporated into the initial clinical work-up are the symptom checklist scales and the Graded Chronic Pain Scale, described earlier.

Patient Self-Assessment The reason that such self-evident considerations as chief complaint, pain description, and treatment history are included as part of the

TABLE 20–5.	**Biobehavioral Assessment of TMD Patients: Major Domains**		
Patient Self-Assessment	**Jaw Disability and Parafunctional Behavior**	**Psychological Status**	**Psychosocial Status**
Chief complaint Pain description Treatment history Explanatory model	Diurnal clenching, grinding Nocturnal clenching, grinding Other oral habits	Depression Anxiety Nonspecific physical symptoms (somatization)	Chronic Pain Grade Social support Use of health care

biobehavioral assessment is to emphasize the integrated way in which clinical data are used to arrive at a clinical physical diagnosis (e.g., masticatory muscle, internal derangement, arthralgia disorder, either singly or in combination) *and* a clinical biobehavioral assessment—the latter shedding light on the patient's adaptation to pain, the patient's beliefs about the origin of the condition and the type of treatment that may be efficacious, the relationship of symptom description to known physiologic mechanisms, and the patient's compliance with prior treatment. Taken together, the self-perceived and self-appraised historical elements and current beliefs or explanatory models yield an integrated picture of the patient's physical problem and its current impact on his or her thinking, behavior, emotional status, and treatment seeking.

Jaw Disability and Oral Parafunctional Behaviors The RDC/TMD Axis II also includes a measure of jaw disability, whose psychometric properties have not been studied extensively. The assessment of this domain seeks to identify the presence of oral habits and postures habitually assumed by the stomatognathic system that may be deleterious to its health. Specific concerns revolve around the persistence of maladaptive parafunctional behaviors, such as jaw clenching and bruxism, to which dentists are well sensitized. Since publication of this Axis II measure, other workers[43] have produced comparable scales of the biobehavioral impact on jaw function associated with TMD. These scales have better-known psychometric properties, and we recognize the need to compare the reliability, validity, and clinical utility of our jaw dysfunction scale with comparable measures reported in the TMD clinical literature.[43]

Psychological Status and Psychosocial Status The concepts and methods associated with psychological and psychosocial aspects of the biobehavioral assessment of TMD patients have been amply discussed in the preceding section. Here it is necessary only to reemphasize that it is not the objective of this biobehavioral assessment to arrive at a formal diagnosis of the psychological status of the patient, which is beyond the training of most dentists and surgeons and beyond their need for managing TMD cases. The intent here is to give the surgeon or any other biomedical clinician a systematic yet practical way to screen for potential

misinformation, lack of clarity about treatment aims, and potential noncompliance; to determine the extent to which the presenting problem interferes with normal functioning of the person; and to gain a clinical sense of the presence, if any, of emotional disturbance. When the assessment process uncovers a potentially serious or debilitating psychological status, such as marked depression or highly irrational statements concerning causes of or cures for the presenting condition, the surgeon should consider referral to a mental health specialist, just as other specialists are used to obtain specialized images of the TMJ or more specialized clinical medicine studies. Indeed, it makes sense that the patient should be evaluated by a mental health specialist to the same degree that the joint is evaluated by an imaging specialist when the clinical history and examination so indicate. The accompanying box, adapted from materials produced by the University of Washington's Multidisciplinary Pain Center, summarizes some practical suggestions as a guide to dentists gathering a biobehavioral assessment of TMD patients.[44]

INDICATIONS FOR PSYCHOLOGICAL EVALUATION OF CHRONIC PAIN PROBLEMS

1. Pain persists beyond normal expected healing time without clear evidence of ongoing nociception from physical defect and *significantly* disrupts normal functioning in one or more of the following areas: ambulation, self-care, work, home care, recreational activities, marital or family relationships, or social activities.
2. Patient exhibits signs or symptoms of significant psychological distress (e.g., depression, anxiety).
3. Disability greatly exceeds that expected on the basis of physical findings.
4. Patient excessively uses the health care system; patient persists in seeking tests or treatments that are not indicated on the basis of the physical findings.
5. There is excessive or prolonged use of opioid or sedative-hypnotic medications, alcohol, or other substances for pain control.

The biobehavioral assessment should be structured as follows:

1. The first stage requires the dentist to review the patient-provided information obtained from the history questionnaire. The major domains of biobehavioral assessment that are incorporated into the history questionnaire and patient-provided database are summarized in Table 20–5. Note that much of the information reviewed at this stage is clinically relevant to both Axis I and Axis II evaluation.

2. The second stage consists of a clinical interview and discussion with the patient, based on data from the written information. The dentist's objective is to elicit, for each of the domains of biobehavioral assessment, as clearly as possible what the patient is intending to communicate. It is generally preferable to begin with more open-ended questions (e.g., "On the questionnaire you indicated that TMD pain limits you; can you tell me more about that?" perhaps followed by a more specific question, "How does pain affect your ability to eat or talk?" or a summary question, "So your pain worsens during the day?").

To determine the importance of biobehavioral factors in a chronic pain problem, ask the following questions:

1. What activities are you doing more of now compared with before your pain began? Look for increases in avoidant behaviors, such as extensive rest and neglecting responsibilities at work, home, or school.

2. What activities are you doing less of now compared with before your pain began? Look for decreases in "healthy" behaviors, such as less exercise or less social interaction.

3. What effect has the pain had on your ability to work? How have things been going at work? Look for inability to work because of pain, stresses at work, prior poor work history.

4. What body movements do you avoid because of fear of increased pain? Look for guarding or phobic avoidance, in the belief that pain equals damage.

5. How would your life be different if the pain were cured? Look for realistic appraisal of increased capabilities versus unrealistic resolution of life problems well beyond the impact of the pain or disability.

6. What do significant others do when your pain is bad? Look for expressions of concern or sympathy, cautions to avoid activity, offers to take over tasks, or suggestions to call the doctor, take medications, or take "time out" from stress or conflict.

7. Are you involved in litigation related to your pain? Are you receiving or have you applied for disability compensation? Look for financial implications of continued disability versus return to normal functioning.

8. What kinds of stresses have you had recently besides your pain problem? Have you had any problems, such as the death or serious illness of someone close to you, marital problems, problems with your children, financial problems, or just a lot of hassles? Look for major life stresses or daily hassles.

A useful bottom line is to ask yourself: How well do I know where this patient is coming from with regard to his or her TMD? Are there any expectations I need to be careful about? Are both the patient's psychological status and the TMD's impact on the person consistent with my clinical examination findings, or do I detect more anxiety, depression, or pain interference than I would have suspected? Finally, ask yourself: Can I put all these factors together so that a coherent picture would emerge if I were describing this patient to a colleague?

Biobehavioral Treatment

Psychologically based treatments directed at conditions in which both physical and emotional or biobehavioral factors loom large, such as chronic pain conditions, have followed two broad divisions into which most current psychotherapies can be placed. One school of psychodynamic psychotherapy, derived from Freud, seeks to accomplish its objectives of changes in thinking, emotions, and behavior by allowing enhanced personal insight. This approach, involving so-called talking therapies such as psychoanalysis, object-relations, or interpersonal psychotherapy, seeks to facilitate the patient's increased understanding of the origins and meanings of the personal conflicts that have resulted in physical and emotional symptoms, such as pain and depression. Such therapies focus on past events and seek to connect childhood and later occurrences, such as abandonment, abuse, or emotional trauma, with current psychological disturbances that prevent adaptive modes of thinking, feeling, and behaving from emerging.

From the broadest perspective, the most common alternative approaches, derived originally from Pavlov's elaboration of stimulus-response conditioning, encompass such psychotherapeutic modalities as behavior modification or biobehavioral therapy and cognitive-behavior therapy. This group of therapies focuses much more on the here and now, delves much less deeply into the emotional past of the patient, and often incorporates educational components to help the patient evolve more rational and practical patterns of thinking and feeling to help adapt to or cope with current physical and emotional problems.

General agreement has emerged in the scientific literature that biobehavioral and educational modalities are useful and effective in the management of chronic pain conditions.[45–48] These treatment modalities constitute a component of virtually every reported chronic pain treatment program.[45] The majority of studies establishing the efficacy of psychologically based treatments for chronic pain have focused on the two most common chronic pain conditions: back pain and headache. The management of TMD has benefited from such biobehavioral interventions as well.[46]

The label "biobehavioral" has gained acceptance as a collective term to refer to treatment approaches for chronic pain derived from the application of biobehavioral science theories and methods to change the perception and appraisal of pain and to ameliorate or eliminate the personal suffering and psychosocial dysfunction that often accompany persistent pain conditions.[45, 46] The biobehavioral pain management modalities are drawn more specifically from the field of psychotherapy; those methods most heavily investigated and scientifically validated derive largely from cognitive-behavioral and biobehavioral psychotherapeutic approaches. The efficacy of psychodynamic and psychoanalytic treatment approaches for the management of chronic pain has not yet been as fully validated. The biobehavioral interventions cited in this section are viewed as safe, reversible, and noninvasive, and for the most part, they emphasize strategies under the patient's control.

The label "biobehavioral treatments" encompasses a large collection of treatment modalities. Overwhelmingly, these methods emphasize self-management and the acquisition of self-control over not only pain symptoms but also cognitive attributions or meanings given to those symptoms, as well as the maintenance of a productive level of psychosocial function, even if pain is not totally absent.[47, 49] It is well beyond the scope of this chapter to offer how-to approaches, and oral and maxillofacial surgeons will not provide such psychologically based therapies. Instead, a review of salient findings and features associated with biobehavioral therapies commonly used for chronic TMD is presented to facilitate better-informed referrals to mental health care providers if the biobehavioral assessment of candidates for TMD surgery indicates that specific patients might benefit from such complementary therapies.

COMMON BIOBEHAVIORAL THERAPEUTIC MODALITIES FOR CHRONIC PAIN

- Biofeedback
- Relaxation
- Hypnosis
- Cognitive-behavioral therapy
- Education

Whenever biobehavioral therapy components are deemed potentially useful, whether delivered by the surgical team or by a psychiatrist or clinical psychologist, such biobehavioral therapy should be integrated into the planned surgical care to achieve maximal benefit. It is highly advisable that a clear description be given to both the patient and the treating mental health care provider of the oral and maxillofacial surgeon's therapeutic objectives, along with information regarding what the surgeon expects by way of complementary and integrated treatment from the biobehavioral domain. The objectives of biobehavioral therapy before TMD surgery might include reducing depression, developing a more rational set of outcome expectancies, instituting adaptive pain coping strategies, and defining a clear postoperative plan with regard to future use of health care and medications.

Several workers, including Rudy,[50] Fricton,[51] Krogstad,[52] Kinney,[53] and McCreary[13] and their respective colleagues, have demonstrated clear relationships between biobehavioral, psychological, and psychosocial risk factors and TMD treatment outcome. Especially salient were the presence of depression, somatization, low self-esteem, and anxiety, which were identified as predictors of outcome for treatment of TMDs. Although these studies varied in methodologic rigor and sophistication of statistical analyses, they all concluded, whether for U.S. or Scandinavian clinic samples, that for many patients, management of biobehavioral and psychological factors is a requirement if long-term management of TMD is to be successful. Conversely, it is fair to conclude from the scientific literature that there are no studies demonstrating that physical pathology variables are better than psychological variables for predicting positive TMD treatment outcome—as is similarly acknowledged for headache and back pain.

A recent National Institutes of Health Technology Assessment Conference proceeding, entitled "Integration of Behavioral and Relaxation Approaches into the Treatment of Chronic Pain and Insomnia," is the best available summary of the state of the art concerning the suitability of biobehavioral methods to ameliorate chronic pain and its debilitating psychosocial sequelae.[46] With regard to TMD, reference is made to specific studies establishing the relative efficacy of relaxation, biofeedback, hypnosis, and cognitive-behavioral methods in their management.

It is clearly not intended for oral and maxillofacial surgeons to diagnose psychiatric disorders or provide extensive biobehavioral management. Table 20–6 summarizes do's and don'ts with regard to biobehavioral assessment and management of TMD patients. Table 20–7 is an outline of suggested approaches for making a referral to a biobehavioral clinician (either a psychiatrist or a clinical psychologist).

Summary

By and large, when biobehavioral treatments are used in the management of TMD, effects are virtually always positive and in the hypothesized beneficial direction, although the effects are often moderate in size. However, these biobehavioral methods, especially those subsumed under the label "cognitive-behavioral," appear to have the potential for producing long-lasting benefits that exceed those observed with the usual clinical treatment for TMD. Increasingly, conservative, noninvasive approaches to TMD management are being advocated as the preferred overall treatment approach for this hard-to-understand chronic pain problem.[54] These so-called conservative treatments generally incorporate many of the same elements (e.g., relaxation, stress education, habit behavior modification) found in cognitive-behavioral and biobehavioral therapies for TMD. Thus, both the usual clinical treatment for TMD and biobehavioral treatment use multimodal approaches, and it is not yet possible to determine which components are most efficacious. If one method were to be singled out, relaxation emerges as a consistently effective method for chronic pain management in a wide variety of pain conditions and a wide variety of clinical settings. However, of the combined biobehavioral methods commonly used in clinical practice and in research, no one method has been proved superior to another.

It is important to note that the same is true with regard to biomedically based TMD treatments. There is no strong scientific evidence to substantiate the superiority of invasive versus noninvasive treatments or pharmacologic treatments emphasizing analgesics versus those stressing antidepressants or muscle relaxants. It is the absence of compelling evidence to the contrary that has led many clinical researchers to advocate conservative, reversible therapies for the largest number of TMD patients.

TABLE 20–6.	Do's and Don'ts in Assessing and Managing Chronic Pain

Do's

1. Tell patients that you believe their pain is real.
2. Treat chronic and acute pain differently. Strategies that may be appropriate for acute pain (immobilization, rest, opioid medications) are usually counterproductive for chronic pain.
3. Listen to patients. Ask them what they think may be causing the pain and what needs to be done to assess and treat the problem, and respond to their opinions.
4. Try to resolve ambiguity regarding the cause versus maintenance or "flare-ups" of patients' pain as much as possible and as quickly as possible. Spend time going over test results with patients, explaining the purpose of each test and the implications of findings. To the extent possible, tell patients what factors you think are contributing to persistence of their pain.
5. Adopt a rehabilitation rather than curative model toward persistent pain complaints that have been adequately studied diagnostically. Make improved function rather than disappearance of the symptom the therapeutic goal.
6. Ask patients about their emotional state, life stresses, work situation, and symptoms of depression and anxiety. Dysphoria may not be obvious, so ask about loss of interest and pleasure, sleep and appetite disruption, loss of energy and libido, and hopelessness. This may yield important information about factors that may be impeding recovery and may require psychological or psychiatric assessment and treatment. Antidepressants and cognitive-behavioral therapies are especially useful in pain patients.
7. Let patients know that you will stick with them and continue to see them, even if their pain persists.
8. Use time-contingent, rather than pain-contingent, schedules for medications and reactivation. Once you have done adequate diagnostic studies to determine that pain is not signaling an ongoing destructive process, send this message clearly and definitively to the patient. Pain-contingent schedules label pain as dangerous as well as aversive.
9. Turn as much as possible of the responsibility for getting better back to patients. You can guide them, but the patients must work by following a regular program to improve their health, comply with medication regimens, and so forth.
10. Involve patients' family members when possible. They may provide important information about factors contributing to the problem and may be allies in treatment.

Don'ts

1. Don't think of chronic pain as either somatogenic or psychogenic. *All* pain is *both*.
2. Don't oversimplify patients' questions about the origins of pain. These are often really questions about the legitimacy of suffering. Restate questions about the origin of pain as questions about the nature of appropriate treatment. "Just because the radiograph does not show something wrong with your TMJ does not mean that your pain is all in your head. It means that our crude tools cannot see what is wrong and other crude tools (surgery) would not make it better. Let's find something that will work."
3. Don't continue opioid and sedative-hypnotic medications beyond the first week or so after injury just because the pain continues. Begin a rehabilitation program if there are no contraindications. If you meet resistance, seek psychological or psychiatric consultation.
4. Don't instruct patients to "do what you feel you can; let pain be your guide," and don't instruct patients to take opioid or narcotic analgesics on an as-needed basis.
5. Don't abandon patients because they do not need a specific curative dental or biomedical intervention. Regular visits and a commitment to care can prevent doctor shopping and iatrogenic injury.
6. Don't wait too long before referring dysfunctional patients to an appropriate specialized pain center. The longer such patients are entrenched in patterns of disability, disuse, and opioid and/or sedative medication use, the more difficult it will be to reverse these patterns.

A great deal more research is needed before it is possible to adequately evaluate how biobehavioral interventions achieve their desired effects and which components of the multimodal approaches now in common use are most potent. Perhaps of greatest interest is the need to develop treatment approaches tailored to both the physical and the biobehavioral status of the patient, as recently advocated with the introduction of the RDC/TMD.[39]

Typically, treatment of TMD is driven largely by the physical diagnosis alone, without addressing the personal or psychosocial impact of TMD pain or the patterns of coping used by TMD patients. Although TMD is regarded by many as a condition in which psychosocial factors influence the course of disease,[50, 55–57] little attention has been paid to assessing how psychological or psychosocial factors influence treatment outcome and whether successful clinical outcome is associated with improved psychosocial function. It is fair to say that outcome assessment for TMD, except for self-reports of pain, is focused almost exclu-

TABLE 20–7.	Guidelines for Making a Biobehavioral Referral

Discussing the Referral with the Patient

1. Good rapport with the patient is essential before discussing referral ideas.
2. Emphasize that the patient's pain is "real."
3. A multidimensional condition requires multidisciplinary care.
4. Discuss referral early (multiple discussions may be required).
5. Dispel misconceptions about abandonment.
6. Involve the patient in the referral decision.
7. Develop a good referral network.

Choosing a Practitioner

1. Practitioner's philosophy
   Has specialty training
   Uses cognitive-behavioral methods
2. Practitioner's knowledge
   Chronic pain management
   Temporomandibular disorders
3. Practitioner's communication strategy
   Supports two-way communication
   Provides an initial evaluation
   Furnishes progress and treatment summaries

---

sively on physical factors (e.g., range of jaw motion, joint sounds); the few exceptions have been cited here.

Historically, psychologically based therapies for the medically ill have been met with some resistance among some patients and some health care providers. The resistance to incorporating biobehavioral treatments has been largely resolved by the medical profession, as evidenced by the large number of psychologists and biobehavioral medicine specialists employed in scientific research and the rehabilitation of stroke, cardiac, cancer, and other chronic disease patients, including chronic pain patients treated in major multidisciplinary pain centers. But no review of the efficacy and potential role of biobehavioral interventions incorporated into the management of TMD would be complete without at least acknowledging that resistance to such approaches remains.

Too often, well-documented resistance still accompanies a recommendation for the inclusion of psychologically based treatment for TMD. For some, such recommendations carry the negative and clearly undesirable implication that TMD problems must be "all in the head" or somehow "psychological,"

and hence "not real." No such destructive implication is ever intended when biobehavioral medicine specialists advocate a biobehavioral treatment. TMD-related pain and distress are as real as the distress associated with any other chronic condition, and people will vary in their capacity to endure, let alone thrive, under such difficult physical conditions. It is unfortunate if unhealthy and unwarranted negative misapprehensions prevent any TMD patient from being helped through the use of readily available, scientifically sound, and safe methods that integrate biomedical and biobehavioral treatments for TMD.

REFERENCES

1. Dworkin SF: Behavioral and educational modalities. Oral Surg Oral Med Oral Pathol Oral Radiol Endod 1997;83:128–133.
2. Fordyce WE, Roberts AH, Sternbach RA: The behavioral management of chronic pain: A response to critics. Pain 1985;22:113–125.
3. Rugh JD, Dahlstrom L: Psychological management of the orofacial pain patient. In Stohler CF, Carlsson DS (eds): Biological and Psychological Aspects of Orofacial Pain. Ann Arbor, University of Michigan Press, 1995, pp 133–147.
4. Turner JA, Romano JM: Psychological and psychosocial evaluation. In Bonica JJ (ed): The Management of Pain, vol 2, ed 2. Philadelphia, Lea & Febiger, 1990, pp 595–609.
5. Fordyce WE: Behavioral Methods in Chronic Pain and Illness. St. Louis, CV Mosby, 1976.
6. Ohrbach R: Patient evaluation in temporomandibular disorders: Overview. In Zarb G, Carlsson G, Sessle BJ, et al (eds): Temporomandibular Joint and Masticatory Muscle Disorders. Copenhagen, Munksgaard, 1994, pp 391–405.
7. Ohrbach R: History and clinical examination. In Zarb G, Carlsson G, Sessle BJ, et al (eds): Temporomandibular Joint and Masticatory Muscle Disorders. Copenhagen, Munksgaard, 1994, pp 406–434.
8. LeResche L, Dworkin SF: Facial expressions of pain and emotions in chronic TMD patients. Pain 1988;35:71–78.
9. Craig KD: Emotional aspects of pain. In Wall PD, Melzack R (eds): Textbook of Pain, ed 2. Edinburgh, Churchill Livingstone, 1989, pp 220–230.
10. Prkachin K, Mercer SR: Pain expression in patients with shoulder pathology: Validity, properties and relationship to sickness impact. Pain 1990;39:257–265.
11. Bradley LA, McDonald Haile J, Jaworski TM: Assessment of psychological status using interviews and self-report instruments. In Turk DC, Melzack R (eds): Handbook of Pain Assessment. New York, Guilford Press, 1992, pp 193–213.
12. Deardorff WH: TMJ Scale. In Conoley JC, Impara JC (eds): The Twelfth Mental Measurements Yearbook. Lincoln, Buros Institute of Mental Measurements, University of Nebraska–Lincoln, 1995, pp 1070–1071.
13. McCreary CP, Clark GT, Oakley ME, et al: Predicting response to treatment for temporomandib-

ular disorders. J Craniomandib Disord Facial Oral Pain 1992;6:161–169.

14. Derogatis LR: SCL-90-R: Administration, Scoring and Procedures Manual—II for the Revised Version. Towson, MD, Clinical Psychometric Research, 1983.

15. Buckelew SP, DeGood DE, Schwartz DP, et al: Cognitive and somatic item response pattern of pain patients, psychiatric patients, and hospital employees. J Clin Psychol 1986;42:852–860.

16. Dworkin SF, Von Korff M, LeResche L: Epidemiologic studies of chronic pain: A dynamic-ecologic perspective. Ann Behav Med 1992;14:3–11.

17. Dworkin SF, Von Korff MR, LeResche L: Multiple pains and psychiatric disturbance: An epidemiologic investigation. Arch Gen Psychiatry 1990;47:239–244.

18. Dworkin SF, Wilson L, Massoth DL: Somatizing as a risk factor for chronic pain. In Grzesiak RC, Ciccone DS (eds): Psychologic Vulnerability to Chronic Pain. New York, Springer, 1994, pp 28–54.

19. List T, Dworkin SF, Harrison R, et al: Research diagnostic criteria/temporomandibular disorders: Comparing Swedish and U.S. clinics [abstract]. J Dent Res 1996;75(special issue).

20. Turk DC, Rudy TE: Toward an empirically derived taxonomy of chronic pain patients: Integration of psychological assessment data. J Consult Clin Psychol 1988;56:233–238.

21. Rudy TE, Turk DC, Zaki HS, et al: An empirical taxometric alternative to traditional classification of temporomandibular disorders. Pain 1989;36:311–320.

22. Rudy T, Turk D, Kubinski J, et al: Efficacy of tailoring treatment for dysfunctional TMD patients. J Dent Res 1994;73(special issue):439.

23. Pilowsky I: Abnormal illness behaviour: A review of the concept and its implications. In McHugh S, Vallis TM (eds): Illness Behavior: A Multidisciplinary Model. New York, Plenum Press, 1986, pp 391–396.

24. Bergner M, Bobbitt RA, Carter WB, et al: The Sickness Impact Profile: Development and final revision of a health status model. Med Care 1981;19:787–805.

25. Keefe FJ, Gil KM: Behavioral concepts in the analysis of chronic pain syndromes. J Consult Clin Psychol 1986;54:776–783.

26. Brown GK, Nicassio PM: Development of a questionnaire for the assessment of active and passive coping strategies in chronic pain patients. Pain 1987;31:53–64.

27. Lazarus RS: Coping strategies. In McHugh S, Vallis TM (eds): Illness Behavior: A Multidisciplinary Model. New York, Plenum Press, 1986, pp 303–308.

28. Lennon MC, Dohrenwend BP, Zautra AJ, et al: Coping and adaption to facial pain in contrast to other stressful life events. J Pers Soc Psychol 1990;59:1040–1050.

29. Gatchel RJ, Baum A: Pain and pain management techniques. In An Introduction to Health Psychology. New York, Random House, 1983, pp 259–277.

30. Levitt SR, Lundeen TF, McKinney MW: Initial studies of a new assessment method for temporomandibular joint disorders. J Prosthet Dent 1988;59:490–495.

31. Levitt SR: Predictive value: A model for dentists to evaluate the accuracy of diagnostic tests for temporomandibular disorders as applied to the TMJ Scale. J Prosthet Dent 1991;66:385–390.

32. Levitt SR: Predictive value of the TMJ Scale in detecting clinically significant symptoms of temporomandibular disorders. J Craniomandib Disord Facial Oral Pain 1990;4:177–185.

33. Levitt SR, Lundeen TF, McKinney MW: The TMJ Scale Manual. Durham, NC, Pain Resource Center, 1994.

34. Rugh JD, Woods BJ, Dahlstrom L: Temporomandibular disorders: Assessment of psychosocial factors. Adv Dent Res 1993;7:127–136.

35. Glaros AG, Glass EG: Temporomandibular disorders. In Gatchel RJ, Blanchard EB (eds): Psychophysiological Disorders. Washington, DC, American Psychological Association, 1993, pp 299–356.

36. Fricton JR, Schiffman EL: The craniomandibular index: Validity. J Prosthet Dent 1987;58:222–228.

37. Rugh JD, Ohrbach RK: Occlusal parafunction. In Mohl ND, Zarb GA, Carlsson GE, et al (eds): A Textbook of Occlusion. Chicago, Quintessence, 1988, pp 249–261.

38. Merskey H: Classification of chronic pain: Descriptions of chronic pain syndromes and definitions of pain terms. Pain 1986;3(suppl):1–8.

39. Dworkin SF, LeResche L: Research diagnostic criteria for temporomandibular disorders: Review, criteria, examinations and specifications, critique. J Craniomandib Disord Facial Oral Pain 1992;6:301–355.

40. Diagnostic and Statistical Manual of Mental Disorders, Fourth Edition. Washington, DC, American Psychiatric Association, 1994.

41. Von Korff M, Ormel J, Keefe FJ, et al: Grading the severity of chronic pain. Pain 1992;50:133–149.

42. Wilson L, Dworkin SF, Whitney C, et al: Somatization and pain dispersion in chronic temporomandibular pain. Pain 1994;57:55–61.

43. Stegenga B, de Bont LGM, de Leeuw R, et al: Assessment of mandibular function impairment associated with temporomandibular joint osteoarthrosis and internal derangement. J Orofacial Pain 1993;7:183–195.

44. LeResche L, Dworkin SF, Massoth D, et al: Comprehensive Assessment and Management of Temporomandibular Disorders: Dentist's Handbook (revised). Seattle, University of Washington, 1997.

45. Gallagher RM: The comprehensive pain clinic: A biobehavioral approach to pain management and rehabilitation. Presented at Integration of Behavioral and Relaxation Approaches into the Treatment of Chronic Pain and Insomnia, NIH Technology Assessment Conference, Bethesda, MD, 1995, pp 1–34.

46. National Institutes of Health: Integration of Behavioral and Relaxation Approaches into the Treatment of Chronic Pain and Insomnia. NIH Technology Assessment Conference, Bethesda, MD, 1995.

47. Turk DC, Meichenbaum D: A cognitive behavioral approach to pain management. In Wall PD, Melzack R (eds): Textbook of Pain, ed 2. London, Churchill Livingstone, 1989, pp 1001–1009.

48. Turk DC: Customizing treatment for chronic pain patients: Who, what, why. Clin J Pain 1990;6:255–270.

49. Turner JA, Clancy S, McQuade KJ, et al: Effectiveness of behavioral therapy for chronic low back pain: A component analysis. J Consult Clin Psychol 1990;58:573–579.

50. Rudy TE, Turk DC, Kubinski JA, et al: Differential treatment responses of TMD patients as a function

of psychological characteristics. Pain 1995;61:103–112.

51. Fricton JR, Olsen T: Predictors of outcome for treatment of temporomandibular disorders. J Orofacial Pain 1996;10:54–65.

52. Krogstad BS, Jokstad A, Dahl BL, et al: Relationships between risk factors and treatment outcome in a group of patients with temporomandibular disorders. J Orofacial Pain 1996;10:48–53.

53. Kinney RK, Gatchel RJ, Ellis E, et al: Major psychological disorders in chronic TMD patients: Implications for successful management. J Am Dent Assoc 1992;123:49–54.

54. Clark GT, Seligman DA, Solberg WK, et al: Guidelines for the treatment of temporomandibular disorders. J Craniomandib Disord 1990;4:80–88.

55. Dworkin SF: Illness behavior and dysfunction: Review of concepts and application to chronic pain. Can J Physiol Pharmacol 1991;69:662–671.

56. Marbach JJ, Lennon MC, Dohrenwend BP: Candidate risk factors for temporomandibular pain and dysfunction syndrome: Psychosocial, health behavior, physical illness and injury. Pain 1988;34:139–151.

57. McGlynn FD, Gale EN, Glaros AG, et al: Biobehavioral phenomena in dentistry: Some research directions for the 1990's. Ann Behav Med 1990;12:133–140.

Index

Note: Page numbers in *italics* refer to illustrations; page numbers followed by t refer to tables.